SHAKESPEARE &
CLASSIC WORKS

in the

CLASSROOM

Teaching pre-20th Century Literature at KS2 and KS3

Dennis Carter

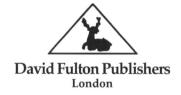

David Fulton Publishers
London

David Fulton Publishers Ltd
Ormond House, 26–27 Boswell Street, London WC1N 3JZ

www.fultonpublishers.co.uk

First published in Great Britain in 2002 by David Fulton Publishers

British Library Cataloguing in Publication Data
A catalogue record for this book is available from the British Library.

ISBN 1 85346 810 X

Typeset by Textype Typesetters, Cambridge
Printed in Great Britain by The Cromwell Press Ltd, Trowbridge, Wilts.

Contents

Acknowledgements

First, I want to thank all the children who were involved in the case study projects, particularly those in Taliesin Junior School, Shotton, Flintshire; Gwersyllt Junior School, Wrexham; Ysgol Estyn, Hope, Flintshire; Wood Memorial CP School, Saltney, Flintshire; Ewloe Green CP School, Ewloe, Flintshire; The Alun High School, Mold, Flintshire; Bryn Offa High School, Wrexham; Connah's Quay High School, Flintshire; and Dinas Bran High School, Llangollen, Denbighshire. In addition I want to thank the children I worked with at Tarvin CP School, Cheshire, and Redhills Combined School, Exeter, Devon, because many of my ideas were first developed in those two schools.

I want to thank the following individuals who have done so much to support various aspects of the work described in the case studies: Simon Richey of the Calouste Gulbenkian Foundation for sponsoring the Four Branches Project; Terry Tully for her work on The Odyssey Project and The Gerard Manley Hopkins Centenary Project; Catherine Carter for her work on 'Hamlet in Gwersyllt' and The Gerard Manley Hopkins Centenary Project; Kevin Lewis former director of Outreach Theatre Company for his superb production of *The Tempest* and for our exciting collaborations; Christopher Parry formerly of the University of Wales; Keith McDonogh former Director of Education for Clwyd for his generous support of all my work.

I want finally to thank the Wales Arts Council for its substantial financial support throughout my work for Clwyd County Council and the Clwyd Poetry Project; also The Crafts Council for supporting The Odyssey Project.

CHAPTER 1

Bringing Shakespeare and classic works to children

Introduction

Apart from occasional encounters I came to great literature late in my own education. There was grandfather's memorisation of Gray's 'Elegy written in a country churchyard' and 'The Rubaiyat of Omar Khayyam'. Sometimes, if we were lucky, he would speak a few verses out loud just to prove he knew them 'off by heart' and we would listen attentively to this boiler-maker's relish for poetry. But these were private pursuits for him. His well-worn Palgrave's *Golden Treasury of English Verse* was kept on his bedside table. His daughter, my mother, also liked to recall being Rosalind in a school production of *As You Like It*, even naming my sister after that character. Or she would provide brief snippets of the plots of *The Merchant of Venice* with 'that villain Shylock' or of *Twelfth Night* with 'that drunken rascal Sir Toby'.

As with many people it was a single teacher who enabled me really to be touched by great literature, a man in his twenties called Wilf Kimber, at Prenton Secondary Modern School, Birkenhead. I was in the GCE stream and Mr Kimber fired me up about Shakespeare's *Julius Caesar*, Dickens's *Great Expectations* and poems by Wordsworth, Tennyson and Browning. I can particularly remember the lines 'dry clashed his harness in the icy caves and all to left and right the bare, black cliffs clang'd round him as he based his feet on juts of slippery crag that rang sharp smitten with the dint of armed heels', from Tennyson's 'Idylls of the King'. Those lines jump straight out of my head almost without my thinking. It was one of the quotes we learnt to impress the examiners with our knowledge of assonance, alliteration and onomatopoeia. More importantly, its sound moves me powerfully even now.

Although I passed the exam, like many of my contemporaries from the working classes of Merseyside, I had to find employment at the age of sixteen. Then the practicalities of earning a living pushed King Arthur, the noble Brutus, the cunning Cassius, Pip, Miss Havisham and Estelle into the background. Yet the richness of these stories, the intimacy I had developed with the characters and the resonance of the language that carried them bubbled on underneath the surface. Consequently, I felt I was lucky when I heard many of my contemporaries saying that they hated Shakespeare or that Charles Dickens was boring. I had been taught by someone special.

Wilf Kimber manifested a love for the novels, the plays and the poems he taught. When reading passages to us you could tell he did. He was no Lawrence Olivier, but you knew he was putting his best into it. He relished speaking Cassius' lines with a mean voice or Pumblechook's with a pompous one. Through him I had been touched by the greatness of literature. In the words of the Italian critic Italo Calvino in *Why Read the Classics?*,[1] my youth had endowed those readings 'with a unique flavour and significance'. Perhaps the experiences with Wilf Kimber in the first floor of an old, downtown school had 'given a form or shape to [my] future experiences, providing them with models, ways of dealing with them, terms of comparison, schemes for categorising them, scales of value, paradigms of beauty' (Calvino 1999: 4).

Long after favourite films and television programmes had faded from my memory I could recollect the thrilling speech by Mark Anthony at the funeral of Caesar or identify with Pip's falling expectations when Magwich appears at his home one night to identify himself as Pip's true benefactor. Although these classics had been read, in Calvino's words, 'out of a sense of duty or respect', because of the GCE paper, I had really been reading them 'for love' (*ibid.*: 6). But wasn't this a fortunate accident? What if I had gone to a different school and my experience had been of a droning bore or a rigid taskmaster only interested in getting more A-grade passes than anyone else? Might I have hated Shakespeare, too? Might I also have found Dickens boring?

When training to be a primary teacher I discovered a pleasure equal to that of sitting in Wilf Kimber's classes. I found that the sharing of enthusiasms with children is as great as pursuing those enthusiasms for oneself. Asked to prepare lessons on Tudors in history for teaching practice with a Year 4 class I was soon teaching *A Midsummer Night's Dream* and directing a production of the rude mechanicals' scenes and the children adored it! So did the class teacher and my supervisor. But wasn't I working on a mere hunch? What was the relevance of this? What were the aims and objectives? How did I know I was doing the right thing?

Luckily for me such questions were not asked with the same sort of intent in the 1960s and I was able to follow my literary enthusiasms with children for many years to come. I grew ambitious. It seemed that so much great literature was suitable for children alongside the children's literature they were reading themselves or sharing as a class. My canon expanded to include Shakespeare, Chaucer,

Dickens, Milton, Swift and a range of poems from most periods of English poetry and much in translation.

I was attempting to generate that feeling of love of great literature and help the children endow their reading of such works 'with a unique flavour and significance'. I realised that secondary school might be too late for many children to have significant experiences of great literature and that the context of examinations was more likely to put them off than turn them on. There are not many Wilf Kimbers around.

However, the climate in schools has changed radically since I was experimenting in primary and middle schools in the 1960s, 70s and 80s. The Educational Reform Act of 1988 and subsequent initiatives have tended to stop hunches, experimentation, and the pursuit of the ideas argued by Italo Calvino. 'Entitlement' was the buzzword in the late eighties and nineties as if a national curriculum, testing and inspection could guarantee good provision throughout the land. This process has been taken much further with the 'nuts and bolts' of literacy laid out in detail in the National Literacy Strategy and in the Key Stage 3 Framework for Teaching English. But such programmes cannot guarantee that children will endow their reading 'with a unique flavour and significance'. Indeed, the danger is that they may have the opposite effect. Children are more likely to read great literature, if they read it at all in their schools, 'out of a sense of duty or respect' rather than reading it 'for love'. There is even the danger that they might learn to hate the works or find them one more boring set of steps through school.

In this book I offer my own enthusiasm for great or classic works of literature to students and teachers and my enthusiasm for sharing it with children in the middle years of schooling. I realise, however, that this is not enough. I therefore share more than thirty years of experience of teaching classic works to children in Key Stages 2 and 3, many years of organising large-scale projects in primary and secondary schools and my researches into the field. This chapter and Chapter 2 develop reasons for doing this kind of work and ways of doing it using the creative arts. The other five chapters provide case studies and projects for teachers to try. At the end of the book there are ten tables, which show the objectives covered in the National Curriculum for both Key Stages 2[2] and 3,[3] the National Literacy Strategy Framework for teachers[4] and the Key Stage 3 National Strategy Framework for teaching English.[5]

Great literature and creativity

Much of the thinking which led to the 1988 Act and subsequent developments was notable for a deep scepticism towards child-centred education and creativity. There was and still is a belief that knowledge, skills and abilities were neglected in pursuit of individual self-expression. Everybody in education is aware of this argument, notably through the many controversial pronouncements made by the previous Chief Inspector of Schools throughout the 1990s.

Yet this negative attitude towards the ideology which dominated educational thought for more than 30 years had been growing for much longer. It surfaced in the mid-1970s in the Black Papers, and many prominent thinkers articulated versions of it. For instance, in an interview with the Director of the Shakespeare and Schools Project, Dr Rex Gibson, Dr Jonathan Miller expressed great concern at what he perceived to be 'a general movement against literacy' in our schools:

> Speaking verse, knowing poetry, learning verses of the Bible off by heart and being acquainted with the literature of the past is something which has given way to what I believe to be a slightly suspect subject: creativity. The emphasis is put upon the child's creativity rather than the achieved creativity of the great reputations of the past.[6]

The feeling that children were having little or no experience of great art works and classical texts was widespread. It led to the establishment of the Shakespeare and Schools Project in the mid-eighties and to arts projects funded by such bodies as the Gulbenkian Foundation and the Leverhulme Trust. An article in the TES in 1990, by Adrian Greeves of Westminster College, Oxford, was fairly typical of this attitude. Greeves specifically identified child-centred education as the cause of the loss of great works in the primary school:

> It is a long time since I heard in a primary classroom the larger sounds of poetry or prose not written expressly for children: child-centred learning has won the day so triumphantly that we are in danger of producing child-restricted learning.[7]

But wasn't Greeves, like Miller, aiming his criticisms at the wrong target? Surely, it was not the child-centredness of the pedagogy which was to blame so much as the limited vision of what children are capable of understanding and handling. He continued, 'in addition to the revolution in children's literature we need to have a revolution in literature for children'. Greeves was right in this. A powerful and rich resource for the development of children's understanding of the world was and still is being neglected. Greeves saw this as a form of impoverishment of children's imaginations and saw more exciting possibilities: 'A child's reach should exceed his grasp or what's an education for? It's good to be allowed to play with pussy-cats; but it is enlarging as well as challenging to confront the dazzle of the "Tyger"' (Greeves 1990). Such concerns are just as pressing in 2002 as they were in 1990 and I address them positively and practically in this book.

Culture and the individual

There would be, however, grave dangers in a move away from self-expression, creativity and child-centredness towards engagement solely with great literature of the past. It would be folly to advance the cause of the classics so far that the individual needs of children were moved to the margins of education. But it seems that, according to Miller and Greeves, so long as we get children hearing and speaking 'Tyger', Shakespeare, *The Rime of the Ancient Mariner* and the King James Bible, 'culture' will stick to them willy-nilly.

There has to be a balance. An exclusive focus on great literature would be inadequate. There is also a need to focus on the individual, on creativity and expressiveness and those things Miller and Greeves were so suspicious about. The most productive way forward, I believe, is for teachers to concentrate on the individual frequently operating his creativity within great works. Such an enterprise involves a great deal more than making 'the larger sounds of poetry or prose' resound in the classroom or 'learning verses of the Bible off by heart and being acquainted with the literature of the past'. It requires the movement of feeling and involves teachers in a more subtle, demanding and responsible vocation than getting children to perform other people's plays, to do recitations for concerts, Eisteddfodau or school assemblies. Such practices, which are important parts of the cultural lives of children in schools, are simply not enough.

A fuller literary and cultural experience consists of personal and shared encounters in the outside world which, in childhood, are manifested in various forms of play. However, an individual's relationship with the culture begins with the inner world of the individual and not with the culture itself. Without using their inner worlds children would be virtually unable to act at all within the culture, let alone respond to its great works. Children's cultural activity, therefore, depends upon an actively developing inner world, and the agent of such activity is sensibility. Without the engagement of sensibility within the culture an individual's experience of cultural forms will be more to do with consumption than personal enrichment.

Creative literacy

There need be no actual conflict between Dr Miller's wish to engage children with the great works of art of the past and a wish for them to exercise creativity. Indeed, it is quite clear that the proper engagement of children with the works of great artists such as Shakespeare *depends upon* the exercise of individual creativity. In this way the child-centred approach to education is seen to have a new importance.

Ironically, at the same time as the child-centred approach was being so contemptuously debunked by politicians and schools inspectors, educational theorists were advocating reader-response theory. This, crudely, claims that the reader is at least the equal of the writer in relation to any text. Richard Andrews, for instance,[8] makes the analogy with music and theatre, that 'the score or script [text] is but a mere template for the performance' of the reader reading it (Andrews 2001: 71). Citing the work of Wolfgang Iser, Andrews writes that 'the act of reading is as creative as the act of composition', and continues:

> For the reader, the act of reading is a constructive, compositional one in which he or she brings not only his/her experience of the world, but also experience of reading other texts. For the text, the embedded affective possibilities are not released until the reader releases them – and then they may not be the same concoction as was released before . . . It is the interaction between reader and text that is the key to the interpretative act. (*ibid.*: 72)

Obviously, taken to the extreme, this theory relegates the importance of the literature itself and might encourage the unrestricted subjectivism of an 'anything goes' attitude. But it usefully adjusts the balance away from the view of the reader as a mere receiver of the pearls of wisdom from writers, and of the texts as objects with fixed meanings completely owned by the writers. In terms of the education of children, it also implies that great literature might essentially be used to assist their intellectual and emotional development. Andrews also considers reader-response theory to be liberating both for teachers and for children:

> Most significantly, emphasis upon the reader allows for pedagogical invention in that it opens up the possibility of multiple meanings mediated by readers. The business of teaching a book becomes not so much a matter of exegesis or leading one's students to 'appreciate' the qualities of a work, but enabling access to it and allowing the readers to make their own versions of it. (*ibid.*: 81)

This is a very persuasive argument with exciting implications for the classroom.[9] It turns great literature from untouchable monoliths into what I have elsewhere called 'old forges' where things can be made by children (Carter 1976: 3). This idea of creative activity is what I will be concerned with throughout this book, the idea that teachers lead children to engage their sensibilities with great literature, rather than merely learning about it. I will attempt to demonstrate the value of children having their creative imaginations honed and trained by regular engagement, as artists, with works of literature. Furthermore, it will be implicit throughout this book that the engagement of children with great literature through the exercise of creativity or expressiveness is not only important for the understanding of works of art but, more importantly for the child, it also develops that child's creativity itself.

The texture of the words

A vital ingredient in the training of creative literacy is substantial experience of the kind Dr Miller mourns the loss of: 'speaking verse, knowing poetry'. However, this needs to be part of a more ambitious enterprise in which genuine attempts are made to assist children to make meanings out of the words they are speaking. Greeves's 'incomprehensible though meaningful encounters' simply will not do for the majority of our children. Our expectations for them should be much higher than this. One of the outcomes of creative literacy is the emergence of children who are flexible in their writing, who can operate as successful writers in many genres and for all kinds of purposes.

The issue of the words, the medium, the text, the language of the great writer is nowhere more important than in a child's engagement with Shakespeare. I do not concur with Dr Miller's view, expressed in that same interview, that 'an enormous amount of Shakespeare is a bad, cheap airport nouvelle' transformed by the language. But it usefully emphasises the vital importance of Shakespeare's language. Any school's work on Shakespeare which does not substantially involve children in listening to, reading and speaking Shakespeare's words is more like 'Shakespearian storytime' than a serious attempt to introduce Shakespeare to children.

All three activities involving the words – listening, reading and speaking – are important and this was why I brought actors into the three projects which I undertook during my associateship with The Shakespeare and Schools Project, based on *Twelfth Night*, *Julius Caesar* and *Macbeth*.[10] So, for instance, a whole class took part as either conspirators or witnesses of the death of Caesar on the steps of the Capitol. Caesar, played by a visiting actor, was assassinated by one group which had been waiting for him and rehearsing for the moment of his death for weeks! Crucially, however, the children knew the significance of their words. Those who played the conspirators Metellus, Brutus and Cassius knew full well that their pleas for the release of Publius Cimber from banishment were only a device to set up the assassination. When it happened, Shakespeare's words carried the action and his 'real' words assisted the 'willing suspension of disbelief'. The children were not playing at killing someone in a playground game. Shakespeare's words placed the assassination far away in a different time and place and context. They gave it its taste and texture as an experience, and more importantly, they gave it its definition, its confines. It was a ritual with the incantation of Shakespeare's words as its text.

Cultural paradigms

Words of great or classic literature such as the plays of Shakespeare, the poetry of Chaucer, the novels of Dickens or the epics of Homer provide a culture with its paradigms and its universals. Such works are not so much parables offering simple moral truths to be followed as uniquely individual patterns for us to hold up and contemplate and measure our humanity against. According to Italo Calvino they also 'exercise a particular influence, both when they imprint themselves on our imagination as unforgettable, and when they hide in the layers of memory disguised as the individual's or the collective unconscious' (Calvino 1999: 4).

Classic works of literature carry, for instance, much greater power than the models provided by great lives or great events in history. They transcend events and individual lives. Thus Shakespeare's *Richard III* is very different from the monarch who ruled for a time in the fifteenth century, not because Shakespeare was telling lies about him but because he was fictionalised by the process of art. Shakespeare's dramatic techniques, of which his poetry is foremost, take an actual king out of his actual context and put him on stage with motives to be worked through in three hours and five acts. Success, in this enterprise, is not measured by historical accuracy but by what Witkin has called the 'intelligence of feeling'.[11] The former satisfies our enquiring minds, but the latter fulfils our enquiring humanities. The difference is one of compass and scale. A.J.P. Taylor pleases me intellectually. Shakespeare shakes me to the foundations of my being.

Imagine, for instance, Shakespeare's *Macbeth* in Act I, Scene vii of the play:

> If it were done, when 'tis done, then 'twere well
> It were done quickly. If th'assassination
> Could trammel up the consequence, and catch
> With his surcease, success; that but this blow
> Might be the be-all and the end-all here –
> But here upon this bank and shoal of time –
> We'd jump the life to come. But in these cases
> We still have judgement here, that we but teach
> Bloody instructions, which being taught return
> To plague th'inventor . . .

Macbeth, here, is not the stuff of history. He is of now, speaking directly to us. He is embodied, the fiction accepted. We are present at his crisis and share it. Although he is talking about the projected murder of the King of Scotland, Duncan, he speaks for all ages. At one and the same time these words are particular and general. They are particular to this work of art, to its structure and to the protagonist's thinking, which results in the committing of a particular murder. They are general in that they speak directly to us about the human condition, about its weakness faced with irresistible temptation and how we 'rationalise' such a temptation. We are affected powerfully by such language because it penetrates the inner recesses of our minds and feelings. No other forms of writing affect us in quite this way and it is not altogether surprising that a phrase such as 'the be-all and the end-all' remains embedded in our use of our language some 400 years after its composition. It speaks to us all of the powerlessness of even the most powerful.

Relevance

The power of Shakespeare's language to transform the ordinary as well as the extraordinary into art has important implications for children living in an age of instant, popular culture and important implications for our idea of relevance. The notion of relevance, so strong in the1970s, was misguided not in principle but in application. Those who argued the case for 'relevance' had in mind a narrow social application for the term. They certainly didn't have in mind the sense of 'other worlds' different from our own or the world of dreams and fantasies. Their application of the concept of relevance did not extend much to the pupils' psychological development. Dr Miller is, quite rightly, uncompromising about this sort of approach when he says:

> The notion of relevance has partly invaded all areas of modern life: things are only interesting in so far as they can be mapped onto current problems, current issues . . . If children don't get history, literature, then Shakespeare dropped into the middle of it simply ruptures it, like a cannonball dropped into a cobweb. It just has no support . . . If you've got to make Shakespeare 'relevant' then junk it. It should be self-evidently relevant with a very short introduction. (Gibson 1987)

Now Macbeth and Bill Sykes from *Oliver Twist* are self-evident villains, and the evil which drives their behaviour is present in the behaviour of the villains of today, both in fact and in fiction. We might then ask why it is important to contemplate such villains when we have more than enough from our own time to stalk and haunt the imaginations of our children. Alternatively, we might take a superior position and attempt to replace certain villains by pouring scorn on the fictions which they inhabit. Thus we might tell children that they ought not to be watching *Eastenders*, and thereby eliminate Phil Mitchell from their rogues' galleries. The former view dismisses high art, the latter dismisses popular culture. However, the slavish adherence to the searching-out of relevance often makes false links between the two.

In a child's imagination Phil Mitchell, Osama Bin Laden, Macbeth and Bill Sykes can coexist without any contrivance on the part of teachers, and it is quite possible that children may identify the villainy in Macbeth and Sykes because of their knowledge of contemporary villains. Similarly, by inhabiting the worlds of those two great literary protagonists children may be more educated explorers of the contemporary villains and the worlds they inhabit. Shakespeare, Dickens and the contemporary thereby become mutually inclusive. Common ground exists and should be recognised. The teacher can broaden the children's imaginary worlds by introducing them to works they might not otherwise meet. There can be fruitful coexistence between classics and soaps if the teacher seizes on ground already tilled. More children are conversant with adult issues, for instance the greed for money, than ever before. Such awareness, which is often highly developed even in nine- and ten-year-old children, can be turned to good effect as 'preparation', for, say, works of literature such as Chaucer's *Pardoner's Tale*, which is presented in Chapter 4.

However, there is a more pressing kind of relevance, which exerts greater power. That is the relevance to the children's unconscious, to their dream worlds, to that part of them which responds to folk and fairy tales, myths and legends. Some of the force of a play such as *Hamlet* depends on its foundation in legend, and this is the starting point of its relevance to children. The importance of the unconscious to the development of children is great and such stories as are found in fairy and folk tales, legend, and myth provide encouragement and structure for the welter of impressions which exists there.

Children are damaged by the repression or tight control of such impressions, but these stories provide a validation for them and what Bruno Bettelheim calls 'an emotional quality of truth' which goes beyond everyday relevance.[12] *Hamlet*, for instance, which is relevant to contemporary issues affecting children, also has that deeper appeal to struggles in their unconscious. One of childhood's more significant struggles, for instance, is against regressive behaviour, of doing anything but the thing one needs to do. By engaging with that struggle in a work of art such as *Hamlet* the problem is recognised, rather than repressed, and worked through in the child's imagination. Furthermore, if that working-through is extensive and essentially aesthetic, this whole process will be enhanced and its effects deepened.

The other worlds of literature

In his book *Fictional Worlds*, Thomas Pavel sees works of literature as kinds of 'possible worlds' with their own territories and boundaries, which are related to the real world that we live in.[13] The implication of this simple concept to me is that, instead of viewing a work of literature merely as an interesting formation of words for us to read and interpret, we need to accept and enter into it.

For instance, we need to pretend that an ordinary man like Lemuel Gulliver *has* landed on an island populated by six-inch-tall people and that their behaviour and his response to it are actually happening while we read Part I of *Gulliver's Travels*. Or, when we see Othello smothering his innocent wife with a pillow, we need to accept the illusion of it while it is happening on stage. This doesn't mean that, like one theatre-goer in the mid-west many years ago, we go and shoot Othello or even shout out to Desdemona to watch her back! But for full engagement we have to believe the make-believe or, as Coleridge famously argued, allow ourselves 'the willing suspension of disbelief'.

Pavel obviously has in mind narrative worlds, the worlds of stories, but other writers have applied similar ideas to lyric poetry. Samuel Levin, in *Metaphoric Worlds*, for example, invites the reader of lyric poetry to forget the analysis of language and accept the concept they contain, however strange or 'deviant' it may be.[14] He writes: 'An expression like "The trees were weeping", say, might be construed to mean that the trees were dripping moisture, shedding their leaves, exuding sap, or something similar' (Levin 1988: 1).

But such an interpretation, which is obviously a valid one from the perspective of the language itself, does not take us fully into the new world which the poet is trying to create. Levin suggests that we accept the concept literally and 'try to conceive of trees – those very things – as weeping'. If we do this, he argues, it is no longer the language which is metaphoric, it is the world of the poem. In other words, the poet has created a 'metaphoric world'.

The ideas of Pavel and Levin might seem like sophisticated forms of hair-splitting, but they imply a major shift in the way we might read stories and poems. They imply a somewhat deeper experience of literature in which stories and poems might take over our imaginations while we read. Indeed, they imply that when we read we detach ourselves from the real world and live in the imagined world. I labour the point here because it suggests to me that when we involve children in great or classic works of literature something active and all-involving is necessary, and the arts are the perfect vehicle for such an enterprise.

Renaissance in the classroom

Classic literature provides fictional or metaphoric worlds of a highly wrought kind, and children's involvement in such worlds can have considerable life-enhancing effects upon them. In terms of the cultural life of a school, the overall effect of regular involvement in these worlds can be akin to a renaissance, a rebirth or a renewal. By using the highly charged cultural word 'renaissance' I may appear fanciful, but the process I am advocating bears similarity with the explosion of cultural activity which began in fifteenth-century Italy. This 'renaissance' was sparked by the discovery of great works of literature and art from Greece and Rome. These works, having been read and found to have profound meanings for life in those times, led to a rush to emulate. The discovery of these works led to a flowering of literature across Europe. But this flowering was not exotic; it was not a new flowering of Greek or Latin literature. New works were by writers such as Dante, Cervantes and Shakespeare in their own languages.

What I am promoting here is the idea that classic works of literature, introduced into schools in the right way, can fire 'renaissance' for the children. Children can be enabled to make such works their own through artistic activity. So, children 'discover' great works of the past – from other cultures as well as their own – and use them as a sort of motor force for their development as readers, writers and people. Ways can be found to give children access to the richness of Shakespeare, Chaucer, Swift, Coleridge, Dickens and others despite the difficulties they present.

Even before the Renaissance, when people were more dependent on their communities than we are, stories and songs were celebrated communally. They were accepted as visions of wisdom to be enacted by the people. Sharing such visions as those provided by, say, the *Mahabharata*, the *Odyssey* or *Beowulf* could animate and uplift them, strengthening their resolve in times of adversity. Great literature can be celebrated in this way by children and teachers in schools.

The teacher's interventions in such ambitious projects is catalytic and may take many forms. The more successful of these usually involve artistic activity of one kind or another. By this I do not mean a few rare geniuses engaging as an exclusive group with something reserved for their special minds alone. I mean a far more democratic activity, one which is all-inclusive. The many case studies reported in this book provide copious examples of this inclusivity.

Developing the strands of language

One key benefit of such involvement in the worlds of the classics will be in children's growth as writers. The process leading to this is sometimes called 'creative mimesis'. 'Mimesis' is the Greek word which gave us the words 'mimic' and 'imitation', but those words carry merely the surface meanings of what the Greek word meant. A third English word from that root, 'mime', is closer to it. 'Mime' is an art form in which the artist does not merely copy pieces of behaviour, but interprets them into his or her own framework. Often this framework is comic, even mocking and satirical, often tragic.

'Creative mimesis' involves the grafting of personal response onto that which is being imitated. In terms of writing a useful image for this is provided by T.S. Eliot in his introduction to the translations of Ezra Pound:

> In each of the elements or strands there is something of Pound and something of some other . . . and the strands go to make one rope . . . good translation . . . is not merely translation, for the translator is giving the original through himself and finding himself through the original.[15]

If the work of literature has made a deep enough impression upon the child so that chords are plucked and the child can respond directly, then that response may approximate to translation in the sense Eliot means. 'Strands' is a useful word in this respect, 'strands' as threads to be spun together, to be plucked or teased out. Consider, for example, this poem by an 11-year-old written during a project based on James Reeves's retelling of Cervantes' *Don Quixote*:

> *Don Quixote and his books*
> A trap of dreams killing off reality.
> The dust of long years in wait of reading.
> But as this man of imagination turns
> the dead pages, the book seems to breathe
> a crackly breath of life that is the words.
> His house once the talk of the village.
> But now it is an old age books home.

The act of processing various strands of Cervantes' novel using her own sensibility has caught strands of this child and spun them into the rope of the poem. Having had the first two chapters read to her by the teacher, with enactments in drama, invitations to paint and to write, she decided to focus on Don Quixote sitting in his library. This decision was also the result of seeing an engraving by Gustave Dore in which Quixote is sitting in his library reading a book with characters flying about the room, being released by the process of the words in the book upon Quixote's imagination.

The child makes an intuitive selection of strands, the outcome of that part of the text and the Dore engraving probing her imagination. Quixote's books, which put strange notions into his head, are reworked as a 'trap'. She sees dreams as traps which kill off reality, a succinct summary of the trouble Quixote makes by trying to live out his fantasies. She sees words as having magic powers once they are read; they make dead ideas come alive. This is a strand vibrating both with Cervantes' narrative and with Dore's engraving. Finally, she sees a once-magnificent house becoming no more than a library for books, 'an old age books home'. This is her most original addition to Cervantes, bringing to bear the modern concept of special homes for old people.[16]

Secondary and tertiary worlds

The poet W.H. Auden, like Pavel and Levin, also thought of works of literature as other worlds. He also had a clear idea of the human value which such worlds have. In his essay *Secondary worlds*[17] he wrote:

> Present in every human being are two desires, a desire to know the truth about the primary world, the given world outside ourselves in which we are born, live, love, hate and die, and the desire to make new secondary worlds of our own or, if we cannot make them ourselves, to share in the secondary worlds of those who can. (Auden 1954: 1)

But 'sharing' is an insufficient description for the kinds of involvement I am advocating in this book. I am proposing something more active, exuberant and creative than receiving a portion of something. What was happening in 'Don Quixote and his books' was that the child was entering imaginatively into the world of a great, old work translated from Spanish and was creating something of her own. Out of the secondary world of Cervantes' novel, she has created something new again.

There is, therefore, a third dimension to this kind of work. When children engage with works of literature with the emphasis on the creative arts, they may make something new *again*. If they do, then they can be said to be creating tertiary worlds. I would claim 'Don Quixote and his books' as a work of art in its own right, a creative act of reading and writing made from the secondary world of another. Furthermore, the process which children go through will lead to real and tangible personal growth for the child as both reader and writer.

So my proposition is that literature can be the source of a contemporary renaissance and flowering of literature and the arts in schools, providing that it is based mainly in aesthetic activity. This aesthetic activity will take many forms and be expressed with varying degrees of intensity. It will take place in private as well as public ways, driven by the sensibilities of the children. But what kind of teaching and learning approaches would be necessary to embody these ambitions, bearing in mind the demands of the National Curriculum, the National Literacy Strategy and Key Stage 3 National Strategy? I will attempt to answer this question in Chapter 2.

References

1. Calvino, I. (1999) *Why Read the Classics?* London: Vintage Classics.
2. DfEE (1999) *The National Curriculum Handbook for Primary Teachers*. London: DfEE.
3. DfEE (1999) *The National Curriculum Handbook for Secondary Teachers*. London: DfEE.
4. The National Literacy Strategy Framework for Teachers.
5. Key Stage 3 National Strategy Framework for Teaching English.
6. Gibson, R. (1987) 'Jonathan Miller on Shakespeare', *Shakespeare and Schools*, Newsletter No. 3. Cambridge: Cambridge Institute of Education.
7. Greeves, A. (1990) 'For adult eyes only', *TES*, 20 April.
8. Andrews, R. (2001) *Teaching and Learning English*. London: Continuum.
9. Carter, D. (1976) *The Old Forge*. Unpublished dissertation, University of Exeter.
10. Carter, D. (1987) *Something Rich and Strange*. Mold: Clwyd County Council.
11. Witkin, R. (1974) *The Intelligence of Feeling*. London: Heinemann.
12. Bettelheim, B. (1976) *The Uses of Enchantment*. London: Thames and Hudson.
13. Pavel, T. (1986) *Fictional Worlds*. Cambridge, MA: Harvard University Press.
14. Levin, S.R. (1988) *Metaphoric Worlds*. New Haven, CT: Yale University Press.
15. Eliot, T.S. (1928) 'Introduction 1928', in *Ezra Pound: Selected Poems*. London: Faber.
16. Ruzika, J. (1974), *Gustave Dore Illustrations to Don Quixote*. London: Academy.
17. Auden, W.H. (1954) *Secondary Worlds*. London: Faber.

CHAPTER 2

Teaching and learning processes

Planning and preparation

Planning should be more a conscious rehearsal of actions than a bureaucratic treadmill, and the right kind of preparation and planning usually leads to creative and successful projects using classic literature. Such rehearsals of actions may lead directly to the teacher being an inspiration to her children and will have much to do with her feelings. The teacher's feelings about the literature must direct the course of any classic literature project.

It is, therefore, essential that the teacher choose a work which has moved her in the past, so that it produces an animation of rediscovery when she visits it again. One of Calvino's reasons for reading classic literature is that 'each rereading offers as much of a sense of discovery as the first reading'. To this he adds that the classic work 'has never exhausted all it has to say to its readers'. If the teacher chooses a work she loves she is more likely to bring inspiration to her teaching of it through her obvious animation when presenting it to children.[1]

Presenting or performing texts to children

One of the teacher's main concerns is the text and how much of it to use. On the one hand most texts appear to be too difficult to use with children, on the other a work of literature is great mainly because of its text. Text is, therefore, vital to the teaching of classic literature to children. For instance, Gulliver's adventures in Lilliput would appear more as a quaint folk tale without Swift's storytelling style, and Romeo and Juliet's love affair might look more like Mills and Boon without Shakespeare's poetry.

Let us imagine, for instance, that we are planning a project involving Shakespeare's *Hamlet*. The story is simple. Its greatness is in the way it is transformed into art. Some of this is achieved by Shakespeare's structuring of the material for the stage, but more through the power of the language. If we base our Shakespeare project on retellings we lose much of the essence of *Hamlet*. Approaches based on retellings distort, misinterpret or exaggerate because of the different demands made on the writer by the medium of narrative fiction. *Hamlet* is open to interpretation whereas, say, Leon Garfield interprets it for us because he is writing a prose version in the past tense.

We have to find a compromise which presents the work clearly and understandably, but with sufficient real text to connect the children with the true nature of the work. In a Shakespeare project there are two approaches to this: either

- read from a retelling of the story – preferably a retelling prepared by the teacher which uses the present tense – and recite key extracts from the text; or
- tell the story in the present tense and recite key extracts from the text.

The second method is preferable to the first because it is more flexible and brings the teacher's presentation a little closer to a sense of performance. The disadvantage, however, is that the teacher needs to know the plot well and be confident enough to take risks with it.

Applied to a project on *Hamlet* this latter approach might proceed as follows. The teacher

- prepares a poster showing the *dramatis personae* with the characters grouped to indicate their relationships (e.g. Ghost linked to Gertrude by a broken line, Gertrude linked to Claudius with an unbroken line) and the children learn these names and relationships;
- holds a copy of the play in one hand with the extracts she intends to recite already marked;
- starts at the very beginning, telling the children that this is Act I, Scene i, and saying 'A guard called Francisco is on the battlements of Elsinore Castle in Denmark. It is night time and the guard is changing. Bernardo, an officer, enters in the dark and says, "Who's there?"';
- recites Shakespeare's words until the entrance of Horatio and Marcellus, who are introduced so: 'Another officer called Marcellus enters with Prince Hamlet's friend Horatio. Francisco hears them and says, "I think I hear them. Stand ho! Who is there?"'
- recites Shakespeare's words again to the end of the scene.

So this approach combines storytelling with recitation and can be varied to suit any age group and the requirements of teacher, children and situation. For this flexible method cuts are made for several reasons:

- The language may be too difficult for the children.
- The scene may be too long to maintain their interest.
- The subject matter may be beyond the children's understanding.

There will also need to be short asides, explanations, questions and digressions, which bring the teacher out of role. For instance, in Act I, Scene i of *Hamlet*, the teacher, on speaking the line, 'Touching this dreaded sight, twice seen of us', might expect the pupils to be able to describe what that sight might be, having studied the *dramatis personae* chart. The children will also be filled with speculations as to why King Hamlet is a ghost at all.

At these early stages the presentation will get discursive with the teacher in and out of role and explaining many things. For instance, 'ambitious Norway' must be explained as 'ambitious [king of] Norway' and the speech of Marcellus, in which he questions the warlike preparations which are taking place, will need to be explained in terms of what has gone before. However, by the end of the first session the children will be buzzing with ideas, questions and speculations. They will have been touched deeply by the strange force of the language.

As the project ripens the teacher might feel compelled to draft children into her presentation by the sheer force of words and action combining. For instance, after the players have performed 'The murder of Gonzago' and Claudius goes to his room the children will be powerfully moved by a sense of outrage and a deep desire for revenge. They will see Claudius at prayer and will desperately want Hamlet to obey the ghost's instructions for revenge.

When I presented this scene to a class of Year 5 and 6 children I simply had to have one of the children at prayer on the edge of the group. I left the room. There was a stony silence. I re-entered clutching an invisible sword, and saying, 'Now might I do it pat, now 'a is a-praying.' I advanced right up behind Claudius. I raised the sword. The children gasped as if a sword was really there. I *was* going to do it. There were despairing sighs as I lowered it saying, 'And so am I reveng'd?' The words were forked lightning at this point. Human experience was more than illuminated by words. Words embodied deeds. The logic behind Hamlet's backing-off was clear, but more so the futility of it. They knew Claudius could not pray even while Hamlet was behind him: 'My words fly up, my thoughts remain below.' The whole scene was revealed as a missed opportunity leading directly to the killing of Polonius.[2]

This method should be sparing in its cuts. All scenes stay in their correct order. So the pupils get Shakespeare partially interpreted for them. They are, in the main, audience, but gradually becoming performers in preparation for drama work later. The children will savour the sense of performance and be roused to greater heights of enthusiasm. The immediacy will spill over into all aspects of their response.

Of course, the teacher's presentation of prose fiction, narrative and lyric poetry will not follow the process described above in some of its details. However, the sense of the dramatic through storytelling and recitation in varying measures should be a feature of a teacher's presentation and performance of all works of great literature, whether they be epics like *Beowulf*, narrative poems like *Sir Patrick Spens* or prose fiction like *Gulliver's Travels*. Obviously, lyric poetry requires a different approach and is dealt with separately in Chapter 7.

Children at work

So much depends on the first encounters with an episode, throughout a project on Shakespeare or other great literature. These encounters must 'disturb' the children rather than merely delivering the story or poem. Disturbance will be easy to see in the behaviour of the pupils: animated expressions; hands shooting up; gasps of air denoting a desperation to speak; up on knees or even standing; a torrent of verbal response, often accompanied by actions. These are the clear signals of motivation. As a project develops, this excitement comes under the control of a variety of works, some individual, some collaborative.

I offer, in this chapter, ideas for using all the five main arts: drama, dance, music, writing and visual art, as well as for literacy, particularly text level work. But what are the likely processes that children ideally will pass through for a full experience of Shakespeare or other classic literature? The following simple model embodies these processes from the point of view of children's experiences rather than teachers'.

1. **Meeting**. The children listen to the teacher's initial presentation/performance of a part of the work of literature, ask and answer questions, discuss ideas and begin to apply their imaginations to it.
2. **Knowing**. The children achieve increasing levels of knowledge and feeling about the work through activities such as recitations of extracts of text, planned discussions and writing.
3. **Transforming**. The children make various kinds of responses in the arts both individually and as members of a group, thereby transforming their increased knowing into new objects or tertiary worlds, such as:

    - a play about the Lilliputians finding Gulliver,
    - a poem such as 'Don Quixote and his books',
    - a dance about Sir Patrick Spens's sea voyage,
    - a bust of Caliban in *The Tempest*,
    - a musical setting of Blake's 'The Tyger'.

4. **Publishing**. The children communicate their work to others in the following ways:

    - talk about it with others,
    - display it on a wall or in a class book,

- perform or present it to an audience, either formally or informally,
- have multiple copies made and distributed.[3]

Writing

Writing can lead to the assimilation and accommodation of new ideas and help children to spin strands of their knowing and feeling in with these new ideas. This spinning process, when working well, can transform the new into personal expression. Writing is, therefore, a primary way for children to process the new sensations arising out of an episode in a project based on classic literature.

Consider, for instance, this line from a poem about Claudius at prayer (*Hamlet*, III. iii) by a Year 6 child:

> A fist of my brother's blood is my guilt.

This line has taken the idea in 'What if this cursed hand were thicker than itself with brother's blood?' then added the notion of Claudius's aggressive ruthlessness with 'fist' for 'cursed hand' and an evaluative commentary in the use of 'guilt'. This was not part of a conscious intention by the child but arose from instant response to the teacher's presentation. The child's subconscious processed it so that something of the child was fastened onto Shakespeare's idea. This is sensibility at work on culture leading to transformation.[4]

Looking over a large range of writings in response to classic literature projects I find that they reveal a remarkable consistency, with four clearly identifiable kinds of writing and a clear scale of complexity as follows.

1. Reportage

Here children re-write an incident in their own words, often feeling safe writing this way, particularly at the early stages of a project. Some, however, rarely stray from its security. A useful example is afforded by this extract in response to Act I, Scene i in *Hamlet*:

> Every midnight the ghost of Prince Hamlet's father appears
> in the same clothes as he wore on the same day he killed
> Fortinbras of Norway.

Although straightforward, this piece brings together information which the child has absorbed from different parts of the scene:

- the ghost wears the clothes he wore in the Norwegian wars
- he killed Fortinbras.[5]

2. Commentary

Here children mix opinion, personal response and facts, sometimes in a conversational tone, and sometimes with a poetic turn of phrase as in this from a *Twelfth Night* project:

> Sir Toby and Andrew they like some good fun
> They try to make everything into a pun.
> Maria tries to make them behave
> But fun swallows her up too, like a cave.

Comment here is in the assessment of Maria's role, in how flimsy are her attempts to tame the others whose riot is huge and dark like a cave.[6]

3. Reconstruction

At this stage children remake a writer's idea, for instance a Year 5 child invents the speech Ophelia might have made to her father after he had given his advice about her liaison with Hamlet (II. i):

> Father Polonius why all the advice? Please leave me alone.
> For I love Prince Hamlet. Laertes gave advice like yours.
> Please retain yourself and let me love him.

Then she gives Polonius's reply:

> Ophelia how can you say such things to your father?
> Yet I love you no matter what you say. You are
> my daughter. But stay away from him although
> you love Prince Hamlet.

The child ends the piece with a generalised comment about the state of Denmark:

> On the battlements bababa ba ba baaaa coming from
> the hall. Denmark is a drunken old place.

Her personal response is at its highest in these last lines.[7]

4. Transformation

There is a point at which a child's absorption of the work leads to a response which is transformed into something new. For instance, a Year 6 child imagines Gloucester's suicide in *King Lear* (IV. vi):

> Falling, he thinks he's falling,
> Down the suicidal cliffs.
> Edgar has saved him from the gates of Hell.
> Screams from the gulls,
> Thinking if he's alive.
> Or has he reached his destination.

> Shallowy pits as the sea rushes past.
> Edgar says, 'Look up yonder, can't you see
> The great white cliffs?'
> 'I can't. All I can see is solitude darkness.'

The child has transformed the ideas coming into her during the teacher's performance of this episode with five 'strands' of personal response:

- The cliffs are 'suicidal' as the place from where the fall was thought to have been made.
- The 'gates of Hell' invest the act with its Christian significance, damnation being the punishment for suicide.
- The 'gulls' are introduced as players in the drama with their commentary.
- The sea, also, has a part to play with the allusion to Hell in its 'shallowy pits'.
- The child has imagined Gloucester's isolation with 'solitude darkness'.

Yet all this personal response is spun in comfortably with the play's original strands to make a thread which has much unity.[8]

Art

In his book *Realms of Meaning*[9] Philip Phenix writes:

> In the esthetic realm . . . the object of knowledge is the singular, particular form. The primary concern is not with types of things – not with kinds and classes of things – but with unique individual objects. Essentially, every esthetic object is incomparable. (Phenix 1964: 141–2)

This is important throughout every stage of a project but is more important when using visual art, which can become no more than the creation of pretty pictures. For instance, in a project based on *The Tempest* it is easy to be side-tracked into stormy sea pictures. These might be gorgeous but have very little to do with Shakespeare's *The Tempest*. They may be types of things. They may be about any storm, but not *The Tempest*.

To make transformations out of the storm in *The Tempest* we must turn to the text itself. What is unique about the storm in *The Tempest*? To answer this we should look at the characters on board the ship and at what Ariel says *about* the storm, which he has raised. Ariel was on board the ship and 'flam'd amazement'. It is in this sort of image that the particularity will be found and, therefore, this is where the most fruitful way of making transformations in art must lie.

Children are also more aware through their sense of sight than through any other sense, registering visual images instantaneously. Once an image has registered it is difficult to replace. For instance, the art possibilities could have been restricted in my *Hamlet* project by the children seeing the painting on the front cover of the

Arden edition, in which Hamlet is shown in doublet and hose with a ruff. This image of Hamlet became fixed in the children's imaginations and I had to find a way to develop the art with it in mind. I chose to challenge the children to make visual images directly out of the imagery in Shakespeare's words.

A positive way of developing art response to classic literature texts is by making use of art history. One secondary teacher, for instance, working on *The Tempest*, brought to his class a range of images, including African masks. There were several exciting developments from these masks, particularly in portraits and busts of Caliban. One of these was particularly powerful, a bust of Caliban which was a transformation of influences absorbed from the descriptions of Caliban by Prospero and Miranda and those absorbed from the masks. The piece has the simplicity of design found in masks, but with statements about his deformity in grotesque mouth and eyes, and about his evil in the single horn on his head, a powerful, arresting image.[10]

In my experience children move through three distinct stages on their way to making transformations of great literature into art as follows:

1. Representation

In a Hamlet project, for instance, a Year 5 child responds to these lines from one of Hamlet's soliloquies

> For in that sleep of death what dreams may come
> When we have shuffled off this mortal coil
> Must give us pause.

On black paper she paints wraithlike human outlines in white, which swirl and corkscrew off the page. They are literally a 'mortal coil', a coil of human bodies. Her image is a diagrammatic representation of one idea.[11]

2. Interpretation

A Year 6 child makes a picture in response to Hamlet's self-disgust at his failure to avenge his father in Act II, Scene ii:

> I should ha' fatted all the region kites
> With this slave's offal.

He paints a wall with kites flying down it and a selection of objects – a bloodstained crown, a broken bottle, a ring, a heart, an ear and blood – at the bottom. It is his particular selection, which reveals his interpretation. This showed he was beginning to transform ideas in the play:

- The bloody crown off the head of Claudius reveals what Hamlet feels he should have done – killed the king.

- The broken bottle could be two things: the poison bottle or a wine bottle to signify the decadence of the Danish court.
- The ring next to the amputated hand signifies the severing of the marriage of Claudius to Gertrude and the amputated hand a punishment visited on the hand that poured the poison in the ear.
- The ear itself resonates with two possible meanings: an ear for an ear, or the ear that has done so much listening behind the arras, the spying ear.

In this picture the child has interpreted two lines in terms of a swathe of context in the play, expressing his own perception.[12]

3. Transformation

A Year 5 child was interested in the idea of Hamlet as a split personality and worked on the opening lines of the soliloquy in Act I, Scene ii:

> O that this too, too sullied flesh would melt
> Thaw and resolve itself into a dew.

He painted Hamlet wearing doublet, hose and ruff, half in black, half in white. The costume identifies Hamlet but the colour makes the transformation. Black represents the present, white the desired state: to be melted, 'thawed into a dew'. Though living, Hamlet is unhappy in black and in the black part the child gave him a downturned mouth. In the desired state of thawing, Hamlet is happy and, therefore, has an upturned mouth. It is a clear example of a child's transformation of great literature.[13]

Dance

It appears to me that there are two main ways in which dance can offer opportunities for children to transform great literature. These I will call naturalist and symbolist.

Naturalist

Dance can be made from

- the plot or story, the sequences of happenings;
- the characters, how they look, behave and relate with others.

The possibilities of making dances from plots are obvious. But how can dances be made from characterisations? A good example is afforded by Feste in *Twelfth Night* when he asks Sir Andrew and Sir Toby, 'Did you never see the *picture* of "we three"?' The question is then one of 'How should the characters look? How should they look in relation to each other?' Naturalist explorations can focus on this. Children might make dances about the relationship between Feste, Sir Andrew and Sir Toby starting with that 'we three'. In a kind of gallery portrait they might explore the dominance of one over the other, how they conspire against the common enemy, how one succeeds and the other fails embarrassingly in shapes and movements.

The work, focused on the physical shape and movement of characters, will continually be re-informed by the narrative and can gather fresh resonance when used as accompaniment to the words themselves. Thus the words are underlined and the action takes on the feeling associated with ritual. A good example of this is provided by a dance about the murder of Cinna the poet during a *Julius Caesar* project.

Two actors had appeared as Brutus and Anthony in a rehearsal of Act III, Scene ii with a Year 6 class who had learnt their parts. However, poor Cinna was almost trampled to death before he could attempt to answer the questions fired at him by the mob. The problem was solved by dance accompanying the words. With Cinna at their centre the class made a circle and each question was an incantation accompanied by an advancing movement until a tight circle was made, enclosing Cinna. This was the signal for the mob to take up snarling wolf positions leading to a second wave of questions. When Cinna finally divulged his name the mob rose over him snarling and spitting out the final words. At a clap the mob dispersed leaving the crumpled form of Cinna.[14]

Symbolist

Getting deeper into a great work requires a penetration into its themes and imagery. The use of dance here is likely, therefore, to be symbolist, as in this example based on Hamlet's two soliloquies, 'To be or not to be . . .' and 'O that this too, too sullied flesh'. The session began with an exercise on the notion of melting, as in 'O that this too, too sullied flesh would melt / Thaw and resolve itself into a dew.' These lines were actually used as a mantra for the meditation, which led to relaxation. The children were then invited to focus on the ideas contained in:

- 'For in that sleep of death what dreams may come;'
- 'The undiscover'd country, from whose bourn
  No traveller returns.'

The children then told a friend about what they had seen in their reverie. This exchange led them to movement sequences being developed to embody them.

- The 'undiscover'd country' extract led to:
  1. A traveller carrying a rucksack and disappearing through a barrier. A hand reached out of a lake, which turned into a grave and pulled the traveller down into it.
  2. A traveller disappearing in a mist and reappearing as a skeleton.
  3. A hand pouring something from a bottle onto the grass and all of the grass dying away into a wasted, barren ground.

- The 'sleep of death' extract led to a king lying down in an orchard. The weeds grabbed him in their embrace. The ground then turned over and all was normal again, except that the king had gone.[15]

These led to dreamlike dances, which illustrated how a few lines of text will draw in ideas from the surrounding hinterland of the play. Transformations such as these go beyond the words themselves into themes in the play. Such 'floating images', to use Caroline Spurgeon's words, contain the metaphysical basis of the whole work and, by guiding children to engage in these symbolic ways, the enterprise extends beyond story and character.[16]

Drama

Drama is most fruitfully used when the elements of story, character and language are made available to the children as tools and materials. Middle-years children are not able to play the part say of King Lear as written, but can play *with* it, approaching it through their natural ability to play dramatically. So, in a drama lesson, a boy might fetch a rolled-up paper, stretch it on the floor and say to the girl playing Cordelia, 'Do you see all those lands over there? Well, you're not having any!' By so doing he is finding, in a small way, an expression for his feelings about Lear's treatment of Cordelia, using the device of a teasing game, which he might use in real-life situations. He is bringing this familiar game to the new material and assimilating Lear's behaviour into his scheme of things.[17]

Work such as this only comes about when children are immersed in the theme, plot and characters of the play. They need to:

- hear, speak and discuss the language regularly;
- talk and write;
- be attracted to certain elements of plot and language and explore the themes.

To enable them to transform these things into personal expressions in drama the teacher needs to set up well planned individual and pairs work in movement and speech before groups make plays. For instance, the theme of being trapped or enslaved, from Act I of *The Tempest*, might be explored in a variety of ways before improvising a play about how Ariel was imprisoned in the pine tree or Caliban was turned from adopted son into beast of burden. The children might improvise in small groups, using their own language, but with fragments of Shakespeare introduced as and when they feel them to be useful.

If pupils are working towards some kind of performance more and more fragments of the original, even whole speeches or short scenes, gradually find their way into what becomes a well-crafted piece of spontaneous playing. Consideration then has to be given to presentation techniques as the children prepare their plays for performances. At this stage also there is enormous value in using professional actors. The children then engage in performances which more closely resemble those of the theatre. The various skills associated with performance may be developed quickly and dynamically through contact with the special skills of actors. A good example of this use of actors is provided in the *Tempest* case study in Chapter 5.

Music-making

The more obvious opportunities for music-making in a project are provided by any song lyrics to be found in the work itself. In a play such as *The Tempest*, for instance, songs are vital to the action and theme. Middle-years children are capable of 'setting' these to music, whether this be in the form of accompaniments to readings or the composition of tunes for singing the lyrics.

There is more to the musicality of literature, however, than any songs which may be there. For instance, Homer's *Odyssey* was sung to the lyre and drum and *Sir Patrick Spens* is a ballad. To realise the possibilities of this, much can be learnt from the way composers of opera have approached literature. Giuseppe Verdi, for instance, was attracted to characters such as Macbeth, Othello, Iago and Falstaff, and his focus on characterisation as a source of composition is a productive one for children. The idea of characters having a sort of signature tune is rich with potential, and this was how Verdi approached characters. So, for instance, the baritone enters as Macbeth, Iago or Falstaff, with his deep voice and his own orchestration, and eventually the audience knows he is going to enter because of these musical clues. This principle can lead to musical transformations in a Shakespeare play by children, using the simplest of techniques.

The signature tune works through familiarisation, each character being associated with a particular tune or motif, and these motifs subsequently evoke the characters even in their absence. Its potential in a literature project is great indeed, and children easily understand the idea. Once they are familiar with the characters they can create musical motifs to represent them. This might involve the use of key lines from their speeches; for instance, with a child making a doleful figure on chime bars based on the words 'To be or not to be', and these lines may then be chanted or sung.

Such a focus on characters having their own music might lead to interesting musical encounters. Once children have worked out signature tunes the challenge is to invent sounds and motifs to represent encounters between them. How, for instance, can Malvolio's spoiling of Sir Toby's party be represented in a pattern of non-verbal sounds? Such a challenge may lead a group of children to probe not only what happens but also why it happens. It may also lead to the realisation of the importance of the words themselves. Malvolio's 'gabble like tinkers at this time of night' contains musical ideas both in its rhythms and in the image it conjures up, which might provide great opportunities.

Musical explorations of character and story will be limited if the language is neglected, because so much is in the rhythm of the words. Our concern here is with the prominence of the sounds of a work, but it is not merely a matter of looking for 'nice noises'. It is also to do with exploring meanings implicit in the work. This may seem a tall order, but it has simple beginnings in the speaking of the words, often called choral speaking or recitation.

Choral speaking is the root of oratorio and is a fruitful way of exploring intrinsic music in a work. Key scenes, incidents, passages or movements can be used as libretti for oratorios. Thus, for instance, the children who have so enjoyed incantating all the witches' chants in *Macbeth* can use this technique on some of Macbeth's lines such as 'Tomorrow, and tomorrow and tomorrow' and reveal the influence of the witches on his behaviour. This perception of the language as a libretto can gain further interest by adding sound effects. This may simply be with a drum or may involve the full range of a school's musical resources, involving those who are learning musical instruments.

Publishing

The process is not complete without some kind of presentation or sharing of work, because the child's learning process requires the testing of ideas and inspirations within a sympathetic community. This is obviously more pressing with drama, dance and music-making, which are instant and usually unrecorded forms of art. However, all kinds of achievement deserve celebration, and a literature project deserves some kind of communal expression. Classic literature projects ought to end in some kind of event which brings everything together and towards which the children shape their works. So, the classroom becomes a gallery and a performance space is set aside. A concert may carry the bulk of the performance pieces, or, maybe, several events might take place over a number of days.

It is vital for the self-esteem and communication skills of all children that their art and writing be shared and published, perhaps in multiple copies so that they become part of a school's cultural heritage alongside professionally made work. Even the most unpromising communities can accept and participate in the cultural pursuits described and argued for throughout this book. Shakespeare and classic literature, often considered the preserve of the clever and the wealthy, can enter any community as a creative force to enhance the vitality of its children and their parents and friends.

References

1. Calvino, I. (1999) *Why Read the Classics?* London: Vantage Classics.
2. Carter, D. (1989) 'A country discovered', *Cambridge Journal of Education* 19(3): 333–50.

3. This model, which is used in Chapters 3, 4, 5, 6 and 7 as a means to present children's work, is based on a model presented in Ross, M. *et al.* (1993) *Assessing Achievement in the Arts*. Buckingham: Open University Press.

4. Carter 1989.

5. *Ibid.*

6. Carter, D. (1987) *Something Rich and Strange*, Associate's Report for the Shakespeare and Schools Project. Cambridge: Cambridge Institute of Education.

7. Carter 1989.

8. Carter, D. (1986) '*King Lear* in the junior classroom', *English in Education* 20(1): 44–7.

9. Phenix, P.H. (1964) *Realms of Meaning*. New York: McGraw-Hill.

10. Carter, D. (1990) *The Isle is Full of Noises*. Project Report. Mold: Clwyd County Council.

11. Carter 1989.

12. *Ibid.*

13. *Ibid.*

14. Carter 1987.

15. Carter 1989.

16. Spurgeon, C. (1935) *Shakespeare's Imagery*. Cambridge: Cambridge University Press.

17. Carter 1986.

CHAPTER 3

Epics and myths: *The Odyssey* and *Beowulf*

Introduction

In this chapter many of the ideas discussed in Chapters 1 and 2 are seen in action in a real project involving a class of Year 4, 5 and 6 children with several teachers and arts workers. Teachers will be able to judge for themselves the value of these ideas by considering the outcomes produced by the children in this ambitious project based on Homer's *The Odyssey*.

The Odyssey Project is followed by a project on the Old English epic *Beowulf*.[1] This is designed for Years 4, 5, 6 and 7. As well as substantial suggestions for various genres of writing this project strongly features work in combined performing arts.

Case study: *The Odyssey*

The project

- A class of Year 4, 5 and 6 children in an urban junior school engaged with Robert Fitzgerald's verse translation of Homer's *The Odyssey* for five months.[2]
- A student, three specialist teachers and three craftspeople supported the teacher.
- The aim was to explore *The Odyssey* as a source for literacy development and expressive response in the arts.
- The language of 'The Odyssey Project' was the language of Homer as provided by Fitzgerald, and children's work was based in it, which gave the project its particular character.
- Each member of the team made working plans for their own contributions with the key criterion that their ideas be based in the Fitzgerald text.
- Considerable planning went into the project but it was not divided into detailed objectives.

The text

The Odyssey is difficult for children, and careful editing was necessary so that a version could be assembled which would contain extensive but digestible tracts of Fitzgerald's Homer within a clear narrative structure. One problem was in the sequencing. All children's versions of *The Odyssey* are re-sequenced to conform to chronological time, which takes away much of the narrative impact of the poem. We had to conserve this sequence and were rewarded as this is exactly how it worked on the children in the project. There follows a synopsis of the story.

Parts One and Two

In Ithaka suitors for the hand of Penelope, Odysseus's wife, have gathered during his long absence. They treat his house without respect, eat his food and drink his wine. They game, swear and act like louts. Telemakhos, his son, frets, feeling unable to act. Pallas Athena, the goddess chosen by Zeus to save Odysseus, persuades Zeus to have him released from his imprisonment with the beautiful Kalypso. Athena goes to Ithaka, disguised as Mentes, to activate Telemakhos, who then goes in search of information about his father to Nestor and Menelaus, two of Odysseus's comrades in the Trojan wars.

Parts Three and Four

Pallas Athena sends Hermes to persuade Kalypso to release Odysseus. He sets sail for home but Poseidon the ruler of the seas, who hates Odysseus, sends a great storm. Odysseus is shipwrecked, naked, on Skheria. Nausikaa, the princess, whilst supervising the washing of clothes in the river, sees him, dresses him and invites him to the court of her father Alkinoos. It is here that Odysseus recounts his adventures since he left Troy.

Part Five

After the games, in which Odysseus is the best athlete, to Laodamas's shame, he tells his story to King Alkinoos. He cries many tears as he yearns for home. In one adventure he meets the Lotus-Eaters with their deadly property to induce forgetfulness. However, a worse fate awaited them on the island of the Kyklopes, the one-eyed giants where Polyphemus ate many of Odysseus's men. Here Odysseus showed the same cunning which made the wooden horse. He tricked and blinded Polyphemus and escaped but without many of his comrades.

Part Six

After surviving another storm, caused by another mistake by Odysseus, they reached Aiaia, the island of Kirke the witch. His next mistake was to kill a noble stag for meat to feed his crew. Kirke eventually turned half his men to swine.

Odysseus escaped by taking 'molu' supplied by the god Hermes. Kirke relented, released his men and helped him leave the island. But before journeying home he had to visit the Island of the Dead.

Part Seven

Odysseus and his men went to 'Persephone's deserted strand' and found the 'crumbling homes of the dead'. Odysseus dug the votive pit, poured libations, sacrificed lamb and ewe with oaths and let the black blood pour into the pit. The souls of the dead gathered out of Erebos: Elpenor, who died in Kirke's island; Antiklea, Odysseus's mother; Teiresias, Prince of Thebes; Epikaste, the mother of Oedipus; Persephone; Agamemnon; Minos; Tantalos; and Sisyphos.

Part Eight

Odysseus returned to Aiaia, made a funeral pyre for Elpenor, met Kirke again and was warned about the Sirens. She told the men to plug their ears with wax and bind Odysseus to the mast. She warned of the monster Skylla and the whirlpool Charybdis. Odysseus left and met those perils, losing more men. They reached the island of Helios, rich in cattle, but Kirke warned them not to kill these sacred beasts. Odysseus's men swore that they wouldn't, but their oaths were broken, with fatal consequences.

Parts Nine to Twelve

The Phaiacians of Skheria deliver Odysseus safely. But Poseidon, annoyed at this, turns the men and their ships into stone. Pallas Athena turns Odysseus into an old beggar and he meets Eumaios, the swineherd. Eumaios takes care of him. Odysseus meets Telemakhos and discloses the secret of his disguise. Eumaios tells Penelope of Telemakhos's homecoming. Odysseus goes home in this disguise and is the only man who can bend the great bow, firing an arrow through the neck of the arrogant suitor Antinoos. All the weapons in the house have been removed, so Odysseus and Telemakhos slaughter every suitor and Odysseus reclaims his hearth.

Homer's structure was followed, as were the Greek spellings of characters' names: Kirke not Circe, Poseidon not Neptune. The class teacher presented the text with a combination of storytelling and reciting extracts of text.

Teaching and learning processes

Meeting and knowing

The student immersed the children in stories of the gods and mortals and the causes and outcomes of the Trojan Wars, enabling them to understand the beliefs of the ancient Greeks. They learnt the complicated names of characters and places with the music specialist, who used them as the basis for clapping and chanting games. They relished the sounds and remembered them easily as a result.

Storytelling groups were established, in which the children would retell each episode to each other and stand to be corrected. This introduced a strong discipline into the children's thinking. When they came to improvise extracts of the narrative their work was better informed because of this. Their interest accumulated with each successive episode so that the concentration on its themes made them eager to master new ways of working. Often, skills were quickly learnt because of the intensity of the engagement.

Transforming: Writing
The children's writing demonstrated their ability and maturity to handle material which has helped to shape Western civilisation. They met and understood issues, situations and characters which have shaped the imaginations of poets, artists and musicians and playwrights down the ages. Much of it has helped define social and psychological understanding too, entering the language and informing a range of concepts.

For instance, a reluctant writer fixes in writing the situation of Oedipus and Epikaste, which has given definition to the psychological condition known as the Oedipus Complex:

> Epikaste's evil son got Epikaste to marry him, so he will get the power to rule and to be king of the land. Well his conscience knows of the murder which took place that night when his father died. He knows but does not care. Epikaste says 'I can live no longer with that shame'. She commits suicide. She hung herself and her body swings for all time among the spirits.

Another child, assuming the role of Odysseus, pinpoints Odysseus's emotions when trying to make contact with his mother on the Island of the Dead:

> I feel deep sorrow in my heart. But each time I go to reach out to her to touch her it's very painful. There's a thick lump in my throat. It feels like I am going to burst out crying. Everything inside me is a muddle. My heart is ready to EXPLODE.

Throughout the project writing, along with discussion, helped the children assimilate the epic. Homer's words were daily brought to life. Many pieces are improvisatory. The writer of the next piece, for instance, imagines she is one of Nausikaa's maids present when Odysseus is discovered naked on the island:

> Look at this dirty sheet. I wouldn't be surprised if it had been under this couch for a god's century. Still I mustn't grumble. It will be a good day out . . . What's that I hear? My mistress asks her father, the great sea-king Alcinoos for a mule to pull the cart she promised to use. Phew, as least I won't have to walk. When dawn spread out her fingertips of rose we stood outside the palace . . .
> The greeny blue glossy river bed does its work well. The thick dust floats downstream . . .

What is it? A wild man. At least he holds an olive branch to cover his nakedness. I bet he is ashamed, a middle-age man in his prime.

Here the child gets into the role by focusing on the dirty sheet, a commonplace, producing a stream of consciousness in what she assumes to be the maid's chatty voice. This is a fine perspective for the poem's more significant event at this stage, the discovery of Odysseus. She also gives life to the circumstance of that discovery, creating the details which prove her total involvement in her role: 'The greeny blue glossy river bed does its work well. The thick dust floats downstream'.

This strand of personal response spins very easily with Homer's formulaic lines, which she happily re-uses:

> 'When dawn spread out her fingertips of rose . . .'
> 'the great sea-king Alcinoos . . .'

Homer's use of such stock phrases is an important part of his oral formula. This child adopts his style, and this is seen again in her moralistic description of the naked Odysseus, 'a middle-age man in his prime'. So, although this child explores a character without real importance, the strength of her piece depends on these aspects of the text.

The children found it particularly easy to enter certain parts of *The Odyssey*. The visit to the cave of Polyphemus was relished by all, and they were quick to assume any role, for instance of Odysseus, in their writing:

> What an appalling sight to see. I was sick to my stomach. The giant tore them apart like chicken pieces and ate them. He bashed out their brains on rocks. My heart sickened for a while. A sudden pain came over me. Would it be me next? Would it be me? . . . We rammed the scorching stick into the crater eye. Hearing that bellowing cry many Cyclops were awakened. They bellowed from outside of the cave 'What's the matter? What is all the fuss about?' Polyphemus the Cyclops answered 'Nobody is killing me!' The Cyclops neighbours moved away. 'Then if nobody's killing you, you won't need our help.'

Another appealing incident was on the island of Aiaia with the witch Kirke. While relishing it for its spookery, the children also revealed an appreciation of the subtleties of the place, as in this piece in which much is compressed into the delicious expression, 'A sparkle went into her head.'

> A goddess called Kirke said to the friendly lions
> and tigers 'SCAT! I want to see him on his own.'
> She said, 'What is your name and what brings you here?'
> 'Odysseus is my name.' A sparkle went into her head.
> 'He is the one who always gets on the Gods' nerves.'

The children developed diversity in their writing, and this was given further impetus when the teacher invited them to collaborate in pairs. They had to discuss their ideas onto a tape and then write them as in the following lyrics for the Sirens (Cyrenes) and Odysseus, in which two children went into role to compose this song, one playing the Sirens, the other Odysseus:

> Come nearer, come nearer, come on, come on.
> Join us, join us, hear our song.
>
> You have heard our song, you have heard our song.
> Let us sing another one.
>
> Stop, stop you hurt me a lot, please, please
> or my heart will freeze.
>
> You have heard our song, you have heard our song.
> Let us sing another one.
>
> Draw nearer, draw nearer, we plead, we plead.
> If you don't respond our hearts will bleed.
>
> You have heard our song, you have heard our song.
> Let us sing another one.
>
> I beg, I beg. Let me go, let me go.
> For if you don't, I will kill you so.
>
> You have heard our song, you have heard our song.
> Let us sing another one.

Transforming: Art

Large folders were made by hand, using carefully cut card and linson with wax resist, ink-washed Greek motifs. These made handsome containers for the children's written work and provided an opportunity for using bookbinding skills already well developed.

Most of the art, however, was carried out by three craftspeople: potter, fabric worker and theatre designer. Each had the challenge of introducing a set of skills which were largely unfamiliar to the children and making these skills work for them.

The potter:

- talked about Greek pottery, explaining how it was produced and its influence;
- demonstrated basic techniques: relief work based on flat, rolled-out shapes; three-dimensional work; the making of reliefs by indenting; plain pot construction; and the use of self-made templates to create patterns in glazes;
- got the children to draw favourite Odyssey images as starting points for their work in clay.

The children

- made drawings which were appropriate for working in clay, for instance a domed Kalypso's cave, writhing snakes on a plate, faces of the gods and a ship for Odysseus and his men;
- discussed their pictures and how they might be made in clay, based on the techniques already demonstrated;
- played with clay, knocking out its air bubbles;
- worked their drawings in clay.

Clay proved to be a particularly responsive and satisfying medium for the children to use, and the time between the conception and realisation of an image was very short. The children found it easy to express their ideas, as in one piece which was a relief sculpture of Polyphemus. It is a twisting figure which conveys horror and tragedy at the same time. In the face of the figure the child expresses her impressions of Polyphemus, and in the body records information she has acquired.

Transforming: Other art work
The children made

1. Six large dyed and embroidered fabric panels of various islands for the walls of the school with the fabric artist.
2. Large sculptures of the various monsters with the theatre designer as follows:
   - 3-foot-long flying Siren with voluptuous but disastrous lips, claws and colourful wings;
   - Odysseus bound to the mast;
   - 5-foot-high Kyklopes in his chicken wire cave;
   - an enormous eagle sent by Zeus as a punishment.

Transforming: Dance
1. The dance specialist based her work on Odysseus's visit to the Island of the Dead. She discussed with the children the idea of seeing a loved one but not being able to touch, of ' the souls not being able to communicate' and explored this in three stages:
   - Not being able to touch.
   - One moving, the other following.
   - Escaping from touch, remembering that Odysseus longed to touch his mother.
2. She had the children imagining the 'Valley of Death' and how Odysseus and his crew might feel on entering it.
   - They thought of atmospheric words then created them in movement.
   - As this was difficult she had them standing absolutely still then moving their

heads only to look around the room, slowly and smoothly, then quickly.
- This idea of focus was then used in movement and levels.
- Music was introduced and this improved the quality and feeling in the movements.

3. The idea of bodiless souls, which could not be touched, was explored.
   - The children were divided into two groups: the souls and Odysseus's men.
   - The souls made movements to match the characters they had been in life.
   - Odysseus's men entered the valley to the music, then moved among the souls who were still.
4. The work moved into ritual, the children working on the idea of circles (the pit for the blood to be poured into) and leading towards a 'spiral effect, finishing in an enclosed circle'.

Transforming: Music
1. The music specialist based her work on Odysseus in Skheria and Aiaia.
2. Three groups worked on Kirke's song as she weaves at her loom, creating three different effects:
   - words of the text, 'low she sang / in her beguiling voice, while on her loom / she wove ambrosial fabric sheer and bright', leading to phrases on the auto harp;
   - a rocking rhythm on the large glockenspiel using notes D and A with soft beaters;
   - voices making 'oooo' sounds with a rocking rhythm and movements down the scale.
3. The children discussed ways of changing the mood as Kirke weaves her spell, suggesting that mounting tension and increasing volume should be created.
4. The three pieces were put together so that from the spoken introduction there was an unbroken sequence of sound depicting Kirke at her loom changing from beautiful weaver of cloth into menacing weaver of spells that turn men into swine.

Publishing
There were many audiences for the various kinds of work produced similar to those described elsewhere in this book. Here I describe a particularly valuable one.

1. Her Majesty's Inspectors in Wales had organised a residential course for primary teachers and invited the Odyssey children to attend for the afternoon of one of their days and present their work.
2. Firstly, the children spent half an hour with the teachers in small groups, showing their portfolios of Odyssey work and discussing the project. There was no inhibition because they were confident about their knowledge, experiences and work.

3. Next the children and their teacher made a 50-minute presentation which combined telling the story and reciting their written work. The audience of sixty teachers was enthralled by their assured and well articulated presentation.[3]

Project: *Beowulf*

The project

- For children in Years 4 (Term 2), 5 (Term 2) and 6 (Term 2) in primary schools and Year 7 in secondary schools.
- To be used as part of a focus on storytelling in poetry, particularly of epics.
- To demonstrate how form affects meaning.
- To show how a text from more than a thousand years ago can still be significant.
- To develop skills and knowledge in literacy, art, dance, drama and music.

The text

Beowulf is the most important work of literature from the Anglo-Saxon period. Although it was written down in the tenth century it was developed as a work in the oral tradition for hundreds of years before. It was probably composed in its present form by the end of the eighth century. However, the stories in it are from fifth-century Scandinavia and were brought over by the Vikings.

Although there are several important digressions in the poem, the main story tells of the hero Beowulf who, as a young man, rescues his father's friend King Hrothgar from the monster Grendel. After ridding Hrothgar's palace, Heorot, from Grendel, Beowulf kills the monster's mother under a lake. Much later when he is an old man and king in Geatland, Beowulf has to fight a dragon. He kills it but is killed himself.

Beowulf is the only epic poem to have survived from the Old English period in English literature. It is a genuine epic poem and enjoyed a growing reputation throughout the latter part of the twentieth century. Its most notable recent achievement is to have won a major literary award for the latest translation by the Irish poet Seamus Heaney.

In the text presented here I attempt to provide a storytelling script with highlights from Heaney's translation. I focus my attention entirely on Beowulf's exploits in Denmark and largely omit the digressions. I recommend that teachers requiring more of the original text turn to Heaney's brilliant translation published by Faber in 1999.

Beowulf in Denmark

1. The poet recalls the fame of the kings of Denmark, beginning with Scyld Shefing, who became a great king despite his humble childhood. When Scyld

Shefing died he was given a great ship burial, sailing out for the last time in a boat laden with treasures. Scyld's son Beow, who was famous for his bravery, ruled after him. He was succeeded by Beowulf the Dane and, later, Healfdene his son.

It was when Healfdene's own son Hrothgar became king that troubles began. Hrothgar was a mighty warrior king and vanquished all his foes. He became rich with the duties paid to him and built the greatest hall ever known in those parts. It was called Heorot, and here Hrothgar showed his generosity by giving presents to his followers and friends. Heorot became a place of feasting, music-making and storytelling. But there was an evil monster living nearby, which hated to hear all this merry-making.

The monster's name was Grendel and he lived in fens and marshes. He was said to have descended from the sons of Cain along with other monsters, ogres and evil-ones.

> So, after nightfall, Grendel set out
> for the lofty house, to see how the Ring-Danes
> were settling into it after their drink,
> and there he came upon them, a company of the best
> asleep from their feasting, insensible to pain
> and human sorrow. Suddenly then
> the God-cursed brute was creating havoc:
> greedy and grim, he grabbed thirty men
> from their resting places and rushed to his lair,
> flushed up and inflamed from the raid,
> blundering back with the butchered corpses.
>
> Then as dawn brightened and the day broke
> Grendel's powers of destruction were plain:
> their wassail was over, they wept to heaven
> and mourned under morning. Their mighty prince,
> the storied leader, sat stricken and helpless,
> humiliated by the loss of his guard,
> bewildered and stunned, staring aghast
> at the demon's trail, in deep distress.
> He was numb with grief, but got no respite
> for one night later merciless Grendel
> struck again with more gruesome murders.
> Malignant by nature, he never showed remorse.
> It was easy then to meet with a man
> shifting himself to a safer distance
> to bed in the bothies, for who could be blind
> to the evidence of his eyes, the obviousness

of that hall-watcher's hate? Whoever escaped
kept a weather-eye open and moved away.

(Lines 115–43)

Grendel then fought against goodness and ruled in Heorot, which stood empty at night for twelve years. The news of Hrothgar's sufferings spread through songs. Nothing could be done about it. Grendel continued to stalk the night and strike. He would even sleep the night in the hall. Daily meetings were held to search for an answer. Prayers and offerings to the old gods were even made. But the nightmare continued unabated.

2. This news came across the seas to Beowulf, a young Geat. He was a mighty warrior without equal in those days. At once he had a boat built and announced that he would go and help Hrothgar. The elders of the Geats encouraged him and Beowulf chose the best men he could find to come with him. There were fourteen, and they boarded the ship with their captain.

Time went by, the boat was on water,
in close under the cliffs.
Men climbed eagerly up the gangplank,
sand churned in the surf, warriors loaded
a cargo of weapons, shining war-gear
in the vessel's hold, then heaved out,
away with a will in their wood-wreathed ship.
Over the waves, with the wind behind her
and foam at her neck, she flew like a bird
until her curved prow had covered the distance
and on the following day, at the due hour,
those seafarers sighted land,
sunlit cliffs, sheer crags
and looming headlands. The landfall they sought.
It was the end of their voyage and the Geats vaulted
over the side, out on to the sand,
and moored their ship. There was a clash of mail
and a thresh of gear. They thanked God
for that easy crossing on a calm sea.

(Lines 210–28)

A watchman saw them land. He was impressed with them, particularly with Beowulf, but also worried by their appearance and questioned them. Beowulf reassured the watchman, saying he was the son of the great warrior Ecgtheow and was come to help Hrothgar overcome his enemy. The watchman believed Beowulf's words so he led them to Heorot.

At Heorot Beowulf and his men laid aside their weapons and met Wulfgar, herald to Hrothgar. Beowulf explained his purpose and Wulfgar went in to Hrothgar to pass it on. Hrothgar was delighted. He knew Beowulf from when he was a boy. He had also heard that Beowulf now had the strength of thirty men. He thanked God and sent his herald to bring Beowulf in with his men.

Beowulf entered the hall and made a great speech. He said that he knew of Grendel and of Heorot being empty at night and that the wise men of his people had urged him to come and help. He said also that these wise men well knew of his strength and how he had already fought and killed giants and sea serpents. Beowulf then asked Hrothgar to give him permission to cleanse Heorot. He added that, as Grendel never used weapons, he would fight him with his bare hands and if he should die Hrothgar should send his battle-shirt to King Hygelac in Geatland.

Hrothgar answered Beowulf's fine speech with one of his own, recalling Beowulf's father's exploits and how he, Hrothgar, had helped him. Hrothgar then talked of his own troubles at the hands of Grendel. He spoke of his disappointment that many of his men tried to fight with Grendel but met their ends. He invited Beowulf and his men to banquet with him and a space was cleared for them.

3. During the banquet many stories were told. One man, Unferth, who was jealous of Beowulf, said that Beowulf was not as brave as he claimed and told a story to prove it. Beowulf told the true story to disprove it, adding that, if Unferth was so brave, why hadn't he killed Grendel?

Hrothgar grew ever more confident in Beowulf. Wealtheow, his wife, offered Beowulf the mead cup first and greeted him. Beowulf vowed to her that he would rid them of their enemy. There were more speeches and songs, salutations and good wishes before the Danes left Heorot in the hands of Beowulf and his Geats.

Beowulf took off his coat of mail and handed his sword to an attendant. He told his men he would fight Grendel without these things and lay down on a bench to await his enemy. Outside, Grendel was on his way across the moors and approaching the shining hall. Desperate for blood, he tore off the door. A light was in his eyes as he trod across the floor. He was delighted when he saw the ranks of sleeping men. Little did he know what was in store for him that night. Beowulf was watching as Grendel seized a man off a bench, bit into him and gorged himself on lumps of flesh. Then he approached Beowulf.

> Venturing closer,
> his talon was raised to attack Beowulf
> where he lay on the bed, he was bearing in
> with open claw when the alert hero's
> comeback and armlock forestalled him utterly.
> The captain of evil discovered himself

in a handgrip harder than anything
he had ever encountered in any man
on the face of the earth. Every bone in his body
quailed and recoiled, but he could not escape.
He was desperate to flee to his den and hide
with the devil's litter, for in all his days
he had never been clamped or cornered like this.
Then Hygelac's trusty retainer recalled
his bedtime speech, sprang to his feet
and got a firm hold. Fingers were bursting,
the monster back-tracking, the man overpowering.
The dread of the land was desperate to escape,
to take a roundabout road and flee
to his lair in the fens. The latching power
in his fingers weakened; it was the worst trip
the terror-monger had taken to Heorot.

(Lines 745–65)

Beowulf and Grendel wrestled on, crashing around the walls of Heorot and smashing mead-benches. Then a fearful scream went up. It was Grendel wailing in agony as Beowulf held onto him tightly. Beowulf's men tried to help, poking their swords into Grendel, but did not realise that no sword could cut into Grendel's hide. But Grendel's powers began to falter as Beowulf exerted his handgrip.

The monster's whole
body was in pain, a tremendous wound
appeared on his shoulder. Sinews split
and the bone-lappings burst. Beowulf was granted
the glory of winning; Grendel was driven
under the fen-banks, fatally hurt,
to his desolate lair.

(Lines 814–20)

The proof of Beowulf's victory was plain to see. Grendel's whole arm from talon to shoulder was torn off and hung on the wall just below the roof. Everybody flocked to see it next morning. Meanwhile, Grendel staggered off to the mere, making the water red where he dived, his life ebbing away. Those who rode away from the scene of Beowulf's triumph sang his praises, comparing his heroic deeds with those of Sigemund the dragon-slayer.

4. So great was Hrothgar's joy that, after heaping honours on Beowulf, he said that he would give him anything he wanted. He said that Beowulf's deed would make

his name live forever. Beowulf answered that he would have been better pleased if Grendel's body were lying on the floor and regretted his escape. Unferth had nothing to say. Everybody inspected the arm and saw how like barbed steel were the nails.

Men and women busied themselves in the great hall, refurbishing it and decorating the walls. They prepared a banquet and filled the benches with a great company, who ate hungrily. The mead flowed and the time soon came for Hrothgar to present gifts to Beowulf. Hrothgar was generous. He gave a gold standard with embroidered banner; special breast mail, helmet and sword; and eight horses with gold bridles. Hrothgar also gave out gifts to Beowulf's men and paid compensation for the Geat killed by Grendel.

The song of the Frisian King Finn was sung to the tune of the harp, a tale of battle and loss, but victory for the Danes. The stewards brought more mead around and Wealtheow, the queen, came and sat among the Geats. She thanked and praised Beowulf and gave him more gifts. One was a torque, which Beowulf would give to his king, Hygelac. Then it was bedtime and the men slept in the hall with their weapons and armour at the ready.

But Grendel had a mother and she wanted revenge for her son's fatal wound. She came down to Heorot to have it. The warriors snatched up their swords and frightened her.

> The hell-dam was in panic, desperate to get out,
> in mortal terror the moment she was found.
> She had pounced and taken one of the retainers
> in a tight hold, then headed for the fen.
> To Hrothgar, this man was the most beloved
> of the friends he trusted between the two seas.
> She had done away with a great warrior,
> ambushed him at rest.
>   Beowulf was elsewhere.
> Earlier, after the award of treasure,
> the Geat had been given another lodging.
>
> (Lines 1293–1302)

Grendel's mother grabbed her son's arm off the wall as she left. Heorot was in turmoil, Hrothgar's most loyal man taken. Beowulf was soon with him, listening to the woeful tale of the loss of Aeschere, Hrothgar's chief adviser. Hrothgar said that he had often heard that there were two monsters at large, one like a woman. He told Beowulf of the haunted mere where the monsters lived, which even frightened wild animals. He offered more treasure to Beowulf if he would settle this feud once and for all.

Beowulf tried to reassure Hrothgar and promised that he would go and get Grendel's mother even if she were under the ground or at the bottom of the ocean.

At once Hrothgar organised an expedition to the mere. As they approached the mere, one of the company found Aeschere's head. Then they looked into the mere and saw hot blood bubbling there along with all kind of monsters. Beowulf shot one of them, a disgusting creature, then armed himself with special armour and a sword called Hrunting, lent to him by Unferth.

5. With a speech of goodbye and praises for Hrothgar Beowulf dived into the mere. He swam for most of the day until he saw the bottom. Grendel's mother had sensed that a human was coming and was waiting. She caught him in her grasp, but his armour protected him. Her claws could not penetrate Beowulf's chainmail.

At the bottom of the mere she dragged him into her den. He caught sight of her and swung the sword down on her head. The sword made no mark on her. This mighty sword was useless. Beowulf threw it away in anger and relied on his mighty arms, grabbing her by the shoulder and throwing her to the floor. But she was quickly up and grabbed him in a tight embrace. Beowulf fell down and felt vulnerable. She drew a sharp knife and stabbed him, but, again, his chainmail saved him. God was surely protecting him. Then Beowulf found another weapon.

> Then he saw a blade that boded well,
> a sword in her armoury, an ancient heirloom
> from the days of the giants, an ideal weapon,
> one that any warrior would envy,
> but so huge and heavy of itself
> only Beowulf could wield it in battle.
> So the Shieldings' hero, hard-pressed and enraged,
> took a firm hold of the hilt and swung
> the blade in an arc, a resolute blow
> that bit deep into her neck-bone
> and severed it entirely, toppling the doomed
> house of her flesh; she fell to the floor.
> The sword dripped blood, the swordsman was elated.
>
> A light appeared and the place brightened
> the way the sky does when heaven's candle
> is shining clearly. He inspected the vault:
> with sword held high, its hilt raised
> to guard and threaten, Hygelac's thane
> scouted along the wall in Grendel's wake.
> Now the weapon was to prove its worth.
> The warrior determined to take revenge
> for every gross act Grendel had committed –
> and not only for that one occasion

> when he'd come to slaughter the sleeping troops,
> fifteen of Hrothgar's house-guards
> surprised on their benches and ruthlessly devoured,
> and as many again carried away,
> a brutal plunder. Beowulf in his fury
> now settled that score: he saw the monster
> in his resting-place, war-weary and wrecked,
> a lifeless corpse, a casualty
> of the battle in Heorot. The body gaped
> at the stroke dealt to it after death:
> Beowulf cut the corpse's head off.

(Lines 1558–91)

Hrothgar's men, watching the water, saw blood surge up to the surface and thought it was Beowulf's. Later they left with their king, but Beowulf's men stayed, hoping to see their leader. Down below Beowulf watched the mighty sword melt and saw many treasures, but he was only interested in the jewelled handle of the sword and Grendel's head. He took these things and swam to the surface. His men saw him break the surface and thanked God as they advanced to meet him.

Beowulf took off his helmet and armour and the mere settled darkly down. It took four men to lift Grendel's head onto a spear and carry it to Heorot, where it was hauled across the floor to the amazement of the company. Beowulf offered it to Hrothgar as a trophy and told of his dire struggle with Grendel's mother. He praised God and described how the ancient sword helped him then melted with Grendel's blood on it. Handing the jewelled handle of the sword to Hrothgar, Beowulf promised that his troubles were finally over.

Hrothgar admired its golden patterns and runes and praised Beowulf's goodness and bravery, saying that his fame was widespread. He also spoke of the difficulties of fame, power and pride and how danger is always waiting. Finally, he praised God for the end of his troubles and promised more treasures to Beowulf. The whole company feasted again then went to bed.

Next morning Beowulf and his men made preparations to return home to Geatland. Beowulf thanked Hrothgar for his great hospitality and promised that he would return if ever needed. Hrothgar praised Beowulf and added that one day he would make a great king. He presented more gifts then embraced Beowulf with tears in his eyes. They went down to their ship.

> Right away the mast was rigged with its sea-shawl;
> sail-ropes were tightened, timbers drummed
> and stiff winds kept the wave-crosser
> skimming ahead; as she heaved forward,
> her foamy neck was fleet and buoyant,

> a lapped prow loping over currents,
> until finally the Geats caught sight of coastline
> and familiar cliffs. The keel reared up,
> wind lifted it home, it hit the land.

(Lines 1905–13)

Beowulf and his men strode up the shore in the sunlight, their treasure was carried off the ship and Hygelac the king of the Geats was told of their arrival. A feast was held and Beowulf told his king of his adventures in Denmark. He shared his treasures with Hygelac, who gave Beowulf a great sword and many lands. Years later, after Hygelac fell in battle, Beowulf became king of the Geats and ruled the people wisely for fifty years.

Teaching and learning processes

Meeting and knowing
1. Tell the children that:
   - Long before there were any books there were stories, poems and songs and that these were memorised by poets who would tell or sing them at feasts and other special occasions.
   - Some of these were eventually written down and are as skilfully crafted as any works written in later years and that *Beowulf* is one of them.
   - *Beowulf* was composed in the eighth century by Anglo-Saxon poets and written down 200 years or so later.
   - They will work with about two-thirds of this poem in the translation by Seamus Heaney.
2. Establish discussion groups to
   - compare and contrast Heorot with Grendel's cave;
   - find, compare and contrast adjectives used to describe Beowulf and Grendel;
   - compile a list of features in *Beowulf* which show that it is a legend;
   - find and make a list of interesting-sounding words and phrases in the extracts;
   - discuss the different moods and feelings in the story.

Meeting and knowing: Additional work for Year 7 children
3. Teach the children the basics of the form of *Beowulf* as follows:
   - Each line of the original is divided into two parts with a *caesura* or break in the middle as in this example:

> *Swa fela fyrena*   *feond man-cynnes*
> *atol an-gengea,*   *oft gefremede*

(Lines 164–5)

which literally means

So many crimes   the enemy of mankind,
the dread lone-walker,   often brought about

There is a sense here of units of sound, two to the line, with a slight silence in the middle.[4]

- Each half line or unit of sound contains two stressed and two or more unstressed syllables:

Swa fela fyrena   feond man-cynnes
atol an-gengea,   oft gefremede

- Each line carries an alliterative sound in the stressed syllables, which unites the two units. So in line 164 the alliterative sound is the consonant *f* as in *fela* and *fyrena* in the first half of the line and *feond* in the second half.

4. Explain to the children that it is difficult for a translator to get all this exactly right, but that Seamus Heaney's lines are divided into two units of sound with stressed and unstressed syllables even though he doesn't always put in the alliteration.

5. Ask the children in small groups to explore the extracts of Heaney's text for examples of these aspects of form and to record them in their English books.

6. Finally, explain that this form indicates that the poem was orally composed, being so based on a distinct rhythmic pattern with clear rules. This would help the performer to maintain the momentum of his performance throughout the whole story.

7. Tell the story and recite the extracts in the five episodes indicated in the text, taking about five weeks for it.
   - When reciting the extracts try to convey the rhythm of the piece so that they sound distinctly different from the storytelling parts.
   - Ask the children to retell the plot to a partner after each episode.
   - After the episode in which Beowulf fights Grendel in Heorot ask them to predict the outcome of the entire story.
   - Use the extracts as recitation scripts for the children to work up into performances.
   - Encourage them to emphasise the rhythmic pattern.

Transforming: Writing
1. Settings.
   - In their own words children to write descriptions of Heorot, the sea which Beowulf sails across, the fen which Grendel crosses, the mere and Grendel's underwater den.
   - Encourage them to use vivid language as in the original.

- Invite more confident writers to write their descriptions as poems in the style of the original.
- Year 7 children should attempt to write their descriptions using stressed and unstressed syllables and alliteration.

2. Character sketches.
   - Attempting to imitate the style of the original, the children to write poems about the main characters: Hrothgar, Grendel, Beowulf and Grendel's mother.
   - Year 7 children should attempt to write their descriptions using stressed and unstressed syllables and alliteration.

3. Narratives.
   - There are many digressions in Beowulf, in other words other stories outside of the story of Beowulf defeating Grendel and his mother. The most interesting ones are:
     (a) Beowulf and Breca. Best friends, these two have a swimming contest across the ocean, which goes very wrong and leads to dangers and adventures.
     (b) Sigemund the dragon-slayer. As a young man Sigemund enters alone into the much-feared dragon's cave in order to gain its treasure-hoard. Later he is betrayed and ambushed.
     (c) Hildeburh and Finn. Hildeburh is a Danish princess. Finn is the Frisian king. They are married and have a son. Denmark and Frisia are often enemies. At a feast a fight breaks out. Princess Hildeburh's brother and her son are killed.
     (d) Heremod. Heremod is the very opposite of Beowulf. He rises to power through death and destruction and never gave out presents at feasts.
     (e) Beowulf and the dragon. After he has ruled for fifty years a dragon causes havoc in Geatland. Beowulf is the only man brave enough to fight with it.
   - Children to choose one plot from this list of digressions to plan and write a narrative which
     (a) has a dramatic opening which sets the plot in motion;
     (b) uses vivid sometimes figurative language;
     (c) portrays the main characters clearly.
   - Encourage the confident writers to write their narratives in the style of the original.
   - Year 7 children should attempt to write their narratives using stressed and unstressed syllables and alliteration.
   - Children to review and edit their narratives after reading them to friends and yourself.

Transforming: Art

1. Settings.
   - Using sketchbooks for recording, children to

    (a) research the exteriors and interiors of Anglo-Saxon and other Dark Ages buildings, with particular focus on large, important buildings;

    (b) explore and imitate the work of the expressionists Munch, Derain, Kokoschka, Marc, early Kandinsky, Chagall and Soutine for ways of representing nature.

- Using the ideas in the sketchbooks children to make paintings of
  - (a) Heorot,
  - (b) the sea which Beowulf sails across,
  - (c) the fen which Grendel crosses,
  - (d) the mere, or
  - (e) Grendel's underwater den.

2. Characters.
   - Using sketchbooks for recording, children to:
     - (a) research the clothing worn by Dark Ages people, particularly fighting men and the nobility;
     - (b) explore twentieth-century portrait painting for ways of representing people, particularly their faces, and imitate favourites;
     - (c) explore and imitate pictures of freaks and monsters.
   - Using the ideas in the sketchbooks children to make paintings of Hrothgar, Grendel, Beowulf or Grendel's mother.

3. Murals.
   - Divide the children into groups and set them the task of producing large murals of one of the following scenes in *Beowulf*:
     - (a) the building of Heorot,
     - (b) Grendel ravaging Heorot,
     - (c) Beowulf and his men travelling across the sea,
     - (d) Beowulf fighting Grendel,
     - (e) the feast with the gift-giving,
     - (f) Grendel's mother taking Aeschere,
     - (g) Beowulf in the mere,
     - (h) the fight in the underwater cave.
   - Try to assemble a mural for each scene, which can be arranged in sequence on a wall.
   - Children to refer to their researches into settings and characters and to make smaller, preliminary sketched versions in chalk or charcoal.

Transforming: Dance, drama and music

1. With all four age groups use Igor Stravinsky's *The Rite of Spring*, Part 1, 'The adoration of the earth' as a sort of film score for a sequence of five lessons, one after each week's episode.

2. Before using the music, familiarise the children with it as follows:

- Play the music frequently in class.
- Ask them in their discussion groups to describe, discuss and evaluate the entire section.

3. Divide the story into the following five scenes:
   - *Scene 1.* Grendel ravaging Heorot, the hall being empty and Hrothgar grieving
   - *Scene 2.* Beowulf and his men travelling across the sea and offering to help
   - *Scene 3.* Beowulf fighting Grendel, including the preparations
   - *Scene 4.* The feast with the gift-giving then Grendel's mother taking Aeschere
   - *Scene 5.* Beowulf in the mere and the fight in the underwater cave

4. In the sequence of lessons explore the contrasts between
   - triumph and despair,
   - celebration and disruption,
   - speech-making and fighting,
   - characters being alone and in large groups.

5. Introduction. Children to
   - Lie down and slowly rise up, join together in a mass then separate to all parts of the hall as apart from each other as possible.
   - Repeat with one child causing the separation of the mass and making the separation quick and hectic, even violent.
   - Repeat then make building movements.

6. Celebration. Children to
   - Explore the movements the people in Heorot would make when celebrating (e.g. swigging drinks, waving across tables, standing up to make speeches or sing songs, being served and eating).
   - Make their movements a little larger and slower than in real life.
   - Make smaller celebration scenes in which one child is left outside and doesn't like it.

7. Travelling and fighting. Children to
   - Explore the movements associated with travelling in the story: marching, sailing, riding, swimming and Grendel coming to Heorot and hurrying away.
   - Work out fight scenes in which they never make contact with each other but simulate contact and make movements larger and slower than in real life.

8. Using the music. Children to
   - Help to choose suitable extracts of *The Rite of Spring* for use in each scene and re-record the extracts required onto tape for use when building the scenes. (Some motifs will probably be essential for almost every scene, others particular to certain scenes.)

9. Using the text. Children to
   - Introduce each scene of the dance drama by telling and reading extracts of the story. (Year 7 children to find and edit extracts of the speeches and integrate these into the drama.)

10. Using masks and spotlights. Children to
    - Create outrageous effects for Grendel and his mother and a sense of mayhem in the fight scenes by using a spotlight.

Publishing

1. Display the sequence of murals in sequence in a public space in the school. On tables or shelves underneath them lay out the stories, perhaps in a whole class anthology, and the sketchbooks.
2. If the dance, drama and music lessons have been successful, consider mounting a production of the work for parents and friends of the school.
3. Include a tour of the gallery and stories as part of the event.

References

1. Heaney, S. (trans.) (1999) *Beowulf.* London: Faber.
2. Fitzgerald, R. (trans.) (1961) Homer, *The Odyssey.* London: Heinemann.
3. Carter, D. (1987) *The Odyssey Project.* Mold: Clwyd County Council.
4. Wrenn, C.L. (ed.) (1953) *Beowulf.* London: Harrap.

CHAPTER 4

Narrative poetry

Introduction

In this chapter the main ideas in the book are given further exemplification by a project in which a teacher follows his enthusiasm for Coleridge's *The Rime of the Ancient Mariner* with his class of Year 5 and 6 children, with substantial work in writing, art, dance and drama.

Two projects are then offered to teachers. The first, based on the well-known ballad *Sir Patrick Spens*, is for Year 6 and 7 children. As well as the many suggestions for writing it strongly features work in combined performing arts of dance, drama and music.

The second, based on Chaucer's *Pardoner's Tale*, is for Years 4 and 5 and Year 8. There is a history focus for both age groups and, as well as extensive suggestions for writing, there is a strong focus on art and drama.

Case study: *The Rime of the Ancient Mariner*

The project

A class of Year 5 and 6 children worked with their class teacher on *The Rime of the Ancient Mariner*, as part of their normal literacy and arts curriculum.

The text

The teacher used the Dover Publications copy of the text with whole page illustrations by Gustav Dore (1970). These illustrations fill every other page of the book and are evocative, haunting responses to Coleridge's verses. The illustrations etched by Dore are from his late period and were published in 1875. Dore drew for his inspiration on the medieval districts of Paris, and on the characters and clothes that he observed in the Paris streets. The illustrations are theatrical, particularly those which include groups of characters. The text in the book is well laid out in large, bold print with Coleridge's prose summaries of the action at the side. It is the ideal text to use with children in the middle years.[1]

Teaching and learning processes

Meeting and knowing

The illustrations proved to be of enormous value to the project, particularly as an aid to the teacher's presentation of the text to the children. He read every verse of the poem in short episodes every other day or so, showing the pictures as he went. He asked and answered questions and drew the children's attention to archaisms and other textual matters. For instance, on reading the verse,

> Alone, alone, all, all alone,
> Alone on a wide, wide sea!
> And never a saint took pity on
> My soul in agony.

the teacher asked, 'What do you notice about the language in that verse?' The children noticed the repetition of 'alone' and 'all'. The teacher then asked why might Coleridge have repeated words like that, and received answers such as, 'Because he wanted to make the loneliness seem to go on forever.'

At the beginning and end of each episode the children helped the teacher reconstruct the plot. The teacher would simply say, 'So let's see what has happened so far' and the children would start to retell it in their own words.

Groups of children also took part in recitations of favourite verses, which they would learn by heart and rehearse prior to performing them to the class and sometimes to the school in sharing assemblies. This work was initiated by a written request from the teacher as follows:

- Read the verses as a group several times using your voices in different ways.
- Try to find the rhythm in the lines.
- Work out a performance which catches the atmosphere in the lines.
- Use sound effects if you want to.

The groups also had regular sessions in which they discussed the meanings and features of certain verses, often the ones that were being performed. Then they reported back to the whole class. This discussion work followed these guidelines:

- Are there any words you don't know the meaning of? If so, use the dictionary.
- What is happening in these verses? What do they mean?
- Make sure everyone has the chance to pass an opinion.
- Try to reach an agreement and make notes of the main points.

- Note any different opinions.
- Practice presenting your ideas, ready for sharing.

Transforming: Writing

There were vivid moments in the poem with particular appeal for the whole class:

- The ship frozen into the sea. It was 'The ice was here, the ice was there' which caught their imaginations in these early stages.
- The albatross. They loved the idea of the albatross being like a magic wand, which makes the sea melt and the wind fill the sails. They were as appalled as the crewmen when the Mariner shot it.
- The spectre-bark. The children were attracted by the image of a ship of death sailing towards the Ancient Mariner's ship with Death and 'The nightmare Life-in-Death' on board casting dice for the souls of the seamen.

Many poems were written about these scenes. The teacher also asked the children to write poems in response to certain lines of the poem. The two most productive of these were:

- 'The ice was all around', and
- 'Water, water everywhere'.

The children's poems were reconstructions, as discussed in Chapter 2, but many children transformed original lines into their own individual expressions. In this first example a Year 5 child reconstructs the part in which 'the spectre-bark' appears. He writes:

> It glitters and shines in the sun's rays.
> But what is this?
> Death in a cloak as black as burnt ash.
> And Life-in-Death playing games with our souls.
> And thrusting her sails like a raging torrent
> Did bellow but no wind did whistle.
> The ship so fine, like the lightest note
> It glides the surface. Our hopes did fall
> To a bottomless pit and our faces
> Did crack with horror and fear.
> And she came closer with a vile smile.

This child here has selected those parts of the original which most appeal to him. He has, for instance, mainly ignored the descriptions of Death and Life-in-Death, confining himself to his blackness and her 'vile smile'. His main interest is the movement of the ship despite the lack of wind. There is a fine contrast between that movement and the downward motion of the sailors' hopes.

In the next example a Year 6 child takes the original elements much further. He imagines the albatross coming to the ship and describes it in his own way:

> Gliding, swooping, slashing the air
> As he glides through.
> The albatross is a world-wide
> Poem bird hunting for food.
> He sees the ship in the distance.
> As he lands he flip-flops
> The runway and a man stops him.
> Playing flying high in the light blue sky.
> And then the Ancient Mariner shot
> The poor albatross in the air.
> He hit the deck and was dead.

This poem is a mixture of fragments from the child's imagination and his retelling of the story. By retelling the story he senses the beauty of the albatross, expressed in the phrase 'world-wide poem bird', yet its clumsiness when on its feet in 'he flip flops the runway'. This is a perceptive contrast.

The poems with the most perceptive lines and which reveal the process from reconstruction into transformation were the ones arising directly from Coleridge's lines rather than the story. The most fascinating of these was written by a Year 6 child who had had learning difficulties in his early education, but who had overcome them. He was alive to the possibilities of language and delighted in the challenge of reading and writing. This child was attracted to the lines beginning 'Water, water everywhere' and all that they implied:

> Water water everywhere.
> Neck brittle and still.
> No chin wagging
> Or a joyful laughing.
> Instead a dismal
> sheen of silence.
> As dry as a stone
> A ghost ship is becalmed.

There is a unity to this child's perceptions which is infrequent in poetry written by children of this age. In the poem the lack of water to drink, powerfully contained in Coleridge's verse: 'Water, water, every where / And all the boards did shrink. / Water, water, everywhere / Nor any drop to drink' is the same as the lack of movement of people and the ship and the lack of sound. It is as if all the senses are shut down because there is no water to drink. Thus there is no conversation and no laughter. All is 'brittle' and, 'dry' and therefore, 'dismal'. This is a profound transformation of a fragment of classical literature in which the child has made the work full of meaning for himself.

Transforming: Art

Painting was a favourite way of responding to the poem. During previous years in the school the children had built up a sketchbook approach to the formulation of ideas and composition. They had experimented with colour and line and enjoyed the freedom to develop their own ideas. They were well used to working big and working collaboratively.

There was a wide range of response to parts of the poem, including both large- and small-scale work. Much of the work was representational with paintings of albatrosses, ships in storms and locked in ice, Death and Life-in-Death. One picture is typical of this representational work. This is a large collaborative effort about two metres square. The background is of an ice blue sea daubed in thick paint with white icebergs. A huge iceberg, painted separately and cut out, is mounted in the foreground, and a ship in full sail is in the background. An albatross flies from behind the large iceberg. It made a dramatic focal point for a display of children's written work and paintings.

Many children showed a greater degree of interpretation and transformation in their work. For instance, one child created a ghostly impression in his painting of the 'spectre bark'. There is a deep blue sea and a lighter blue sky, again, thickly painted. The top half of an enormous orange setting sun occupies the whole of the right side of the painting with bird shapes across sky and sun. In the foreground is a skeletal ship in black. Everything on the ship is skeletal, even the sail which stretches right across the picture with the mast reaching to the top. It is a striking interpretation of the sense of the unreal in this part of the poem.

Some children took their interpretations further than this, transforming the ideas, images and language of the poem into personal expressions. Two paintings are particularly interesting in this respect. They are abstract and diagrammatic.

The first of these works is painted on a piece of card about a metre square. The background is bisected by a line which runs from the middle of the top of the painting diagonally into the left-hand corner at the bottom. The larger shape is painted uniform black, the smaller uniform red. At the bottom of the red is a curved line to represent the sun's globe. Across the black shape, near the top are three lines of asterisks to represent stars. Each asterisk has lines running to the right to show that the stars are moving. Running along the bottom of the picture is a series of five ships in full sail. These are identical cut out shapes made with a template, designed by the child. The child is depicting the voyage of the ship through night and day, but there is a strong feeling of foreboding in it. The series of white ships seems to be crushed by the huge black and red shapes above.

In the second of these abstract paintings the child reveals just how deep children's thinking and feeling can go when their perceptions are sufficiently activated. He was attracted to the stanza:

> The souls did from their bodies fly –
> They fled to bliss or woe!
> And every soul it passed me by,
> Like the whiz of my crossbow.

(lines 220–23)

The painting, however, reaches beyond this stanza in its statement, for the child has picked up on the notion in two earlier lines:

> And I had done a hellish thing,
> And it would work 'em woe.

(lines 91–2)

Perhaps the word 'woe' sparked the idea which leads the child to represent hell with a tunnel of red at the foot of the picture. Through this tunnel crossbow bolts move, emerging into the blue and proceeding towards an albatross in the top left corner. This is the 'hellish thing' – the firing of the bolt – and the bolts gather as feathers along the tail and left wing of the bird, from where they are fired at the ship as a punishment visited upon it. This is in terms of the original action of the Mariner because lines 222–3 suggest the relationship between soul of Mariner and 'whiz' of bolt. The souls in bliss are pink, drifting upwards and merging with a second albatross in the right corner. So, bliss is a heavenlier bird with which to merge. The souls which 'fled' to 'woe', on the other hand, are the black ones falling downwards. These turn into bolts and join the others in the tunnel of hell at the foot of the picture to complete the cycle.

Now this painting is so much more than an act of comprehending the stanza, although it does reveal the utmost comprehension of Coleridge's lines. It goes outwards from the four lines to the whole Christian structure of the poem. The child has perceived the spiritual meanings in the poem, and his process of conceptualisation approximates to Coleridge's. He has thought about the cyclical nature of sin, punishment, damnation and atonement and made this work out of the play of his sensibility on four lines. There is a sense in which the child is adding to Coleridge. It grows out of Coleridge's poem generally and lines 220–3 in particular. But there are significant additions. The most significant of these is the conversion of the souls fleeing to woe into crossbow bolts, the external objects of the poem's hellishness.

Transforming: Dance and drama

Dance and drama were used in two main ways during the project. Firstly, the teacher decided to use dance as the means for getting the children into the mood of the poem, into its inner feeling. For his early lessons in the hall he used a recording of the first movement of Vaughan Williams's *Sinfonia Antartica*. There were three stages to his lessons:

1. Individual work on sailing then freezing, then melting and sailing again.
   - The children make full sail body-shapes and move slowly forward with regular steps.
   - The teacher emphasises the word 'smooth' for these movements.
   - The children show great contrast between smooth movement and the freezing of movement.
   - The teacher suggests that when they move they are gentle and when frozen up they are harsh.
2. Pairs work on the characters on board ship.
   - The idea is to show the contrasting attitudes of the mariners towards the arrival of the albatross and the Ancient Mariner's subsequent shooting of it.
   - This work is closer to mime than dance.
   - One scene shows a seaman feeding and petting the albatross while another rejects it.
   - Another shows one shooting the albatross and the other making menacing gestures towards him.
   - Ways of showing people rejecting other people were explored at some length.
   - Group work about the first part of the poem using *Sinfonia Antartica* for mood and rhythm was carried out.
3. Children made dances to show
   - The ship sailing out and freezing.
   - The albatross arriving and the ship sailing again.
   - The Ancient Mariner shooting the albatross and being treated with contempt as a result.

Publishing

The Rime of the Ancient Mariner was shared with the rest of the school as follows:
- One child played the Ancient Mariner, another the Albatross.
- Four speakers told the story and recited verses.
- There were four dances:
  - (a) Ship sailing and being frozen in the ice.
  - (b) Mariners working on board the ship.
  - (c) Albatross dance and the happiness he brings to the mariners.
  - (d) Shooting the albatross and facing the consequences.
- Several children read their own poems as part of the dramatic performance. For instance, when the scene freezes in (a), children read their poems about this part of the story.

Project 1: *Sir Patrick Spens*

The project

- For children towards the end of Year 6 in primary schools and Year 7 of secondary schools;
- to be used as part of a focus on storytelling in poetry, particularly the ballad form;
- to develop skills and knowledge in literacy, art, dance, drama and music.

The text

Sir Patrick Spens is a ballad that comes from the English oral tradition from the border area between England and Scotland.[2] It is thought to be based on the following two incidents in early Scottish history:

> In the reign of Alexander III of Scotland, his daughter Margaret was escorted by a large party of nobles to Norway for her marriage to King Eric; on the return journey many of them were drowned. Twenty years later, after Alexander's death, his grand daughter Margaret, the Maid of Norway, was heiress to the Scottish throne, and on the voyage to Scotland she died.[3]

The ballad was sung by travelling minstrels and others from the Middle Ages onwards, and there are several versions of it. Most of these vary only in some of the spellings, although there is a much longer version. This includes much detail from the return voyage from Norway. As the various spellings can get in the way of an appreciation of the poem by children I have modernised them below. Apart from this minor change the poem is exactly as found.

Sir Patrick Spens
Adapted by Dennis Carter

The King sits in Dunfermline town
Drinking the blood-red wine:
'O where will I get a good sailor
To sail this ship of mine?'

Up and spoke an older knight,
Sat at the King's right knee:
'Sir Patrick Spens is the best sailor
That sails upon the sea.'

The King has written a broad letter
And signed it with his hand;
And sent it to Sir Patrick Spens
Who's walking on the sand.

The first line that Sir Patrick read
A loud laugh laughed he:
The next line that Sir Patrick read
The tear blinded his eye.

'O who is this has done this deed
This ill deed done to me;
To send me out this time of the year
To sail upon the sea?

'Make haste, make haste my merry men all,
Our good ship sails at dawn.'
'O say not so, my master dear,
For I fear a deadly storm.

'Late yesterday I saw the new moon
With the old moon in his arm,
And I fear, I fear my dear master,
That we will come to harm.'

O our Scots nobles were right loath
Their cork-heeled shoes to drown,
But long before the play was played
Their hats they swam around.

O long, long may their ladies sit
With their fans held in their hand
Before they see Sir Patrick Spens
Come sailing to the land.

O long, long may their ladies sit
With their gold combs in their hair,
Waiting for their own dear lords,
For they'll see them no more.

Go over, go over to Aberdeen –
It's fifty fathoms deep;
And there lies good Sir Patrick Spens
With the Scots lords at his feet.

Teaching and learning processes

Meeting and knowing

1. To prepare for the project ask the children to find a story about a real tragedy and bring it into class. In the first lesson children to
   - tell the main events of their story to a partner;
   - say where they got it from;
   - compare the way each of the partners told it.

2. Share a few of these stories as a whole class, then discuss the various ways stories can be told:
   - on television and radio
   - in newspapers and magazines
   - in story and poetry books
   - in the theatre and by a storyteller
   - in conversations
   - in songs.

3. Tell the children that stories have always been told and that we can still read stories which were told by our distant ancestors, for instance Greek myths, legends and fairy tales.

4. Tell them that one of the oldest kinds of stories are ballads sung by minstrels, and that they
   - are songs that tell a story but not the whole story;
   - concentrate on the most dramatic parts;
   - present the speech of characters within a series of incidents;
   - have a simple rhyme scheme, usually arranged in four line verses (quatrains)
   - often have a chorus for the audience to join in with;
   - use well-known phrases or clichés (e.g. 'milk white steed', 'rosy-red lips');
   - sometimes leap from one scene to a completely different one.

5. Make a large version of the poem or provide individual copies.
   - Read it to them as rhythmically and expressively as you can.
   - Invite them to respond freely to the reading and keep notes of the things they say.
   - Divide the class into groups of two or three and allocate a verse to each group. Allow a few minutes for them to rehearse recitations of their verses, then run through the whole poem group by group. Continue working in this way until it sounds right.

6. Ask the groups to
   - discuss what their verses mean;
   - describe what they see in their imaginations, the place, the characters, all the details;
   - record their discussions and present to the class;

Discuss which parts of the story are actually told to us, and which parts we have to fill in for ourselves (e.g. we are told in some detail about the letter and reactions to it, but nothing about what happened to the ship).

7. Rehearse a whole class recitation involving larger groups as narrators and individual children for the King, Sir Patrick and his speaking sailor.

Transforming: Writing

1. Ask the children to learn the stories they brought to the class and to tell them to each other in small groups. The emphasis here should be on good quality performances, so the children will need time to rehearse with partners. The partners should act as trusted critics.

2. Remind the children that the *Sir Patrick Spens* poet only wrote in detail about selected parts of the story, but that we knew the things he missed out by guessing or inferring. Then ask them to think about their stories and which parts they would like to write about in detail and which parts they could safely miss out.

3. Children to write their ballads, attempting to imitate the rhythm of *Sir Patrick Spens* but avoiding rhyme at this stage. The objective should be to get the raw material of a ballad written: the story, the rhythm and the pattern of language.

4. With their partners the children to
   - read their ballads;
   - make any necessary changes through discussion.

5. Children to redraft their ballads
   - using the thesaurus to find alternatives to words that they wish to replace;
   - attempting to make rhymes if they want to.

Transforming: Art

1. Talk to the class about how colour, light and shade can create a mood in a painting even before any details are painted into it.

2. Show examples from the work of the following expressionist artists: Edvard Munch, Wassily Kandinsky, Oskar Kokoschka and Marc Chagall and invite discussion.

3. Children to choose and think about one of the following couplets in the ballad:
   - The King sits in Dunfermline town / Drinking the blood-red wine
   - The first line that Sir Patrick read / A loud laugh laughed he
   - To send me out this time of the year / To sail upon the sea?
   - Late yesterday I saw the new moon / With the old moon in his arm
   - But long before the play was played / Their hats they swam around
   - O long, long may their ladies sit / With their fans held in their hand
   - And there lies good Sir Patrick Spens / With the Scots lords at his feet

4. Children to think about the setting for these lines. Where is it taking place (e.g when Sir Patrick laughs his 'loud laugh' he is 'walking on the sand')? The setting will

determine the colours to be used to a certain extent (e.g. the 'loud laugh' painting will require yellow for the sand). However, the mood of the poem should also determine colour as well as shade and the amount of light and dark (e.g. the 'loud laugh' represents Sir Patrick's realisation that doom awaits him and his men and, therefore, suggests some darkness gathering in the sky, in the sea and even on the sand).

5. Children to
   - decide on and mix their colours;
   - set up the painting on a large piece of strong drawing paper;
   - draft out in chalk the areas where the colours will be applied;
   - do the painting.

6. Children to
   - Decide what features, figures or details they want on their paintings (e.g. for Sir Patrick and the letter, perhaps some pebbles and shells or a harbour wall and a distant ship for the 'loud laugh').
   - Draft these in charcoal on a separate piece of paper then redraft onto the painting itself in chalk.
   - Paint them, when the children are satisfied with the size and where they are placed on the background.
   - Experiment with colour, which is important to the mood and meaning in the lines and whole poem.

Transforming: Dance and drama

1. Children to explore the following shapes, gestures and movements:
   - writing a letter and sealing it;
   - opening a letter, reading and responding to it;
   - new moon holding the old moon;
   - a crowd gathering then preparing a ship;
   - walking in high heels (i.e. 'cork heels') and hats, then being swept away;
   - sitting upright and fanning;
   - swirling down to the bottom of the sea.

2. The emphasis of these explorations should be on establishing motifs or signs that stand for action. (e.g. scattered people hurriedly gathering for the response to Sir Patrick's 'Make haste, make haste my merry men all, Our good ship sails at dawn').

3. Children to improvise the following scenes using their own words:
   - the king at dinner with the lords and ladies asks for the best sailor and Sir Patrick's name is volunteered;
   - Sir Patrick down at the shore when a messenger brings the letter;
   - Sir Patrick tells his crew to prepare for a voyage and one of them tries to persuade him not to.

4. Build a dance/drama by integrating the three improvised scenes into the series of seven shapes, gestures and movements.

Transforming: Music
1. Children to choose recorded music to create the mood for
   - the king in Dunfermline and Sir Patrick on the sand;
   - preparing the ship and the lords coming on board;
   - the ladies waiting for their husbands;
   - Sir Patrick and the Scots lords 'fifty fathoms deep'.
2. Or groups of children to:
   - choose pitched and non-pitched instruments which are suited to the mood of their scene (including instruments which some children are learning to play);
   - discuss the mood of each scene (helped by the similar work in Art);
   - work out tunes or sound effects to be used and practise playing them;
   - blend the instruments to make an overall pattern of sounds, which can be repeated;
   - perform their compositions – ask each group to play them in sequence.

Publishing
1. Set up an exhibition of the paintings and use the couplets which the paintings were based on for titles at the bottom. Display the children's ballads, illustrated with smaller drawings, in a class book alongside the paintings.
2. Children to perform:
   - The new ballads in class;
   - The recitation of *Sir Patrick Spens* and the dance/drama with the musical pieces to the whole school, perhaps inviting parents and friends and including a visit to the exhibition.

Project 2: *The Pardoner's Tale*

The project

- For children in Years 4 and 5 in primary schools and Year 8 in secondary schools.
- For Years 4 and 5 to be used as part of a focus on classic poetry, longer classic poetry, including narrative poetry and couplets.
- For Year 8 to be used for the study of a substantial text by one poet, to identify links between literary heritage and their time (the Middle Ages) and how it reflects the culture of that time.
- To develop skills and knowledge in literacy, art and drama.

The text

In *The Canterbury Tales* Geoffrey Chaucer retells stories from many sources, within a framework of an imaginary journey by pilgrims to the shrine of Thomas Becket in Canterbury Cathedral. Pilgrimages were a very common pastime in the Middle

Ages and provided an ideal theme to unite the stories. Chaucer also tells us a great deal about the pilgrims themselves and makes social commentaries on his times. For instance, the Pardoner is a greedy cheat, delivers a sermon against the seven deadly sins then tells a story about greed being the root of all evil.

Pardoners were confidence tricksters. They travelled around pretending to be holy men and claiming they could pardon people's sins on the authority of the Pope in Rome. They preached like real holy men and carried fake decrees, known as papal bulls, as evidence of their authority. They also carried bags full of bones and other bits and pieces such as locks of hair or pieces of cloth, claiming that these were from saints or even Christ himself. They sold them to whoever was gullible enough to buy them. This worked because in the Middle Ages everybody believed in Christ and his resurrection. They were keen to have their sins forgiven and to be granted good fortune.

The Pardoner who tells the story makes no attempt to disguise the fact that he is a cheat. Ironically, he is very honest in his self-assessment:

> 'What! Do you think, as long as I can preach
> And get their silver for the things I teach,
> That I will live in poverty, from choice?
> That's not the counsel of my inner voice!
> No! Let me preach and beg from kirk to kirk
> And never do an honest job of work'

This pardoner is so brazen that he spends the first 374 lines of the poem giving a sermon on the seven deadly sins. However, *The Pardoner's Tale* is a moral story. I tell it here with extracts from Nevill Coghill's translation.[4]

1. Once in Flanders there were three riotous young men who spent their time boozing, gambling, swearing, eating too much and misbehaving. Early one morning they were sitting in a pub having a drink when they heard the clinking of a hand bell. A coffin was being carried to a grave and the three rioters wanted to know whose body was in it. The barman told them:

> 'Two hours before I came here I was told.
> He was a friend of yours in days of old,
> And suddenly, last night, the man was slain,
> Upon his bench, face up, dead drunk again.
> There came a privy thief, they call him Death,
> Who kills us all round here, and in a breath
> He spears him through the heart, he never stirred.
> And then Death went his way without a word.
> He's killed a thousand in the present plague,

> And, sir, it doesn't do to be too vague
> If you should meet him; you had best be wary.
> Be on your guard with such an adversary,
> Be primed to meet him everywhere you go,
> That's what my mother said. It's all I know.'

The landlord joined in, telling the three young men that Death had recently killed a whole village, including the children, and that Death probably lives near that village. The three decided that they would 'kill this traitor Death' and swore an oath 'to live and die for one another'. In a 'drunken rage' they left the pub swearing and shouting threats.

2. When they had walked no more than half a mile and were about to climb a stile,

> They came upon a very poor old man
> Who humbly greeted them and thus began,
> 'God look to you lords, and give you quiet!'

But the three were in no mood to show good manners and their answer was rough:

> To which the proudest of these men of riot
> Gave back the answer, 'What, old fool? Give place!
> Why are you all wrapped up except your face?
> Why live so long? Isn't it time to die?'

The old man said he'd never met anyone who would exchange their youth for his age and not even Death would take his life. He said he often asked the earth the question, 'When will these bones be laid to rest?' but was still left alive. The old man also complained to them, saying,

> 'But it dishonoured you when you began
> To speak so roughly, sir, to an old man,
> Unless he had injured you in word or deed.
> It says in holy writ, as you may read,
> "Thou shalt rise up before the hoary head
> And honour it." And therefore be it said
> "Do no more harm to an old man than you,
> Being now young, would have another do
> When you are old" – if you should live till then.
> And so may God be with you, gentlemen,
> For I must go whither I have to go.'

The boldest of the three young rioters continued being rough and rude. He accused the old man of being a spy for Death who was bent on killing young people.

The old man then told them where they could find Death. 'Turn up this crooked way,' he said,

> 'Towards that grove, I left him there today
> Under a tree, and there you'll find him waiting.
> He isn't one to hide for all your prating.
> You see that oak? He won't be far to find'

3. The three young men ran to the tree and immediately found

> A pile of golden florins on the ground
> New-coined, eight bushels of them as they thought.

This changed their whole attitude so that they forgot about seeking Death,

> For they were all so thrilled to see the sight,
> The florins were so beautiful and bright,
> That down they sat beside the precious pile.

The three thought it was their lucky day. But there was a problem. How could they get the gold back to their houses without being seen? If they were seen they might be accused of stealing the money. So they made a plan. One of them said,

> 'No, we must bring this treasure back by night
> Some prudent way, and keep it out of sight.
> And so as a solution I propose
> We draw for lots and see the way it goes;
> The one who draws the longest, lucky man,
> Shall run to town as quickly as he can
> To fetch us bread and wine – but keep things dark –
> While two remain in hiding here to mark
> Our heap of treasure. If there's no delay,
> When night comes down we'll carry it away,
> All three of us, wherever we have planned.'

So they drew lots and the youngest drew the longest straw. Straightway, he went to the town, to get the bread and wine. As soon as he was gone the others talked about how much richer they would be if the golden coins were divided between the two of them rather than three. One of them suggested:

> 'Now look; when he comes back, get up in fun
> To have a wrestle; then, as you attack,
> I'll up and put my dagger through his back
> While you and he are struggling, as in game;
> Then draw your dagger too and do the same.

Then all this money will be ours to spend,
Divided equally of course, dear friend.'

4. Meanwhile the youngest also thought about the golden coins. He thought how much better if he had them all himself and made his own plot. He went to the chemist and said,

'Sell me some poison if you will,
I have a lot of rats I want to kill
And there's a polecat too about my yard
That takes my chickens and it hits me hard'

The chemist had the very thing the young man wanted and he described it:

'If any living creature eat or drink
A mouthful, ere he has the time to think,
Though he took less than makes a grain of wheat,
You'll see him fall down dying at your feet;
Yes, die he must, and in so short a while
You'd hardly have the time to walk a mile,
The poison is so strong you understand.'

The youngest friend bought the poison at once, got three bottles, put poison in two of them, then went and got them filled up with wine. When he returned, things happened very quickly:

They fell on him and slew him, two to one.
Then said the first of them when this was done,
'Now for a drink. Sit down and let's be merry,
For later on there'll be a corpse to bury.'
And, as it happened, reaching for a sup,
He took a bottle full of poison up
And drank; and his companion, nothing loth,
Drank from it also, and they perished both.

The three riotous young men found Death and the moral of the story was spoken in Latin by the Pardoner, 'Radix malorum est cupiditas', which means 'Greed is the root of all evil.'

Teaching and learning processes

Meeting and knowing: Years 4 and 5
1. Children to find and learn a story with a moral in it such as a fable and bring it into class, then:

- tell the story to a partner;
- say where they got it from;
- identify what the moral of the story is.

2. Share a few of these stories as a whole class and talk about stories which teach us lessons or which have morals in them.
3. Familiarise yourself with the text written above. Tell the children that it is a narrative poem, a poem that tells a story; then:
   - Tell the story and recite the extracts or read it as it stands.
   - Before reading out the moral of the story ask the children to work it out first.
   - Discuss then write the Latin on the board with its translation.
   - Using the notes above tell the children about *The Canterbury Tales* and the Pardoner.
   - Ask the children for their opinions about the story the Pardoner tells compared to what he is like himself.
4. Divide the children into groups of four and allocate a section of the story to each. Groups to
   - read their part through, looking up any words which create problems;
   - rehearse a recitation, making sure that they have more or less equal parts and that there are different voices for the spoken parts.
5. Groups then to
   - work out the rhyme scheme in their extracts (i.e. rhyming couplets);
   - clap out the number of syllables (beats) in each line (i.e. ten);
   - discuss what they notice about how the story changes when it is in verse.
6. Groups then to
   - discuss what might be an alternative ending for the story;
   - discuss what was the old man's importance in the story;
   - consider if they know any other stories like this one;
   - share their ideas.

Meeting and knowing: Additions for Year 8

1. Set the following research tasks on CD-Rom, Internet and reference books for a homework or follow-up activity in class:
   - Chaucer's Pilgrims – who they were, what they were like, how they are described.
   - Pilgrims and pilgrimages – why people went on them – the famous sites in Europe – what the pilgrims found when they got there.
   - The Christian church in the Middle Ages.
2. Discuss the Christian concept of sin and, in particular, the seven deadly sins: Pride, Wrath, Envy, Lust, Gluttony, Avarice and Sloth. Children to decide on the relative sinfulness of each.
3. Create groups and allocate copies of the story to each.

4. Groups to
   - read the story silently;
   - divide it into parts: Narrator, Three rioters, Barman, Old Man and Chemist;
   - have a more or less equal part each;
   - rehearse a dramatic recitation of the whole story.
5. Next groups to turn their recitations into plays for voices, by
   - creating greater variation between voices;
   - adding music and sound effects;
   - recording onto a tape and performing to the class.
6. When the recitations are good enough allow each group a performance time. Then discuss the different approaches of the groups.

Transforming: Writing
1. Children to imagine the following locations in the story:
   - the tavern;
   - the stile where they meet the old man;
   - the place where they find the gold.
2. What do they see? Can they describe it? Children to write a short description of each (no more than two or three short sentences). Share some of these and discuss their effectiveness as introductions to the scene in the story.
3. Children to think about the main characters: the three friends and the old man. Are there any differences between the three? Discuss, then ask them to create differences themselves.
4. Children to write short introductory descriptions for each of them as follows:
   - Describe each of the friends in such a way as to evoke dislike.
   - Describe the old man in such a way as to evoke sympathy.
5. Children to write an alternative ending to the story in which the three friends get the gold back to their houses, but nothing good comes of it.
6. Taking into account the work done on settings and characters, children to write the stories they brought to the first session.

Transforming: writing (Variations for Year 8)
1. Teach the children that this story is written in a special verse form called iambic pentameters, in which every line has ten beats to it. Ask them to check the text to see if this is always true, then discuss the effect this has on the telling of the story. Emphasise that it gives the story the momentum of a clear rhythm.
2. Children to tell their own stories again, then attempt to write them using iambic pentameters. This is not as difficult as at first appears.

Transforming: Art
1. Children to research medieval costume and the interiors of medieval buildings.

2. Children to find and draw
   - the clothes that the innkeeper, the three friends, the old man and the chemist might have worn;
   - the interiors of inns and taverns.
3. Groups to make a series of drawings of the following scenes, labelling them with a suitable, short quotation from the text:
     (i)   in the tavern;
     (ii) the funeral procession;
     (iii) the three friends meet the old man;
     (iv) they find the gold coins;
     (v)   the two friends plot to kill the youngest;
     (vi) the youngest buys poison from the chemist;
    (vii) the two kill the youngest;
   (viii) they drink the poisoned wine and die.

Transforming: Drama
1. Using their own words, groups to improvise the following scenes:
   - Three friends drinking in the tavern see the funeral passing by and ask the barman about it.
   - They are rude to the old man.
   - They find the gold, choose lots, the youngest leaves for town and the other two plot to kill him.
   - The youngest buys the poison, buys food and wine and poisons two of the bottles.
   - The three meet their deaths.
2. Make a class play out of these scenes and with the following extras:
   - a chorus of several children who take it in turns to speak the part of Narrator;
   - new scenes to take place in the tavern;
   - a funeral procession scene with mourners, funeral director and grave scene;
   - a scene in which a family catch the plague one by one.

Transforming: Music
1. Play CDs of original medieval music and ask the children to choose pieces to accompany the scenes in their plays. Children to give sound reasons for their choices.
2. Alternatively, children to choose recordings of contemporary music they think would serve the same purpose. Children to give sound reasons for their choices.

Publishing
1. Make a class anthology of the children's written versions of stories with a moral.
2. Make classroom displays of their storyboards.
3. Record their radio plays on audio-cassette.
4. Perform their improvised plays to the whole school or a wider audience.

References

1. Coleridge, S.T. (1970) *The Rime of the Ancient Mariner*, with illustrations by Gustav Dore. New York: Dover Publications.
2. Kinsley, J. (ed.) (1969) *Sir Patrick Spens*, in *The Oxford Book of Ballads*. Oxford: Oxford University Press.
3. www.tnellen.com
4. Coghill, N. (trans.) (1951) Chaucer, *The Canterbury Tales*. Harmondsworth: Penguin Books.

CHAPTER 5

Shakespeare

Introduction

Two very different case studies are presented. The first, based on *Hamlet*, records a project undertaken by a teacher of Year 5 and 6 children with the help of a professional artist. The teacher managed the whole project and developed work in writing, drama, dance and music. The artist developed work in visual art. This project shows what can be achieved on a small scale.[1]

The second project, based on *The Tempest*, records a large-scale project involving several of a local authority's agencies and many primary and secondary schools. This project shows how classic literature can be given a high profile with the right kind of collaboration and organisation.[2]

A project for teachers based on *Twelfth Night* is then presented with a wide range of suggestions for work in literacy and the arts. This project is intended for Key Stage 2 teachers working with their own classes on a small budget and for Key Stage 3 teachers working in collaboration with colleagues in the art, music and PE (dance) departments.

Case study 1: *Hamlet*

The project

Year 6 children explored *Hamlet* through literacy and the arts. An artist worked alongside the class teacher, helping to develop the drawing and painting. The teacher developed writing, music-making, dance and drama. The project lasted eight weeks.

The class teacher's objectives were for the children to

- enjoy a work of Shakespeare;
- understand the play and the relationships of the characters within it;

- explore the emotions of the characters at different times;
- engage with key images through a variety of art forms;
- work individually and in small/large groups.

The artist's objectives were for the children to develop

- a process for turning perceptions into paintings;
- response to imagery through painting;
- the skills of drawing and painting;
- response to ideas from art history.

The text

The teacher's presentation of text was through present-tense storytelling with extracts of text quoted. The extracts were copied from the Arden edition and the children recited them in preparation for setting some to music.[3]

Teaching and learning processes

Meeting and knowing

The project began with a look at Shakespeare's theatre and information about Shakespeare himself. When the teacher said she was going to share *Hamlet* many children quoted the first few lines of the 'To be or not to be' soliloquy and there was widespread enthusiasm. Some children went to the library in their spare time and one child told the class the story of *The Merchant of Venice*, learnt from her father.

First responses to episodes were expressed in group discussions, during which the children often showed insight. For instance, one child commented on Polonius's relationship with his children: 'He has brought them up not to behave badly and to obey him, but he puts them in awkward positions, like when he tells Ophelia she couldn't see Hamlet again.'

The children became more confident with Shakespeare's language as implied by the teacher's record:

> I had prepared some quotes that we had focused on since the beginning of the play and with a few minutes to spare at the end of the day wondered if they could guess 'who said what'. They could. I picked out more from the book, even ones they hadn't heard and I was amazed the way they tried to work out who it could be.

Transforming: Writing

Writing developed out of presentation and discussion and the majority of pieces were examples of reconstruction, as discussed in Chapter 2, in which the children grafted response onto Shakespeare's original. For instance, having worked on the

'Get thee to a nunnery' scene, many children wanted to write lines for the 'To be or not to be' soliloquy.

One child wrote, 'to find yourself floating about in the sins of your head', reflecting well Hamlet's sense of guilt. Another, preoccupied with the idea of the undiscover'd country, wrote: 'I may be in that lost bit of world.'

Many children also identified with Ophelia's plight in Act IV, Scene vi and to the report of her subsequent death (Act IV, Scene vii) and some of this work is particularly interesting for the use of the iambic pentameter, as in:

- My father's been murdered and my heart too.
- She's trapped in a timeless struggle of murder.
- I have picked these flowers for you father.
- My father has died in the queen's bedroom.
- My sorrow lies in my mind forever.

Most pieces like these came from situations, dilemmas and actions, others from the images and themes of the play. This latter work led to transformations. After the second episode, for instance, about Hamlet still grieving, the children considered the following images during discussions:

- 'Good Hamlet, cast thy nighted colour off'
- 'Do not seek . . . for thy noble father in the dust'
- 'all that lives must die, Passing through nature to eternity'
- 'O that this too, too sullied flesh would melt, Thaw and resolve itself into a dew'
- ''Tis an unweeded garden That grows to seed'
- 'Would the night would come. Till then sit still my soul.'

After the discussions the children were invited to write about Hamlet or in the role of Hamlet, and many transformed the material easily. One child, for instance, wrote:

> Death after victory.
> Victory for me, no.
> Clothing night, mind night.
> Spirit of death beyond the walls.
> Queen and new king,
> bright, recovered.

The writing during this lesson was notable for its dwelling on the notion of darkness, the children inferring this from the imagery. Although one child's 'Hamlet is in a very dark world' is more commentary than reconstruction or transformation, other children took greater possession of the imagery. One evokes the trumpet as well as the image of darkness, the trumpet, which announces the entrance of Claudius and Gertrude:

> I feel lonely and sad,
> there's a trumpet playing a hard
> and a dark song in my mind.

This child has responded at that intuitive level. He is preoccupied by the lonely, brooding prince; the sound of the trumpet; and the image of darkness. His use of the trumpet is remarkable. He has perceived the irony of the situation. The trumpet announces what should be a happy occasion but for Hamlet, dwelling in darkness, the trumpet has a hard and dark sound.

At the end of the project the teacher asked the children to think about the whole play and write their thoughts; an invitation to summarise and evaluate, a different kind of writing. Many children were accomplished at doing this, too, as in these examples:

> You were there, you were there love, but now you have gone.
> Hamlet dies and so do all the rest, but
> We never forget what Hamlet might have been.
> An old king, a good king.
> A new king, a bad king.
> A ghost walking,
> Talking of murder.
> Hamlet confused,
> Guilt was what he found.

Transforming: Art

The artist established sketchbooks for first ideas and three main areas for painting:

1. Textual interpretation.
   - Extracts of text were chosen by the teacher and the artist to be used as stimuli for drawings and paintings. These were copied out onto cards and the children responded to the imagery with drawings and paintings.
   - Thus a worried mind – 'a mote to trouble the mind's eye' – was a head filled with scribbles and rough, bold colour.
   - Many children made single pieces of text the main focus of all their art, teasing out meanings and following up initial responses.
2. Exploring themes.
   - These themes were identified as central to the play: mortality, immortality, sickness and decay; and they were explored using abstract expressionism.
   - The artist showed the children abstract expressionist artists and invited them to work collaboratively on large pictures.
   - He taught them that colour can represent emotion and established the saying, 'Image for Foreground and Emotion for Background'.
   - He urged them to make the surface of the paintings work as a whole,

background and foreground in harmony to make the meanings of the work. For instance, one child painting Hamlet's 'sea of troubles' showed the figure of Ophelia drowning in a sea with the sun, planets and stars all in the wrong places. This idea of the visualisation of emotions enabled the children to transform rather than merely interpret fragments of the work.

3. Portraits.

- The main characters were studied in terms of what they say and what other characters say about them, and their portraits were drawn and painted at various stages of development.
- The expressionist ideas had an effect on the painting of characters, the artist emphasising the need to create mood and atmosphere, even in the picture of a character's head.
- He showed examples of Celtic, Viking and Saxon faces, gargoyles and masks and portraits by artists as diverse as Modigliani and Rembrandt.
- When they made their portraits they operated within a cultural context provided by *Hamlet* and the images of the human face.
- The work of a group, painting Ophelia's portrait, illustrates the process.
    - (a) They found a book on Matisse and the Fauves and were impressed by the brushwork, colours and strong black lines in many of the pictures.
    - (b) They decided to use this idea to express, in the background, the madness which engulfs Ophelia. In their picture the background is deliberately graded and toned, from light into dark, to express Ophelia's descent into madness.
    - (c) The relationship between background and foreground is successfully achieved with the darkening background reflecting in her face as if she were victim of the background of events over which she has no power.

4. Finished work.

Most individual paintings showed great variation in technical skill and maturity, reflecting the wide range of ability in the class. More importantly they show the widespread perceptual ability of the children to interpret and transform the material which interests them. The following are examples of this fascinating development:

- King Hamlet sits against a tree in a garden that is unweeded. His brother Claudius is one of the things 'rank and gross in nature', sweeping down from the tree as a serpent to sting his life. Gertrude is looking on from behind the tree. King Hamlet already appears ghostly. His colouring is unusual, a blue-glowing pink. On a brooding background weeds are represented expressionistically too, with two huge leaves and an enormous creeper opposite the figure of the king.
- King Hamlet's face dominates the whole picture. There is a small figure, Prince Hamlet. The painting is a response to Hamlet's words on the battlements,

If it assume my noble father's person
I'll speak to it though hell itself should gape
And bid me hold my peace.

Hamlet is in a dilemma. From the sides hell's forces pour towards him while overhead is the gigantic figure of his father demanding revenge. It's as if the full weight of Hamlet's revenge responsibility is represented here. He is isolated at the top of a white ladder. Although the visual achievement of the piece is in the splendid King Hamlet, it reveals great perception in the positioning of Hamlet alone and besieged in that no-man's land.

- Claudius's rise to power is represented as a schoolboy in a modern school setting. At bottom left is a smiling schoolboy, innocently happy. Soon he has ambitions, conveyed in a thought balloon. Finally, he achieves these, wearing the crown and backed by Gertrude. The background, which works with the foreground, results from the abstract expressionist work and features squiggles and zig-zags to interpret the lines,

The serpent that did sting thy father's life
Now wears his crown.

Transforming: Dance, drama and music

Dance, drama and music were not separated in the project but used together. It was exploratory at first, but developed so well that the children were confident enough to perform an improvised play for the whole school and guests in the school hall at the end of the project. This development went as follows.

1. The children responded strongly to the dramatic nature of the literature:
   - During the third class lesson, for instance, the teacher grouped the children in threes and gave each group a copy of Act I, Scene i, lines 1 to 54.
   - She asked them to practise speaking the parts of Marcellus, Barnardo and Horatio and to create music to accompany it.
   - The musical pieces were noticeable for sounds like clanking of armour as a response to the Ghost's 'warlike form' stalking. One child even learnt the part of Barnardo and when she spoke the words 'looks 'a not like the king?' she bowed and crossed herself.
2. Sessions in the hall were exploratory and collaborative and led to a unity in the class:
   - In the first session, based on the encounter between Hamlet and the Ghost on the battlements (Act I, Scene iv) the teacher created a mysterious mood using a recording of Miles Davis's *Aura* and urged the children to try to imagine which parts of the scene the music could accompany.
   - One group made a play about the death of King Hamlet in the garden, then his body being placed in the coffin and rising up.

- The whole class then took up the theme of King Hamlet rising from the dead to his unpurged sins, 'to fast in fires'.
- The children spun extracts of the text with their own words. Phrases such as 'all that lives must die' from a child playing Gertrude fitted comfortably with 'phoney king' from one playing Hamlet.

3. The teacher's warm-ups were very effective as a means for the children to interpret the characters and as a preparation for improvisation:
   - For Act II, Scenes i and ii, the children were asked to walk like different characters and greet each other in role as characters, for instance, 'Pick up a book and walk like Hamlet,' or 'Greet Rosencrantz and Guildenstern as if you are Claudius.'
   - The teacher noted how the children had portrayed some of these characters: 'Hamlet was generally portrayed as sad and thoughtful; Polonius as a fusser who darts about; Ophelia as someone very pretty and obedient.'
   - This led to improvisations about Rosencrantz and Guildenstern's arrival in Elsinore, and it was clear just how easily the children were picking up inferences directly from the text.
   - They realised that Hamlet's schoolfellows were not very good friends. In one improvisation Hamlet offers them money if they will tell him the truth, and the word 'snitch' was applied to them by many children.

4. This work on characterisation was not only demonstrated in improvised drama, but also in creative music-making:
   - Using untuned instruments together with xylophones, glockenspiels and keyboards, the groups composed signature tunes for Polonius, Ophelia and Hamlet.
   - Polonius's tune was fussy, moved quickly, then paused as if Polonius were formulating a new idea, then darted off again.
   - Ophelia's was beautiful and haunting with gently played notes, conveying sadness.
   - Hamlet's was slow and melancholy with a series of confused sequences in it.

5. The children's ability to understand the play, the motives of the characters and the implications for what was to come was revealed when they were invited to make up a play that could be performed for Claudius:
   - The teacher gave them the quote 'to prick the conscience of the king' as a title.
   - They had not yet met the actual play within a play (Act III, Scene ii) but each group made a play about the murder of a king or important person.
   - When each group shared their play the others were invited to go into role as the audience in the court of Elsinore, and the child playing Claudius took over the proceedings from the teacher, calling for quiet, and the groups bowed to him before performing.

- During one group's performance the child playing Claudius actually rushed out of the hall.
- The children had anticipated the actual scene because of their understanding of the play and the characters.

6. Autonomy and innovation was present in the children's movement work.
    - For the scenes in which Hamlet encounters Claudius at prayer and visits his mother (Act III, Scenes iii and iv), the teacher chose four quotations of text, which suggested 'shape' or 'movement'.
    - She allocated one quotation to each group, reminding them of their interpretations in art and music where a brushstroke or a sequence of notes can convey a certain feeling or express something in the text.
    - One group of six children used Gertrude's

        > O Hamlet, speak no more.
        > Thou turnest mine eyes into my very soul
        > And there I see such black and grained spots
        > As will not leave their tinct. (Act III, Scene iv)

    - In their sequence a character speaks the words while the others move:
        (a) The character stands in the middle of their circle, which turns in on her.
        (b) The five in the circle stretch their hands and press her down and she turns as she goes down.
        (c) Those in the circle turn sideways and sink to represent the black and grained spots, which then lay outstretched on their sides, toe to head.
        (d) The central child also stretches lengthways on the floor in the centre.
    - This sequence revealed a natural ease with the imagery. Gertrude, played by the standing child, is brought down by what is in her soul, represented by the circle. That circle turns out to be composed of the black and grained spots.
    - Such work as this is intellectual adventure, in which the children, as artists, accept the premise contained in a metaphor and explore the implications in it; creative literacy at its best.

Publishing

1. The classroom and the spaces outside were a gallery and forum for daily sharing of work.
2. There was a performance of drama, dance, music and readings of poems at the end of term to which other children, teachers, governors and parents were invited.
3. The audience was told the story of Hamlet with
    - the improvised scenes;
    - the children's own words;

- extracts of Shakespeare;
- musical compositions, songs, poems and choral speaking.

4. During the summer holidays paintings were framed and hung in the local arts centre.

Case study 2: *The Tempest*

The project

Year 4, 5 and 6 children in 14 primary schools and Year 7 and 8 children in six secondary schools in Clwyd explored *The Tempest* through literacy and the arts prior to the performance by a theatre-in-education company in the schools. The Arden edition of the play was used.[4]

This arts collaboration was organised by the Arts in Schools Project and Outreach Theatre Company and involved 35 teachers, 11 student teachers, five arts workers, staff of two TVEI centres and about 1,200 children. The authority's arts coordinator and theatre-in-education director wanted to develop a challenging theatre-based arts project which would cross the key stages and involve primary and secondary teachers sharing ideas and experiences.

The key aims were to

- Extend Clwyd's work on middle years Shakespeare, established in previous years.
- Promote the value of Shakespeare in the middle years.
- Develop multidisciplinary approaches to the arts in schools.
- Demonstrate good arts teaching approaches.
- Involve student teachers in arts education.
- Generate excitement, enlightenment and joy in the education process.

Teaching and learning processes

Meeting and knowing: preparations

The teachers and students were involved in two days' training as follows:

- A practical introduction to the play and its context by a university lecturer.
- Visual arts workshops, exploring a range of media.
- Music workshops, based on the rhythms of the language, the setting of the songs, the speaking of the iambic pentameters and the composition of tone poems.
- Dance and drama workshops focusing on games or imaginative playing; the exploration of underlying themes (e.g. changing from worse to better); dramatisation of the stories which are told but not enacted (e.g. Sycorax's story); using the text for choral speech and mime and developing dances to accompany the songs.

- Writing workshops based on alternative stories (e.g. Caliban's story when he is left alone on the island); alternative plays (e.g. the night when Prospero and Miranda are forced aboard the ship), poetry about the special properties of the island and the inner preoccupations of the characters (e.g. Ariel's real feelings).

The teachers worked in their schools as follows:

- The primary teachers worked in all art forms with help from students and arts workers.
- The secondary teachers had to persuade colleagues in the various arts departments to collaborate. The extent of their success varied from school to school. In all cases English and drama colleagues collaborated. Some music and art departments were involved.

Outreach Theatre Company rehearsed a cut-down performance of *The Tempest*.

- Four actors acted all the parts from a text reduced by about a third.
- The actors were challenged by the diversity of the roles. For instance, Miranda doubled as Stephano, Ariel as Trinculo, and Caliban as Ferdinand.
- The performance was in the round with costume changes made outside the circle.
- The children, therefore, experienced many aspects of theatre craft.

Meeting and knowing: presenting plot, character and text

Most teachers presented *The Tempest* as a 'once upon a time' story rather than as a play with a dramatic present-tense approach.

- Some story-told but others read from retellings.
- Almost all incorporated extracts of Shakespeare's text into their presentations.

The teachers consolidated the story in various ways.

- One played a Radio-vision tape/slide version.
- Others showed a BBC dramatisation on video.

Whatever method, the children in every school knew the story thoroughly by the time Outreach Theatre Company performed for them.

Every class from Year 4 to Year 8 also engaged with extracts of text to some extent, including children with special educational needs.

- Most children learnt short extracts by heart and some learnt whole speeches.
- The most popular passages for learning and working with were the songs.
- The teachers chose passages they felt the children could understand and treated such passages as material to do things with. Words were not learnt just for the sake of it.

The language was an essential part of the experience and gave particularity to the work that was undertaken. Children enjoyed using this language, which was rewarded when the children heard the actors speaking it. One teacher, for instance, reported on a 'less able' child who had played the role of Trinculo in a workshop at school: 'Seeing him glance at me when the Outreach Company enacted that particular scene; that glance said, 'That's my scene. I know it.' Another teacher reported that three girls were out in the rain and sheltering under one coat and one of them said, 'Misery acquaints a man with strange bedfellows.'

Secondary children made greater use of the text than primary children. They:

- Learnt parts for whole scenes and performed them to audiences.
- Chose pieces of text to accompany paintings they were working on.
- Played chanting games with the material.
- Were pleased to find that with practice they could read 'Shakespeare perfectly'.

Teaching and learning processes

The description of processes and products may seem somewhat fragmentary in this case study because of the sheer scale of the project, and it is difficult to be representative. Here I describe a few of the many examples of good practice and creative response.

Transforming: Writing

The vast quantity and extensive range of written work was convincing evidence of the self-confidence of the teachers in setting up situations which led to expressive writing. The strategies were many and covered most modes of writing. Some writing was of the 'write about' kind but most was expressive in various ways. This falls into three types: poetry, play scripts and narrative prose. The play-scripts are discussed under 'Performances and scripted dramas'.

Transforming: Writing (Poetry)

1. Several teachers developed their children's ability to make images by setting up exercises.
   - For instance some provided children with a model phrase such as 'Sycorax **was so** wicked **that** . . .' and this led directly to similes and metaphors as in this by a Year 4 child:

   > Miranda was so beautiful that
   > her golden hair looked like
   > a great waterfall plunging
   > into a deep pool.

   - Another good example is this by a Year 5 child:

> Ariel is a green ghost.
> Ariel is a blue floating gas.
> Ariel is a golden glass
> filled with silver ice-cubes.

2. Several primary teachers used lines of text as starting points for writing, which led to many quality lines.

- For instance, a Year 6 child focused on Caliban's line, 'The isle is full of noises,' and this led her to adopt the role of Caliban pacifying Stephano and Trinculo:

> The island is full of noises.
> Don't worry I hear them every day.
> This island is home to thee.

- The 'Full fathom five' song was particularly valuable in this way, as in this by a Year 5 child:

> nails turn to diamonds
> shining through the seaweed.
> His heart turns to a big red ruby.
> It attracts fishes' eyes

- And this by a Year 6 child, which uses rhyme effectively:

> Full fathom five thy father stay.
> Nothing of him that doth decay

- Such appropriation of Shakespeare's language led another Year 6 child to write a poem which is a clear transformation into a personal response:

> But changes into something weird.
> His hair is now a rock's flowing beard.
> His money-soft fists are now stones.
> That is coral that was his bones.
> His skin has changed into a silky ray.
> All this because to his dismay
> The boat began to crack and sway
> Then broke out a violent storm
> And now your father is reborn.

- This writer manages to maintain the rhythm of Shakespeare's original, and there are many moments of real insight, such as the 'rock's flowing beard' with its implication that the seabed itself is also transformed, and the final line, which concludes the piece delightfully.

3. Many teachers and children were interested in curses and insults, and many examples of this kind of writing reveal the influence of the dramatic nature of Shakespeare's poetry.

- The following curse by Caliban on Prospero, written by a Year 7 child, is particularly powerful:

> My mama will get her cauldron
> And search the isle for tarantula's
> Silver home, covered with poisonous dew.
> And I will give her your special book,
> So you will lose your power.
> And ripple like a crook.
> So disease will cast on you
> Cos my Sycorax is power.

- This child has transformed the formula of the curse to make something which is at one and the same time very much her own and true to the model.
- The same skilful balance is present in this poem by a Year 8 pupil:

> Caliban will be cursed
>   on this dark night.
> Under my feet he will
>   lie tonight.
> Ripped and scratched by
>   beasts of the dark.
> Stung by bees and
>   Stitch marks.
> Even though he is in pain
>   He will always live again.

4. One of the students suggested that her Year 6 children should 'cast spells with words'. This was particularly effective when they were writing spells to make storms as in:

> Mystery and magic,
> Magic and mystery,
> Make me a storm
> To go down in history.

5. Most teachers set poetry-writing tasks based on the characters and some of these were remarkable for their use of imagery and rhythm.
   - For instance, a Year 8 child writes of Prospero's thoughts about his brother Antonio:

> He is the nightmare
> Of all my dreams.
> He is the cat among the birds.

- The next example shows an assured use of rhythm and rhyme in a portrait of Ariel:

> Fairy flying, golden wings
> Such a sweet song Ariel sings
> In a tree the spirit lies
> Tears of water as he cries.
>
> Free at last no curse on him
> Thunder, lightning at his whim
> Waves surging o'er the boat
> Sailors stranded on the coast.

6. The island was a source of inspiration for all teachers and children, and the variety of response was wide.
   - Here, for instance, is a delightful rhyme in which a Year 5 child assumes the role of Ariel:

> As I walk along the beach
> Roughing up the sand
> I hear the sound of music
> Everywhere around
> Lurking on this island
> Is a magic spell of mine.

   - Many poems convey a sense of Utopia or paradise, like this from a Year 4 child:

> The sound of trees buzzing in the air.
> The sounds of monkeys chattering together.
> The palm trees wave side to side like the wind.
> The smell of the sweet flowers
> And mouth watering fruits
> The sights of fluttering butterflies.

Transforming: Writing (Narrative prose)

1. The most expressive use of prose was in its use for retelling the story. A good example is 'Ariel's release', written from Caliban's point of view by a Year 6 child:

I was asleep in the Elm tree on the west side of this island when the slow thud of footsteps awakened me. It was he, Lord of the Island, Prospero, who slowly came unto the cloven pine tree where Ariel lay in slumber. Prospero whispered some words and then bellowed 'I release thee Ariel on the count thee will serve me.' The tree shuddered, creaked and moaned as the breeze grew stronger and whirled round the tree as bright flashes of light shot out of the bark and out tumbled the tormented spirit, Ariel.

The strength and originality of this piece is in its attention to detail, 'the thud of footsteps' and the contrasts in Prospero's voice, but particularly in those cataclysmic happenings in the 'cloven pine'.

2. Some teachers invited their children to invent their own islands, and this led to some interesting writing. Here, for instance, is an extract from 'Tritanic Glytanica' by a Year 7 child, whose island is divided according to usage: education, accommodation and entertainment.

> The first section is used by youths to educate them. The ages are between five and sixteen. NO homework is allowed on this island. The learning system also has a medical room where people from the island go to be cured. The learning goes on in one great room which by the push of a button changes into other rooms. These consist of a gymnasium, a hall, a canteen (which is like a posh restaurant) . . .

Here is the Year 7 child's heart's desire: not having to traipse around from one room to the next for lessons. At the push of a button the rooms traipse after the pupil!

Transforming: Art

1. The teachers were less confident in their use of art, and here I describe the successful, exciting work, which showed two influences:
   - the expressionist approaches demonstrated by the artist during the in-service session;
   - close focus on Shakespeare's text.

2. One class of Year 4 and 5 children produced a series of powerful stormy sea paintings, in which the sea and the sky were evoked abstractly. For instance:
   - One has thin lines of red that appear to be flying off the centre across a heavily yellow-flecked black background.
   - The idea of Ariel in 'I flam'd amazement' is represented in another painting by a huge glistening yellow serpent line that crackles like fireworks across a shining cobalt and orange background.

3. A primary teacher successfully used Picasso's *Crying Woman* as a stimulus for painting, inviting the children to make portraits of characters in imitation of this style.
   - Prospero's mysteriousness, for instance, is shown in a picture which looks like a puzzle. A series of purple, blue, black, red and yellow shapes tesselate, but Prospero is only revealed when one follows certain lines. The overall effect is Prospero the wizard, a sort of Merlin.

4. A secondary art teacher also made use of art history, bringing to his Year 8 class a range of images from African mask pictures to paintings of the human form throughout art history.

- The mask pictures led to clear-cut, distinctive paintings of Ariel and Caliban, ranging from portraits which were like mask designs through to whole figures with masklike faces.
- There was also a magnificent bust of Caliban in clay, which was influenced by Shakespeare's text as well as the masks. The idea of Caliban as innocent and good at first then mischievous and dangerous later is conveyed by a tragic expression in the mouth and eyes, but a vicious weaponlike tusk. (See Chapter 2 for a more detailed description.)

5. Many techniques were used in the primary and secondary schools:
   - relief pictures in plaster and scraps;
   - dyed and embroidered fabrics;
   - collages using many materials.

Transforming: Drama

Most teachers used improvisation as a way of exploring not only actual encounters in the text but also possible encounters implied by the text. For instance, one class enacted a possible encounter between Ariel and Prospero, which led to Ariel's release from the pine tree. Several teachers developed scenes about the early relationship between Prospero, Miranda and Caliban. Many of the children in these classes focused on the idea of one character teaching the other useful knowledge. So Prospero was shown by Caliban useful things to eat and Caliban was taught how to name some of these things.

Many teachers worked with their children on performance pieces or programmes of items, including poetry and prose. Some groups of schools organised sharing events involving work across all the arts. The following are three examples of the drama performances.

1. Years 5 and 6

A play involving half a class in the children's own words:

- Prospero tells Ariel to make a tempest. Ariel asks what a tempest is.
- The scene becomes a ship at sea. Ariel, dressed in net with strips of seaweed, dances to music composed and played by the children.
- This dance becomes a sequence, in which Ariel takes each mariner by the hand and places him in a different part of the island.
- The sounds of voices crying 'Help me, I'm drowning' and so on are heard.
- Prospero calls for Ariel and asks, 'Where is the king?'
- The chanting of 'Full fathom five' begins and Ferdinand enters. Ariel takes Ferdinand to meet Prospero and Miranda.
- The play concludes with the announcement, 'After a few months they get married.'
- In this play there was a strong sense of the tempest being something that does no harm, underlined by the fact that Ariel takes each mariner by the hand.

2. Year 6

Groups performing a set of polished improvisations of favourite scenes.

- Many involved Stephano, Trinculo and Caliban, particularly the clothesline scene, but some did less obvious ones.
- One group chose Act II, Scene i and the dialogue between Antonio and Sebastian which leads to the drawing of swords. Here is an extract of that dialogue:

ANTONIO: Sebastian, listen, if we kill Alonso then you can be King of Naples.

SEBASTIAN: Yes and with you Duke of Milan and me King of Naples we could plot together.

ANTONIO: Yes, well I don't mind killing them but I'm not going to draw my sword first.

SEBASTIAN: Don't look at *me*. I'm not.

(Pause)

ANTONIO: There's only one other thing we *can* do.

SEBASTIAN: What's that?

ANTONIO: Draw them together.

SEBASTIAN: Sounds fine to me.

This is a straightforward paraphrase of the parts of the scene but it is interesting that the children inferred from the text that Sebastian is reluctant to take the initiative.

- Another group worked on part of Act IV, Scene i, in which Prospero entertains the young lovers. Here is an extract:

PROSPERO *(to Ferdinand and Miranda)*: Watch!

(Three children dance)

FERDINAND: This is a most majestic vision!

PROSPERO: Wait!

(Signals to dancers to go)

Caliban! I forgot. *(Pause)*

Goddesses for lovers. A banquet for kings. But fine clothes for drunkards.

The interest here is Prospero's summary of what he provides for lovers, kings and drunkards, which is an intelligent distillation and successfully transforms the ideas in the plot into a personal response.

3. Year 8

A group of Year 8 children worked in a video suite with technicians to produce a piece of television out of Act III, Scene i, in which Miranda sees Ferdinand carrying wood.

FERDINAND: That old man gave me so much work, I feel like dying. But I'll do anything to be near Miranda. It does upset her, seeing me work like this.

(*Enter Miranda with music*)

MIRANDA:	Oh, dear Ferdinand, I can't bear to see you work so hard. I'd have preferred the logs to have burned than see you carry them. You have a rest while Father is studying.
FERDINAND:	It'll be sunset soon. I've got to carry on.
MIRANDA:	Sit down, love, I will carry the logs for you.
FERDINAND:	No, I would rather break every bone in my body than see you work while I rest.
MIRANDA:	I could do it a lot more quickly and I would look as good doing it as you.
PROSPERO(*from the side*):	Poor little thing. She's mad about him and this just shows it.
MIRANDA:	You look tired.
FERDINAND:	Never, with you near. What is your name, my dear?
MIRANDA:	Miranda.
FERDINAND:	Ah, Miranda. You are so wonderful. The best woman I have ever seen
MIRANDA:	I wouldn't know. I've never seen any other women . . . or men. But you seem pretty good to me.
FERDINAND:	Although I am probably king now, and shouldn't be doing jobs like this, I don't mind because I'd do anything for you
MIRANDA:	Do you love me then?
FERDINAND:	More than anything in the world.
MIRANDA:	I love you too and will be your wife if you want me.
FERDINAND:	With all my heart and we will be so happily married.
PROSPERO:	Ferdinand has come through my test well and I think they will be happy together. They have my blessing.

This tracks the key issues in Shakespeare's text effectively in the children's own words. They made the scene their own, particularly in

- Miranda's 'I could do it a lot more quickly and I would look as good doing it as you', with its hint of sexual equality;
- Ferdinand's inferred knowledge of the role of kings in 'Although I am probably king now, and shouldn't be doing jobs like this'.

Transforming: Music

1. A student concentrated on the music that could be made from everyday objects, starting with the children's own bodies and mouths.
   - The children explored the tapping and banging of furniture and classroom objects then drew graphic scores for each other.

- They made musical impressions of characters; for instance, Ariel represented by a set of pipes made from bottles containing different levels of water and with fingers rubbed around the edges of water-filled glasses. A haunting melody was produced this way.

2. One made good use of the children's abilities with tuned instruments. These children were asked to compose music to accompany readings of the song lyrics and try to capture the mood of the song in their compositions.

Transforming: Movement

1. Movement was used as a way of getting children into the play.
   - There were explorations of ship movements accompanied by sound effects.
   - The line 'We split! We split!' was used by one teacher as a signal for her class to fall away in different directions.
   - Another class worked on flame movements based on extracts of Ariel's speech to Prospero in Act I, Scene ii with the lines 'sometime I'd divide / And burn in many places'.
2. The characters, particularly Caliban, were explored in movement.
   - Some children sculpted Caliban, one child manipulating another's body to represent the character.
   - Others made the shapes of the different characters, then moved like them, attempting to show contrast, for instance, between Caliban and Ariel.

Publishing: Exhibitions

One primary school developed a splendid gallery of work in the foyer, with

- a large paper and fabric sculpture of Ariel emerging from the 'cleft pine';
- a paper bust of Prospero;
- many drawings, paintings and murals;
- handmade and properly bound folders and books of children's writings with handwriting in beautiful calligraphic script.

This teacher had involved her children in a major literary experience, which would stay with them for many years. They were

- experiencing great literature as active and enactive, as something which deserves to be worked at with your hands as well as your brain;
- investing it with feeling, experiencing it through their senses.

All the schools had effective, if smaller, displays of work.

Publishing: Performances and workshops

The Outreach Theatre Company's performances and workshops were the ultimate conclusions to the project and were immensely successful.

After the first performance of the play to an audience of more than 60 Year 4, 5 and 6 children, the director was highly animated. He talked about the deep attention of these children – not a shuffle, no eyes straying – for the one hour twenty minutes of the play all in Shakespeare's words. They knew the play 'inside out', judging by their responses in the workshop, asking pertinent questions, articulating their views knowledgeably and taking part energetically in the activities.

This continued for performance after performance. Even the youngest children were heard quietly speaking the text at appropriate moments. One of these, who had played Trinculo in his class's play, looked at his teacher knowingly when the Outreach Trinculo said, 'A most ridiculous monster, to make a wonder of a poor drunkard!'

The teachers were struck by their children's level of involvement.

- Many teachers told of children outraged by Prospero's attitude towards Caliban.
- When Prospero was hot-seated children would ask questions such as, 'Don't you think you have responsibility for him?'

The main workshop activities devised by Outreach were as follows:

- Children made *tableaux vivants* of Caliban's happiest and saddest moments.
- Scenes were frozen and children asked to say if the actors were in the right places in relation to each other.
- Scenes were frozen and members of the audience invited to stand by characters and say what they might be thinking.
- Whole audiences were divided into those on Prospero's side and those on his brother Antonio's side and a debate conducted about the rights and wrongs of each.

The project demonstrated a great deal to all those involved. It proved the value of

- the arts approach to learning in literature;
- collaboration between different agencies.

None of the children involved could have enjoyed the opportunities they had without such collaboration and, despite the changed climate, such opportunities can still be created. Local authorities still have arts coordinators, there are still many theatre-in-education companies at work and there are more funding opportunities available now than ever.

Project: *Twelfth Night*

The project

The project is for Year 5 and 6 children in primary schools and Year 7 and 8 in secondary schools. The aims are for the children to

- enjoy a play by Shakespeare;
- understand the story of *Twelfth Night* and the relationships between the characters within it;
- engage with extracts of the language;
- develop storytelling and recitation skills;
- develop discussion skills;
- develop response to story, characters and imagery through the arts, particularly writing and drama.

The text

The suggested method for the teachers to present *Twelfth Night* is a combination of storytelling and recitation of extracts of text, although teachers might prefer to recite the storytelling sections. Here I combine the plot for every act and scene with extracts of text for the children to hear, read and work on. I recommend that the present tense be used throughout.[5]

The Characters in Twelfth Night
ORSINO, Duke of Illyria
VALENTINE, a gentleman attending Orsino
CURIO, a gentleman attending Orsino

VIOLA, a shipwrecked lady
SEBASTIAN, her twin brother
CAPTAIN of the wrecked ship
ANTONIO another sea captain

OLIVIA, a countess
MARIA, her waiting-gentlewoman
SIR TOBY BELCH, her uncle
SIR ANDREW AGUECHEEK, his friend
MALVOLIO, Olivia's steward
FABIAN, one of her servants
FESTE, her jester
A priest
A servant
Musicians, lords, sailors, attendants

ACT I
Scene i
- Orsino, Duke of Illyria, is listening to sad music. He says to the musician,

> If music be the food of love, play on,
> Give me excess of it, that, surfeiting,
> The appetite may sicken, and so die.
> That strain again! It had a dying fall.
> O, it came o'er my ear like the sweet sound
> That breathes upon a bank of violets,
> Stealing and giving odour.

- Orsino's sadness makes him moody. 'Enough, no more!' he says to the musician, ''Tis not so sweet now as it was before.' Curio suggests they go hunting for the 'hart' or deer.
- Orsino, lovesick for Olivia, says he's already hunting for the 'heart', meaning Olivia's love.
- Valentine returns from Olivia bringing bad news. She mourns the death of her brother and won't speak to Valentine.
- Orsino wonders if she will ever be able to fall in love. If she did it would be like 'sweet beds of flowers'.

Scene ii

- Viola is saved from shipwreck by the Captain but fears her brother, Sebastian, is drowned.
- The Captain says he saw Sebastian holding onto the ship's mast and that they are in his birthplace, Illyria, which is ruled by Orsino, who loves the 'fair Olivia',

> A virtuous maid, the daughter of a count
> That died some twelvemonth since, then leaving her
> In the protection of his son, her brother,
> Who shortly also died; for whose dear love,
> They say, she hath abjured the sight
> And company of men.

- Viola says she would like to help Olivia. She gives gold to the Captain for helping her to dress as a man, so she can go and offer to serve Orsino.

Scene iii

- Olivia's gentlewoman Maria is telling off Sir Toby, Olivia's uncle, for going to bed late and drunk every night and for bringing the foolish knight, Sir Andrew, to woo Olivia.
- Sir Toby says Sir Andrew is tall and rich and good at lots of things.
- Maria says that he's foolish, quarrelsome and gets drunk every night with Sir Toby.
- Sir Toby says they get drunk by drinking to Olivia's good health.
- Sir Andrew enters and Sir Toby introduces him to Maria. They joke around, trying to outwit each other. Maria makes a fool of both of them and leaves.

- Sir Andrew is dull and easy to make fun of, misunderstanding most things people say.
- Sir Toby makes fun of him again.
- Sir Andrew says he's going back home tomorrow because Olivia won't even see him.
- Sir Toby persuades him to stay longer and have fun.

Scene iv

- Viola, disguised as the young man Cesario, is at Orsino's court, and Valentine is telling her that the Duke likes her.
- Orsino joins them and asks Viola to go to Olivia to speak of his love for her.
- Viola says she may not be allowed in, and what should she say anyway?
- Orsino says,

> O, then unfold the passion of my love.
> Surprise her with discourse of my dear faith.
> It shall become thee well to act my woes

- Viola agrees to do it, but has already fallen in love herself with Orsino.

Scene v

- Maria is scolding Feste the clown. She wants to know where he has been.
- He answers with jokes and riddles.
- She joins in the joking but tells Feste to prepare a good excuse for Olivia. She leaves.
- Olivia enters with her steward Malvolio and attendants.
- Feste jokes but Olivia is bored with him and says, 'Take the fool away.'
- Feste answers, 'Do you not hear, fellows? Take away the lady.'
- Olivia's annoyed but agrees when Feste asks her to allow him to prove that she is a fool.
- Feste says, 'Good madonna, why mourn'st thou?'
- Olivia answers 'Good fool for my brother's death.'
- The proof goes like this:

FESTE: I think his soul is in hell, madonna.
OLIVIA: I know his soul is in heaven, fool.
FESTE: The more fool, madonna, to mourn for your brother's soul, being in heaven. Take away the fool, gentlemen.

- Olivia asks Malvolio what he thinks of Feste.
- Malvolio calls Feste a 'barren rascal'.
- Olivia is not pleased with this and says, 'O, you are sick of self-love, Malvolio'.
- Maria enters and says a young man wants to speak to Olivia.
- Olivia sends Malvolio to speak with the young man, saying that if he's from Orsino she is 'sick or not at home'.

- Sir Toby enters 'half drunk' and says the young man is a 'gentleman'. He cracks a few jokes and leaves with Maria.
- Olivia tells Feste to look after Sir Toby because he's 'drowned' with drink.
- Malvolio returns saying that the young man will not be put off with excuses and will not go without seeing Olivia.
- She asks Malvolio what he's like.
- Malvolio says he's half way between a boy and a man, and 'One would think his mother's milk were scarce out of him.'
- Olivia decides to see the young man, who is really Viola disguised as Cesario (Viola/Cesario we will call her for now).
- Viola/Cesario enters, asking to see the 'honourable lady of the house'.
- Olivia says, 'Speak to me.'
- Viola/Cesario starts making a speech.
- Olivia keeps interrupting.
- Maria then tries to lead Viola/Cesario out but she refuses to go.
- Olivia sends Maria away and continues interrupting Viola/Cesario's speech.
- Viola/Cesario gets cross and calls Olivia 'the cruellest she alive' and 'too proud' but says her master, Orsino, loves her,

> With adorations, fertile tears
> With groans that thunder love, with sighs of fire.

- Olivia says she 'cannot love him' and he should have known that 'long ago'.
- Viola/Cesario cannot understand why Olivia 'cannot love him'.
- Olivia starts fancying Viola/Cesario. She says she doesn't want any more offers of love from Orsino but would like to see Viola/Cesario again and even tries to give money.
- Viola/Cesario refuses rudely and as she leaves says

> I am no fee'd post, lady; keep thy purse.
> My master, not myself, lacks recompense.
> Love make his heart of flint, that you shall love,
> And let your fervour like my master's be
> Placed in contempt. Farewell, fair cruelty!

- Olivia fears that she is in love with Viola/Cesario and observes,

> Even so quickly may one catch the plague?
> Methinks I feel this youths perfections,
> With an invisible and subtle stealth,
> To creep in at mine eyes. Well, let it be!

- She calls for Malvolio and asks him to take a ring to Viola/Cesario, pretending that he left it by mistake and to ask him to return tomorrow.

ACT II

Scene i

- Viola's twin brother Sebastian is saved from drowning by Antonio a sea captain. He thinks his sister has been drowned. He tells Antonio who he is and that he is from Messaline.
- Antonio asks to be Sebastian's servant.
- Sebastian thanks him but refuses, saying, 'I am bound to the Duke Orsino's court. Farewell.'
- Antonio has enemies in Illyria but follows Sebastian anyway.

Scene ii

- Malvolio tries to give Viola/Cesario the ring and says Olivia wants no more messages from Orsino. She refuses the ring.
- Malvolio leaves, tossing it on the ground and saying, 'If it be worth stooping for, there it lies in your eye; if not, be it his that finds it.'
- Viola/Cesario realises what it is going on, saying to herself

> I left no ring with her; what means this lady?
> Fortune forbid my outside have not charmed her!
> She made good view of me, indeed so much
> That – methought – her eyes had lost their tongue,
> For she did speak in starts, distractedly.
> She loves me, sure, the cunning of her passion
> Invites me in this churlish messenger.
> None of my lord's ring? Why, he sent her none.
> I am the man! If it be so – as 'tis –
> Poor lady, she were better love a dream.

- Viola/Cesario is in a difficult situation. Her master, Orsino, loves Olivia, Viola, disguised as a man, loves her master and Olivia loves her, thinking she is Cesario, a man. She says,

> O time, thou must untangle this, not I!
> It is too hard a knot for me t'untie.

Scene iii

- Sir Toby and Sir Andrew are up late again.
- Feste enters and says, 'Did you never see the picture of We Three'.
- They talk in riddles and Sir Toby asks Feste to sing a love song.
- Feste sings,

> O mistress mine! Where are you roaming?
> O, stay and hear: your true love's coming,
> That can sing both high and low.

Trip no further little sweeting;
Journeys end in lovers meeting;
Every wise man's son doth know.

What is love? 'Tis not hereafter;
Present mirth hath present laughter,
What's to come is still unsure.
In delay there lies no plenty –
Then come kiss me, sweet and twenty,
Youth's a stuff will not endure.

- Sir Toby persuades the others to join in a noisy song called 'Hold thy peace'.
- They sing loudly and Maria comes to shush them, saying Olivia might get Malvolio to sort them out.
- Sir Toby starts another noisy song, 'O the twelfth day of December'.
- Malvolio enters full of self-importance, saying,

My masters, are you mad? Or what are you? Have you no wit, manners, nor honesty, but to gabble like tinkers at this time of night? Do you make an ale-house of my lady's house, that ye squeak out your coziers' catches without any mitigation or remorse of voice? Is there no respect of place, persons, nor time in you?

- Sir Toby, who is Olivia's uncle, replies, 'We did keep time, sir, in our catches. Sneck up!'
- Malvolio, really only a servant of Olivia, gets above himself and says,

Sir Toby, I must be round with you. My lady bade me tell you that, though she harbours you as her kinsman, she's nothing allied to your disorders. If you can separate yourself and your misdemeanours, you are welcome to the house. If not, an it would please you to take leave of her, she is willing to bid you farewell.

- Sir Toby sings another noisy song and Feste joins in.
- Maria says, 'Nay, good Sir Toby!'
- Sir Toby continues, singing, then says to Malvolio,
  Art any more than a steward? Dost thou think, because thou art virtuous, there shall be no more cakes and ale?
- He adds for good measure,

Go, sir, rub your chain with crumbs!'

- He asks Maria for more wine.
- Malvolio, stiff with indignity, looks at the jug of wine and as he leaves says,

Mistress Mary, if you prized my lady's favour at anything more than contempt, you would not give means for this uncivil rule. She shall know of it, by this hand!

- Maria is tired of Malvolio's pomposity and calls after him, 'Go, shake your ears.'
- Sir Andrew says how good it would be to challenge Malvolio to a duel.
- Sir Toby says he should do it.
- Maria says that Malvolio is a puritan type of person, full of his own importance, who thinks everybody loves him, and that she has a plan to get back at him.
- She will write a love letter to Malvolio in Olivia's handwriting, saying she admires his features. She will drop the letter where he is bound to see it and where Sir Toby, Sir Andrew, Feste, herself and Fabian can hide and watch. They are delighted with her plan.
- Sir Toby says Sir Andrew could win Olivia but that he needs to send home for more money.
- Sir Andrew says he will and Sir Toby invites him carry on drinking until the morning.

Scene iv
- Orsino demands to hear the song he heard the day before but Feste is not there.
- Curio goes to look for Feste.
- Orsino talks to Viola/Cesario about love. Orsino guesses that she also is in love.
- He asks 'What kind of woman is't?'
- Viola/Cesario answers, 'Of your complexion.'
- He asks how old the woman is.
- Viola answers, 'About your years, my lord.'
- Orsino says she is too old because the man ought to be older than the woman. It is clear that Viola/Cesario is in love with Orsino but he has no idea. He thinks she is a man.
- Curio leads Feste in to sing the love song that Orsino wants,

> Come away, come away, death,
> And in sad cypress let me be laid.
> Fie away, fie away, breath!
> I am slain by a fair, cruel maid.
> My shroud of white, stuck all with yew,
> O, prepare it!
> My part of death, no one so true
> Did share it.
>
> Not a flower, not a flower sweet
> On my black coffin let there be strewn.
> Not a friend, not a friend greet
> My poor corpse, where my bones shall be thrown.
> A thousand, thousand sighs to save,
> Lay me, o, where

Sad true lover never find my grave
To weep there.

- Orsino gives money to Feste, who speaks in riddles then leaves.
- Orsino sends everyone else away except Viola/Cesario.
- He asks her to go to Olivia and tell of his love 'more noble than the world'.
- Viola/Cesario says, 'But if she cannot love, sir?'
- Orsino ignores this and says his love is 'as hungry as the sea'.
- Viola gives hints to Orsino that she loves him, saying that if she were a woman she might love him. She even makes up a story about a woman who loved a man but 'never told her love'. In the end she agrees to return to Olivia with a jewel.

Scene v
- Sir Toby, Sir Andrew and Fabian are in Olivia's garden, looking forward to the trick they will play on Malvolio.
- Maria joins them. She has seen Malvolio walking in the garden and tells them to hide behind the hedge while she drops a letter on the grass.
- Malvolio enters, talking to himself, pretending that Olivia fancies him.
- Behind the hedge Sir Toby and Sir Andrew cannot keep their mouths closed, particularly when they hear Malvolio say, 'To be Count Malvolio'.
- Fabian tries to shut them up, but they can't, particularly when they hear Malvolio say, 'Having been three months married to her, sitting in my state'.
- Sir Toby says, 'O for a stone-bow to hit him in the eye!'
- Malvolio continues, 'Calling my officers about me'.
- 'Fire and brimstone!' says Sir Toby.
- Fabian says, 'O Peace, peace!'
- Malvolio makes this impossible by saying 'to ask for my kinsman Toby'.
- 'Bolts and shackles', says Sir Toby.
- Malvolio says, 'Toby approaches, curtsies there to me . . .'
- 'Shall this fellow live?' asks Sir Toby.
- It continues like this for some time and it is a wonder that Malvolio doesn't hear the babble behind the hedge. But he doesn't.
- Malvolio sees the letter, picks it up and recognises Olivia's handwriting. The letter is full of riddles, particularly the letters M.O.A.I.
- But Malvolio is certain it is a love letter to him from Olivia. He realises that M.O.A.I. are letters from his name, rearranged as part of the riddle.
- The letter encourages Malvolio's hopes and expectations. It says, '*In my stars I am above thee, but be not afraid of greatness. Some are born great, some achieve greatness, and some have greatness thrust upon them.*'
- It tells him to be rude to Sir Toby and 'surly with the servants'.
- It suggests that he wear clothes in a fashion which is out of date, '*Remember who commended thy yellow stockings and wished to see thee ever cross-gartered.*'

- Finally, it says, '*If thou entertainest my love, let it appear in thy smiling, smiles become thee well. Therefore in my presence still smile, dear my sweet, I prithee.*'
- Malvolio is a serious, unsmiling man. This will make him look ridiculous, particularly with the cross-gartered yellow stockings!
- As he leaves Malvolio says that he will smile and do everything the letter commands.
- Fabian, Sir Toby and Sir Andrew are delighted. When Maria returns they heap praise on her.
- She asks if the trick worked. She need not have asked.
- She tells them to be present when Malvolio first approaches Olivia, for 'He will come to her in yellow stockings, and 'tis a colour she abhors; and cross-gartered, a fashion she detests; and he will smile upon her, which will now be so unsuitable to her disposition'.
- They leave anticipating great fun.

ACT III
Scene i
- Viola/Cesario meets Feste at Olivia's house.
- Feste finds a funny meaning for everything Viola/Cesario says to him.
- Viola/Cesario gives him money for his jokes and when he is gone realises how clever he is, saying, 'This fellow is wise enough to play the fool.'
- She meets Sir Toby and Sir Andrew, who also make jokes, then sees Olivia and Maria. Olivia sends them all away except Viola/Cesario.
- Olivia asks Viola/Cesario questions, which all show that she fancies her/him but doesn't like Orsino.
- She reminds Viola/Cesario of the ring she sent to her/him last time she came and Viola/Cesario says 'I pity you.'
- The conversation gets difficult but in the end Olivia admits her feelings,

> Cesario, by the roses of the spring,
> By maidenhood, honour, truth and everything,
> I love thee so that, maugre all my pride,
> Nor wit nor reason can my passion hide.

- Olivia has fallen in love with a woman, thinking she's a man!
- Viola/Cesario is in love with a man, who also thinks she's a man!
- It's so confusing and Viola/Cesario's reply to Olivia's declaration of love is confusing too,

> By innocence I swear, and by my youth,
> I have one heart, one bosom, and one truth.
> And that no woman has, nor never none
> Shall mistress be save I alone.

- Olivia is so in love she tells Viola/Cesario that she might change her mind about Orsino,

> Yet come again; for thou perhaps mayst move
> That heart, which now abhors, to like his love.

Scene ii

- Sir Toby and Fabian are trying to persuade Sir Andrew to stay longer at Olivia's, but Sir Andrew wants to leave because he's had no encouragement from Olivia. He says he saw Olivia showing more favour to Orsino's servingman (Viola/Cesario).
- The others say Olivia did this to make him jealous. Sir Toby even suggests that Sir Andrew challenge Viola/Cesario to a duel, saying that if Sir Andrew hurts Viola/Cesario this will make Olivia admire him for his valour.
- Sir Andrew agrees and goes to write a challenge, which Sir Toby will take to Viola/Cesario.
- Sir Toby and Fabian make fun of Sir Andrew when he's gone.
- Maria comes and leads them off to see Malvolio with Olivia, dressed in cross-gartered yellow stockings and smiling!
- She says, 'He does smile his face into more lines than is in the new map with the augmentation of the Indies.'

Scene iii

- Antonio catches up with Sebastian and says he wants to help him find his way around Illyria because it is often 'rough and inhospitable'.
- Antonio wants to get Sebastian some lodgings but Sebastian wants to see the sights.
- Antonio says he once fought against Orsino's men. He offers Sebastian his purse and tells him to lodge at The Elephant, where they will meet later.

Scene iv

- Olivia asks Maria 'Where's Malvolio?'
- Maria says, 'He's coming madam, but in a very strange manner. He is sure possessed madam.' She says, 'he does nothing but smile' and adds that Malvolio is 'tainted in his wits' and maybe dangerous.
- Olivia sends Maria to get Malvolio.
- Malvolio enters smiling and saying, 'Sweet lady! Ho! Ho!' as if they share a secret.
- Olivia says he shouldn't be smiling at such a sad time.
- He answers that he could be sad for 'this does make some obstruction in the blood, this cross-gartering'.
- Olivia, thinking he's unwell, says, 'Wilt thou go to bed, Malvolio?'
- This makes his smile bigger. He replies, 'To bed! Ay, sweetheart, and I'll come to thee!'

- Maria asks him why he's come to Olivia in such a silly way.
- He quotes from the letter, saying 'Be not afraid of greatness –' and 'Some are born great –' and 'Some achieve greatness –' and 'some have greatness thrust upon them.'
- He reminds Olivia about the yellow stockings and cross-gartering.
- Olivia is amazed, and says, 'Why, this is very midsummer madness', even though, of course, Twelfth Night is in the middle of winter.
- A servant comes to tell Olivia of Viola/Cesario's arrival.
- Olivia tells Maria to 'Let some of my people have a special care of' Malvolio for she fears harm might come to him. Olivia and Maria leave.
- Malvolio is alone talking to himself. He thinks that Olivia has proved her affection for him by saying words like 'fellow'. He thinks he is made.
- Sir Toby, Fabian and Maria come looking for Malvolio.
- Fabian asks Malvolio how he is, but Malvolio says, 'Go off.'
- Maria tells Sir Toby that Olivia wants him to 'care for' Malvolio.
- Malvolio thinks this is yet more proof that she loves him.
- Sir Toby and Fabian start making fun of Malvolio.
- Fabian says, 'The fiend is rough.'
- Sir Toby calls him a 'bawcock'.
- Maria joins in, asking Sir Toby to get Malvolio to say his prayers.
- Malvolio turns on them and on his way out says,

Go, hang yourselves all. You are idle, shallow things; I am not of your element. You shall know more hereafter.

- Sir Toby and Fabian can hardly believe how well the plot is working, but Maria wants them to keep goading Malvolio to make sure it keeps developing.
- They agree and Sir Toby says they will keep him in a dark room like a madman.
- Sir Andrew comes in with his letter, challenging Viola/Cesario to a duel.
- It is a silly, badly written letter but Sir Toby and Fabian praise it.
- Maria tells Sir Andrew that Viola/Cesario is with Olivia now.
- Sir Toby tells him to go into the orchard and draw his sword as soon as he sees Viola/Cesario. Sir Andrew does as he is told.
- Sir Toby says he will go to Viola/Cesario but instead of delivering the letter will issue the challenge by word of mouth and say how brave and fierce Sir Andrew is. He thinks that Viola/Cesario and Sir Andrew will be terrified and will just stare at each other.
- Sir Toby and Fabian hide and overhear the conversation between Olivia and Viola/Cesario
- Olivia admits that she has already 'said too much' and that Viola/Cesario has 'a heart of stone'. She's a little ashamed of herself but cannot help it.
- Viola/Cesario compares this to Orsino's situation.

- As she leaves Olivia gives Viola/Cesario a locket with her picture in and asks her/him to return next day.
- Viola/Cesario says she will come but only to try to win her love for Orsino.
- Olivia says she has already pledged her love to Viola/Cesario.
- Sir Toby and Fabian come out of their hiding place and greet Viola/Cesario.
- Sir Toby warns her/him about Sir Andrew,

> That defence thou hast, betake thee to't. Of what nature the wrongs are thou hast done him, I know not; but thy intercepter, full of despite, bloody as the hunter, attends thee at the orchard end. Dismount thy tuck; be yare in thy preparation; for thy assailant is quick, skilful, and deadly.

- Viola/Cesario is terrified and says she has no quarrel with any man.
- Sir Toby says it is 'otherwise' and that she should prepare herself for a fight.
- Viola/Cesario asks what sort of man her enemy is.
- Sir Toby says he's 'a devil in a private brawl' and has already killed three men.
- Viola/Cesario asks Sir Toby to find out how she has offended the knight.
- Sir Toby says he will and leaves Viola/Cesario with Fabian, who repeats that the knight is a skilful and bloody opponent, but says he will try to make peace between them.
- Sir Toby then tells Sir Andrew that Viola/Cesario is a skilful swordsman and very angry.
- Sir Andrew doesn't want a fight. He says he's prepared to give his best horse to his opponent to 'let the matter slip'.
- Sir Andrew and Viola/Cesario are brought to opposite ends of the orchard. Sir Andrew draws his sword.
- Viola/Cesario says, 'I do assure you, 'tis against my will.'
- Just then Antonio comes into the orchard, hears this and thinks it is Sebastian (Viola's twin brother) so offers to fight the duel.
- Officers of the law come into the orchard.
- Viola/Cesario asks Sir Andrew to put up his sword.
- Sir Andrew is relieved and says she can have the horse.
- The officers arrest Antonio for what he did in the fight years before.
- Antonio asks Viola/Cesario for his purse back, thinking she is Sebastian.
- Viola/Cesario doesn't know him and offers to lend him money for helping her.
- Antonio cannot believe her ingratitude and tells her so.
- She says she doesn't know him.
- Antonio is furious and tells everyone that he saved her/him from drowning.
- As he is dragged off by the officers, he shouts a few last words at Viola/Cesario,

> Thou hast, Sebastian, done good feature shame.
> In nature, there's no blemish but the mind;

> None can be called deformed, but the unkind.
> Virtue is beauty; but the beauteous evil
> Are empty trunks o'er-flourished by the devil.

- Viola/Cesario is confused and says, 'He named Sebastian'. She realises her brother might be alive after all, saying, 'Tempests are kind, and salt waves fresh in love!'
- Sir Toby, Fabian and Sir Andrew leave the orchard saying that Viola/Cesario is 'a coward' for 'leaving his friend here in necessity and denying him'.

ACT IV
Scene i
- Feste has been sent to bring Viola/Cesario to Olivia, but meets Sebastian instead.
- Sebastian tells Feste to go away, saying 'vent thy folly somewhere else'.
- Feste likes this phrase 'vent thy folly' and says,

> Vent my folly! He has heard that word of some great man, and now applies it to a fool. Vent my folly! I am afraid this great lubber the world will prove a cockney. I prithee now, ungird thy strangeness, and tell me what I shall vent to my lady? Shall I vent to her that thou art coming?

- Sebastian offers Feste money to go away and threatens to 'give worse payment' if he doesn't leave at once!
- Sir Andrew, Sir Toby and Fabian enter.
- Sir Andrew hits Sebastian, thinking he is Viola/Cesario.
- Sebastian hits Sir Andrew with the handle of his dagger.
- Sir Toby tells Sebastian to stop it or else.
- Feste runs off to tell Olivia what has happened.
- Sir Toby grabs hold of Sebastian, but Sir Andrew wants to leave and threatens to sue Sebastian 'for battery' even though he struck the first blow himself.
- Sebastian breaks free of Sir Toby's grasp and draws his sword.
- Sir Toby draws his sword.
- Olivia enters just then and tells Sir Toby to stop. She scolds him and says he's 'fit for the mountains and the barbarous caves' and to get 'out of my sight'.
- Sir Toby, Sir Andrew and Fabian leave.
- Olivia also thinks Sebastian is Viola/Cesario and says to him:

> I prithee gentle friend,
> Let thy fair wisdom, not thy passion, sway
> In this incivil and unjust extent
> Against thy peace. Go with me to my house,
> And hear thou how many fruitless pranks
> This ruffian hath botched up, that thou thereby
> Mayst smile at this. Thou shalt not choose but go;

> Do not deny. Beshrew his soul for me!
> He started one poor heart of mine, in thee.

- Sebastian can't believe it. He wonders if he's mad or dreaming but goes with Olivia.

Scene ii

- Maria has fetched a disguise for Feste to pretend to be Sir Topas, a holy man.
- She then goes to get Sir Toby.
- Feste puts on the gown and beard.
- Maria returns with Sir Toby. He is pleased to see Feste in disguise.
- They go and stand outside the cell where Malvolio is being kept.
- Malvolio hears something and shouts 'Who calls there?'
- Feste replies 'Sir Topas, the curate, who comes to visit Malvolio the lunatic.'
- Malvolio is desperate and says 'Sir Topas, never was man thus wronged. Good Sir Topas, do not think that I am mad. They have laid me here in hideous darkness –'.
- To make Malvolio think he is mad Feste pretends that the room is not dark.
- Malvolio says it is dark, that he is abused and asks Feste to test whether he is mad or not.
- Feste asks him a silly question and when Malvolio tries to answer it Feste says his answer proves he's mad.
- Sir Toby and Maria are pleased with Feste's performance.
- Sir Toby asks him to go into the room without his disguise to find out what state of mind Malvolio is really in. Sir Toby has had enough of this trick and is worried about Olivia's disapproval. He and Maria leave.
- Feste enters the dark room singing a song.
- Malvolio calls him a fool and asks for pen, ink and paper to write a letter to Olivia.
- Feste asks Malvolio how he became mad.
- Malvolio says 'I am as well in my wits, fool, as thou art.'
- Feste replies, 'Then you are mad indeed, if you be no better in your wits than a fool.'
- Next, Feste pretends to be Sir Topas again, saying to Malvolio, 'Endeavour thyself to sleep and leave thy vain bibble-babble.'
- He then goes from one voice to another just to confuse Malvolio.
- Malvolio wants pen, ink, paper and some light so he can write to Olivia and promises to 'advantage' Feste if he gets it.
- Feste agrees to get it, sings another song and leaves.

Scene iii

- Sebastian has just received a present from Olivia, a pearl, and can't believe his luck.
- He's tried to find Antonio 'at The Elephant' but Antonio isn't there.

- He stands in wonder at his good fortune.
- Olivia comes to him with a priest and asks him to marry her!
- Sebastian agrees and they go off to get married.

ACT V

Scene i

- Fabian wants Feste to show him the letter he's carrying to Olivia from Malvolio.
- Feste refuses.
- They meet Orsino, Viola/Cesario and others.
- Feste speaks riddles to Orsino.
- Orsino enjoys them and gives Feste gold.
- Feste says, 'I would you could make me another.'
- Orsino gives him another gold coin.
- Feste asks for another saying, 'the third pays for all'.
- Orsino says he'll only give Feste more if he goes and fetches Olivia.
- Feste leaves.
- Poor Antonio, who rescued Sebastian from the storm and who now thinks Viola/Cesario is Sebastian, is brought in by officers.
- Orsino recognises him as the captain of the ship who once attacked his fleet.
- One officer reminds Orsino of this and says Antonio is arrested for fighting in the streets.
- Orsino asks Antonio why he has come to Illyria.
- Antonio replies that he's not some pirate, adding

> That most ingrateful boy there by your side
> From the rude sea's enraged and foamy mouth
> Did I redeem; a wrack past hope he was.

- Antonio says he came into the town to help this 'ingrateful boy' but was denied by him.
- Viola/Cesario does not understand.
- Orsino asks Antonio when he first arrived in Illyria.
- Antonio says, 'Today, my lord'.
- Orsino says Antonio's words are madness because Viola/Cesario has been with him for three months. He tells the officers to take him to one side because Olivia has enterered with some of her servants.
- Olivia is looking for Viola/Cesario, who she thinks is now her husband. She sees her/him and says 'Cesario, you do not keep promise with me.'
- Orsino interrupts with 'Gracious Olivia'.
- Olivia says she doesn't want to hear him if it is 'the old tune'.
- Orsino is upset again and asks her what he should do.
- She tells him to do what he pleases.

- Orsino gets very upset, calling her 'the marble-breasted tyrant' and threatening never to let her see Viola/Cesario again.
- Viola/Cesario says she will willingly come with him.
- This upsets Olivia. She says, 'Where goes Cesario?'
- Viola/Cesario replies, 'After him I love.'
- Olivia cannot believe it. The man she thinks is her new husband wants to be with Orsino.
- She sends for the priest and calls Viola/Cesario 'husband'.
- Orsino is amazed and says to Viola/Cesario 'Her husband, sirrah?'
- Viola/Cesario denies it.
- Olivia says Viola/Cesario is too frightened to admit it.
- The priest comes and confirms that the two were married two hours ago.
- Orsino turns on Viola/Cesario, saying, 'O thou dissembling cub!' and 'Farewell, and take her.'
- Viola/Cesario denies it.
- Sir Andrew comes in calling for a surgeon and saying, 'He's broke my head across, and he's given Sir Toby a bloody coxcomb too.'
- Olivia asks Sir Andrew who did it.
- Sir Andrew says it was Cesario. He sees Viola/Cesario and says, 'You broke my head for nothing; and that that I did, I was set on to do't by Sir Toby.'
- Viola/Cesario denies this, too.
- Sir Toby and Feste come in.
- Orsino asks them how they are.
- Sir Toby says he's been hurt, but adds, 'and there's the end on't'.
- Olivia tells a servant to look after Sir Toby and asks who is responsible for the fighting.
- Sir Andrew offers to help Sir Toby.
- Sir Toby calls him 'asshead', 'coxcomb' and 'thin-faced knave'.
- Sir Toby and Sir Andrew leave with help from Feste and Fabian.
- Sebastian arrives, apologising to Olivia for hurting Sir Toby. He says to her lovingly, 'Pardon me, sweet one.'
- Orsino is amazed by Sebastian's appearance, saying

> One face, one voice, one habit, and two persons!
> A natural perspective, that is and is not.

- Sebastian then sees Antonio and says

> Antonio! O, my dear Antonio!
> How have the hours racked and tortured me
> Since I have lost thee!

- Antonio looks at Sebastian and then at Viola/Cesario and says,

> How have you made division of yourself?
> An apple cleft in two is not more twin
> Than these two creatures. Which is Sebastian?

- Olivia says, 'Most wonderful!'
- Sebastian says he never had a brother but had a sister who is drowned and asks Viola/Cesario who she is.
- She says she's from Messaline, that her father was Sebastian and her brother too.
- Sebastian says that if she were a woman she would be Viola, his sister.
- Viola says, 'My father had a mole upon his brow.'
- Sebastian says, 'And so had mine.'
- Then she admits that she's not a man. She's a woman and her name is Viola.
- Orsino is delighted because he loves Viola. He says,

> If this be so, as yet the glass seems true,
> I shall have share in this most happy wrack.
> Boy, thou hast said to me a thousand times
> Thou never should'st love woman like to me.

- Viola says it's true.
- Orsino takes her hand and asks her to go and get into woman's clothes.
- Viola says the captain who saved her has her clothes and is with Malvolio.
- Olivia sends for Malvolio just as Feste enters with the letter from Malvolio.
- She asks Feste how Malvolio is and Feste says he's mad and reads the letter to her in a mad, fast voice because it is from a madman.
- Olivia stops him, snatches the letter and gives it to Maria to read.
- The letter describes what Malvolio has suffered: being put into darkness and being ruled over by Sir Toby, receiving a letter supposedly from Olivia and so on.
- Olivia sends Fabian to release and bring Malvolio to her, then asks Orsino to think of her as a sister and suggests that they should celebrate their good fortune.
- Orsino agrees, then says to Viola,

> Your master quits you; and for your service done him
> So much against the mettle of your sex,
> So far beneath your soft and tender breeding,
> And since you called me master for so long,
> Here is my hand; you shall from this time be
> Your master's mistress.

- Malvolio comes in with Fabian and says

> Madam, you have done me wrong;
> Notorious wrong.

- Olivia denies it.

- Malvolio hands over the letter he found in the orchard, saying

> Why have you given me such clear lights of favour?
> Bade me come smiling and cross-gartered to you,
> To put on yellow stockings, and to frown
> Upon Sir Toby and the lighter people?

- Olivia says that the writing in the letter is not hers even though it looks like it but is Maria's. She remembers also that Maria was first to say that Malvolio was mad. She promises to punish those responsible.
- Fabian tells her about the trick they pulled on Malvolio. He says that they did it because of Malvolio's attitude and adds that Sir Toby has married Maria for setting it all up.
- Olivia looks at Malvolio and says, 'Alas, poor fool! How have they baffled thee!'
- Feste shouts,

Why, 'Some are born great, some achieve greatness, and some have greatness thrown upon them.'

- Feste admits his role in the trick, as Sir Topas, but reminds her of Malvolio's attitude, particularly calling Feste 'a barren rascal' and adds that 'the whirligig of time brings in his revenges'.
- Malvolio storms off, shouting, 'I'll be revenged on the whole pack of you.'
- Olivia says that Malvolio has been 'notoriously abused'.
- Orsino says that peace needs to be made between them all.
- They all leave, Orsino and Viola hand in hand, and Feste sings this song to end the play:

> When that I was and a little tiny boy,
> With hey-ho, the wind and the rain;
> A foolish thing was but a toy,
> For the rain it raineth every day.
>
> But when I came to man's estate
> With hey-ho, the wind and the rain;
> 'Gainst knaves and thieves men shut their gate,
> For the rain it raineth every day.
>
> But when I came, alas, to wive,
> With hey-ho, the wind and the rain;
> By swaggering could I never thrive
> For the rain it raineth every day.
>
> But when I came unto my beds,
> With hey-ho, the wind and the rain;

With tosspots still had drunken heads
For the rain it raineth every day.

A great while ago the world began
With hey-ho, the wind and the rain;
But that's all one, our play is done,
For the rain it raineth every day.

Teaching and learning processes

Meeting and knowing

1. Work on approximately one act each week. Act II and Act III may need longer. The activities are for half a term's work.
2. Provide copies of the list of characters. With a partner, children to

- discuss the relationships between the characters:
- practise speaking their names;
- have a who's who test.

3. After each presentation ask partners to retell the story in their own words and bullet point the developments in each scene.
4. Partners to discuss what has happened, what it means and what might happen next.
5. Children in larger groups to practise speaking the quoted passages out loud for a performance later in the project.
6. At the start of each session re-establish what has happened in the story.

Transforming: Writing

Children from both ages to choose from the following writing tasks for each act:

1. Act I
- A poem about lovesick Orsino at court listening to music and receiving a message from Olivia saying she doesn't want to hear about his love.
- The Captain's speech describing to Viola how he saw Sebastian escape from drowning in the storm.
- An account of how Viola makes herself look like a man.
- A love poem from Orsino to Olivia.
- The thoughts of Olivia. Her father and her brother have died. She wears dark clothes. Servants come to her from Orsino with messages of love, but she doesn't like him.
- Viola/Cesario's speech to Olivia telling her about Orsino's love for her.

2. Act II
- The thoughts of Olivia about Viola/Cesario just after she's fallen in love with her/him.

- A poem about Sir Toby Belch, Sir Andrew Aguecheek and Feste the clown at their late-night drinking, singing and dancing.
- Other lines like 'Go, sir, rub your chain with crumbs,' or 'Go, shake your ears,' which could be shouted at Malvolio after he spoilt the party.
- The thoughts of Viola about Orsino now she's fallen in love with him but has to carry his words of love to Olivia.
- A poem about Malvolio in the garden, showing off to himself, finding the letter and thinking Olivia loves him.
- Other lines like 'O for a stone-bow to hit him in the eye!' and 'Bolts and shackles!' to be spoken by those hiding behind the hedge listening to Malvolio.
- A description of Maria and her clever trick to make a fool of Malvolio.

3. Act III
- The words of Olivia's declaration of love to Viola/Cesario.
- The thoughts of Sir Andrew Aguecheek after he's seen Olivia being loving to Viola/Cesario.
- The words of Sir Toby trying to persuade Sir Andrew to stay longer.
- The story of the sea fight Antonio had with Orsino's men years before.
- A poem about Malvolio coming to Olivia in yellow stockings, cross-gartered and smiling.
- Malvolio's thoughts about Olivia, who he loves and of Sir Toby, Sir Andrew and Maria, who he thinks are 'idle, shallow things'.
- A letter from Sir Andrew to Viola/Cesario challenging him to a duel.
- Viola's thoughts after she has been challenged to a duel.
- A description of Sir Andrew as if he's a ferocious fighter, to be feared, then a description of him as he really is.

4. Act IV
- A poem about Sir Toby Belch, what he looks like, the things he likes to do and how he treats others.
- A piece called 'Fights in Olivia's orchard'.
- A description called 'This house is as dark as ignorance'.
- A poem about Feste, the way he speaks, sings and talks in riddles and jokes and his disguise as Sir Topas.
- Other phrases like 'bibble-babble' to mean 'nonsense'.
- Sebastian's words to Antonio in which he might describe his good fortune in Illyria.

5. Act V
- The letter Malvolio sends to Olivia from the dark room.
- Antonio's speech to Orsino describing what he did for 'that ingrateful boy', Viola/Cesario.

- Other lines like 'Live you the marble-hearted tyrant still' which Orsino might speak to Olivia and other phrases like 'O thou dissembling cub' which he might use to Viola/Cesario when he thinks he's married Olivia.
- Other lines like 'an apple cleft in two' to describe identical twins.
- A speech for Viola describing to Sebastian what happened to her in Illyria.
- A speech for Sebastian describing to Viola what has happened to him in Illyria.
- A speech for Malvolio, describing the wrongs done to him by Sir Toby and the others.
- Fabian's speech telling the truth about what they did to Malvolio and why they did it.

Transforming: Art
1. Children to
- Research Tudor costumes, portraits, gardens and buildings, particularly the interiors.
- Make a series of drawings of various kinds of people at different levels of Tudor society, paying particular attention to the clothes they wore.
2. Referring to the material from their researches and sets of drawings, children then to
   (a) Act I
      - Draw Orsino hunting Olivia's 'heart' rather than 'hart' meaning deer.
      - Paint true love as 'sweet beds of flowers'.
      - Draw Sebastian fighting for his life in the stormy waves.
      - Paint a portrait of Sir Toby 'quaffing and drinking' or of Sir Andrew called 'The great quarreller'.
      - Draw Viola dressed as the man called Cesario.
      - Draw a drunken man looking like a 'drowned man, a fool and a madman'.
      - Draw a picture of Olivia called 'Fair cruelty'.

   (b) Act II
      - Draw Antonio rescuing Sebastian from 'the breach of the sea'.
      - Make a diagram showing Orsino loves Olivia loves Viola loves Orsino as a sort of hard knot, which is difficult to 'untangle'.
      - Paint the picture of Sir Toby, Sir Andrew and Feste suggested in 'Did you never see the picture of We Three?'
      - Draw a cartoon showing 'the night-owl' being roused by 'We Three' singing and dancing.
      - Paint a picture showing a lover being 'slain by a fair cruel maid' or showing love 'as hungry as the sea' or showing the following lines:

         She never told her love,
      But let concealment, like a worm I'the bud,
      Feed on her damask cheek.

- Draw Malvolio walking in the garden, showing off to himself or reading the letter to himself.

(c) Act III
- Paint Feste singing songs or cracking jokes.
- Paint Malvolio coming to Olivia smiling and wearing yellow stockings with cross-gartering.
- Draw Viola/Cesario one side of the orchard with her sword drawn and Sir Andrew the other side with his drawn, both terrified.

(d) Act IV
- Paint a portrait of Sir Toby to show him as an 'Ungracious wretch / Fit for the mountains and the barbarous caves'.
- Paint Feste in disguise as Sir Topas in the dark room.

(e) Act V
- Paint Olivia, no longer in her mourning clothes, to represent the description of her as 'Now heaven walks on earth' or as a 'marble-breasted tyrant'.
- Draw Viola and Sebastian as 'An apple cleft in two'.
- Draw Malvolio all in a mess with his letter and complaining to Olivia about the way he has been treated.
- Make a diagram to show 'Some are born great, some achieve greatness, and some have greatness thrust upon them.'

Transforming: Drama and dance

For this work the children should work individually ('individuals'), then with partners ('partners – A and B'), then in groups of four or five ('groups').

1. Act I: Mime and movement.
   (a) Begin with individuals lying or sitting and listening to sad music then walking as in Olivia's 'veiled walk' slowly and sadly around the space.
   (b) Next, individuals to fight for their lives in the stormy sea, then be washed up on the shore.
   (c) Individuals to stand and walk like Orsino, Olivia, Sir Toby, Sir Andrew, Feste and Malvolio.
   (d) Partners to work on the following sequences:
   (e) A helps B to change from a woman into a man;
   (f) B comes to A as if pleading for something and A sends B away.

2. Act I: Improvisation.
   (a) Partners to work on the following encounters:
      - Viola asks the Captain about Illyria and the Captain helps her disguise herself as a man.

- Sir Toby complains to Maria about Olivia still dressed in mourning clothes. Maria scolds him for drinking and enjoying himself noisily late at night.
- Orsino tells Viola/Cesario of his love for Olivia and asks him to take a message to her.
- Viola/Cesario tries to win Olivia's love for Orsino but only succeeds in making Olivia love him/herself.

(b) Groups to work on the following scene:

- Malvolio comes to Olivia saying that Viola/Cesario won't take no for an answer; Olivia tells him to let her/him into the house; Viola/Cesario speaks of Orsino's love, leaves and is followed by Malvolio with the ring.

3. Act II: Mime and movement.
    (a) Repeat and improve 1, 2 and 3 from Act I'.
    (b) Partners to try and look like each other. A makes a facial expression and B copies it. B poses and A copies it and so on.
    (c) Make threes then create 'the picture of We Three', Feste, Sir Toby and Sir Andrew.
    (d) Groups to mime:

    - Sir Toby, Sir Andrew, Feste and Maria singing, dancing and joking, then Malvolio coming in and telling them all off.
    - Sir Toby, Sir Andrew, Feste and Fabian hiding behind the hedge, then Malvolio coming in, showing off, finding the letter then showing off even more.

4. Act II: Improvisation.
    (a) Partners to work on the following encounters:

    - Sebastian tells Antonio who he is and where he is from and that he has a sister called Viola; Antonio asks to be his servant but is refused.
    - Malvolio gives Viola/Cesario the ring in a rude manner.
    - Orsino once again talks to Viola/Cesario about love and asks her/him to go to Olivia.

    (b) Groups make up a play in which identical twins are mistaken for each other.

5. Act III: Mime and movement.
    (a) Individuals to make fencing poses and movements.
    (b) Partners to work out fencing dances, ensuring that when A attacks, B defends, and vice versa.
    (c) Groups to mime:

    - Malvolio coming to Olivia smiling in yellow, cross-gartered stockings, watched by Maria then Sir Toby and Fabian.
    - Sir Andrew and Viola about to fence when Antonio stops them and is held back by officers.

6. Act III: Improvisation.
   (a) Partners to work on the following encounters:
       - Viola/Cesario tells Olivia his name and tries to tell her about Orsino's love; Olivia says she loves him/her.
       - Sir Andrew says he's leaving because Olivia doesn't like him; Sir Toby persuades him to stay longer.
       - Sir Toby tells Viola/Cesario to prepare him/herself for a fight with Sir Andrew and says what a ferocious fighter Sir Andrew is; Viola/Cesario wants to know why.
   (b) Groups make up a play in which identical twins cause a potentially serious situation, but which is resolved in the nick of time.

7. Acts IV and V: Mime and movement.
   (a) Partners show Feste, disguised as Sir Topas, going into the dark room, where Malvolio is imprisoned and asking for help.
   (b) Groups to make a sequence in which Sebastian is attacked and fights back against Sir Toby and Sir Andrew, then goes off with Olivia and the priest to be married.

8. Acts IV and V: Improvisation.
   (a) Partners to work on the following encounters:
       - Olivia asks Sebastian to marry her. He agrees and speaks to himself about his good fortune.
       - Feste goes to Malvolio in the dark room and says he's mad; Malvolio says he's not, complains about what has happened and asks for pen, ink and paper.
   (b) Groups make a play about one of the following:
       - Love at first sight, which sometimes works and sometimes doesn't.
       - Identical twins being shipwrecked on an island.
       - On Twelfth Night some people want fun and others want to get back to normal.

Transforming: Music
Divide the children into groups of four or five. Using tuned and untuned instruments as well as voices and everyday objects, music groups to compose, rehearse and perform:

- A piece for sad lovers like Orsino, with 'a dying fall' motif going down the scale.
- Signature tunes for Sir Toby Belch, Sir Andrew Aguecheek, Feste, Malvolio and Olivia.
- Tunes for the songs.
- Percussion accompaniment to one of the speeches (e.g. Malvolio scolding Sir Toby and the others for making a noise at night).

Publishing

1. Compile an anthology of the children's best writing, covering the full range and organised act by act.
2. Illustrate this with a selection of the children's best drawings.
3. Children to select and mount/frame their best paintings and set up a gallery exhibition.
4. Select the most effective mimes, dances, improvisations and musical compositions; polish, rehearse and perform to an audience.

References

1. Carter, D. (1994) *Hamlet in Gwersyllt.* Mold: Clwyd Poetry Project.
2. Carter, D. (1990) *The Isle is Full of Noises.* Mold: Clwyd County Council.
3. Jenkins, H. (ed.) (1982) *Hamlet.* London: Methuen.
4. Kermode, F. (ed.) (1954) *The Tempest.* London: Methuen.
5. Mahood, M.M. (ed.) (1968) *Twelfth Night.* Harmondsworth: Penguin Books.

CHAPTER 6

Prose fiction

Introduction

The chapter begins with the description of an unusual project. Year 4, 5 and 6 children in four schools made stories into versions of the oratorio form. The stories, from *The Mabinogion*, are cornerstones of Welsh culture and required reading in the schools of Wales. The project sought to recognise and celebrate this and explore the oratorio form. The children wrote poems and storytelling scripts from the orally transmitted stories.

A project based on all four parts of Swift's *Gulliver's Travels* is then offered to teachers of Years 5, 6, 7 and 8 children. As well as extensive suggestions for work in writing there are many ideas for art and drama. Suggestions for work in history are also set down.

Case Study: The Four Branches of the Mabinogi

The project

The project was part of 'Arts in Schools Week' at a local theatre, and its aim was to develop Year 4, 5 and 6 children's compositional skills in writing, music-making and storytelling in response to *The Four Branches of the Mabinogi* and to create four oratorios. Four schools were chosen. The objectives were to:

- give the children a fluent working knowledge of their story;
- develop storytelling skills;
- write song lyrics and storyteller's scripts;
- make the lyrics into songs;
- compose tone poems;
- create four oratorios from the scripts, songs and tone poems.

A poet and a musician were appointed to work in the schools to help the teachers and children to develop lyrics, storytelling scripts, songs and tone poems.

The text

The Four Branches of the Mabinogi are four stories with the same group of central characters: Pwyll, Prince of Dyfed; Branwen, Daughter of Llyr; Manawydan, Son of Llyr; and Math, Son of Mathonwy. The work is written in Welsh but the English translation by Gwyn Jones and Thomas Jones was used.[1]

Teaching and learning processes

The focus for the project was the performance of four oratorios, one for each branch of the Mabinogi, in the local theatre. As the project developed, writing, storytelling and musical composition became more and more intertwined. I will, therefore, briefly list the teaching approaches of the poet and musician, then describe the learning processes of the three arts together.

Meeting and knowing: writing

The poet began work after the children had been told their story. Her first priority was to consolidate it and work it into lyrics and a narrative line which could carry them. Her approaches were as follows:

- Establish that children know the story.
- Analyse characters and their relationships.
- Establish a narrative chart in the shape of a tree with the time-sequence growing from root to top with poems attached as 'blossoms'. This was useful, as the project developed, to see where there were gaps in the developing oratorio scripts.
- Write and redraft poems individually and in groups about favourite parts of the story.
- Introduce the idea of writing to tell the story, reflect on vivid parts of it and set it to music.
- Commission various groups and individuals to do the work, collate it, then build a script.
- Make a first draft of the whole work, edit and allocate parts.

Meeting and knowing: music

The musician's first priority was to get the children to compose tone poems and to teach them how to set the poems to music. Her initial approaches were as follows:

- Locate musical resources and discover the special musical abilities the children had.
- Discuss the musical aims – the oratorio form – and demystify the composition process.

- Establish the fundamentals of music – sound and rhythm – through workshops.
- Explore responses to story situations in music – sound effects, tone poem/film score.
- Work on individual poems, based on the metre of each line of the poem, after demonstration lessons, and establish a process for composition as follows:
  (a) clap the rhythms in the lines;
  (b) sing the lines on one pitch;
  (c) attempt to sing tunes to them;
  (d) explore possible tunes on the glockenspiel.
- Musician to write the tunes produced.
- Discuss the elements of music: rhythm, melody, timbre.
- Add instrumental accompaniments to the songs.
- Explore motifs for characters, using the rhythms in the names.
- Assemble a musical score in collaboration with the poet's script.
- Rehearse and perform.

Transforming: Building the oratorios

Four oratorios were created, which accorded with many of the traditions of the oratorio form, although the children spoke rather than sang the stories. Their songs were reserved for heightened emotional moments, like arias. Another departure from oratorio was that the children found it difficult to convey the drama of their stories without enacting parts using their bodies. The performances were, therefore, hybrids of oratorio, musical and storytelling

No child had composed a song. It was a challenge because the poems had firstly to emerge from stories before becoming songs, entailing two changes of form. Consequently, the poet and the musician had initial problems. Some children were happy writing poems, but found it difficult to set them. Others were far more comfortable exploring the poems of others on the glockenspiel than writing their own. So the work was divided according to interest.

Composition in any medium can be laborious, but it can also seem to happen by magic. One child, working on the story of Pwyll, imagined what it must have been like when her husband (who, through magic, was someone else in disguise) didn't kiss her any more. She wrote, 'I wondered if my hair had lost its shine', but she only had one line and went to the poet with it. The poet gave the line strong praise and asked her to think of other examples. This was a crucial intervention, which affirmed the initial idea and provided further challenge. The child built the line into an ideal song lyric and by so doing transformed this part of the story for herself:

> I wondered if my hair had lost its shine.
> I wondered if I'd got all crinkly lines.

> I wondered if I'd lost my sense of touch.
> I wondered if my voice was shrill and rough.
> I wondered if my eyes had lost their glow.
> I wondered if my body was too slow.
> I wondered if Arawn no longer loved me.
> I wondered, could he see the real me.

The process of turning this poem into a song also happened as if by magic. As the children tapped out the rhythm on various notes, one tune soon emerged as the right one but it took the musician's affirmation of this before the children felt it was right. She also wrote out the notes, giving formality to the tune and making it available to other instrumentalists and the singer. Eventually, it was sung as a solo by the child playing Rhiannon in 'Pwyll Lord of Dyfed', accompanied on violin and recorder.

There is a half-way house between unsung poem and song. I am reminded of my days in the choir in a High Anglican church when the rector 'gave' the congregation the Nunc Dimittis in a half-spoken, half-sung monotone because he was a dreadful singer! There is a species of poem/song, which is almost the equivalent of the sort of singing in an opera that leads into a full song: the recitative. Another name for this is 'chant'.

Several 'songs' in this project were of this basic kind, the most obvious of which came from a poem about the digression story in the Pwyll myth about Gwawl being transformed into a badger, which is then bagged and beaten:

> I am a badger in a bag
> kicking, cracking and crying.
> I am badger in a bag
> yelping, people are laughing.
> I am a badger in a bag
> battered, bruised and bleeding.
> I am a badger in a bag
> mouth watering because of food.
> I am a badger in a bag
> being crushed and pushed.
> I am a badger in a bag.
> I am a badger in a bag.
> I am a badger in a bag.
> I am a badger in a bag.

The formula for this chant is simple but effective. The incident it embodies is violent and the chant form is exactly right. In performance, as a choral piece for the whole class, it was stunning: loud, staccato and rising to a tumult.

These examples show the process of poems arising out of incidents. Other songs came through the poet's focus on characters. This led to some fascinating innovations towards the oratorio form. The work on characters in 'Manawydan', for instance, led to collaboration between two children. One had written about Manawydan through the eyes of his lover, Rhiannon, the other about Rhiannon through Manawydan's eyes, which led to a delightful duet accompanied on glockenspiel and percussion. The words of the song were intended as thoughts:

MANAWYDAN:	Rhiannon is so beautiful like a mystic unicorn.
RHIANNON:	Manawydan is clever, crafty as a fox.
MANAWYDAN:	Rhiannon is intelligent; she could rule the world.
RHIANNON	Manawydan's a cautious man but he's still very quick.
MANAWYDAN:	Rhiannon's strawberry blonde hair glistens, glimmers in the sun.
RHIANNON:	Manawydan tall and dark is the perfect match for me.
MANAWYDAN:	Rhiannon is a very loving woman I wish that she could love me.
RHIANNON:	Manawydan seems a kindly man I think I'll let him marry me.

These words were sung from two different places on the stage to denote the separation of the characters, a device used in a duet on a different theme from the story of 'Branwen'. Branwen is imprisoned in Ireland at the behest of her husband and thinks of her brother across the sea. She trains a starling, puts a message on its wing and sends it to him. Her brother, Bran, receives the message. The duet begins with their thoughts about each other:

BRANWEN:	I wonder how my brother is. Is he still the king?
BRAN:	I wonder how my sister is. The mightiest ever queen.
BRANWEN:	My strongest brother is far away in my old homeland.
BRAN:	How I miss my lovely sister – white crow proud and grand.
BRANWEN:	I hope he comes to save me from this gloomy prison.
BRAN:	She'll be sitting on her throne clotted in jewels that glisten.
BRANWEN:	He could be feasting in a tent with pleasure and with joy.
BRAN:	She could have had a darling child, could even be a boy.

Each singer then sings an aria, beginning with Branwen's:

> Starling comes to me each day,
> flies into my hand,
> nudges its head against my arm
> and twitters in my ear.
> I try to teach it how to speak,
> it sings in tune for me.
> Tie a message to its foot
> to Bendigeid from me.

Bran, having received the letter via the starling, sings his aria:

I've just received a message from a starling,
told me that from Branwen came bad news.
Don't believe it. Won't believe it
and anyway – How can a starling speak?

I open up the letter,
crush the paper in my fist,
fell to dust.

In terms of oratorio the duet and the arias were very successful: a simple musicality which supported the lines in the poems, conveying feeling with subtlety and force. Bran's aria shows great verbal skill in the way rhythms are varied to suit feelings. The Branwen sequence of seven songs is an impressive body of work composed by children who had never composed before.

The composition of the narrative script and the integration of the songs within it was a major undertaking. Groups of children wrote the narrative, but each group operated differently – some had specialists, others collaborated – and the scripts were uneven in length. The poet had to edit many times, but this led to four tight, dramatic narrative scripts. The songs had to be integrated so that there would be a fair spread, a problem because some songs, such as the Branwen sequence, were so strong they had to be included. Much time was spent trying different fits. This extract from 'Math' demonstrates how song was integrated with narrative:

STORYTELLERS: Pryderi was so pleased [*with Gwydion and Gilfaethwy, who were in disguise as storytellers*] he asked how he could reward them. Arawn, the king of the underworld, had just given Pryderi some new animals called pigs and it was these that Gwydion asked for. But Pryderi, although he wished to please his guests, had promised that he would not let the pigs go until they had doubled in number. In the dead of night, Gwydion took a toadstool and slowly and silently began to weave a magic spell. As the spell grew and grew twelve horses appeared with golden saddles and bridles, then came twelve hounds with golden collars and twelve shining shields, beautiful things glittering in the moonlight.

SINGER: Waking up at midnight
I got out my magical wand
and with all my might
and a shining bright light
myself Pryderi conned.

I charmed twelve horses,
hounds and shields
all sparkling like

corn-fested fields.
Pryderi says, 'Let me have these,
you have the pigs
with disgusting fleas.'

Now back up north I go
through the forest
by the midnight glow.

Songs heighten the emotional importance of an incident or reinforce the qualities of a character. In this example the incident was given colour as the various light-sounding instruments such as glockenspiels, chime bars and high notes of keyboard introduced and accompanied the song with its rich-sounding words. The songs dwelt on things, drawing the audience's special attention to them. But the division between narrative and song was seamless at its best. The overall effect was of the story being taken to a higher level of significance by the lift received from tunes and sounds and characters singing instead of speaking.

Publishing

One of the chief aims was for the oratorios to be performed, and it was essential that they be fully rehearsed so that everything was as near perfect as possible. Eventually, therefore, four oratorios emerged and were publicly performed on two occasions to large audiences.

About 350 people attended these performances, and the atmosphere was particularly exciting and dramatic at the local theatre with the full benefit of professionally prepared lights and sound system. We felt that the children performed impressively and that the works were powerful in terms of storytelling, songs and tone poems. These were evenings of vivid colour, splendid diction, compelling storytelling and sweet songs.[2]

Project: *Gulliver's Travels*

The project

- For children in Years 5 (Term 1) and 6 (Term 1) in primary schools and Years 7 and 8 in secondary schools.
- To be used as part of a focus on classic fiction.
- To demonstrate how form affects meaning.
- To show how a text from more than 250 years ago can still be significant.
- To explore the link between a text and its culture and times.
- To develop skills and knowledge in literacy, art and drama.

The text

Jonathan Swift's satire *Gulliver's Travels* is a key work of English literature. Although written as a political satire, the simplicity of its story, the clarity of its prose and the universal appeal of its theme have made it important not only for adults but also for children.

Swift's prose style, which he aimed to make simple enough for ordinary people to read, is quite accessible to the whole age range suggested above (i.e. nine to thirteen years). I recommend that teachers make their own cuts according to their knowledge of their children and the aims and objectives they have for the project. Parts I and II are suitable for all four year groups, but Parts III and IV are more suited to Year 7 and Year 8 children.

In order to assist in the making of choices I now provide a synopsis of the story in each of the four parts of the work. Each synopsis is followed by an extract of Swift's text. Although some of the activities are based on each part as a whole, more detailed activities are based on the extracts.[3]

The text: Part I, 'A Voyage to Lilliput'

1. Synopsis

Gulliver is shipwrecked on an uncharted island and recovers consciousness to find that he has been tied down with a network of fine cords. There is a six-inch-high man-like creature standing on his chest, and from the high-pitched voices around he guesses that there must be many more nearby. He tries to escape, pulling up the cords one by one, but is stung by a warning volley of arrows and has to stop. Gulliver is taken to the capital city, where he learns the people's language. The name of the island is Lilliput and their name for him is Quinbus Flestrin or Man Mountain.

The Lilliputians are amazed by the things Gulliver has in his pockets, especially his pocket watch. Gulliver does his best to behave gently and win their trust, and they bring him food. In time they allow him a great deal of freedom. He is, however, a great drain on their resources, eating as much as 1,724 Lilliputians. In return for his keep he agrees to help Lilliput in its war against the neighbouring island of Blefescu.

The strait dividing the islands is shallow, so he wades across, captures the entire enemy fleet and brings it back to Lilliput. Having seen the effectiveness of Gulliver as an ally, this is not enough for the Lilliputian emperor. He wants Gulliver to defeat and conquer Blefescu. Gulliver refuses and loses popularity. When he puts out a fire in the royal palace by urinating on it this only increases his unpopularity with the emperor. Distrusting Gulliver's loyalty and tired of his presence the emperor plans to have him blinded by arrows. Gulliver escapes to Blefescu, where a normal-sized ship's boat has drifted ashore. He leaves both islands to be rescued and brought home by an English ship.

2. Extract from pages 64 to 65.
Gulliver, his leg fastened to a stake by a long chain, receives a visit from the Emperor.

The Emperor was already descended from the tower, and advancing on horseback towards me, which had like to cost him dear; for the beast, although very well trained, yet wholly unused to such a sight, which appeared as if a mountain moved before him, reared up on his hinder feet: but that prince, who is an excellent horseman, kept his seat, till his attendants ran in, and held the bridle, while his Majesty had time to dismount. When he alighted, he surveyed me round with great admiration, but kept beyond the length of my chain. He ordered his cooks and butlers, who were already prepared, to give me victuals and drink, which they pushed forward in a sort of vehicles upon wheels till I could reach them.

He is taller by almost the breadth of my nail, than any of his Court, which alone is enough to strike awe into the beholders. His features are strong and masculine, with an Austrian lip and arched nose, his complexion olive, his countenance erect, his body and limbs well proportioned, all his motions graceful, and his deportment majestic. He was then past his prime, being twenty-eight years and three quarters old, of which he had reigned about seven, in great felicity, and generally victorious.

His dress was very plain and simple, the fashion of it between the Asiatic and the European; but he had on his head a helmet of gold, adorned with jewels, and a plume on the crest. He held his sword drawn in his hand, to defend himself, if I should happen to break loose; it was almost three inches long, the hilt and scabbard were gold enriched with diamonds. His voice was shrill, but very clear and articulate, and I could distinctly hear it when I stood up.

The text: Part II, 'A Voyage to Brobdingnag'

1. Synopsis

During his next voyage Gulliver is stranded on an unknown island. He strikes inland and finds himself in a field of corn some forty feet high. It is being harvested by giants as tall as church steeples and he is afraid that they will accidentally tread on him. He manages to attract their attention, is picked up by one of them and taken to the farmer's house. The farmer's nine-year-old daughter, who is forty feet tall, looks after him as kindly as she can and he begins to learn the language of the giants. He calls her Glumdalclitch or little nurse. The country is called Brobdingnag.

In this giant world he loses independence and dignity. He also witnesses many everyday events, such as people going to the toilet, which disgust him. The farmer sees an opportunity for personal gain and exhibits Gulliver as a freak. Soon the king hears about Gulliver and sends for him. At court he is made a great pet.

Gulliver continues to be amazed and often distressed by what he sees. Although they may seem as attractive to each other as ordinary human beings are, to his eyes the Brobdingnagians are often physically disgusting, for instance the pores of their skin are like great pits and their nostrils huge caverns. More disturbing is the fact that he can never feel safe for ordinary creatures such as bees are monsters compared to him.

The king, in turn, is surprised and repelled by what Gulliver tells him about the government and customs of Europe. He is appalled, for instance, when Gulliver offers to teach him how to make gunpowder so that he can kill his enemies.

Gulliver leaves Brobdingnag when a giant bird seizes the box in which he is carried and drops it in the sea. He is rescued and taken home to England.

2. Extract: The opening paragraph of Chapter 2, pages 133 to 134
Gulliver, brought home from the fields by a giant farmer, is given to his daughter to look after.

My mistress had a daughter of nine years old, a child of forward parts for her age, very dexterous at her needle, and skilful in dressing her baby. Her mother and she contrived to fit up the baby's cradle for me against night: the cradle was put into a small drawer of a cabinet, and the drawer placed upon a hanging shelf for fear of the rats. This was my bed all the time I stayed with those people, though made more convenient by degrees, as I began to learn their language, and make my wants known. This young girl was so handy, that after I had once or twice pulled off my clothes before her, she was able to dress and undress me, although I never gave her that trouble when she would let me do either myself. She made me seven shirts, and some other linen, of as fine cloth as could be got, which indeed was coarser than sackcloth; and these she constantly washed for me with her own hands. She was likewise my school-mistress to teach me the language: when I pointed to anything, she told me the name of it in her own tongue, so that in a few days I was able to call for whatever I had a mind to. She was very good-natured, and not above forty foot high, being little for her age. She gave me the name *Grildrig*, which the family took up, and afterwards the whole kingdom. The word imports what the Latins call *naunculus*, the Italians *homunceletino*, and the English *manikin*. To her I chiefly owe my preservation in that country: we never parted while I was there; I called her *Glumdalclitch*, or 'little nurse': and I should be guilty of great ingratitude if I omitted this honourable mention of her care and affection towards me, which I heartily wish it lay in my power to requite as she deserves, instead of being the innocent but unhappy instrument of her disgrace, as I have too much reason to fear.

Teaching and learning processes for Parts I and II

Meeting and knowing: Background information
Tell the children that:

- *Gulliver's Travels* was written in the early eighteenth century when explorers were still discovering new lands in the world. Travel stories were very popular, and most of these were true, sometimes in the form of journals or log books.
- Jonathan Swift set out to write a book which would attack the things he thought were wrong with people in the early eighteenth century. His way of attacking was through making fun of them, making them seem ridiculous. He did this sometimes by making up characters, who were like them, but exaggerated. For instance, the Emperor of Lilliput is a version of King George I. This is called 'satire' and was very popular in the eighteenth century.
- He wanted the book to seem like a true account of sea voyages and to be easy to read, so the style is plain and clear.

Meeting and Knowing: Reading, speaking and listening
1. Establish small groups for storytelling, reading passages and discussion.
2. After each of your readings ask these groups to consolidate the plot by briefly retelling the story to each other.
3. Groups to read the opening paragraph of Part I and discuss
   - the impression it creates about the kind of story that is to unfold (i.e. it is the stuff of a real autobiography);
   - whether it provides any hints as to the amazing things Lemuel Gulliver will experience.
4. Groups to read the opening paragraph of Part II and compare:
   - Does it still appear to be a true autobiography?
   - Does it provide any hints as to what will happen?
   - When amazing things do happen what effect does the plain and simple style have? (i.e. does it make these things even more amazing because they appear to be true?)
5. Groups to read the passages about the Emperor of Lilliput, then:
   - Discuss what his chief characteristics are, underlining the giveaway lines that show this.
   - Track him throughout the remainder of Part I and assess how his character is developing (i.e. he reveals himself as a tyrant after Gulliver takes the Blefuscan navy)
6. Groups to track the development of other characters as follows:
   - one more Lilliputian character;
   - Glumdalclitch, after reading and discussing the passage from Chapter 2 in Part II;
   - one more Brobdingnagian character.

7. Groups to discuss and find examples of the way Swift makes them form their opinions of the characters, through
   - Gulliver's description of them;
   - what they say;
   - their relationships with other characters.
8. At the end of Chapter 5, Part I, groups to work out how the story of Gulliver's voyage to Lilliput will end.
9. At the end of Chapter 7, Part II, groups to work out how Gulliver will leave Brobdingnag.

Transforming: Writing
1. Children to:
   - Establish character journals for the Emperor of Lilliput, another Lilliputian, Glumdalclitch and another Brobdingnagian.
   - After each chapter make a brief entry about Gulliver's description of the character, what the character said and did and how he or she treated other characters.
   - At the end of each part write an evaluation of a character based on the journal entries.
   - Write a plot summary for one chapter of each part, based on the storytelling session.
   - Draw a line graph to show the most dramatic and least dramatic moments in either the 'Voyage to Lilliput' or the 'Voyage to Brobdingnag'.
   - At the end of Chapter 5, Part I, write an ending for Gulliver's voyage to Lilliput.
   - At the end of Chapter 7, Part II, write an ending for Gulliver's voyage to Brobdingnag.
2. Ask the children to imagine they are one of the Lilliputians who examines the contents of Lemuel Gulliver's pockets and to write that part of the story in the words spoken by that character to his wife (who has never even heard of Gulliver) over dinner that evening.
3. Ask them to imagine they are a character who attends a fair in a Brobdingnagian town and write the entry in that character's diary.

Transforming: Art
1. Using sketchbooks and copying details, children to:
   - Investigate eighteenth-century clothing and costumes, looking for the main fashions of the times for the aristocracy, the middle classes and the working classes.
   - Explore the etchings, engravings and paintings of William Hogarth for images of eighteenth-century people.

- Research eighteenth-century seafaring, mariners, ships and discoveries.
- Draw and paint Gulliver in any scene with Lilliputians and with Brobdingnagians to show their comparative sizes.

2. Children to make any Lilliputian and Brobdingnagian tool or utensil to show their sizes compared with ours (e.g. the Lilliputian emperor's sword, which is 3 inches long, or a Brobdingnagian cup suitable for the mouth of a person as tall as a steeple). If successful, whole class to make a collection of such objects, for instance a set of crockery for the farmer's kitchen.

3. If the sessions in drama require it, children to make properties for the plays.

Transforming: Drama

1. Using pairs and group work explore the concept of bigness and smallness in Lilliput and Brobdingnag.

2. Pairs to imagine and improvise scenes:
   - The first Lilliputians to discover Gulliver lying asleep on the beach.
   - Sent to search, make an inventory of and confiscate the contents of Gulliver's pockets.
   - Clear away Gulliver's mess!
   - The Brobdingnagian farm workers who discover Gulliver lying asleep in the corn.
   - The farmer and his wife, looking at and feeding Gulliver at supper time.
   - Glumdalclitch protecting Gulliver from a rat or a wasp.

3. Groups to build plays through improvisation on the following themes:
   - Discovering and tying down Gulliver, then releasing him.
   - Scholars teaching Gulliver the Lilliputian language.
   - Blefuscans trying to stop Gulliver taking their fleet.
   - The farmer, accompanied by Glumdalclitch, exhibiting Gulliver at a Brobdingnagian fair.
   - Gulliver being taken to see the King.

The text: Part III, 'A Voyage to Laputa, Balnibarbi, Glubbdubbdrib, Luggnagg and Japan'

1. Synopsis

On another voyage, to the Far East, Gulliver is set adrift by pirates and comes to land on a rocky coast, which seems uninhabited. Suddenly it becomes dark and cold because the sun is obscured by an island floating overhead. He watches it moving upwards and downwards and from side to side and sees that people are on it. They let down a chain and he is pulled up onto the flying island, Laputa.

Gulliver is made welcome and shown round. In the vast astronomer's cave he sees the great magnet which provides the force to keep the island in the air and with which it can be steered and controlled.

Laputa houses the court of the King of Balnibarbi, the land below. When the people down there rebel Laputa hovers over them, cutting off light and rain and, in extreme circumstances, threatening to crush them. The inhabitants of Laputa are so distracted by their own speculations that they are hardly aware of everyday events. They require servants, called Flappers, who tap them on the ear if someone wishes to speak to them and on the mouth when it is time to reply.

Later, Gulliver is allowed to visit the capital city, Lagado, which is on the island of Balnibarbi. Here he sees an extraordinary academy where researchers are involved in many bizarre schemes, for instance how to extract sunshine out of cucumbers.

Gulliver leaves this strange country and travels by way of several neighbouring islands, which are similarly unusual. In Luggnagg, for instance, he meets the Struldbruggs who are immortal. This does not make them happy for they are too old to enjoy life and most of them would like to die. Gulliver returns home on a Dutch ship.

2. Extract: Opening of Chapter 2, pages 200 to 201
Gulliver is lifted from the island of Balnibarbi by a ladder up to the island of Laputa.

At my alighting I was surrounded by a crowd of people, but those who stood nearest seemed to be of better quality. They beheld me with all the marks and circumstances of wonder, neither indeed was I much in their debt, having never till then seen a race of mortals so singular in their shapes, habits, and countenances. Their heads were all reclined either to the right, or to the left; one of their eyes turned inward, and the other directly up to the zenith. Their outward garments were adorned with the figures of suns, moons and stars, interwoven with those of fiddles, flutes, harps, trumpets, guitars, harpsichords, and many more instruments of music, unknown to us in Europe. I observed here and there many in the habit of servants, with a blown bladder fastened like a flail to the end of a short stick, which they carried in their hands. In each bladder was a small quantity of dried pease or little pebbles (as I was afterwards informed). With these bladders they now and then flapped the mouths and ears of those who stood near them, of which practice I could not then conceive the meaning; it seems, the minds of these people are so taken up with intense speculations, that they can neither speak, nor attend to the discourses of others, without being roused by some external taction upon the organs of speech and hearing; for which reason, those persons who are able to afford it always keep a *flapper* (the original is climenole) in their family, as one of their domestics, nor ever walk abroad or make visits without him. And the business of this officer is, when two or more persons are in company, gently to strike with his bladder the mouth of him who is to speak, and the right ear of him or them to whom the speaker addresseth himself. This flapper is likewise employed diligently to attend his master in his walks, and upon occasion to give him a soft flap on his eyes, because he is always so wrapped up in cogitation, that he is in manifest danger of falling down every precipice, and bouncing his head against every post, and in the streets, of jostling others or being jostled himself into the kennel.

The text: Part IV, 'A voyage to the country of the Houyhnhms'

1. Synopsis

On his final voyage there is mutiny on the boat on which Gulliver is captain, and once again he is set down on a strange island. It is cultivated and well cared for and he sets out to find the people who live there. In a field he comes across hideous humanlike creatures which attack him, but the creatures run away as soon as they see a horse approaching. Gulliver tries to stroke the horse but is reproved by the horse gently pushing away his hand and shaking its head. A second horse approaches and they seem to converse.

They lead Gulliver to a house where he meets the horse's family: a mare, a colt and a foal. They live as a human family would, while outside in the stables several of the humanlike creatures are tethered. Gulliver learns the language of the horses, or Houyhnhms. The humanlike creatures are Yahoos, which are savage, unintelligent beasts. They are fit only for menial tasks and are completely untrustworthy and do not even deserve any affection.

Gulliver begins to be ashamed of being human because the Yahoos look like humans, even though they are deformed. He tries never to be seen with his clothes off because that would make the likeness more obvious. The Houyhnhms think his clothes are part of his body until they discover him unclothed. They then treat him as if he is a well-developed Yahoo.

Gulliver is increasingly impressed by Houyhnhm society. They are extremely civilised and don't do anything without careful thought and good judgement. Gulliver also gets increasingly disgusted with the Yahoos, especially when one of the females shows interest in him.

Eventually, the Houyhnhms require Gulliver to leave their island, and when he is told he almost faints with unhappiness. They give him time to build a canoe, and as he sails away they call, 'Farewell, gentle Yahoo', which upsets him even further.

When he returns to England this time he cannot bear human company. He buys two horses and spends as much time as possible with them. He never goes to sea again.

2. Extract from Chapter 1, 'Gulliver meets a Houyhnhm', pages 270 to 271
Gulliver is besieged by a herd of Yahoos with his back to a tree trunk.

In the midst of this distress, I observed them all to run away on a sudden as fast as they could, at which I ventured to leave the tree, and pursue the road, wondering what it was that could put them into fright. But looking on my left hand, I saw a horse walking softly in the field, which my persecutors having sooner discovered, was the cause of their flight. The horse started a little when he came near me, but soon recovering himself, looked full in my face with manifest tokens of wonder: he viewed my hands and feet, walking round me several times. I would have pursued my journey, but he placed himself directly in the way, yet looking with a very mild aspect, never offering the least violence. We stood gazing at each other for some time; at last I took the boldness to reach my hand towards his neck, with a design to stroke it, using the common style and whistle of jockeys when they are going to handle a strange horse. But this animal, seeming to receive my civilities with disdain, shook his head, and bent his brows, softly raising up his left forefoot to remove my hand. Then he neighed three or four times, but in so different a cadence, that I almost began to think he was speaking to himself in some language of his own.

Additional teaching and learning processes for Parts III and IV

Meeting and knowing: Reading, speaking and listening
1. Groups to:
   - Compare the voyages that Gulliver has made and decide which they prefer and why.
   - Decide whether or not Gulliver's point of view during his voyages is the same as Swift's.
   - Speculate what opinion the following characters would have of Gulliver: the Emperor and Skyresh Bolgolam in Lilliput, Glumdalclitch and the King in Brobdingnag, a Laputan, the Houyhnhm host and a Yahoo.
2. Using the notes at the back of the book, investigate the background to the stories:
   - Which individuals or types of people are being criticised (e.g. Flimnap in Part I is Sir Robert Walpole, a government minister)?
   - The historical events parodied.

Transforming: Writing
1. Establish writing groups of about five or six children and ask them to make plays for voices out of suitable chapters as follows:
   - List the characters.
   - Decide the most important happenings and cut the rest.

- Use the words in the text for each character, cutting them if too long and making up words if there are none.
- Use the traditional format with the character's name in capital letters on the left and his/her words next to it and descriptions of what happens in italic.
- Create sound effects as appropriate.

2. Invite the children to make a new part or chapter for *Gulliver's Travels* which reflects the way Swift writes (i.e. as if it is an autobiography and in plain, clear language).
   - Make this a large-scale project with plenty of time allowed.
   - Children to plan the project, creating their own island and describing what is special about the inhabitants and how they react to Gulliver.

Transforming: Art

1. Using the material gathered during investigations into eighteenth-century clothing, costume, seafaring and art, children to draw
   - a Laputan with his flapper;
   - an experiment in the Academy at Lagado and a diagram of one of the machines;
   - a Struldbrugg or immortal old man;
   - Gulliver with the Yahoos;
   - Gulliver with the Houyhnhms.
2. Children to develop one of their drawings into a painting.
3. Children to invent a ridiculous experiment then make the diagram for a machine to carry it out.

Transforming: Drama

1. Pairs to imagine and improvise scenes in which they are:
   - Laputans with their flappers;
   - Experimenters in the Academy at Lagado;
   - A Strulbrugg meeting Gulliver;
   - A Yahoo harrassing Gulliver;
   - A Houyhnhm barring his way.
2. Groups to make plays in on the following themes:
   - Gulliver is lifted onto Laputa and meets the Laputans.
   - He visits the Academy.
   - Houyhnhms compare Gulliver to a Yahoo.
   - Gulliver visits a new island, which the children invent themselves.

Publishing

1. Make a new book of *Gulliver's Travels* which contains the children's own stories.
2. Display written work alongside drawings and paintings.

3. Make a gallery in the school to exhibit paintings and artefacts.
4. Record the plays for voices and make them available for others to listen to.
5. Perform the plays to others.
6. Make the improvised plays into scripts collected in a file.

References

1. Jones, G. and Jones, T. (1949) *The Mabinogion.* London: Dent.
2. Carter, D. (1995) *The Four Branches Project.* Mold: Clwyd Poetry Project.
3. Swift, J. (1967), *Gulliver's Travels.* Harmondsworth: Penguin Books.

CHAPTER 7

Lyric poetry

Introduction

A project is described in which Year 5 and 6 children in two primary schools celebrated the centenary of the death of Gerard Manley Hopkins. This ambitious project led to written work, which was in the best sense imitative. In one school it also stimulated exciting responses in art and dance.

This is followed by a project for each of Years 4, 5, 6, 7 and 8 as follows:

- Year 4, writing and art on John Clare's 'Autumn'.
- Year 5, writing and music on Wordsworth's 'I wandered lonely as a cloud'.
- Year 6, history, drama and dance on Hardy's 'Roman Road' and Kipling's 'The way through the woods'.
- Year 7, writing, art, dance and music on Blake's 'The Tyger'.
- Year 8, history, writing and music on Marvell's 'Bermudas'.

Case study: Gerard Manley Hopkins

The project

Year 5 and Year 6 children in two schools engaged with poems by Hopkins as part of Clwyd's centenary celebration of Hopkins's death.[1] The teaching and learning processes developed by two teachers with different approaches are compared and contrasted:

1. Teacher A focused on 'Spring' and 'Pied beauty', and her work led entirely to written outputs from the children.
2. Teacher B focused solely on 'Inversnaid', but her work was much wider in scope. She used the poem to provide a different dimension to the river theme in geography and followed a multidisciplinary arts approach to the poem.

The texts

1. Teacher A used 'Spring' and 'Pied Beauty'

Spring

Nothing is so beautiful as spring –
When weeds, in wheels, shoot long and lovely and lush;
Thrush's eggs look little low heavens, and thrush
Through the echoing timber does so rinse and wring
The ear, it strikes like lightnings to hear him sing;
The glassy peartree leaves and blooms, they brush
The descending blue; that blue is all in a rush
With richness; the racing lambs too have fair their fling.

What is all this juice and all this joy?
A strain of the earth's sweet being in the beginning
In Eden garden. – Have, get, before it cloy,
Before it cloud, Christ, lord, and sour with sinning,
Innocent mind and Mayday in girl and boy,
Most, O maid's child, thy choice and worthy the winning.

Pied beauty

Glory be to God for dappled things
– For skies of couple-colour as a brinded cow;
For rose-moles all in stipple upon trout that swim;
Fresh-firecoal chestnut-falls; finches' wings;
Landscape plotted and pieced – fold, fallow, and plough;
And all trades, their gear and tackle and trim.

All things counter, original, spare, strange;
Whatever is fickle, freckled (who knows how?)
With swift, slow; sweet, sour; adazzle, dim;
He fathers-forth whose beauty is past change:
Praise Him.

2. *Teacher B used 'Inversnaid'*

Inversnaid

This darksome burn, horseback brown,
His rollrock highroad roaring down,
In coop and in comb the fleece of his foam
Flutes and low to the lake falls home.

A windpuff-bonnet of fawn-froth
Turns and twindles over the broth

Of a pool so pitchblack, fell-frowning,
It rounds and rounds Despair to drowning.

Degged with dew, dappled with dew
Are the groins of the braes that the brook treads through,
Wiry heathpacks, flitches of fern,
And the beadbonny ash that sits over the burn.

What would the world be, once bereft
Of wet and of wildness? Let them be left,
O let them be left, wildness and wet;
Long live the weeds and the wilderness yet.

Teaching and learning processes

Meeting and knowing

The text was central to the work of both teachers and was at the front of the children's minds because they learnt their poems by heart.

1. Teacher A did not begin with the poems. She took the children on a walk in local lanes one sunny afternoon in May to find signs of spring through their senses. The children were also invited to play games in and around the bushes and invent stories to go with them. There was much innovation with words and ideas arising simply out of this playing which made it an important starting point. The children were asked to keep their ideas in their memories or notebooks.

   Back at school, they talked about what they had seen, heard and touched and the games they played. A plenary followed and the session finished with the children writing about their favourite things of the afternoon. She read 'Spring' to them and they discussed what was important in spring to Hopkins. She asked questions such as 'Have you experienced that?' Discussions ranged over words, phrases, rhymes, vision and feelings in the poem. Next the groups concentrated on sections of the poem and worked out the meanings.

   After reading and talking about the poems, including a digression on tongue-twisters as a way of understanding the compounding of words, the children wrote poems. The 'favourite things' writing was the source material for this. The teacher talked about what Hopkins did with his experiences and how they could do something interesting with theirs.

   At the redrafting phase thesauruses were introduced and the children were invited to try and use rhyme and rhythm in their work. This redrafting produced a new range of original phrases and notions such as one child's 'corn-ranks' and another's 'the blurr of fur as dog chases cat'. One child acquired a tape of a thrush's song to accompany the reading of his poem.

Before half-term the class experienced 'Pied beauty' in a similar way and were invited to look for shapes, patterns and colours in the natural world with a view to more writing after the holiday. Each child compiled a personal list of 'dappled' and 'stippled' words. On returning to school the teacher got the children to look at pictures of natural objects for patterns prior to the writing.

2. Teacher B began her work by reading 'Inversnaid' to the children
   - In pairs, groups or as individuals the children were to 'work the poem out'.
   - The children recited the poem. At the end of this they knew the poem by heart and were relishing its rhythms and ideas.
   - They were invited to choose any phrase or idea in the poem and interpret it visually in two or three dimensions, individually or in small groups. As a result of the prolonged exposure to the poem through oral work their ideas were fertile.
   - They were asked to choose suitable musical instruments and attempt to represent the river musically as it moved from source to estuary. This also prepared them for a trip to the River Conwy at the end of the project.
   - Three dance sessions led to one large group working out a dance for performance in a sharing event at the end of the term. After the trip to the Conwy the children worked on their written notes and many of the poems were also read at the sharing event.

Transforming: Writing (Teacher A)

School A's poems are imitations of Hopkins's models and are remarkable. The children were assured at all stages of a very thorough writing process from the formulation of ideas, first drafts and meticulous redrafting. Each poem is somewhat different yet reveals the influence of Hopkins. Each is quite highly structured, yet strands of personal feeling and response are clear. The redrafting is grafting in which the new is added to the old rather than replacing it. These graftings are found in new words from the thesaurus and quite sophisticated rhyme schemes and patterns of scansion. In most cases these new elements are not obvious, but harmonise with the original conceptions.

The following example, for instance, is an achievement for its rhyme scheme alone. Its a/bb/aa/bb/a is complex and echoes Hopkins's scheme. Line 5 is a bold departure from the scansion, which is mainly derived from its model and emphasises the sheer joy which the child clearly feels about spring.

> Nothing is as busy as Spring
> When birds fill the air with music unfurled
> The sun lights the colours in a brand new world
> And the air itself makes you want to sing
> Spring Spring Spring.
> And all new flowers are slightly curled

All new colours are brilliantly whirled
Into a kaleidoscope land. All this is Spring.

The next poem is not so metrically accomplished, but is perhaps more memorable for the images it paints. The close relationship between egg and song in Hopkins's poem is clearly a strong notion for this child, so she takes it a stage further into the hatching of chick. The metaphorical conception of poor 'Old Winter' defeated and crying among the exploding cow parsley buttons is memorable in that it constructs the personification of a whole season out of an observation she made during the walk.

Nothing is so dazzling as Spring
When the sound of birds ring
and shake in the drums of your ears.
A chick first flutters its fragile wings for flight.
Old Winter breaks out in tears
as cow parsley buttons burst out and appear.
Grass grows long lush and fresh.
Spring at last has arrived.

Every child produced at least one memorable line. A boy with learning problems wrote:

With delight the racing season passes by
Is it not a sign of sinning to let it miss your eye?

There is much delight in the sound of words, a sense of power and control and joy in discovering just what language can do, as in

Wild white horses with racing foals
like blossom over shifting grass.

There is conscious awareness of what can be achieved by taking an idea from a different context, for instance, in the following line. The use of the word 'dating' is appropriate because spring is the time when males and females meet at a time and a place. But its urban, post-war context makes it strange:

Birds singing with a *dating* tune once more.

There is also a sense of cultural continuity being fostered in a very precise way in the following redevelopment of Hopkins's delicious line, 'When weeds in wheels shoot long and lovely and lush':

As dry winding brambles around your legs cling
And claw the weeds creeping over the grassy floor.

The work arising out of 'Pied beauty' writing also demonstrates personal experience being given sharper focus by the Hopkins model, as in the next poem in which the child assembles new examples of the theme:

> Glory be to God for dappled things.
> A small spotted egg blue and black blending in
> with marbled fossils.
> And the sea falls into a whitish wave and
> washes up the shell off a turtle's back.

The children in School A experienced a rigorous and exciting relationship with two of Hopkins's poems, which was related to sensuous experiences in and around their school. As a result they developed all aspects of their literacy, particularly their writing, to a higher plane than before. The poems, being imitations of models, are reconstructions rather than transformations. Transformation, however, occurs in individual lines and images, some of which are discussed above.

Transforming: Writing (Teacher B)

The initial discussions, for which the children were equipped with dictionaries, produced phrases, which are like little poems in their own right. There was no sense of arid paraphrase or comprehension exercise. The children's ideas were creative responses to the lines of the original:

> a lurky stream, dark, muddy, soil coming
> up from the bottom.

Hopkins's lines were sparking the children's imaginations and creating in them a set of moving pictures which progressed out of the line or phrase or word, as in

> Foaming bubbles at the bottom of the waterfall.
> Water weaving and rushing in and out of
> the hollows making it frothy like a sheep's fleece.

Often in these responses Hopkins's unexpected use of a word was the attraction and led to the child using it again. A good example of this is the use of the coined word 'beadbonny'. In the following the child perceived the additional possibility of the poet's image. The words have a life of their own and 'bead' is seen to have another association other than with the berries:

> Berries on the tree waving over the brook,
> a mountain ash growing by the burn,
> the tree bends over the stream with berries like beads
> the dew beads on the branches of the ash tree.

In these discussions no two groups or pairs said similar things. Particular words, phrases or images sparked particular groups. One group, for instance, was interested in the word 'flutes':

> Flute could be making a swirling, fluttering noise
> as all the air comes out of the little flutes
> or grooves in the foam whistling like a flute.

The children's main poetry writing was in response to the River Conwy in its four main stages of development: as a mountain stream/river in 'Inversnaid' form; as a series of waterfalls and rapids; as a slowly meandering river in its plain; and at its estuary. So, whereas the writing in School A was based on imitation and Hopkins's influence plain to see, the writing in School B was based on an actual river and Hopkins's influence more deeply assimilated.

Several poems were transformations, but where are the influences of Hopkins? The teacher said that the poems about the River Conwy would have been different without 'Inversnaid' at the backs of the children's minds, but what can be attributed to the poem's influence, and how are the various threads spun together and transformed?

Images of foam and froth emerged in different ways in most children's work. These derived from the lines 'In coop and in comb the fleece of his foam' and 'A windpuff bonnet of fawn froth'. Many simply describe it, as in 'Through the foam there is a rush of water', but some make their own metaphors as in 'whipped up beer'.

Although these foam – fleece images were the most common, there were others in 'Inversnaid' which found an echo in a number of pieces of writing. The image of 'falling home', for instance, was absorbed to re-emerge, as in 'It sparkles like stars. Then laughs. Its home.'

Hopkins's use of 'wet' as a noun rather than an adjective found a response in one child's poem. Hopkins implies places which are 'wet' in 'Of wet and of wildness'. Part of the children's playing with 'Inversnaid' in dance had been to move like a river and stay still like its rocks. This may have led to the use of the word in

> I now know what a rock feels like in a river,
> Waiting for water to carry me along
> To the next stop of wet.

Many also attempted to make Hopkinsian compounds. These had impressed the children, particularly 'beadbonny', 'Windpuff-bonnet' and 'horseback-brown'. This enjoyment of word play is seen in 'tea-bag brown', 'moss-covered', 'tower-high' and in the impressive 'deepness-made-waves'.

Attempts were made to use the rhythm of the poem, as in

> This black stream, this rocky stream
> Now as black as a bear.

Hopkins's line 'Degged with dew, dappled with dew' is well echoed in

> Lovely and calm, Low and calm.

The final example is a transformation caused, I believe, by the various experiences the child had with the model. Although it reflects the influence of Hopkins, it is the child's own poem with much of the child's own vision in its overall structure:

River Conwy

Moss-covered rocks
Like hills in flood,
Foam and froth, bubbling
Like everlasting snow.
Yesterday's bridge
Short and strong.
Reeds like trees,
Short and thin.

Needles pointing down
Frothwhite boats crushing.
I now know what a rock
Feels like in a river,
Waiting for water
To carry me along
To the next stop of wet.

Still. Still,
Except the windblown pattern.
Small peaks, ridged,
Still running, twist.

Mini islands swept by winds,
Blends of water blown.
A furrow in the sand
Dispatches its water.
Seagull swoops, dives, soars
As the sea ripples.
Throngs of weeds
Watching seas as they go away.
No more bubbling stream
Failing to stop,
Tumbling, falling down.

Transforming: Art

This close focus on the images of the poem was evident in the children's work in art. Hopkins's images were echoed in the ideas the children made for their pictures and models. Although some of these works lacked finish, they revealed that the children were able to enter the poet's world rather than merely operating at 'text level':

- 'Twindles' was the key word for one child, who had been taken by the concept of twisting, going downwards and getting smaller during one of the dance sessions. This is not an easy sort of problem to solve in art, but this child's solution was ingenious. She cut and painted four strips of card, a centimetre wide and about a metre long. On one end of the first strip she stuck a white fan shape. She then fastened a second strip with a butterfly clip onto the first, part way down it, then the third onto the second and the fourth on to the third. All ends, apart from the one with the fan, had strong cotton attached. With her friend she held the two pieces of cotton tightly. They then made spiral shapes and this turned into a form of dance. So this work started with the word 'twindles', led into dance, on into visual art and back into dance.

- Another child was attracted to ideas arising out of 'comb' and made a long painting with points piercing through it from behind. This was not entirely successful in the execution, but admirable in the attempt to pursue an idea.

- The horse ideas were important for a number of children. One had the surreal notion of a horse galloping with a river pouring from its tail. The pouring pattern – in paint – attempts to embody the basic changes in the river's flow as interpreted from the poem.

Transforming: Dance

The three dance sessions explored the progress of the river's movements as demonstrated in the poem's images of movement. One polished dance emerged from this work, which I attempt to describe here. With the teacher as consultant the children choreographed quite an elaborate 'Inversnaid' dance, using Khachaturian's Flute Concerto, second movement (*andante sostenuto*). The dance had six main phrases or passages:

1. Stream bubbling out of moors: from a large circle each dancer sluggishly jerks a part of her body so that the whole effect is bubbly; but this has no strength and recedes, to reassert itself and 'get out'.
2. Trickling down: they stretch high in the circle, arms raised then down and crossed in front of them, one after the other (follow-the-leader style), and this creates an effect of waviness.
3. Twindling and in and out of rocks: every alternate dancer moves centre circle, leaving the others on the circumference; the centre group then makes a star-patterned comb with upward points; the dancers on the circumference then 'whoosh' between each tooth of the 'comb'.
4. Whirling: the dancers divide into two groups making various twisting, twindling, cooping and combing sequences as follows:
    (a) linear pattern going down, rolling over, one after the other, with heads tossing like horses to show off manes, then getting cooped and into comb shapes;

(b) the dancers twist, then two of them come together in the centre, push hands together, across, rejoin, hold; a third joins and they twist and rush underneath each other; then a fourth joins; they repeat, but the fifth is trapped in cooped position and is unable to progress with the others;

(c) this group then makes a big group comb shape and the other group twists in and out of it; whirls round the outside, followed by the comb-shape group and into spiral.

5. Waterfall: this large spiral becomes a waterfall newly located by one dancer falling flat to the ground and others following in low spread shapes, middle-height spread shapes and others just above that.

6. Falling home to the lake: they are back to the circle and are whirling and twisting as if at the bottom of a whirlpool; they are closing and falling to the lake and home, which is a still, flat group shape.

Publishing

1. The children's poems from these two schools and from another three schools involved in the overall project were displayed in one of Clwyd's arts centres alongside paintings, drawings and biographical material on the poet. This exhibition was later transferred to an exhibition at the International Eisteddfod in Llangollen.

2. A recitation of many of the poems was performed during an English course for primary and secondary teachers.

3. The schools also mounted their own in-house exhibitions of work and performed recitations of the poems to the other children in special sharing assemblies.[2]

Project 1: Year 4, 'Autumn' by John Clare

The project

For Year 4 children in Term 1, working on poems based on common themes in the Literacy Framework. The poem is selected for inclusion with others to provide models for the theme of autumn.

The text

Once the meanings of the archaic vocabulary are understood, Clare's 'Autumn' poem provides a simple model of what 'I love' or like about autumn.

Autumn
By John Clare

I love the fitful gust that shakes
The casement all the day,

And from the mossy elm-tree takes
The faded leaf away,
Twirling it by the window pane
With thousand others down the lane.

I love to see the shaking twig
Dance till the shut of eve,
The sparrow on the cottage rig,
Whose chirp would make believe
That spring was just now flirting by
In summer's lap with flowers to lie.

I love to see the cottage smoke
Curl upward through the trees,
The pigeons nestled round the cote
On November days like these;
The cock upon the dunghill crowing,
The mill-sails on the heath a-going.

The feather from the raven's breast
Falls on the stubble lea,
The acorns near the old crow's nest
Fall pattering down the tree;
The grunting pigs, that wait for all,
Scramble and hurry where they fall.[3]

Glossary
fitful – irregular
casement – window
rig – roof
cote – shelter, nesting and roosting place for doves and pigeons
dunghill – heap of animal droppings used for manure
mill-sails – windmill sails
lea – meadow

Teaching and learning processes

Meeting and knowing
1. Before looking at the poem.
   - Children to keep a record of autumn observations.
   - Practise reciting the poem so that you convey its rhythm but not mechanically.
   - Prepare a large version of the poem or one copy for each child.
   - Go through the glossary, ensuring that every child knows what the words mean.

2. Reciting the poem.
   - Children to read the poem silently.
   - Teacher to recite the poem to the class.
   - Divide children into four groups, allocate a verse to each and work on a class recitation of the poem, each group performing their verse.
3. Understanding.
   - Groups to
     (a) discuss what John Clare loves about autumn and to make a list;
     (b) discuss what they notice about the structure of the poem;
     (c) discuss what they notice about the language;
     (d) make notes of the discussion and report to the class.
   - Draw the children's attention to the details with which John Clare develops each idea in his poem as follows:
     (a) Nouns usually have adjectives, for instance 'gust' is '**fitful**'.
     (b) Some nouns have verbs, for instance the 'gust' '**shakes** / The casement'.
     (c) Ideas are developed further, for instance the 'gust shakes / The casement **all the day**'.
   - Groups to find modern poems about autumn, then
     (a) practise reciting them;
     (b) discuss what they mean;
     (c) find comparisons and contrasts with John Clare's 'Autumn';
     (d) share this work with the class.
   - Ask the children how John Clare's poem compares and contrasts with modern poems.

Transforming: Writing
1. Children to
   - Read their notes of autumn observations.
   - Write their own poems about the things they like or love about autumn.
2. Tell them that their poems don't have to rhyme, that it is Clare's way of building an idea that you are interested in.
3. Children to
   - Recite their poems to a partner to test if they sound right and make necessary changes.
   - Decide if they can improve their poems by trimming or extending lines or by using more effective adjectives and verbs.

Transforming: Art
1. Collect drawings, engravings and paintings from the late eighteenth and early nineteenth centuries, depicting country life, for instance work by Bewick, Turner, Constable and Linnell.

2. Using their sketchbooks, children to
    - copy favourite images from this collection;
    - illustrate ideas in the poem;
    - illustrate ideas in their own poems;
    - select their favourite illustrations and make fully developed works.

Publishing

1. Make a class book of autumn, including critical evaluations of Clare's poem, comparisons with modern poems, the children's own poems and illustrations to go with them.
2. Select from this material for a display.
3. Hold recitation sessions, in which the children read the poems they found in anthologies and their own poems.

Project 2: Year 5, 'I wandered lonely as a cloud' by William Wordsworth

The project

For Year 5 children in Term 1, working on poems by significant authors in the Literacy Framework. The poem should be included with other poems about flowers and natural observations both classic and modern.

The text

This is the most well known of Wordsworth's poems and is important not only for its description of the daffodils by the side of a lake but also for its insight into the way Wordsworth composed. He composed after the event, lying on his couch recollecting in tranquillity.

> *I wandered lonely as a cloud*
> By William Wordsworth.
>
> I wandered lonely as a cloud
> That floats on high o'er vales and hills,
> When all at once I saw a crowd,
> A host, of golden daffodils;
> Beside the lake, beneath the trees,
> Fluttering and dancing in the breeze.
>
> Continuous as the stars that shine
> And twinkle on the milky way,
> That stretched in never-ending line

Along the margin of a bay:
Ten thousand saw I at a glance
Tossing their heads in sprightly dance.

The waves beside them danced; but they
Outdid the sparkling waves in glee:
A poet could not but be gay,
In such a jocund company:
I gazed – and gazed – but little thought
What wealth the show to me had brought:

For oft when on my couch I lie
In vacant or in pensive mood,
They flash upon that inward eye
Which is the bliss of solitude;
And then my heart with pleasure fills,
And dances with the daffodils.[4]

Glossary
o'er – over
vales – valleys
host – a large number
sprightly – lively and brisk
glee – triumph and delight
gay – carefree and merry
jocund – merry or cheerful
pensive – thoughtful
bliss – perfect happiness
solitude – being alone

Teaching and learning processes

Meeting and knowing
1. Before looking at the poem.
   - Children to look at late summer/early autumn flowers and to record their observations.
   - Practise reciting the poem so that you convey its rhythm but not mechanically.
   - Prepare a large version of the poem or one copy for each child.
   - Go through the glossary, ensuring that every child knows what the words mean.
2. Reciting the poem.
   - Children to read the poem silently to themselves.
   - Recite the poem to the children.

- Divide them into four groups, allocate a verse to each and work on a class recitation of the poem, each group performing their verse.
- Tell the children about Wordsworth's method of composition (see above). Point out that this method is referred to in the fourth verse.

3. Comprehension
   - Groups to
     (a) discuss what William Wordsworth sees in each of the verses and to make lists;
     (b) discuss what they notice about the structure of the poem;
     (c) discuss what they notice about the language;
     (d) report back to the class.
   - Draw their attention to the way Wordsworth develops his poem.
     (a) The first three verses open with figurative language, verses one and two with similes ('lonely **as** a cloud', 'Continuous **as** the stars') and verse three with a metaphor ('The **waves** beside them **danced**').
     (b) In verses one and two he describes the daffodils in detail, where they are and how they move ('Fluttering', 'dancing', 'Tossing their heads').
     (c) In verses three and four he describes his reaction or response to the daffodils ('I gazed', 'my heart dances with the daffodils').
     (d) The dancing metaphor is extended: the daffodils, the waves and finally the poet dance.
   - Groups to
     (a) find modern poems about flowers, particularly daffodils, in anthologies;
     (b) practise reciting them;
     (c) discuss what they mean and find comparisons with 'I wandered lonely as a cloud';
     (d) decide what are the most distinctive features of the poems;
     (e) decide which they prefer and why;
     (f) share with the class.

Transforming: Writing

1. Children to
   - Read their notes of observations of flowers and recall the experiences, which they record.
   - Write their own poems about flowers.
2. Tell them that their poems don't have to rhyme, that it is Wordsworth's approach to the subject matter that you are interested in.
3. Children to
   - Recite their poems to test if they sound right and to make changes as necessary.
   - Work out if they can improve their poems by imagining the flowers again and finding better similes and metaphors and choosing some better words.

Transforming: Art
Children to paint daffodils and other flowers, attempting to reflect the ideas in the poem.

Transforming: Music
1. Talk to the children about Wordsworth's dancing metaphor and the idea that the daffodils are better at dancing than the waves and that they are such good dancers that the poet dances with them in his imagination.
2. Ask them to discuss the following:
   - If daffodils could make music what might it sound like?
   - Would it be different from wave music?
   - What instruments would play daffodil music and wave music?
   - Would the music sound any different when the poet imagined it later on?
3. Groups to:
   - Choose instruments or objects suitable for making the music of the daffodils and waves.
   - Compose a piece of music in four movements:
     (a) The dance of the daffodils.
     (b) The dance of the waves.
     (c) The daffodil dance mingling with and taking over from the wave dance.
     (d) The daffodil dance inside Wordsworth's imagination.

Publishing
1. Make a class flower book, including critical evaluations of Wordsworth's poem, comparisons with modern poems, the children's own poems and the illustrations.
2. Select from this material for a wall display.
3. Hold recitation sessions, in which the children read poems from anthologies and their own poems.
4. Perform the musical compositions to an audience.

Project 3: Year 6, 'Roman Road' by Thomas Hardy and 'The way through the woods' by Rudyard Kipling

The project

For Year 6 children in Term 3, comparing poems by significant poets based on the Literacy Framework. The main poem, 'Roman Road' by Thomas Hardy is selected for comparison with Rudyard Kipling's 'The way through the woods'. A further use for the main poem is as a focus for work on the Romans in history.

The texts

The Roman Road
By Thomas Hardy

The Roman Road runs straight and bare
As the pale parting-line in hair
Across the heath. And thoughtful men
Contrast its days of Now and Then,
And delve, and measure, and compare;
Visioning on the vacant air
Helmed legionaries, who proudly rear
The Eagle, as they pace again
      The Roman Road.

But no tall brass-helmed legionnaire
Haunts it for me. Uprises there
A mother's form upon my ken,
Guiding my infant steps, as when
We walked that ancient thoroughfare,
      The Roman Road.[5]

The way through the woods
By Rudyard Kipling

They shut the road through the woods
Seventy years ago.
Weather and rain have undone it again,
And now you would never know
There once was a road through the woods
Before they planted the trees.

It is underneath the coppice and heath,
And the thin anemones,
Only the keeper sees
That, where the ring-dove broods,
And the badgers roll at ease,
There once was a road through the woods.

Yet, if you enter the woods
Of a summer evening late,
When the night-air cools on the trout-ringed pools
Where the otter whistles his mate,
(They fear not men in the woods,

Because they see so few).

You will hear the beat of a horse's feet
And the steady swish of a skirt in the dew,
Steadily cantering through the misty solitudes,
And though you perfectly knew
The old lost road through the woods . . .
But there is no road through the woods.[6]

Glossary
delve – dig
visioning – imagining
vacant – empty
helmed – wearing helmets
ken – know
thoroughfare – way through

coppice – group of trees growing close together
cantering – between a trot and a gallop
solitudes – lonelinesses

Teaching and learning processes

Meeting and knowing
1. Before looking at the poem,
   - Ask the children if they know or have ever travelled along old roads, Roman roads or overgrown paths or routes through rough country, and invite them to share anecdotes.
   - If possible, organise an outing to such a place during which the children record their observations, or encourage the children to investigate such places during a weekend.
   - If this poem is being used as part of a history project on the Romans, ask the children to research Roman roads.
   - Practise reciting the poems so that you convey their rhythms, but not mechanically.
   - Prepare large versions of each poem or copy them for each child.
   - Go through the glossary, ensuring that every child knows what the words mean.
2. Reciting the poems.
   - Children to read Thomas Hardy's 'Roman Road' silently.
   - Recite this poem to the class.
   - Divide them into four groups, allocating the first verse to two groups and the second verse to the other two, allowing time for practice.

- Work on two recitations of the poem, each group performing their verse. Discuss the best ways of reciting it.
- Groups to work on a verse each of Rudyard Kipling's poem.
- Organise a recitation session to include both poems.

3. Comprehension
   - Groups to discuss what
     (a) is going 'Across the heath';
     (b) the 'thoughtful men' imagine;
     (c) Thomas Hardy remembers;
     (d) they notice about the structure of the poem;
     (e) they notice about the language.
   - Groups report back to the class.
   - Groups then discuss
     (a) What has happened to 'the road through the woods' in Kipling's poem.
     (b) How this contrasts with Hardy's road.
     (c) In 'The way through the woods' what happens if 'you enter the woods / Of a summer evening late'.
     (d) How this compares with the memories people have about Hardy's road.
     (e) The structure of the poem compared with Hardy's.
   - Emphasise the comparison that in both poems the past is conjured up. But point out that whereas in 'Roman Road' it is people's memories ('thoughtful men' and Hardy himself), in 'The way through the woods' there is a sense that ghosts are passing through.

Transforming: Writing
Children to
- Recall an old road, route or path, which they have seen or read about, then
  (a) Imagine the people, animals or vehicles which used it years before.
  (b) Pretend to be seeing and hearing them passing through now as ghostly things.
- Bearing in mind the effectiveness of phrases such as 'the beat of a horse's feet' and 'swish of a skirt in the dew' write a poem about the old road, route or path.
- Regularly watch a local road and record anything interesting that happens or is seen, then
  (a) Write a sequence of poems based on these regular observations.
  (b) Research the past of this road and add poems to the sequence.

Transforming: Dance and drama
- Children to pretend they
  (a) are walking through deep undergrowth in the woods: ducking underneath branches, wading in long grass and ferns, pushing bushes to one side, trying to find an old road or track or way;

    (b) have no weight and float underneath branches, slide through long grass and ferns, slip past bushes and follow the old road or track because they know exactly where it is.
- Children to
  - (a) Research Roman military procedures, particularly how they marched on long journeys.
  - (b) Recreate formations the Romans used when marching and practise marching that way.
  - (c) Play the roles of people visiting a Roman road and comparing the Romans' use of it with how it is used now.
  - (d) Enact a scene in which Romans are resting during a journey.
  - (e) Enact a scene in which modern people are visiting it on holiday.

Publishing
1. Children to redraft and make their sequences of poems into personal collections and make small multiple editions with illustrations.
2. Movement work to be developed into dances.
3. Improvisations to be developed into plays.
4. Both to be performed to the other classes in the school.

Project 4: Year 7, 'The Tyger' by William Blake

The project

For Year 7, working on poems in which form contributes to meaning as in the English Framework. The poem is selected as one of major importance, which has a distinctive form and style.

The text

This is Blake's most well known poem and, possibly, the most important short lyric poem of the Romantic period of English literature.

The Tyger
By William Blake

Tyger! Tyger! burning bright
In the forests of the night,
What immortal hand or eye
Could frame thy fearful symmetry?

In what distant deeps or skies
Burnt the fire of thine eyes?

On what wings dare he aspire?
What the hand dare seize the fire?

And what shoulder, and what art
Could twist the sinews of thy heart?
And, when thy heart began to beat,
What dread hand? And what dread feet?

What the hammer? What the chain?
In what furnace was thy brain?
What the anvil? What dread grasp
Dare its deadly terrors clasp?

When the stars threw down their spears
And water'd heaven with their tears
Did he smile his work to see?
Did he who made the lamb make thee?

Tyger! Tyger! burning bright
In the forests of the night,
What immortal hand or eye
Dare frame thy fearful symmetry?[7]

Glossary
thine – your
aspire – hope
furnace – enclosed chamber containing a very hot fire

Teaching and learning processes

Meeting and knowing
1. Before looking at the poem.
   - Collect copies of William Blake's paintings and engravings on postcards, particularly those for his work 'Visions of the Daughters of Albion'.
   - Practise reciting 'The Tyger' to convey its rhythm, but not mechanically, and to develop a questioning tone in your voice, but not too much.
   - Prepare a large version of the poem or copy it for each child.
   - Ask the children what poems they know and, using their examples, establish that in many poems something is described or a story is told. Involve them in a discussion about this 'voice' that poets often use.
   - Tell the children that the poem you are about to share with them doesn't describe anything and doesn't tell a story.
   - Go through the glossary, ensuring that every child knows what the words mean.

2. Reciting the poem.
   - Children to read William Blake's 'The Tyger' silently.
   - Recite it to the class, then:
     (a) Ask what voice Blake uses in 'The Tyger'.
     (b) Establish that it is a series of questions without answers.
     (c) Discuss why this might be.
   - Divide the class into four groups, allocating one of verses 2, 3, 4 and 5 to each group, with the first and last verses being recited by the whole class.
   - Ask them to develop a questioning tone in their voices, but not too much.
   - Allow for practice.
   - Work on a class recitation of the poem.
   - Discuss the best ways of reciting it.
   - Practise until you get a satisfying performance.
3. Comprehension.
   - Groups to
     (a) Imagine and tell each other what pictures they see in their heads when reciting 'The Tyger'.
     (b) Decide who is being asked the questions.
     (c) List exactly what those questions are.
     (d) Discuss and decide what the poem is really about.
     (e) Work out the structure of the poem.
     (f) Report to the class.
   - Tell the children that William Blake's 'The Tyger' is possibly one of the most important short lyric poems in the English language.
   - Ask them why they think this might be.
   - Tell them also that it was written in the late eighteenth century, more than 200 years ago.

Transforming: Writing
1. For homework children to write
   - a summary of the discussion they had in their groups;
   - an evaluation of why they think the poem is important.
2. Children to find out about William Blake and the background of the poem and make notes for further discussion in the following lesson.
3. Provide each child with a postcard of one of Blake's paintings or engravings and ask them to write a poem in response as follows:
   - Look at the picture, close eyes, look again.
   - Without worrying about spelling, punctuation or correctness, write what comes into your head as you look at the picture.
   - Keep doing this until your imagination is exhausted.
4. Allow them to build a sequence of poems this way.

5. Children to
   - Recite their poems to test if they sound right and to make changes as necessary.
   - Work out if they can improve them by looking at the pictures again and choosing some better words.
   - Correct any spelling or other errors, then redraft.

Transforming: Art
1. Children to draw then make paintings of one or more of the following phrases in the poem:
   - 'forests of the night'
   - 'fearful symmetry'
   - 'What the hand dare seize the fire'
   - 'twist the sinews of thy heart'
   - 'In what furnace was thy brain'
   - 'When the stars threw down their spears'
2. Throughout, allow plenty of opportunity for discussion.

Transforming: Dance
1. Individuals to
   - Chant the words of the first verse and move around the space in time to the rhythm.
   - Imagine they are wandering through a forest in the dark and seeing glimpses of things.
   - Explore the contrast between lifting up on wings and hammering on an anvil.
   - Make hand gestures to represent the words 'seize', 'twist', 'grasp' and 'clasp'.
2. Each group to make a
   - picture to represent 'frame thy fearful symmetry';
   - sequence of movement and still shapes based on the verses they recited.
3. Create a whole class dance as follows:
   (a) All children chant the words of the first verse repeatedly as they move around the space, wander through forests, lift wings, hammer anvils, seize, twist, grasp and clasp.
   (b) They divide into groups and as one group makes its symmetry picture and sequence of movement and still shapes the other children chant the verse several times.
   (c) They finish by repeating (a) and their 'fearful symmetry' pictures.

Transforming: Music
Composition groups to
1. Recite the whole poem then repeat, this time accompanying the recitation with clapping.

2. Discuss the sounds suggested by the poem then choose instruments or other objects to represent them.
3. Using the instruments and reciting, explore the rhythm further.
4. Beat out the rhythm on chime bars, glockenspiel, xylophone or keyboard, attempting to find a suitable tune.
5. Decide on a tune and hum it or la-la it.
6. Try to sing the first verse using this tune.
7. Make variations to the tune if it appears to be monotonous.
8. Work out a sung and accompanied performance.

Publishing
1. Make a class display of the poems alongside the pictures which stimulated their composition. Exhibit the paintings using the phrases which they illustrate as titles.
2. Perform the whole dance and the musical settings of the poems to another class or to the whole year group.

Project 5: Year 8, 'Bermudas' by Andrew Marvell

The project

For Year 8 children, working on substantial texts within the English Framework. The poem is selected as one of the more important texts of the seventeenth century and reflects the religious tensions of the time.

The text

This is a poem or song of praise, an ode in which Andrew Marvell reveals his love of nature and his desire for religious tolerance. Marvell imagines that he hears a Puritan refugee from the religious repression under the Stuarts singing praises to God as he rows along the coast of an island in the Bermudas.

Bermudas
By Andrew Marvell

Where the remote Bermudas ride
In the ocean's bosom unespied,
From a small boat, that rowed along,
The listening winds received this song.
What should we do but sing his praise
That led us through this watery maze,
Unto an isle so long unknown,
And yet, far kinder than our own?

5

Where he the huge sea-monsters wracks,
That lift the deep upon their backs.   10
He lands us on a grassy stage;
Safe from the storms, and prelate's rage.
He gave us this eternal spring,
Which here enamels everything;
And sends the fowls to us in care,   15
On daily visits through the air.
He hangs in shades the orange bright
Like golden lamps in a green night.
And does in the pomegranates close
Jewels more rich than Ormus shows.   20
He makes the figs our mouths to meet;
And throws the melons at our feet.
But apples plants of such a price,
No tree could ever bear them twice.
With cedars, chosen by his hand,   25
From Lebanon, he stores the land.
And makes the hollow seas, that roar,
Proclaim the ambergris on shore.
He cast (of which we rather boast)
The gospel's pearl upon our coast.   30
And in these rocks for us did frame
A temple, where to sound his name.
O let our voice his praise exalt,
Till it arrive at heaven's vault:
Which thence (perhaps) rebounding, may   35
Echo beyond the Mexique Bay.
Thus sung they, in the English boat,
An holy and a cheerful note,
And all the way, to guide their chime,
With falling oars they kept the time.[8]   40

Glossary
Bermudas – islands in the Caribbean Sea
unespied – not seen
maze – complex network
wracks – wrecks
stage – scene of action
prelate – bishop or other churchman of high rank
pomegranate – fruit full of juicy seeds

Ormus – Hormuz in the Persian gulf

apples – pineapples

figs – soft pear-shaped fruit

cedar – species of evergreen tree

Lebanon – country in the middle-east famous for its beautiful cedar trees

ambergris – waxy substance used in making perfume

exalt – praise highly

vault – roof

Mexique Bay –Bay of Mexico in the Caribbean Sea

chime – song

Teaching and learning processes

Meeting and knowing

1. Before looking at the poem.
   - Practise reciting 'Bermudas' so that you convey its rhythm, but not mechanically, and develop a praising tone in your voice, but not too much.
   - Copy the poem, including the glossary, for each child.
   - Discuss the different voices poets use. For instance, they
     (a) describe and express their feelings for people and things;
     (b) tell stories.
     (c) attack what they believe to be wrong.
2. Teach the children that
   - 'Bermudas' is an ode, or poem which praises things, in this case God for the good things he has provided.
   - The ode is an ancient form of poetry developed by the Greeks more than 3,000 years ago, and the first writers of odes usually praised athletes.
   - It was used by poets in Shakespeare's time to praise a wider range of subjects.
   - The ode 'Bermudas' was written during a time when you could be imprisoned or even executed for your religious beliefs.
   - Marvell gives us the words of a possible song that Puritans – such as the ones who sailed to America on the Mayflower – might have sung.
3. Emphasise that under the Tudors and Stuarts there were times when Puritans persecuted Catholics *and* when Catholics persecuted Puritans.
4. Go through the glossary, ensuring that every child knows what the words mean.
5. Recite the poem to the children.
6. Divide them into four groups and in order to get regular changes of voice allocate lines as follows:
   - Group 1 recites the first couplet beginning 'Where the remote Bermudas'.
   - Group 2 recites the second beginning 'From a small boat'.

- Group 3 recites the third beginning 'What should we do'.
- Group 4 recites the fourth beginning 'Unto an isle'.
- Continue changing voices after every couplet.

7. Ensure that there is a distinct change of tone after the fourth line, because these are the lines of a song, and again after line 36, because this is where the song ends.
8. Discuss the best ways of reciting the poem, aiming to create a flowing songlike sound for lines 5 to 36. Rehearse until it is satisfying.
9. Comprehension.
   - Groups to
     (a) Identify and list all the things which Marvell is praising God for providing.
     (b) Decide which ones are their favourites and give reasons.
     (c) Discuss what overall impression or picture the poem creates in their imaginations.
     (d) Work out the form of the poem.
     (e) Report back to the class.
   - Tell the children that Andrew Marvell's 'Bermudas' is an important lyric poem of the seventeenth century and ask them why they think this might be.

Transforming: Writing
1. For homework, children to
   - Write a summary of the discussion they had in their groups.
   - Write an evaluation of why they think the poem is important.
   - Research Andrew Marvell and the background of the poem and make notes for further discussion in the following lesson.
   - Think about a special place, out of doors, which they would like to praise.
2. Once they have identified a special place, ask them to
   - List all the good things they particularly like about the place.
   - Using 'Bermudas' as a model, find a way of describing these good things; for instance, Marvell describes oranges in the shade as 'golden lamps in a green night'.
   - Build as many poetic lines of this kind as possible, not necessarily using rhyme or arranging them in couplets.
   - Read through their lines and make them into a poem.

Transforming: Art
Using whatever materials are available, children to choose their favourite couplet from 'Bermudas' and to work out a cover illustration for a book of Andrew Marvell's poems.

Transforming: Music

Composition groups to

1. Recite part of the poem, then repeat, this time accompanying the recitation with clapping.
2. Discuss the sounds suggested by the poem, then choose instruments or other objects to represent them.
3. Explore the rhythm further using the instruments.
4. Tap out the rhythm on chime bars, glockenspiel, xylophone or keyboard, attempting to find a suitable tune.
5. Decide on a tune and hum it or la-la it.
6. Try to sing some couplets using this tune.
7. Vary the tune if it appears to be monotonous.
8. Work out a performance of the whole poem which is sung and accompanied.

Publishing

1. Make a class display of the children's odes and of their pictures illustrating Marvell's 'Bermudas'.
2. Perform the settings of the poems to another class or to the whole year group.

References

1. Gardner, W.H. (ed) (1953) *Gerard Manley Hopkins: A Selection of his Poems and Prose*. Harmondsworth: Penguin.
2. Carter, D. (1988) *Hopkins Centenary Project*. Mold: Clwyd County Council.
3. Tibble, J.A. and A. (eds) (1965) *John Clare: Selected Poems*. London: Dent/Dutton.
4. Hutchinson, T. (ed.) (1905) *The Poetical Works of William Wordsworth*. London: Frowde.
5. Gibson, J. (ed.) (1976) *Thomas Hardy :The Complete Poems*. London: Macmillan.
6. Kipling, R. 'The way through the woods' in Harrison, M. and Stuart-Clark C. (eds) (1996) *The Oxford Treasury of Classic Poems*. Oxford: Oxford University Press.
7. Plowman, M. (ed.) (1927) *William Blake: Poems and Prophecies*. London: Dent/Dutton.
8. Hutchings, B. (ed.) (1979) *Andrew Marvell Selected Poems*. Manchester: Carcanet.

Appendix: Project tables

The following project tables indicate the intended coverage of National Curriculum 2000 (NC 2000), National Literacy Strategy Framework for Teachers (NLS Framework), Key Stage 3 National Strategy, Framework for Teaching English (NS Framework) if the suggested activities are followed. There are also many incidental objectives covered by these projects.

1. *Beowulf*

Document	Objectives covered
NC 2000	**KS2.** English. *Speaking & Listening.* 4a–d; 8a, b; 9a, b, c; 11a;. *Reading.* 4a–i; 8d, f; *Writing.* 1a–e; 2a–f; 9a, d. Art and Design. 2b; 3a, b; 4–c; 5a, b. PE. 6a, b. Music. 2a, b; 5e. **KS3.** English. *Speaking & Listening.* 1(3); 2(1, 5, 6, 8, 9); 3(3); *Reading.* 1(2, 4); 2(4, 7, 8); 3(3, 5); *Writing.* 1(1, 3, 4, 5, 6); 1(1, 3, 4, 5); 3(1, 8, 9, 10). Art & Design. 1(1–3); 2(1–3);. PE. 3(1, 2) Music. 1(4, 5, 6); 2(1, 2, 3, 6); 3(2, 3, 4).
NLS Framework	**Y4. Term 2.** Reading comprehension: 1, 2, 4, 5, 6, 7. Writing composition: 10, 11, 12. **Y5. Term 2.** Reading comprehension: 1, 3, 4, 5, 6, 7, 8, 10. Writing composition: 10, 11, 12, 13. **Y6. Term 2.** Reading comprehension: 1, 7, 8. Writing composition: 10, 12, 13.
NS Framework	**Y7.** Reading: 19, 20. Writing: 1, 2, 5, 6, 7, 8. Speaking & Listening: 1–17.

2. *Sir Patrick Spens*

Document	Objectives covered
NC 2000	**KS2.** English. *Speaking & Listening.* 4a–d; 8a, b; 9a, b, c; 11a; *Reading.* 4a–i; 8d; *Writing.* 1a–e; 2a–f; 9a, d. Art & Design. 2b; 3a, b; 4a–c; 5a, b; P E. 6a, b. Music. 2a, b; 5e. **KS3.** English. *Speaking & Listening.* 1(3); 2(1, 5, 6, 8, 9); 3(3); *Reading.* 1(2, 4); 2(4, 7, 8); 3(3, 5); *Writing.* 1(1, 3, 4, 5, 6); 1(1, 3, 4, 5); 3(1, 8, 9, 10). Art & Design. 1(1–3); 2(1–3). PE. 3(1, 2). Music. 1(4, 5, 6); 2(1, 2, 3, 6); 3(2, 3, 4).
NLS Framework	**Y6. Term 1.** Reading comprehension: 3, 5. Writing composition: 6, 10. **Term 2.** Reading comprehension: 3, 5, 6. Writing composition: 12, 13. **Term 3.** Reading comprehension: 4. Writing composition: 14.
NS Framework	**Y7.** Reading: 19, 20. Writing: 1, 2, 5, 6, 7, 8. Speaking & Listening: 1–17.

3. *The Pardoner's Prologue and Tale*

Document	Objectives covered
NC 2000	**KS2.** English. *Speaking & Listening.* 4a–d; 8a, b; 9a, b, c; 11a; *Reading.* 4a–i; 8d; *Writing.* 1a–e; 2a–f; 9a, d. Art & Design. 2b; 3a, b; 4a–c; 5a, b. **KS3.** English. *Speaking & Listening.* 1(3); 2(1, 5, 6, 8, 9); 3(3); *Reading.* 1(2, 4); 2(4, 7, 8); 3(3, 5); *Writing.* 1(1, 3, 4, 5, 6); 1(1, 3, 4, 5); 3(1, 8, 9, 10). History. 4a, b. Art & Design. 1(1–3); 2(1–3).
NLS Framework	**Y4. Term 2.** Reading comprehension: 1, 2, 6, 7. Writing composition: 10, 11. **Y5. Term 2.** Reading comprehension: 1, 3, 4, 5, 6,8. Writing composition: 11, 12, 13.
NS Framework	**Y8.** Reading: 2, 13, 14, 15, 16. Writing: 1, 2, 7, 9. Speaking & Listening: 2–16.

4. *Twelfth Night*

Document	Objectives covered
NC 2000	**KS2.** English. *Speaking & Listening.* 4a–d; 8a, b; 9a, b, c; 11a; *Reading.* 4a–i. 8d; *Writing.* 1a–e; 2a–f; 9a, d. Art & Design. 2b; 3a, b; 4a–c; 5a, b. PE. 6a, b. Music. 2a, b; 5e. **KS3.** English. *Speaking & Listening.* 1(3); 2(1, 5, 6, 8, 9); 3(3); *Reading.* 1(2, 4); 2(4, 7, 8); 3(3, 5); *Writing.* 1(1, 3, 4, 5, 6); 1(1, 3, 4, 5); 3(1, 8, 9, 10). Art & Design. 1(1–3); 2(1–3). PE. 3(1, 2). Music. 1(4, 5, 6); 2(1, 2, 3, 6); 3(2, 3, 4).
NLS Framework	**Y5. Term 1.** Reading comprehension: 3, 5, 9, 12. Writing composition: 13, 15, 18, 19. **Y6. Term 1.** Reading comprehension: 1, 3, 4, 5. Writing composition: 6, 9, 10.
NS Framework	**Y7.** Reading: 17, 18, 19, 20. Writing: 5, 6, 7, 8, 9. Speaking & Listening: 1–19. **Y8.** Reading: 13, 14, 15, 16. Writing: 1, 2, 6, 7, 9. Speaking & Listening: 2–16.

5. *Gullivers Travels*

Document	Objectives covered
NC 2000	**KS2.** English. *Speaking & Listening.* 4a–d; 8a,b; 9a,b, c; 11a. *Reading.* 4a–i; 8d; *Writing.* 1a–e; 2a–f; 9a, d. Art and Design. 2b; 3a, b; 4a-c; 5a, b. **KS3.** English. *Speaking & Listening.* 1(3); 2(1, 5, 6, 8, 9); 3(3); *Reading.* 1(2, 4); 2(4, 7, 8); 3(3, 5); *Writing.* 1(1, 3, 4, 5, 6); 1(1, 3, 4, 5); 3(1, 8, 9, 10). History. 4a, b. Art & Design. 1(1–3). 2(1–3).
NLS Framework	**Y5. Term 3.** Reading comprehension: 1,2, 3, 6. Writing composition: 7, 8, 9, 10. **Y6. Term 1.** Reading comprehension: 2, 3, 5. Writing composition: 6, 7, 8, 9.
NS Framework	**Y7.** Reading: 17, 20. Writing: 5, 6, 7, 8, 9. Speaking & Listening: 1–17, 19. **Y8.** Reading: 13, 14, 15, 16. Writing: 1, 2, 6, 7, 9. Speaking & Listening: 1–, 18, 20.

6. 'Autumn' by John Clare

Document	Objectives covered
NC 2000	**KS2.** English. *Speaking & Listening.* 4a–d; 8a, b; 9a, b, c; 11a; *Reading.* 4a–i; 8d; *Writing.* 1a–e; 2a–f; 9a, d. Art and Design. 2b; 3a, b; 4a–c; 5a, b.
NLS Framework	**Y4. Term 2.** Reading comprehension: 4, 5, 6, 7. Writing composition: 10, 11.
NS Framework	————

7. 'I wandered lonely as a cloud' by William Wordsworth

Document	Objectives covered
NC 2000	**KS2.** English. *Speaking & Listening.* 4a–d; 8a, b; 9a, b, c; 11a; *Reading.* 4a–i; 8d; *Writing.* 1a–e; 2a–f; 9a, d. Music. 2a, b; 5e.
NLS Framework	**Y5. Term 3.** Reading comprehension: 6. Writing composition: 9.
NS Framework	————

8. 'Roman Road' by Thomas Hardy and 'The way through the woods' by Rudyard Kipling

Document	Objectives covered
NC 2000	**KS2.** English. *Speaking & Listening.* 4a–d; 8a, b; 9a, b, c; 11a; *Reading.* 4a–f, h, i; 8d; *Writing.* 1a–e; 2a–f; 9a, d. History: 4a, b; 8a. PE. 6a, b. Music. 2a, b; 5e.
NLS Framework	**Y6. Term 3.** Reading comprehension: 2, 3, 4, 6. Writing composition: 12.
NS Framework	————

9. 'Tyger' by William Blake

Document	Objectives covered
NC 2000	**KS3.** English. *Speaking & Listening:* 1(3); 2(1, 5, 6, 8, 9); 3(3); *Reading:* 1(2, 4); 2(4, 7, 8); 3(3, 5); *Writing:* 1(1, 3, 4, 5, 6); 1(1, 3, 4, 5); 3(1, 8, 9, 10). Art & Design. 1(1–3); 2(1–3). PE. 3(1, 2). Music. 1(4, 5, 6); 2(1, 2, 3, 6); 3(2, 3, 4).
NLS Framework	_____
NS Framework	**Y7.** Reading: 19, 20. Writing: 8, 9. Speaking & Listening: 1–14.

10. 'Bermudas' by Andrew Marvell

Document	Objectives covered
NC 2000	**KS3.** English. *Speaking & Listening:* 1(3); 2(1, 5, 6, 8, 9); 3(3); *Reading:* 1(2, 4); 2(4, 7, 8); 3(3, 5); *Writing:* 1(1, 3, 4, 5, 6); 1(1, 3, 4, 5); 3(1, 8, 9, 10). Music. 1(4, 5, 6); 2(1, 2, 3, 6); 3(2, 3, 4).
NLS Framework	_____
NS Framework	**Y7.** Reading: 19, 20. Writing: 1, 2, 7, 9, 19. Speaking & Listening: 2–12.

Select bibliography

Andrews, R. (2001) *Teaching and Learning English*. London: Continuum.

Auden, W.H. (1954) *Secondary Worlds*. London: Faber.

Bettelheim, B. (1976) *The Uses of Enchantment*. London: Thames and Hudson.

Calvino, I. (1999) *Why Read the Classics?* London: Vintage Classics.

Gibson, R. (1987) 'Jonathan Miller on Shakespeare', *Shakespeare and Schools*, Newsletter No. 3. Cambridge, Cambridge Institute of Education.

Carter, D. (1986) 'King Lear in the Junior Classroom', *English in Education*, 20(1).

Carter, D. (1987a) *The Odyssey Project*. Mold: Clwyd County Council.

Carter, D. (1987b) *Something Rich and Strange*. Mold: Clwyd County Council.

Carter, D. (1988) *Hopkins Centenary Project*. Mold: Clwyd County Council.

Carter, D. (1989) 'A Country Discovered'. *Cambridge Journal of Education*, 19(3).

Carter, D. (1990) *The Isle is Full of Noises*. Mold: Clwyd County Council.

Carter, D. (1994) *Hamlet in Gwersyllt*. Mold: Clwyd Poetry Project.

Carter, D. (1995) *The Four Branches Project*. Mold: Clwyd Poetry Project.

Eliot, T.S. (1928) 'Introduction 1928' *Ezra Pound, Selected Poems*. London: Faber.

Greeves, A. (1990) 'For Adult Eyes Only', T.E.S. 20.4.90. London: Times Newspapers.

Levin, S.R. (1988) *Metaphoric Worlds*. New Haven: Yale University Press.

Pavel, T. (1986) *Fictional Worlds*. Cambridge MA: Harvard University Press.

Phenix, P.H. (1964) *Realms of Meaning*. New York: McGraw-Hill.

Ross, M. *et al.* (1993) *Assessing Achievement in the Arts*. Buckingham: Open University Press.

Index

TRANSFUSION
MEDICINE

TRANSFUSION
MEDICINE

JEFFREY McCULLOUGH, M.D.

UNIVERSITY OF MINNESOTA
DEPARTMENT OF LABORATORY MEDICINE
MINNEAPOLIS, MINNESOTA

McGraw-Hill
HEALTH PROFESSIONS DIVISION

New York St. Louis San Francisco Auckland
Bogotá Caracas Lisbon London Madrid
Mexico City Milan Montreal New Delhi San Juan
Singapore Sydney Tokyo Toronto

McGraw-Hill

*A Division of The **McGraw·Hill** Companies*

Transfusion Medicine

Copyright © 1998 by The McGraw-Hill Companies, Inc. All rights reserved. Printed in the United States of America. Except as permitted under the United States Copyright Act of 1976, no part of this publication may be reproduced or distributed in any form or by any means, or stored in a data base or retrieval system, without the prior written permission of the publisher.

1 2 3 4 5 6 7 8 9 0   DOCDOC   9 9 8 7

ISBN 0-07-045113-3

This book was set in Times Roman by York Graphic Services.
Project management was by York Production Services.
The editors were James Morgan and Peter McCurdy;
the production supervisor was Catherine Saggese;
the cover designer was York Graphic Services;
The index was prepared by York Graphic Services;
R.R. Donnelley & Sons was printer and binder

This book is printed on acid-free paper.

Library of Congress Cataloging-in-Publication Data

McCullough, Jeffrey J.
      Transfusion Medicine / Jeffrey McCullough.
          p.   cm.
      Includes bibliographical references and index.
      ISBN 0-07-045113-3
      1. Blood--Transfusion.   I. Title
      [DNLM: 1. Blood Transfusion.   2. Blood Donors.   3. Blood Groups.
4. Blood Banks—organization & administration.   WB 356 M478b 1998]
RM171. M425   1998
615' .39--dc21
DNLM/DLC
for Library of Congress   97–29682
                                                                     CIP

PREFACE

Transfusion medicine and blood banking have come a long way from the landmark discovery of ABO blood groups by Landsteiner in 1900, hemolytic disease of the newborn by Levine and Stetson in 1938, the development of plastic bags for component preparation by Carl Walter in 1950, and the practical application of apheresis in the 1970's. Today's transfusion medicine is sophisticated and complex hemotherapy. Far removed from Landsteiner, Levine, and Wiener, blood group immunohematology involves an understanding of cell membranes, genes, and molecular biology; combines this with fundamental knowledge of the immune system; and extrapolates these into laboratory bench serology to make blood available safely for patients.

Blood component production and therapy is based on a knowledge of blood cell biochemistry and physiology but extends this scientific knowledge to produce blood components for patient therapy at the bedside or in the clinic. Transfusion medicine also depends on the social sciences. Blood donor recruitment involves the analysis and understanding of psychosocial and motivational theories. The collection, testing production, and general blood bank operations have become a complex manufacturing process involving computer control, sophisticated equipment , and modern quality systems that are far removed from the blood bank laboratories of only a decade ago. Blood is a human resource, donated voluntarily, but those who require it seldom have an option about receiving it. Thus, there are considerable social and health policy issues regarding the nations blood supply system that add to the breadth and interest of transfusion medicine.

All of these activities come together in the modern transfusion medicine in that is essential for the care of so many patients ranging from the tiny immature neonate to the patient receiving cancer therapy, undergoing marrow transplantation, cardiovascular surgery or joint replacement, the victim of an automobile accident or the patient with an inherited coagulation disorder. Transfusion medicine brings science and clinical medicine together to provide life-saving therapies made possible by the blood donation of millions of volunteers.

Several excellent large textbooks provide extensive information about all aspects of transfusion medicine. This book is intended to be concise but comprehensive and extensively referenced. The consistency that comes from a single author should create a flow

that makes for easy perusing of sections and a continuity through the book. I hope that this book will be useful not only to those working in transfusion medicine but also valuable to those who use blood and need quick and concise answers to their questions and problems. Thus, practicing hematologists, oncologists, pathologists, surgeons, or anesthesiologists as well as transfusion medicine professionals may find this book to be helpful. The book also can be a nice introduction to our field for hematology or oncology fellows, technologists specializing in blood banking, or others in educational positions who are learning about transfusion medicine.

I am indebted to my colleague Yoon Choo, M.D. who wrote the chapter on HLA and has successfully maintained the style and flow of the book. I thank Jane Ulmann Bester, MS, MT(ASCP) SBB who provided valuable feedback on draft material, and Penny Milne whose typing, organizing, follow-up, and communication was essential in this project. Most of all I am grateful for the understanding and support of my family, Maureen, Mac, and Andy McCullough during the hours devoted to this book.

I hope that this book will be of practical value to all professionals involved in transfusion medicine and blood banking as we go about the daily activities of participating in the care of patients who depend on a safe and readily available blood supply.

CONTENTS

that such blood was effective in animal transfusions.[1] Substances tested for anticoagulation of human blood include ammonium sulfate, sodium phosphate, sodium bicarbonate, sulfarsenol, ammonium oxalate and arsphenamine, sodium iodide, and sodium sulfate.[14,15] The delays in developing methods to anticoagulate blood for transfusion are interesting, because it was known in the late 1800s that calcium was involved in blood clotting and that blood could be anticoagulated by the addition of oxalic acid. Citrates were used for laboratory experiments by physiologists, and by 1915 several papers had been published describing the use of sodium citrate for anticoagulation for transfusions.[1] It is not clear who first used citrated blood for transfusion.[1] It could have been R. Lewisohn,[16] A.S. Hustin, or R. Weil.[17] In 1955, Lewisohn received the Landsteiner award from the American Association of Blood Banks for his work in the anticoagulation of blood for transfusion.

MODERN BLOOD BANKING AND BLOOD BANKS

Major stimuli for developments in blood transfusion have come from wars. During World War I, sodium citrate was the only substance used as an anticoagulant. Dr. Oswald Robertson of the U.S. Army Medical Corps devised a blood collection bottle and administration set similar to those used several decades later[1] and transfused several patients with preserved blood.[18]

Between World Wars I and II, there was increasing interest in developing methods to store blood in anticipation of rather than response to need. It has been suggested that the first "bank" where a stock of blood was maintained may have been in Leningrad in 1932.[1,2] A blood bank was established in Barcelona in 1936 because of the need for blood during the Spanish Civil War.[19] In the United States, credit for the establishment of the first blood bank for the storage of refrigerated blood for transfusion is usually given to Bernard Fantus at the Cook County Hospital in Chicago.[20] The blood was collected in sodium citrate and so it could be stored for only a few days.

CADAVER BLOOD

Cadavers served as another source of blood during the 1930s and later. Most of this work was done by Yudin[21] in the USSR. Following death, the blood was allowed to clot, but the clots lysed by normally appearing fibrinolytic enzymes, leaving liquid defibrinated blood.

The use of cadaver blood in the Soviet Union received much publicity and was believed by many to be the major source of transfusion blood there. Actually, not many more than 40,000 200-mL units were used, and most of them at Yudin's Institute.[1] In 1967, the procedure was quite complicated, involving the use of an operating room, a well-trained staff, and extensive laboratory studies. This was never a practical or extensive source of blood.

THE RH BLOOD GROUP SYSTEM AND PREVENTION OF RH IMMUNIZATION

In 1939, Levine and Stetson published in less than two pages in the *Journal of the American Medical Association*[22] their landmark article, a case report, describing hemolytic disease of the newborn (HDN) and the discovery of the blood group that later became known as the Rh system. A woman who delivered a stillborn infant received a transfusion of red cells from her husband because of intrapartum and postpartum hemorrhage. Following the transfusion, she had a severe reaction but did not react to subsequent transfusions from other donors. The woman's serum reacted against her husband's red cells but not against the cells of the other donors. Levine and Stetson postulated that the mother had become immunized by the fetus, who had inherited a trait from the father that the mother lacked. In a later report they postulated that the antibody found in the mother and subsequently in many other patients was the same as the antibody Landsteiner and Wiener prepared by immunizing Rhesus monkeys.[23] This also began a long debate over credit for discovery of the Rh system.

During the early 1900s, immunologic studies had established that active immunization could be prevented by the presence of passive antibody. This strategy was applied to the prevention of Rh immunization in the early 1960s in New York and England at about the same time.[24,25] Studies of Rh-negative subjects who were given either Rh-positive red cells coated with anti-Rh or anti-Rh only followed by Rh-positive red cells established that this strategy prevented immunization. Subsequent studies established that administration of anti-Rh in the form of Rh immune globulin could prevent Rh immunization and thus almost eliminate hemolytic disease of the newborn. Currently, control of HDN is a public health measure similar to ensuring proper immunization programs for susceptible persons.

COOMBS AND ANTIGLOBULIN SERUM

In 1908, Moreschi[26] is said to have described the antiglobulin reaction. The potential applicability of this in the detection of human blood groups was not appreciated until 1945 when Coombs, Mourant, and Race[27] published their work on studies of the use of rabbit antibodies against human IgG to detect IgG coated red cells. Red cells were incubated with human sera containing antibodies against red cell antigens, washed, and the rabbit antihuman sera used to demonstrate the presence of bound IgG by causing agglutination of the red cells. The availability of antihuman globulin serum made it possible to detect IgG red cell antibodies when the antibody did not cause direct agglutination of the cells. Thus, red cells coated with anti-IgG red cell antibodies could be easily detected, and the era of antibody screening and crossmatching was born. This greatly improved the safety of blood transfusion and also led to the discovery of many red cell antigens and blood groups.

During the mid 1960s, several investigators began to describe the role of complement in red cell destruction. It was established that some red cell antibodies caused red cell destruction by activating complement and that anticomplement activity in antiglob-

ulin reagents could predict accelerated red cell destruction.[28,29] This led to several years of research and debate as to the value of anticomplement activity in antiglobulin reagents.[30]

PLASMA AND THE BLOOD PROGRAM DURING WORLD WAR II

Techniques for collection, storage, and transfusion of whole blood were not well developed during the 1930s. The outbreak of World War II added further impetus to the development of methods to store blood for periods longer than a few days. Although the method of blood anticoagulation was known by the mid-1920s, red blood cells hemolyzed after storage in sodium citrate for 1 week. This limitation also slowed the development of blood transfusion. Although it was also known that the hemolysis could be prevented by the addition of dextrose, the practical value of this important observation was not recognized for over a quarter of a century. Anticoagulant preservative solutions were developed by Mollison in Great Britain.[31] However, when the glucose-citrate mixtures were autoclaved, the glucose caramelized, changing the color of the solution to various shades of brown. The addition of citric acid eliminated this problem and also extended the storage time of blood to 21 days. The advance of World War II also brought an understanding of the value of plasma in patients with shock.[32] In the early 1940s, Edwin J. Cohn, Ph.D., a Harvard biochemist, developed methods for the continuous flow separation of large volumes of plasma proteins. This made possible during World War II the introduction of liquid and lyophilized plasma and human albumin as the first-line management of shock. Initial work using plasma for transfusion was carried out by John Elliott.[32,33] This combination of technological and medical developments made it possible for Charles R. Drew to develop the "Plasma for Britain" program.[34]

PLASTIC BAGS AND BLOOD COMPONENTS

One of the next major developments in blood banking was the discovery and patenting of the plastic blood container, by Carl Walter, in 1950. This made possible the separation of whole blood and the creation of blood component therapy. Dr. Walter's invention was commercialized by the Baxter Corporation (the "-wal" of its Fenwal division represents Dr. Walter's name). One example of the impact of the introduction of multiple connected plastic containers cited by Greenwalt[1] is the increased use of packed red blood cells from 0.8% to 88% during his 12-year tenure as Director of the American Red Cross Blood Program (1967–1978). This separation of whole blood into its components also began to generate enormous amounts of recovered plasma, which made possible the development of large-scale use of coagulation factor VIII concentrates.

CRYOPRECIPITATE AND FACTOR VIII

In 1965, Dr. Judith Pool reported that if fresh frozen plasma (FFP) was allowed to thaw at refrigerator temperatures, precipitate remained that contained most of the coagula-

tion factor VIII from the original FFP.[35] This made it possible for the first time to administer large doses of factor VIII in a concentrated form to hemophiliacs and opened an era in which the bleeding diathesis could be effectively managed. A few years later, reports began to appear describing the use of a concentrated factor VIII prepared using the plasma fractionation technique developed by Edwin Cohn.[36] This further simplified the management of hemophilia, because the ability to store the factor VIII concentrates in home refrigerators enabled the development of home treatment programs involving prophylactic or immediate self-administration of factor VIII.

RED CELL PRESERVATION

The role of 2,3-diphosphoglycerate in oxygen transport by red cells was discovered in the mid 1960s.[37,38] It had been known previously that this compound was better maintained at higher pH, while ATP (which appeared to be involved in red cell survival) was maintained better at a lower pH. The addition of adenine was shown to improve ATP maintenance and prolong red cell survival and storage for transfusion.[39] The next major advance in red cell preservation was the development of preservative solutions designed to be added after removal of most of the original anticoagulated plasma, thus further extending the storage period of red cells.[40]

LEUKOCYTE ANTIGENS AND ANTIBODIES

In 1926, Doan described the sera of some individuals that caused agglutination of the leukocytes from others.[41] Subsequent studies established the presence of leukocyte antibodies, the presence of these antibodies in the sera of polytransfused patients, the occurrence of white cell agglutinins in response to fetomaternal immunization, and the alloimmune and autoimmune specificities associated with these antibodies. These studies, along with studies of the murine histocompatibility system, led to the description of the major histocompatibility system (human lymphocyte antigens [HLA]) in humans and the understanding that there are separate antigenic specificities limited to neutrophils as well.[42] These studies also defined the causative role of leukocytes in febrile nonhemolytic transfusion reactions.[43] Strategies were sought to prevent these reactions by removing the leukocytes from blood.[44]

PLATELET COLLECTION, STORAGE, AND TRANSFUSION

The relationship between bleeding and thrombocytopenia had been known for some time, but the development of the plastic bag system for blood collection made platelets available for transfusion. Several years of work by many investigators—predominantly at the National Cancer Institute during the 1960s—developed the methods for preparing platelets and established that platelet transfusion to thrombocytopenic patients reduced mortality from hemorrhage.[45] Initially, platelets had to be transfused within a

few hours after the whole blood was collected, and thus large-scale application in the general medical care setting was impractical. The seminal report by Gardner and Murphy[46] showing that room temperature allowed platelets to be stored for several days revolutionized platelet transfusion therapy.

GRANULOCYTE TRANSFUSIONS

As the benefits of platelet transfusion for thrombocytopenic patients were recognized, interest developed in using the same strategy to provide granulocyte transfusion to treat infection in neutropenic patients. Initial attempts involved obtaining granulocytes from patients with chronic myelogenous leukemia (CML).[47,48] Transfusion of these cells had clinical benefits,[49] and this led to a decade of effort to develop methods to obtain granulocytes from normal donors.[50] At best, these methods produced only modest doses of granulocytes; improvements in antibiotics and general patient care have supplanted the need for granulocyte transfusions except in very limited circumstances (see Chapter 12).

SUMMARY

Blood banking and transfusion medicine developed slowly during the 1950s but much more rapidly between the 1960s and the 1980s. Some of the important advances mentioned here were understanding blood groups and the identification of hundreds of specific red cell antigens; the development of the plastic bag system for blood collection and separation; plasma fractionation for the production of blood derivatives, especially factor VIII; improved red cell preservation; platelet preservation and transfusion; understanding hemolytic and febrile transfusion reactions; expanded testing for transmissible diseases; and the recognition of leukocyte and platelet antigen systems. Blood collection and storage is now a complex process operated much like the manufacture of a pharmaceutical. Transfusion medicine is now the complex, sophisticated medical-technical discipline described in the remainder of this book.

REFERENCES

1. Greenwalt TJ. The short history of transfusion medicine. Transfusion 1997;37:550–563.
2. Oberman HA. The history of blood transfusion. In: Petz LD, Swisher SN, eds. Clinical Practice of Blood Transfusion. New York: Churchill Livingstone, 1981:11–32.
3. Kilduffe RA, de Bakey M. The blood bank and the technique and therapeutics of transfusions. St. Louis: CV Mosby, 1942.
4. Lyons AS, Keiner M. Circulation of the blood. In: Lyons AS, Petrucelli RJ II, Abrams NH, eds. Medicine: An illustrated history. New York: Harvey N Abrams, 1978:437–459.
5. Lower R. A treatise on the heart on the movement and color of the blood and on the passage of the chyle into the blood. In: Franklin KJ, ed. Special Edition, The Classics of Medicine Library. Birmingham, AL: Gryphon Editions Inc., 1989.

6. Farr AD. The first human blood transfusion. Med Hist 1980;24:143–162.
7. Blundell J. Successful case of transfusion. Lancet 1928–1929;1:431–432.
8. Kuhns WJ. Historical milestones—blood transfusion in the Civil War. Transfusion 1965;5:92–94.
9. Landsteiner K. On agglutination of normal human blood. Transfusion 1961;1:5–8.
10. Isohemmagglutination: recommendation that the Jansky classification be adopted for universal use. JAMA 1921;76:130–131. Miscellany.
11. Hektoen L. Iso-agglutination of human corpuscles. JAMA 1907;48:1739–1740.
12. Ottenberg R. Studies in isohemagglutination, I: transfusion and the question of intravascular agglutination. J Exp Med 1911;13:425–438.
13. Crile GW. Technique of direct transfusion of blood. Ann Surg 1907;46:329–332.
14. Doan C. The transfusion problem. Physiol Rev 1927;7:1–84.
15. Braxton-Hicks J. Case of transfusion: with some remarks on a new method of performing the operation. Guy's Hosp Rep 1869;14:1–14.
16. Lewisohn R. The citrate method of blood transfusion after ten years. Boston Med Surg J 1924;190:733.
17. Weil R. Sodium citrate in the transfusion of blood. JAMA 1915;64:425.
18. Robertson O. Transfusion with preserved red blood cells. Br Med J 1918;1:691.
19. Jorda JD. The Barcelona blood transfusion service. Lancet 1939;1:773.
20. Fantus B. The therapy of the Cook County Hospital: blood transfusion. JAMA 1937;109:128–133.
21. Yudin SS. Transfusion of cadaver blood. JAMA 1936;106:997–999.
22. Levine P, Newark NJ, Stetson RE. An unusual case of intra-group agglutination. JAMA 1939;113:126–127.
23. Levine P, Katzin EM, Newark NJ, et al. Isoimmunization in pregnancy—its possible bearing on the etiology of erythroblastosis foetalis. JAMA 1941;116:825–827.
24. Freda VJ, Gorman JG, Pollack W. Successful prevention of experimental Rh sensitization in many with an anti-Rh gamma 2-globulin antibody preparation: a preliminary report. Transfusion 1964;4:26.
25. Clarke CA, Donohoe WTA, McConnell RB, et al. Further experimental studies in the prevention of Rh-haemolytic disease. Br Med J 1963;1:979.
26. Moreschi C. Neue tatsachen uber die blutkorperchen-agglutination. Zentralbl Bakt 1908;46:49–51.
27. Coombs RRA, Mourant AE, Race RR. A new test for the detection of weak and "incomplete" Rh agglutinins. Br J Exp Pathol 1945;26:225.
28. Sherwood GK, Haynes BF, Rosse WF. Hemolytic transfusion reactions caused by failure of commercial antiglobulin reagents to detect complement. Transfusion 1976;16:417.
29. Petz LD, Garratty G. Antiglobulin sera—past, present and future. Transfusion 1978;18:257.
30. Petz LD, Branch DR, Garratty G, et al. The significance of the anticomplement component of antiglobulin serum (AGS) in compatibility testing. Transfusion 1981;21:633.
31. Loutit JF, Mollison PL. Advantages of disodium-citrate-glucose mixture as a blood preservative. Br Med J 1943;2:744.
32. Elliott J, Tatum WL, Nesset N. Use of plasma as a substitute for whole blood. N C Med J 1940;1:283–289.
33. Elliott J. A preliminary report of a new method of blood transfusion. South Med & Surg 1936;98:643–645.
34. Kendrick DB. Blood Program in World War II. 14-5, Washington, DC: US Government Printing Office, 1964:922.
35. Pool JG, Shannon AE. Simple production of high potency anti-hemophilic globulin (AHG) concentrates in a closed bag system. Transfusion 1965;5:372.
36. Cohn EJ, Oncley JL, Strong LE, Hughes Jr, WL Armstrong Jr. SH, Chemical, clinical, and immunological studies on the products of human plasma fractionation. J Clin Invest 1944;23:417–606.
37. Benesh R, Benesh RE. The influence of organic phosphates on the oxygenation of hemoglobin. Fed Proc 1967;26:673.
38. Chanutin A, Curnish RR. Effect of organic and inorganic phosphates on the oxygen equilibrium of human erythrocytes. Arch Biochem Biophys 1967;121:96.
39. Nakao M, Nakao T, Arimatsu Y, Yoshikawa H. A new preservative medium maintaining the level of adenosine triphosphate and the osmotic resistance of erythrocytes. Proc Jpn Acad 1960;36:43.

40. Hogman CF, Hedlund K, Zetterstrom H. Clinical usefulness of red cells preserved in protein-poor media. N Engl J Med 1978;299:1377.

41. Doan CA. The recognition of a biological differentiation in the white blood cells with a specific reference to blood transfusion. JAMA 1926;86:1593–1597.

42. Lalezari P, Radel E. Neutrophil-specific antigens: immunology and clinical significance. Sem Hematol 1974;11:281–290.

43. Perkins HA, Payne R, Ferguson J, et al. Nonhemolytic febrile transfusion reactions: quantitative effects of blood components with emphasis on isoantigenic incompatibility of leukocytes. Vox Sang 1966;11:578.

44. Greenwalt TJ, Gajewski M, McKenna JL. A new method for preparing buffy coat-poor blood. Transfusion 1962;2:221–229.

45. Freireich EJ, Kliman A, Gaydos LA, et al. Response to repeated platelet transfusion from the same donor. Ann Intern Med 1963;50:277.

46. Murphy S, Gardner FH. Platelet preservation—effect of storage temperature on maintenance of platelet viability—deleterious effect of refrigerated storage. N Engl J Med 1969;380:1094–1098.

47. Morse EE, Carbone PP, Freireich EJ, Bronson W, Kliman A. Repeated leukapheresis of patients with chronic myelocytic leukemia. Transfusion 1996;6:175–192.

48. Morse EE, Freireich EJ, Carbone PP, Bronson W, Frei E. The transfusion of leukocytes from donors with chronic myelocytic leukemia to patients with leukopenia. Transfusion 1966;6:183–192.

49. Freireich EJ, Levin RH, Wang J. The function and gate of transfused leukocytes from donors with chronic myelocytic leukemia in leukopenic recipients. Ann NY Acad Sci 1965;113:1081.

50. McCullough J. Leukapheresis and granulocyte transfusion. CRC Crit Rev Clin Lab Sci 1979;10:275.

THE U.S. BLOOD SUPPLY SYSTEM

In the United States, the blood supply is provided by many different organizations with different organizational structures and philosophies. These organizations function rather effectively to meet the nation's blood needs and thus are referred to here as the nation's blood collection system, although they are not really a unified system. Two comprehensive reports on the nation's blood collection system were prepared several years ago by the Office of Technology Assessment.[1,2] Although time has passed and some details are different today, the general descriptions of the blood collection and supply system in those reports are still valid.

Blood can be collected in two ways: either whole blood can be collected, or only the plasma portion of the blood can be collected, leaving the cellular portion with the donor. These two different collection methods have resulted in the development of two fundamentally different systems in the United States. One system involves the cellular elements and plasma obtained from whole blood, and the other involves large-scale collection of plasma for the subsequent manufacture of plasma derivatives. Whole blood is collected by blood banks, and the cellular products and unprocessed plasma used directly for transfusion are prepared by the blood bank (Fig. 2.1). A separate system and organizations exist that collect only the plasma and use it as raw material to produce plasma "derivatives" that are concentrated forms of selected plasma proteins.

THE WHOLE BLOOD COLLECTION SYSTEM

Whole blood is collected by venipuncture from healthy adults into plastic bags containing a liquid anticoagulant preservative solution. The whole blood is separated into red blood cells, platelet concentrate, and fresh frozen plasma (Table 2.1). The fresh frozen plasma can be (a) used for transfusion, (b) further processed into cryoprecipitate

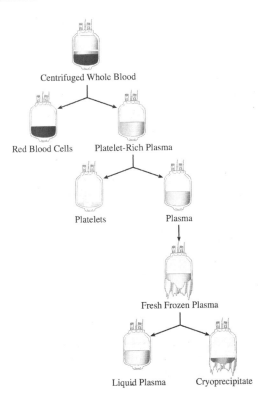

Centrifuged Whole Blood

Red Blood Cells   Platelet-Rich Plasma

Platelets   Plasma

Fresh Frozen Plasma

Liquid Plasma   Cryoprecipitate

Figure 2.1 Schematic diagram showing separation of whole blood into components.

(to be used for transfusion) and cryoprecipitate-poor plasma (which serves as a raw material for further manufacture of plasma derivatives), or (*c*) provided as a source of raw material for subsequent manufacture of plasma derivatives as described below. Blood banks make many modifications to these components to obtain blood products that will be effective for specific purposes. Descriptions of these various blood components and their medical uses are provided throughout this book. A complete list of components that can be produced from whole blood and are licensed by the U.S. Food and Drug Administration (FDA) is provided in Table 2.2. In addition, blood banks distribute many of the plasma derivative products as part of their total supply program for transfusion medicine therapy, but most of these other plasma products are actually manufactured by plasma derivative companies.

The U.S. blood collection system is heterogeneous to some extent, because of the "random development of blood centers without regard . . . to patient referral patterns."[3] In most areas of the United States, there is only one local organization that collects blood; however, in some communities blood may be collected by more than one organization. Blood is collected by blood centers and hospitals. Blood centers are free-

Table 2.1 Components produced by blood banks and their medical uses

Component	Medical use
Red blood cells	Oxygenation of tissues
Platelets	Prevention or cessation of bleeding
Fresh frozen plasma	Cessation of bleeding
Cryoprecipitate	Cessation of bleeding
Cryoprecipitate-poor plasma	Plasma exchange
Granulocytes	Treatment of infection
Frozen red blood cells	Storage of rare blood
Leukocyte-depleted red cells	Prevention of reactions and certain diseases

standing organizations, virtually (possibly) all of which are nonprofit. These centers are governed by a board of local volunteers; their sole or major function is to provide the community's blood supply. Each blood center collects blood in a reasonably contiguous area and supplies the hospitals within the blood collection area. The blood center may or may not supply the total needs of the hospitals in its area and may supply hospitals in other areas as well. The area covered by each center is determined by historical factors and is not developed according to any overall plan. Rather, local interests dictate whether, how, and what kind of community blood program is developed. The entire area of the United States is not necessarily covered by a blood center. There are a total of approximately 180 blood centers in the United States. Approximately 45 of these (25%) are operated by the American Red Cross and the remainder are community blood centers.

The American Red Cross (ARC) is the organization that collects the largest number of units of blood in the United States, collecting slightly less than half of the nation's blood supply. The ARC is a nonprofit, congressionally chartered (but not government sponsored or operated) organization that conducts programs supported by donated funds and/or cost recovery. The Red Cross operates through a network of regional centers. The blood is provided to hospitals and transfusion services, and the Red Cross charges a fee to cover the cost of collecting, testing, processing, storing, and shipping the blood. The areas in which the American Red Cross collects blood are shown in Figure 2.2. In areas not covered by the ARC, blood is collected by one or more community or hospital blood banks.

Some blood is collected by blood banks that are part of hospitals. These blood banks usually collect blood only for use in that hospital and do not supply other hospitals. However, very few hospitals collect enough blood to meet all their needs. They purchase some blood from a local or distant community blood center. Most hospitals in the United States do not collect any blood but acquire all of the blood they use from a community center. Of those that do collect blood, there are no good data available to define the proportion of their needs that they collect. This can be presumed to be quite variable. The author is not aware of any large, major hospital that collects virtually all of the blood and components used in that facility.

Table 2.2 Products produced from whole blood that are subject to license by the U.S. Food and Drug Administration

Cryoprecipitated AHF
Cryoprecipitated AHF irradiated
Cryoprecipitated AHF pooled
Fresh frozen plasma
Fresh frozen plasma irradiated
Liquid plasma
Plasma
Plasma irradiated
Platelet-rich plasma
Platelets
Platelets irradiated
Platelets pheresis
Platelets pheresis irradiated
Red blood cells
Red blood cells deglycerolized
Red blood cells deglycerolized irradiated
Red blood cells frozen
Red blood cells frozen irradiated
Red blood cells frozen rejuvenated
Red blood cells frozen rejuvenated irradiated
Red blood cells irradiated
Red blood cells leukocytes removed
Red blood cells leukocytes removed irradiated
Red blood cells rejuvenated
Red blood cells rejuvenated deglycerolized
Red blood cells rejuvenated deglycerolized irradiated
Red blood cells rejuvenated irradiated
Red blood cells washed
Whole blood CPD irradiated
Whole blood cryoprecipitate removed
Whole blood leukocytes removed
Whole blood modified—platelets removed
Whole blood platelets removed irradiated

AHF: antihemophilic factor A; CPD: citrate, phosphate, and dextrose.

OTHER ACTIVITIES OF COMMUNITY BLOOD CENTERS

Traditionally, blood centers have carried out a variety of activities that provide services in addition to the blood components. These include the following:

Continuing education   Blood centers conduct seminars and symposia to provide updates and continuing education for blood bank technologists and nursing personnel involved in transfusing blood and components. These programs may be offered at the blood center, at community sites, or in hospitals served by the center. Some blood centers sponsor or participate in blood bank specialist (SBB) training programs for medical technologists. A few blood centers have special laboratory areas set aside where

American Red Cross Biomedical Services
Blood Services Areas and Regions

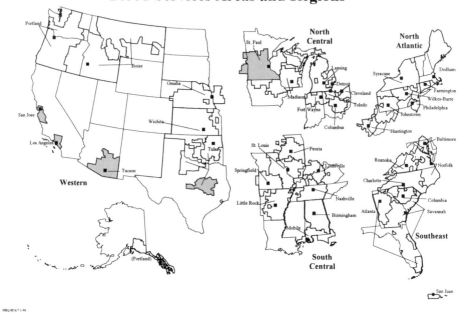

Figure 2.2 Areas of the United States served by the American Red Cross Blood Service.

"wet" workshops are conducted for technologists to update themselves or be trained on new laboratory techniques.

Blood centers commonly provide continuing education programs for physicians in transfusion medicine, therapy, and transfusion-transmitted diseases. Programs are also offered for nurses in transfusion therapy, techniques of blood administration, recognition and management of transfusion reactions, and complications of transfusion.

HLA typing Many blood centers operate HLA typing laboratories to type blood donors and maintain a file of HLA-typed donors for plateletpheresis, to carry out diagnostic HLA typing as a laboratory test service, or to perform typing for solid organ or marrow transplantation as a service to the medical centers they support.

Platelet and/or neutrophil antibody studies and antigen typing Laboratory testing for antibodies to platelets or neutrophils are important in the diagnosis and management of immunohematology and transfusion medicine clinical situations. The techniques are often similar to those used for red cell work, and many blood centers provide these services as well.

Therapeutic apheresis   Because most blood centers operate active normal donor apheresis programs, they are able to utilize the instruments and staff to provide therapeutic apheresis as a service. In this way individual hospitals can have the service available without the need to establish this complex program for use in a relatively small number of patients.

Red cell reference laboratory testing   A natural part of providing blood for hospitals is the operation of laboratories that perform special testing for red cell antibodies to assist the hospitals in evaluating transfusion reactions and in locating compatible blood for patients with red cell antibodies.

Outpatient transfusions   A few blood centers operate outpatient clinics where patients can receive transfusions. In this way the blood center can select blood from its inventory, carry out the compatibility test, and provide the blood all on site. Usually the costs of providing outpatient transfusions at the blood center are substantially less than in the hospital.

Medical consultation for transfusion medicine   Today, transfusion is a complex medical specialty. Most blood centers have knowledgeable physicians available at all times to advise physicians about the use of blood components and the evaluation of complications of transfusion.

In the past, these services were often provided to hospitals and the medical technical nursing community at little or no extra charge because the activities were subsidized by the income generated from the charges for the blood components. However, during the past several years as blood centers have attempted to stabilize or reduce their prices to hospitals, charges for these additional services have increased to make them self-supporting financially. In many situations, hospitals have been unwilling to spend money for the services and, as a result, blood centers are reducing or eliminating these activities.

AMOUNT OF BLOOD COLLECTED

Because the United States has a pluralistic system of blood collection, there is no central repository of data on the number of units of blood collected or on the components produced or transfused. Estimates of the nation's blood production must be developed from various sources, usually involving research studies.

Approximately 190 regional blood centers collect most (about 77%) of the blood supply. The number of community blood centers in the United States declined 4% between 1988 and 1992. During this 5-year period, the average number of units collected by each blood center increased from 64,000 to 68,000 (6%). This suggests that the decline might be due to mergers or consolidations, since the decline was primarily in smaller centers and there was a slight increase in centers collecting larger amounts of blood.[4] In 1992, the 38 centers (21%) that collected 100,000 or more units of blood accounted for 55% of the total blood collection activity.[4]

ARC blood centers collect about 45% and other community blood centers about 42%. A large number of hospitals (more than 600) each collect a small amount of blood to account for 11% of the blood supply; the remaining 2% is imported. In 1992, somewhat more than 12 million units of whole blood and in addition more than 1 million units of autologous blood and 400,000 units of directed donor blood were collected.[5] Thus, the total amount of blood collected in the United States was approximately 13,588,000 units.[5,6] In addition, approximately 206,000 units, representing approximately 1.5% of the U.S. blood supply, were imported from Europe.[5]

There have been several trends in the nation's blood supply during the past two decades, undoubtedly influenced by the AIDS epidemic. From 1971 to 1980, collection of blood by community blood centers increased an average of 4% annually; but then from 1981 to 1992, the increase averaged only 1.6%. During the 5-year period from 1988 to 1992, the increase was only 0.6% annually (Table 2.3).[4] Actually, there was a 7% decrease in the amount of allogeneic blood collected.[6] This was partly counterbalanced by increases of 70% and 25% in autologous and directed-donation blood, respectively.[6] Thus, the active growth rate of blood collections experienced during the 1970s and early 1980s has stopped during the past few years, and blood collection activity appears to have stabilized or begun to decline.

The collection of autologous blood has increased rapidly (23% annually) during the period 1988 to 1992 (Table 2.3). During this 5-year period, the proportion of blood collected by community blood centers that was autologous blood more than doubled, from 2.5% to 5.7%. Interestingly, there appears to be an inverse relationship between the total number of units of blood collected by a blood center and the percentage of those that are autologous units.[4] There is some variation (3.2% to 9.4%) in the percentage of total collections represented by autologous blood in different census regions of the United States (Fig. 2.3). It is not clear whether the proportion of autologous blood in different regions of the United States has any relationship to the prevalence of transmissible diseases such as AIDS or to blood collection activity in general. These figures represent autologous blood collected in the blood centers. Since some hospitals also collect autologous blood, the data do not necessarily reflect the total autologous blood usage in the area. It is possible that factors related to the blood center operation influence the amount of autologous blood reported in the data shown here.

Table 2.3 Units collected by collection source (thousands)

Collection source	1988	1989	1990	1991	1992	Annual growth rate
Total	12,003	12,143	12,344	12,179	12,311	0.6%
Allogeneic units	11,699	11,795	11,894	11,613	11,611	
Percent	97.5%	97.1%	96.3%	95.5%	94.3%	−0.2%
Autologous units	304	348	451	566	700	
Percent	2.5%	2.9%	3.7%	4.6%	5.7%	23.2%

Source: Kindly provided by Mr. John Forbes.

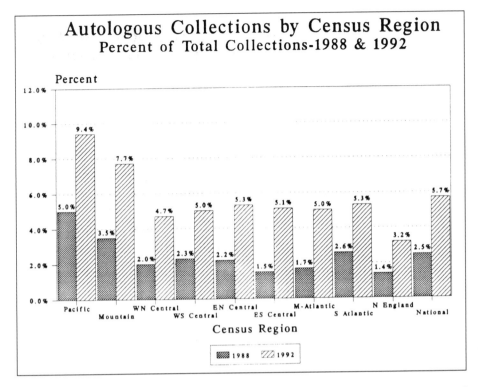

Figure 2.3 Autologous collections by census region: percent of total collections, 1988 and 1992. *(Reproduced with permission from Forbes JM, Laurie ML. The Northfield Blood Collection Report. Community Blood Center Collections, 1988–1992. Evanston, IL: Northfield Laboratories, Inc., August 1993.)*

Blood collection activity varies in different parts of the United States (Fig. 2.4). When analyzed by region, the data show that the South Atlantic region produces the largest portion of the U.S. blood supply (19%), followed closely by the East North Central region (17%). The smallest portions are provided by the New England and Mountain regions (5% each). However, on a per-capita basis, the data are quite different. The West North Central region collects the most blood per population (64 per 1,000), and the Pacific region the least (38 per 1,000) (Fig. 2.4).

The change in blood collection activity during the 1988–1992 period also varied in different parts of the United States.[4] Two census regions (Pacific and New England) experienced negative average annual growth rates, while the remaining regions experienced positive average annual growth rates ranging from 0.2% to 2.9%. The growth rate increased an average 1% annually in the West North Central Region, which had the highest per capita rate of blood donation, but the highest average annual increase (2.9%) occurred in the Mountain Region, which has one of the lowest donation rates per population. Thus, there does not appear to be any relationship between the growth rates and the donation rates.

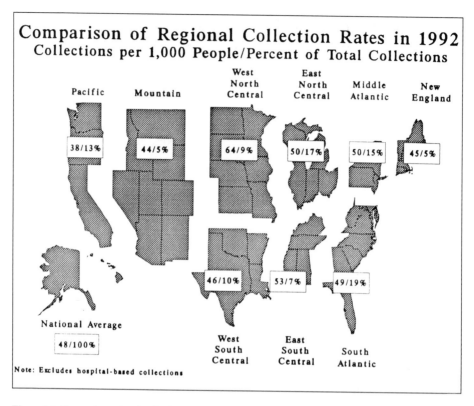

Figure 2.4 Comparison of regional collection rates in 1992: collections per 1,000 people/percent of total collections (excluding hospital-based collections). *(Reproduced with permission from Forbes JM, Laurie ML. The Northfield Blood Collection Report. Community Blood Center Collections, 1988–1992. Evanston, IL: Northfield Laboratories, Inc., August 1993.)*

The adequacy of the nation's blood supply varies at different times of the year and in different parts of the United States.[7] Certain areas of the United States are chronically not self-sufficient in their blood supply. This is discussed in more detail below in the section on blood resource sharing. The extent to which the adequacy of the blood supply is related to the public image of blood banks and the association of blood with AIDS is not clear. This is discussed in more detail in Chapter 3.

Blood Component Production

In 1992 a total of 3,828,000 units of platelets were produced.[6] This represents a 74% increase in the production of platelets between 1989 and 1992.[6] An additional striking trend in platelet production was the shift to single-donor platelets collected by plateletpheresis. Collection of apheresis platelets increased by 72%, while the collection of random platelets prepared from whole blood decreased by 9% between 1989 and 1992.[6] No national figures are available for the production of other blood components.

Nonutilization of Donated Blood

During 1992, approximately 1,500,000 units of allogeneic red blood cells or 11% of the total collected were lost, not used, or unaccounted for.[5] The nontransfusion rate for autologous blood is about 50% and, for directed-donor red cells, about 70%.[5,6] Thus, of all red cells collected, about 18% was not used. This figure can be a bit misleading, because some of the autologous blood would be suitable only for the patient and cannot be considered as part of the generally available blood supply. The proportion of autologous blood that would be suitable for general use is estimated to be 50%, but even this can be misleading because usually the blood is reserved for the patient donor until it is clear that the patient donor has no need for the transfusion. At that point there may be too little time left to use the blood before it becomes outdated.

BLOOD INVENTORY SHARING SYSTEMS

Certain areas of the United States are chronically unable to collect enough blood to meet their local transfusion needs. Some areas of the United States have been able to collect more blood than is needed locally and have provided these extra units to communities in need. The misalignment of blood use and blood collection is a long-standing phenomenon. Blood banks in metropolitan areas that serve large trauma, tertiary, and transplantation centers most frequently experience shortages of whole blood, components, and type-specific blood units. Blood supply to metropolitan areas is especially difficult, if the community blood center does not include a large rural population in their blood service area.

For years, blood banks have participated in systems to exchange blood among themselves to alleviate shortages. To deal with these blood shortages, blood is "exported" from areas of oversupply and "imported" into areas of shortage—a practice called "blood resource sharing." The lack of an adequate local blood supply and the need to import blood causes several difficulties, including possible unavailability of blood or components when needed, complex inventory management, technical disparities, emergency appeal-type donor recruitment, higher costs, decreased independence, and higher risk management costs.[8] Another more recent development is an increased use of blood resource sharing for financial reasons. Some blood centers import blood because they can obtain this blood less expensively than their own costs of production.[9] Other blood centers export blood because the increased volume of collection helps to reduce their own average costs.

Because of the short shelf life of blood, limited access to other blood banks, and restrictions on transportation in the 1950s, resource sharing efforts were primarily local with cooperative agreements among neighboring hospitals and blood centers to better utilize resources among themselves. Resource sharing networks such as these slowly expanded to include communities, states, and regions of the country. In the early 1960s, the American Association of Blood Banks (AABB) established a national clearinghouse so that blood could, if necessary, be moved nationally in response to need. To support the system of blood replacement, financial credits were used by many AABB members

at the time. Most efforts at resource sharing continued to remain local or regional, however. The American Red Cross also developed a system to facilitate resource sharing among its blood centers. Blood was shipped as needed and the exchanges were relatively uncomplicated. As the number of resource sharing networks grew, and the demand for a variety of blood products increased, meeting the needs of all parties—patients, hospitals, other transfusion facilities, and blood centers—became increasingly difficult and exchange practices more complicated.

Today, a considerable amount of blood resource sharing occurs in the United States. A substantial proportion of blood collected by the American Red Cross is actually distributed to hospitals by a regional center different from the region where the blood was collected. In 1991, 46 American Red Cross regions exported to another region at least 3% or 1000 units of the blood they collected for a total of 546,717 units or 9.2% of the total American Red Cross collections for that year. Conversely, 13 regions imported at least 10% of the units they distributed to hospitals. To manage the movement of this amount of blood, the American Red Cross has established a National Inventory Management System. Thus, there is a considerable amount of the nation's blood supply that is shifted from sites of collection to areas of undersupply.

The concept of blood as a national resource slowly gained favor as certain areas of the country (primarily major cities) began to experience critical blood shortages with increasing frequency. To meet the rising demand for blood and blood products, it became apparent that certain blood centers in urban areas required ongoing support to meet their community's blood needs. To protect themselves against constant shortages, these blood banks could no longer rely on the random availability of surplus units from their neighboring blood banks; in addition, to provide blood at a reasonable cost, these same centers could not continue to purchase blood units on an ad hoc basis.

As blood began to be exchanged with increasing frequency, three distinct kinds of blood centers began to emerge. Some blood centers collected the amount of blood needed by their service area; those willing and able to collect more units than their service area needed became known as "exporting" centers, while those blood centers that traditionally required assistance in meeting the community's need became known as "importing" centers. Exporting centers are primarily located in sparsely populated rural areas and importing centers in dense urban areas. The success of resource sharing largely depends on adequately matching these supply centers with demand centers.

One of the major issues in blood resource sharing is the attitude of blood donors. Very few studies have focused on donors' attitudes about being asked to donate more blood than is needed by their local community. In the only study published on this subject,[10] donors to several ARC blood centers indicated a willingness to donate for patients in other areas of the United States as long as their local blood needs were being met.

Exporting Blood Centers

The most common method for a blood center to support the needs of other blood banks or transfusion facilities is to plan to collect more units of blood than the service area typically requires. Besides assisting blood banks that experience frequent shortages,

collecting additional blood units may improve economies of scale and may help to reduce local fees for blood. This usually involves a long-term contractual agreement with centers that experience frequent shortages to provide the needed blood units. Such arrangements permit the exporting center to expand collection operations on a planned basis, better ensuring that contractual obligations will be consistently met at a reasonable cost. In addition to establishing long-term agreements, some exporting centers have surplus blood units available to ship on an ad hoc basis. Depending on the point of shipment and the level of supply, blood purchased on an ad hoc basis may be more costly than blood acquired through long-term contractual agreements. While exporting centers assist immeasurably in helping to meet shortages in certain areas, the normal fluctuations that occur on both the supply and demand sides make a perfect balance very difficult to achieve.

Some agreements for blood shipments are negotiated between the exporting center and the local blood provider (importing center). However, contractual agreements may be arranged directly between a hospital or transfusion facility and the exporting center. In these instances, the exporting center is often able to provide blood units at a processing fee well below that of the local blood provider for a number of reasons. The exporting center provides no reimbursement for unused units. Hospitals therefore use the "drop-shipped" units first, holding the local supplier's units in inventory in the event of shortage and then returning the unused units to the local supplier for credit prior to outdate. The exporting center usually provides only routine units in the shipment. The hospital must continue to rely on the local supplier for special units such as rare blood types, CMV-negative units, or irradiated units. The exporting center does not provide any ancillary services such as medical consultation, special testing, or reference laboratory services. The exporting center most frequently drop-ships in times of excess supply, which may create wide variations in the number of units that the local blood bank must supply. Finally, the exporting center may contract only with large hospitals in the community, where savings are realized as a result of high-volume shipments. While the availability of this lower-cost blood may be appealing to the hospital, it increases the complexity and thus the costs of operating the local community blood center and on balance may not be cost-effective. Some urban hospitals with specialty and emergency centers require a significantly greater number of blood units of a certain group—numbers that exceed the normal distribution of blood groups collected at a routine blood drive. To obtain these units, group-specific recruitment campaigns are necessary, campaigns that are labor intensive and therefore more costly to conduct regardless of the region of the country.

Importing Blood Centers

The majority of blood centers that seek contractual agreements to import blood are either unable to meet the community's need on a routine basis or experience frequent shortages, often of type-specific units. Some importing centers, however, may make a deliberate decision to acquire blood units outside the community for financial reasons. In certain metropolitan areas, high labor costs for recruitment and production personnel and/or inefficient blood collection operations drive up the cost of blood. To control

costs, these centers enter agreements to obtain a certain percentage of blood units from lower-cost areas. Blood centers that experience chronic shortages attempt to establish long-term contracts for additional units whenever possible. Despite the existence of contractual agreements, importing centers must often purchase blood units on an ad hoc basis as well to meet blood needs. One reason for this is that there may be wide fluctuations in demand; another is that the supplying center may not always meet the terms of the agreement. Blood units purchased through ad hoc exchanges may be offered at a higher fee and may not include as favorable a blood group mix as blood units obtained through contractual agreements.

In some areas of the country, the local blood center has not taken responsibility for totally supplying the area's hospitals and transfusion facilities. In such situations, or as a result of frequent shortages, some hospitals have pursued alternatives to meet their blood needs. Where the blood center is a partial supplier or is unresponsive to the needs of its customers, hospitals may establish an in-hospital collection facility, contract with another blood center for blood units, or develop an agreement with the blood inventory management systems.

Currently there is no single national inventory or blood resource sharing system in the United States. Despite the fact that there is not a unified blood banking system, blood banks have made major efforts to utilize blood from areas where it is available in excess. Factors that could further increase blood resource sharing include (*a*) the possibility of the United States becoming self-sufficient in its blood supply, (*b*) the desire to reduce costs by increasing collections in areas of low cost and decreasing collections in areas of higher cost, (*c*) increasing collections in areas with a low incidence of transmissible diseases as a strategy to decrease the risk of disease transmission, and (*d*) an increase in the need for red cells to serve as the raw material for the manufacture of blood substitutes. If the United States requires additional blood, some of this will be collected in areas that already collect in excess of their own needs. This will further increase resource sharing. As cost concerns increase, it may be even more desirable to further increase blood collection in areas of lowest cost, regardless of local needs, rather than increasing or maintaining present collection levels in high-cost areas. This also could increase blood resource sharing activities. Although transmissible disease testing is quite effective, no test is perfect, and some false negatives occur. At least theoretically, the prevalence of transfusion-transmissible diseases in the donor population might be related to the infectivity of the blood supply. Thus, it might be advisable to increase blood collection in areas of low prevalence of transmissible diseases, further increasing blood resource sharing.

THE PLASMA COLLECTION SYSTEM

A method was developed at the beginning of World War II to process large volumes of plasma so that some of the proteins could be isolated in concentrated form and used for medical purposes.[11] This plasma "fractionation" process is the basis for a large industry that provides many medically valuable products generally referred to as plasma "derivatives." The production of these plasma derivatives is a complex manufacturing

process usually involving large batches of plasma up to 10,000 liters or plasma from as many as 50,000 donors.

Plasma Definitions

The FDA uses two terms for plasma that may serve as the starting material for the manufacture of derivatives: *plasma* and *source plasma*. Plasma is "the fluid portion of one unit of human blood intended for intravenous use."[12] This plasma, which is a byproduct of whole blood collected by community blood banks or hospitals, is sold to commercial companies in the plasma fractionation industry who in turn manufacture the plasma derivatives and sell them in the pharmaceutical market. The blood banks' sale of their plasma to the commercial fractionator (manufacturer) may, but usually does not, involve an agreement to provide some of the manufactured derivatives back to the blood bank. Plasma from whole blood collected by the American Red Cross is fractionated through a contract with Baxter Healthcare, who then returns all of the derivatives prepared from that American Red Cross plasma to the American Red Cross for sale by the American Red Cross through their blood provision system.

The amount of plasma obtained from whole blood is not adequate to meet the needs for raw material to produce plasma derivatives. Therefore, much of the plasma that will be made into derivatives is obtained by plasmapheresis.[13] This is called source plasma, which is "the fluid portion of human blood collected by plasmapheresis and intended as the source material for further manufacturing use."[12] Automated instruments are usually used to obtain 650 to 750 mL of plasma up to twice weekly from healthy adult donors. An individual can donate up to about 100 L of plasma annually in the United States, if the plasma protein levels and other laboratory tests and physical findings remain normal. The plasma is used as raw material for the manufacture of the derivatives listed in Table 2.4.

Federally Licensed Plasma Collection and Manufacturing Organizations

Organizations and facilities may need licenses for either plasma collection or the manufacture of derivatives from plasma, or both, depending on the activities they conduct. In 1982, 202 organizations were licensed to produce source plasma at 350 locations, and in 1994, there were 125 organizations licensed to produce source plasma in 433 locations. Although the FDA does not specifically obtain information about the profit status of these organizations, of the 202 organizations in 1982, 183 (91%) were probably for profit and 17 nonprofit. Of the 125 licensees of source plasma in 1994, 115 (92%) were probably for profit and the remaining 10 were not-for-profit.

In 1982, 95 organizations were licensed to produce plasma at 233 locations, and in 1994, 135 organizations were licensed at 253 locations. The profit-nonprofit status of these organizations contrasts with organizations licensed for source plasma. In 1982, 75 (79%) of the organizations licensed to produce plasma were nonprofit community blood centers, three (4%) were government organizations, and 17 (17%) were for-profit organizations. In 1994, 114 (84%) of the organizations were nonprofit community blood centers, three (2%) were government organizations, and 18 (13%) were for-profit organizations. Thus, most of the organizations involved in producing source plasma

Table 2.4 Plasma derivative products and their uses

Albumin	Restoration of plasma volume subsequent to shock, trauma, surgery, and burns
Alpha-1 proteinase inhibitor	Treatment of emphysema caused by a genetic deficiency
Anti-hemophilic factor	Treatment or prevention of bleeding in patients with hemophilia A
Anti-inhibitor coagulant complex	Treatment of bleeding episodes in the presence of factor VIII inhibitor
Antithrombin III	Treatment of bleeding episodes associated with liver disease, antithrombin III deficiency, and thromboembolism
Cytomegalovirus immune globulin	Passive immunization subsequent to exposure to cytomegalovirus
Factor IX complex	Prophylaxis and treatment of hemophilia B bleeding episodes and other bleeding disorders
Factor XIII	Treatment of bleeding and disorders of wound healing due to factor XIII deficiency
Fibrinogen	Treatment of hemorrhagic diathesis in hypofibrinogenemia, dysfibrinogenemia, and afibrinogenemia
Fibrinolysin	Dissolution of intravascular clots
Haptoglobin	Supportive therapy in viral hepatitis and pernicious anemia
Hepatitis B immune globulin	Passive immunization subsequent to exposure to hepatitis B
IgM-enriched immune globulin	Treatment and prevention of septicemia and septic shock due to toxin liberation in the course of antibiotic treatment
Immune globulin (intravenous and intramuscular)	Treatment of agammaglobulinemia and hypogammaglobulinemia; passive immunization for hepatitis A and measles
Plasma protein fraction	Restoration of plasma volume subsequent to shock, trauma, surgery, and burns
Rabies immune globulin	Passive immunization subsequent to exposure to rabies
$Rh_O(D)$ immune globulin	Treatment and prevention of hemolytic disease of fetus and newborn resulting from Rh incompatibility and incompatible blood transfusions
Rubella immune globulin	Passive immunization subsequent to exposure to German measles
Serum cholinesterase	Treatment of prolonged apnea after administration of succinylcholine chloride
Tetanus immune globulin	Passive immunization subsequent to exposure to tetanus
Vaccinia immune globulin	Passive immunization subsequent to exposure to smallpox
Varicella-zoster immune globulin	Passive immunization subsequent to exposure to chicken pox

Source: From information provided by the American Blood Resources Association.

were for profit and most involved in producing plasma were nonprofit. The number of organizations involved in source plasma decreased and the number of locations increased substantially, while the number of organizations involved in plasma increased substantially and the number of locations increased slightly. Thus, in 1994, it appears that there were about 688 locations licensed for collection of plasma either as recovered from whole blood or source material, compared to about 583 in 1982. Although this appears to be an increase, some or many of the locations collecting plasma or source plasma may be the same location, and so the exact change in the number of plasma collection locations has not been summarized. In addition, the number of locations is not necessarily an indication of the amount of plasma collected.

In 1990, there were approximately 95 plasma fraction plants worldwide.[14] The noncommercial community operated 57 plants, while the commercial industry operated 38 facilities. The commercial industry facilities tend to be larger, since they have about 80% of the total plasma fractionation capacity worldwide.

There are 21 FDA-licensable plasma derivatives (Table 2.4). The number of manufacturers licensed to produce each of these ranges from one to six (Table 2.5). In 1982, a total of 11 manufacturers produced one or more of the three derivatives: antihemophilic factor (factor VIII), factor IX, and anti-inhibitor coagulant complex. By 1994, the number of manufacturers had decreased to nine; four had stopped production, and all of these had discontinued producing antihemophilic factor (factor VIII). Two new manufacturers had begun production of factor VIII, resulting in a net of two fewer manufacturers of factor VIII. Four existing manufacturers began production of factor IX. In 1982, ten of the 11 companies involved in derivative manufacture were for profit, and in 1994, seven of nine companies were for profit.

Plasma Collection Activity

Data regarding the plasma derivative industry is proprietary and thus is not readily available. The FDA does not routinely capture data on the nature of plasma donors (paid versus volunteer), the amount of plasma each organization collects, or the number of derivative products produced. According to the American Blood Resources Association (ABRA),[14] the U.S. plasma and plasma products industry employs over 12,000 people nationwide. U.S. plasma collection facilities perform approximately 13 million plasmapheresis donor collection procedures annually. Thus, if an average of 700 mL of plasma is obtained from each donation, it could be estimated that approximately 9 million liters of plasma would be collected annually in the United States by plasma centers. Individuals who donate plasma to support the plasma derivative industry receive between $15 and $20 per donation. According to the ABRA,[14] donors receive compensation of more than $244 million from plasma collection facilities annually. This is in contrast to whole blood donors, who donate voluntarily and do not receive compensation. Thus, 9 million liters would not be the entire volume of plasma used as starting material for derivative manufacture. Much of the plasma obtained from whole blood collected by blood banks is also used for derivative production. The volume of this plasma can be very roughly estimated as follows: approximately 12 million units of whole blood, suitable for use, are collected annually. If

Table 2.5 Partial list of biologic products and number of ABRA member companies that are licensed to manufacture the product

Derivative	Number of manufacturers
Albumin	6
Alpha-1 proteinase inhibitor	1
Anti-inhibitor coagulant complex	1
Anti-hemophilic factor	6
Antithrombin III	1
Coagulation factor IX	1
Factor IX complex	4
Hepatitis B immune globulin	3
Immune serum globulin	5
Intravenous immune globulin	4
Pertussis immune globulin	1
Plasma protein fraction	4
Rabies immune globulin	2
$RH_O(D)$ immune globulin	4
Tetanus immune globulin	5
Thrombin	2
Vaccinia immune globulin	1
Varicella-zoster immune globulin	0

Source: PLASMApheresis 1991;5:71–72.

approximately 2 million units are used for fresh frozen plasma and cryoprecipitate, the remaining 10 million units could produce about 2 to 2.5 million liters of plasma. This combined with the source plasma estimates provide approximately 11 to 11.5 million liters of plasma annually for the production of derivatives, although these are merely the estimations of the author. This is similar to the estimate provided by Blakestone[15] that in 1990 approximately 12 million liters of plasma were consumed in the manufacture of plasma derivatives.

It is estimated[14] that the worldwide sales of plasma derivatives exceed $4 billion annually, with U.S. firms providing more than 60% of the plasma products or $2.4 billion in domestic and export sales. Of the $2.4 billion in domestic and export sales, $645 million is the estimated export revenue from sales in Europe.[14] It is not known how much of the remaining $1.755 billion sales is domestic and what proportion is from other exports.

PROFESSIONAL BLOOD BANK ASSOCIATIONS

There are three major professional associations involved with blood banking. These are the American Association of Blood Banks (AABB), America's Blood Centers (ABC), and the American Blood Resources Association (ABRA). Other organizations such as

the American Medical Association, the College of American Pathologists, the American College of Surgeons, or the American Society of Anesthesiologists may from time to time take positions on blood bank and transfusion medicine related issues and maintain blood bank or transfusion medicine committees. Because the AABB, ABC, and ABRA are the only professional organizations devoted exclusively to blood banking and transfusion medicine, these organizations will be described briefly.

American Association of Blood Banks

The American Association of Blood Banks (AABB) is a professional, nonprofit, scientific, and administrative association for individuals and institutions engaged in the many facets of blood and tissue banking and transfusion and transplantation medicine. AABB member facilities collect virtually all of the nation's blood supply and transfuse more than 80%. Approximately 2,400 institutions (community, regional, and American Red Cross blood centers, hospital blood banks, and hospital transfusion services) and approximately 9,200 individuals are members of the AABB. Members include physicians, scientists, medical technologists, administrators, blood donor recruiters, nurses, and public-spirited citizens. The services and programs of the AABB include inspection and accreditation, standard setting, certification of reference laboratories, operation of a rare donor file, accreditation of parentage testing laboratories, establishment of group purchasing programs, operation of a liability insurance program for blood banks, certification of specialists (technologists) in blood banking, collection of data about the activities of the membership, conduct of regional and teleconference educational programs, provision of professional self-assessment examinations, and conduct of donor recruitment–public education seminars. In addition, the AABB sponsors the world's largest annual meeting where results of new research in blood banking and transfusion medicine are presented; publishes the nation's leading journal reporting scientific, technical, and medical advances in blood banking and transfusion medicine; provides legislative and regulatory assistance to members; develops a wide variety of educational materials for blood bank professionals; participates in the National Marrow Donor Program; and participates in the National Blood Foundation which provides funds for research in transfusion medicine and blood banking.

Institutional members of the AABB are classified either as a community blood center, a hospital blood bank, or a hospital transfusion service. The community blood center collects blood and distributes it to several hospitals but does not transfuse blood. A hospital blood bank both collects and transfuses blood, and a hospital transfusion service transfuses but does not collect blood. Another way of classifying members of the AABB is the corporate structure of the organization. Of the 2,168 institutional members in 1994, 74% were nonprofit, 10% were for profit, and a few were government or other types of institutions.

America's Blood Centers

America's Blood Centers (ABC) is an association of independent (non-American Red Cross) community blood centers that was formed in 1996 as an outgrowth of the

Council of Community Blood Centers (CCBC). The CCBC was established in 1962 to represent the common interests of not-for-profit community blood centers. Efforts to meet the goals of safety, quality, and efficiency in blood services are met through programs such as group purchasing of supplies, services, and liability insurance; efforts to increase volunteer blood donation; effective sharing of blood resources; strengthening of blood center management skills; training programs to ensure compliance with federal regulations; and efforts to ensure fair and balanced resolution of disputes between blood centers and the public they serve. ABC works nationally by helping to shape and influence federal and state regulations, policies, and standards of care that its membership believes are in the best interest of the donors and patients they serve. The association also works to identify and promote needed research and development in blood services; promotes information exchange between members of operational practices; and promotes new programs, policies, and ideas by conducting surveys and meetings of small working groups and by developing workable models. In 1993, the CCBC had 63 institutional members that collected 4,564,714 units of blood (range, 7,617 to 752,273), which represented about 38% of the nation's volunteer donor blood supply. In 1994, every member of the CCBC also held an FDA license.

American Blood Resources Associations

The American Blood Resources Association (ABRA) is a trade association, founded in 1971, to represent the plasma collection and fractionation industry.[14] The fundamental role of ABRA is to educate the public at large about the commercial plasma and plasma products industry. ABRA was founded to serve as the spokesperson for the industry and to represent industry in both federal and state government relations. ABRA's primary purpose is to serve as an advocate for its members, who are engaged in or connected with the collection and manufacture of products derived from human plasma and blood. ABRA's mission is to promote and encourage research, foster and monitor the promulgation of reasonable and just regulations, and institute beneficial projects on behalf of the commercial plasma and plasma products industry. ABRA provides facility and personnel certifications and develops industry manufacturing standards and guidelines. ABRA members operate under a strict code of ethics to ensure the highest standards and quality of its industry. ABRA's members operate over 80% of the U.S. commercial plasma collection facilities and include all of the commercial plasma product manufacturers in the United States and a majority of the manufacturers worldwide. ABRA members manufacture and collect plasma in 42 states across the country.

REGULATION OF THE BLOOD SUPPLY SYSTEM

Federal Regulation

Blood is considered a drug and is regulated by the FDA. The legal basis for this regulation of blood, blood components, and plasma derivatives is provided by two separate but overlapping statutes, one governing "biologics" and one governing "drugs." The

biologics law requires that any "virus, therapeutic serum, toxin, anti-toxin, or analogous product" be prepared in a facility holding an FDA license.[16] A separate law, the Pure Food and Drugs Act, covers drugs intended for the "cure, mitigation, or prevention of disease" and thus includes biologics such as blood and blood components or plasma derivatives.[16] Thus, blood banks are subject to the biologics and the drug regulatory process.

The federal requirements for blood banks are specified in the Code of Federal Regulations. In addition, the FDA publishes "guidelines" that specify the agency's recommendations of specific policies, procedures, or actions regarding any aspect of the acquisition of blood.

FDA law requires that all organizations involved in "collection, preparation, processing, or compatibility testing . . . of any blood product"[16] register with the FDA. This registration allows the organization to collect blood and prepare blood components for its own use. If the organization wishes to ship the components across state lines or engage in commerce by selling the products to other organizations, the organization must obtain an FDA license for this purpose. Thus, for practical purposes, most hospitals that collect blood or prepare blood components for their own use are registered, but not licensed, since they do not ship blood in interstate commerce. Most blood centers are licensed, since they supply multiple hospitals, some of which may be in other states. In addition, blood centers may wish to participate in blood resource sharing with blood centers in other states and thus need to be licensed for interstate shipment of blood.

Federal licensure is intended to ensure that the facility in which the biologic is produced will provide high purity and quality. In addition to licensing the facility or establishment, this law requires that each biologic product itself be licensed by the FDA. Thus, to produce a licensed biologic, an organization must have an establishment license describing the facility in which the product is produced and a product license describing the specific product being produced. Over the years, this law has been specifically amended to include the terms blood and blood component or derivative to make it clear that blood is subject to the biologics regulation.

Blood banks and plasma derivative manufacturers are inspected annually by the FDA and they must submit a report annually to the FDA indicating which products are collected, tested, prepared, and distributed. In 1995, the FDA had licensed 188 organizations at 790 locations for collection and interstate shipment of blood and components. A total of 2,900 locations are registered for collection of blood but not for interstate shipment.

When an organization applies for an FDA license to produce blood components or plasma derivatives, it must provide the credentials of the person in charge (responsible head) and of those responsible for determining donor suitability, blood collection, and laboratory processing and testing. In addition, it must provide blueprints and floor plans of the facility; descriptions of all equipment; indications of any other activities occurring in the facility; provisions for housekeeping, pest control, ventilation, lighting, and water systems; other occupants of the building; activity in adjacent buildings; record maintenance systems; validation of all systems; quality control/assurance programs; procedures for receipt and handling of raw materials; source of starting materials; methods and facilities for any chemical purification; inactivation or transfer steps; formulation and final product preparation; computer systems; and other miscellaneous information.

Along with the establishment license, the organization must file a product license application for each product it plans to produce in the facility. For whole blood and components, the product application involves basic information about the manufacturer (organization), facility, product, standard operating procedures, blood donor screening tests, frequency of donation, donor medical history, presence of a physician, phlebotomy supplies, venipuncture technique, collection technique, allowable storage period, storage conditions, disposal of contaminated units, supplies and reagents, label control processes, procedures for reissue of blood, and a brief summary of experience testing 500 samples. For the manufacture of plasma derivatives, the product license application involves the manufacturer's (organization's) name; the establishment name; procedures for determining donor suitability including medical history, examination by physician, laboratory testing, and methods of preparing the venipuncture site and collecting the plasma; methods to prevent circulatory embolism and to ensure return of red cells to the proper donor; minimum intervals between donation and maximum frequency of donation; techniques for immunizing donors; laboratory tests of collected plasma; techniques of preparing source plasma and storing it; methods to ensure proper storage conditions and identification of units; and label control systems and shipping conditions and procedures.

Other Required Licensure

Blood banks are subject to a number of other requirements or licensure systems in addition to the FDA. The Clinical Laboratories Improvement Act (CLIA) of 1988 established a new section of the Public Health Service Act that requires the Department of Health and Human Services (HHS) to establish certification requirements for any laboratory that performs tests on human specimens and to certify that those laboratories meet the requirements established by HHS. Laboratories participating in the Medicare and Medicaid programs or engaged in testing in interstate commerce must comply with these CLIA requirements. The law makes it possible for HHS to approve certain accreditation bodies and state licensure bodies. Because blood banks carry out testing on human material that is in interstate commerce, and because they provide services to Medicare and Medicaid patients, they must comply with CLIA. Several states also require that blood banks have a license to operate or provide blood in that state. These licenses usually involve a specific application and inspection.

Voluntary Accreditation of Blood Banks

The AABB operates a voluntary accreditation system in which most blood collection and transfusion organizations participate. The AABB Inspection and Accreditation (I&A) program, initiated in 1958, involves a biannual inspection by AABB volunteers. The major intent of the I&A program is to increase the safety in obtaining and transfusing human blood and components. The program is also designed to assist directors of blood banks and transfusion services to determine that knowledge, equipment, and the physical plant meet established requirements to detect deficiencies in practice and to provide consultation for their correction. The I&A program can be used to eliminate duplicate inspections by state governments. Currently the states of Connecticut,

Florida, Illinois, Maryland, Massachusetts, New Jersey, Tennessee, and Wisconsin accept AABB inspection of blood banks and transfusion services to satisfy their licensing requirements. The U.S. Armed Services and Humana, Inc., also maintain an equivalency program with the AABB. The AABB has established a coordinated inspection program with the College of American Pathologists (CAP) in which the CAP and AABB inspections are usually done simultaneously.

CAP Accreditation Program

The CAP, through its Hospital Laboratory Accreditation Program (HLAP), also certifies blood banks and thus involves hospital blood banks but not community blood centers. The LAP was initiated in 1961 with the primary objective of improving the quality of clinical laboratory services throughout the United States. The HLAP has grown considerably in size, complexity, and effectiveness since its inception, but the primary goal remains that of laboratory improvement through voluntary participation, professional peer review, education, and compliance with established performance standards. The CAP accredits approximately 4,300 laboratories throughout the United States, as well as several foreign countries.

The HLAP examines all aspects of quality control and quality assurance in the laboratory, including test methodologies, reagents, control media, equipment, specimen handling, procedure manuals, test reporting, and internal and external proficiency testing and monitoring, as well as personnel safety and overall management practices that distinguish a quality laboratory.

RECENT CHANGES IN THE U.S. BLOOD SUPPLY SYSTEM

Traditionally, blood centers had an organizational culture resembling the practice of medicine and operated somewhat like a clinical hospital laboratory.[17] This involved a patient orientation and individual decision-making for unique situations. Quality control programs were traditional and were designed to test a proportion of the final blood components to assess suitability. Decisions about test results and donor suitability were often individualized, much like patient decision-making. In the late 1980s, public concern about AIDS and blood safety continued to increase even though blood bank professionals believed that blood safety was being improved. As a result of this growing concern, Congress and the media began to increase pressure, and their expectations of blood banks changed. As part of this changing environment, in about 1990, the FDA began citing blood centers for violations of parts of the Code of Federal Regulations that had previously been applied only to the manufacture of pharmaceuticals.[16,18] There were also reports in the media about blood exporting and the financial structures of various blood organizations that cast the blood supply system and the organizations involved in a negative light. FDA citations and public concern mounted, and blood bank organizations began to respond. As a result, during the past decade, the blood collection system in the United States has undergone substantial change.[17] This has been driven primarily by external forces that developed in response to the AIDS epidemic.[18]

Major changes have been made in the medical criteria for selection of donors and in the laboratory testing of donated blood (see Chapters 4 and 8). In addition, more fundamental changes have been implemented in the nature of the organizations that make up the blood supply system. The organizations have adopted philosophies and organizational structures resembling those found in the pharmaceutical industry rather than the previous hospital laboratory and medical model.[17,19] The changes include (*a*) the development and implementation of modern quality assurance systems, (*b*) the introduction of good manufacturing practices like those used in the pharmaceutical industry, (*c*) the development of new computer systems that provide greater control over the manufacturing process, (*d*) the development of training programs designed to implement both the specific changes and also the new organizational philosophy, and (*e*) the revision of management structures to deal with the new kinds of activities and philosophy. The blood supply is safer than ever, and the organizations responsible for the supply use more contemporary practices to ensure its safety.

SUMMARY

In contrast to many other developed countries,[20] the United States does not have a national blood program or a single organization responsible for the nation's blood supply. Most of the supply of blood and components is provided by nonprofit community blood centers; about half is from the American Red Cross. Hospitals collect a small portion of the nation's blood supply. The demand for red cells has leveled off and may be declining, although the demand for platelets continues to increase. A separate set of for-profit organizations collect plasma, almost all of which comes from paid donors. This plasma is manufactured into plasma derivatives such as albumin or coagulation factor VIII that are sold in the national and international market by these for-profit corporations. As a result of the AIDS epidemic, the organizations that collect and provide the blood supply have introduced operations and organizational philosophies resembling those found in the pharmaceutical industry.

REFERENCES

1. Blood Policy & Technology. Washington, DC: Office of Technology Assessment, publication OTA-H-260, January 1985:51–75.
2. Blood Policy & Technology Summary. Washington, DC: Office of Technology Assessment, publication OTA-H-261, January 1985:1–41.
3. Scott EP. Foreword. In: MacPherson JL, ed. Adequacy of the Blood Supply. Proceedings from a national conference held February 18, 1990, sponsored by the American Blood Commission and the Council of Community Blood Centers, Clearwater, FL, August, 1990.
4. Forbes JM, Laurie ML. The Northfield Blood Collection Report. Community Blood Center Collections, 1988–1992. Evanston, IL: Northfield Laboratories, Inc., August 1993.
5. Wallace EL, Churchill WH, Surgenor DM, An J, Cho G, McGurk S, Murphy L. Collection and transfusion of blood and blood components in the United States, 1992. Transfusion 1995;35:802–812.
6. Surgenor D. Longitudinal studies of blood availability. In: Manning FJ, Sparacino L, eds. Forum on Blood Safety and Blood Availability. Blood donors and the supply of blood and blood products. Washington, DC: National Academy Press, 1996.

7. McCullough J. Blood supply fluctuations. In: Manning FJ, Sparacino L, eds. Forum on Blood Safety and Blood Availability. Blood donors and the supply of blood and blood products. Washington, DC: National Academy Press, 1996.

8. Scott EP. Why my blood center imports. In: MacPherson JL, ed. Adequacy of the Blood Supply. Proceedings from a national conference held February 18, 1990, sponsored by the American Blood Commission and the Council of Community Blood Centers, Clearwater, FL, August 1990: 7–12.

9. Anderson K. The economics of importing vs. collecting. In: MacPherson JL, ed. Adequacy of the Blood Supply. Proceedings from a national conference held February 18, 1990, sponsored by the American Blood Commission and the Council of Community Blood Centers, Clearwater, FL, August 1990: 35–37.

10. Bowman R, Clay M, Therkelsen D, et al. Donor attitudes about exporting and importing blood. Transfusion. 1997;37:913–930.

11. Cohn EJ, Oncley JL, Strong LE, Hughes WL Jr, Armstrong SH Jr. Chemical, clinical, and immunological studies on the products of human plasma fractionation. J Clin Invest 1944;23:417–606.

12. Code of Federal Regulations, Subchapter F, 640.60; 1992.

13. Reilly RW. Issues and trends affecting plasma selection for use in further manufacture: worldwide. J Clin Apheresis 1988;4:85–88.

14. Plasma and Plasma Products Industry Economics and Demographics. Annapolis, MD: American Blood Resources Association, 1994.

15. Blakestone MS. Fractionation. Plasmapheresis 1994;5:80.

16. Solomon JM. The evolution of the current blood banking regulatory climate. Transfusion 1994;34:272–277.

17. McCullough J. The continuing evolution of the nation's blood supply system. Am J Clin Pathol 1996;105:689–695.

18. McCullough J. The nation's changing blood supply system. JAMA 1993;269:2239–2245.

19. Zuck TF. Current good manufacturing practices. Transfusion 1995;35:955–966.

20. McCullough J. National blood programs in developed countries. Transfusion 1996;36:1019–1032.

THREE

RECRUITMENT OF BLOOD DONORS

The AIDS epidemic has heightened the concern about blood safety and greatly expanded the requirements for suitability for blood donation. The more stringent donor eligibility requirements (see Chapter 4) and more extensive laboratory testing (see Chapter 8) are excluding an increasing proportion of the population as potential donors. As pointed out in a recent American Association of Blood Banks Think Tank report,[1] as the population ages, blood donation may conflict with people's priorities; geographic and ethnic population shifts may influence blood donation; and the potential donor pool may shrink as a result of increased testing and other requirements. Thus, it is important to understand the motivations of donors and the psychosocial factors that lead to blood donation as a basis for formulating strategies to maintain or increase the number of available donors.

Because of the changes in donor eligibility requirements, concerns about blood safety, and the impact of the AIDS epidemic, it is likely that the characteristics of the donor population are continually shifting. Thus, specific data in this chapter about the demographics or characteristics of donors may not reflect the present situation.

DEMOGRAPHIC CHARACTERISTICS OF BLOOD DONORS

Although most Americans will require a blood transfusion at some time in their lives, less than 5% of the total population or less than 10% of those eligible to donate have ever done so.[2–4] Many donors give once or infrequently, and much of the nation's blood supply comes from a small number of dedicated and frequent donors.[2] Blood donors differ from the general population. A variety of demographic characteristics or other factors have been related to the likelihood of an individual being a blood donor. Some

of these characteristics include age, marital status, gender, educational experience, occupation, peer pressure, humanitarianism, fear of the unknown, apathy, self-esteem, race, social pressure, altruism, convenience, and community service.[2,5–7] These characteristics are described in more detail below.

Gender

There is a preponderance of females among first-time donors,[2,5] but with subsequent donations the ratio shifts to a male preponderance of 60% to 80%.[5,8] In a more recent study from four Red Cross blood centers, males accounted for 46% to 56% of donors, or an average of 52% in the four centers.[9] The greatest loss of female donors apparently occurs at about the fourth to eighth donation. In general, the larger the number of lifetime donations the greater the male preponderance.[8] It seems likely that the shift from female to male donors with increasing numbers of donations is a result of deferral of women in the childbearing age who become iron deficient from menstrual blood loss.[2]

Age

Most donors are 30 to 50 years old, with an average age between 33 and 38.[2,8,9] It appears that the age range of donors may have been shifting during the past few years. In studies mostly from the 1970s cited by Piliavin, only about 2% to 3% of donors were over 60 years of age, whereas in more recent studies 10% of donors were over age 60,[9] and 4% were more than 65 years of age.[8] Among multi-gallon donors, 12% were over 65 years of age.[8] This apparent "aging" of the donor population could reflect a shift in the population age in general; however, during the past few years blood bank professionals have recognized that blood donation is safe for older individuals, and donor age limits have therefore been extended to attract older donors (see Chapter 4).

Race

There are differences in the rate of donation by different ethnic groups. In 1975, whites were 48% more likely to have donated blood during the previous year than nonwhites.[2] By 1989, this figure had increased to 56%. More recent data or data for other ethnic or racial groups are not readily available. Among long-term donors, minority individuals are underrepresented.[8]

Education and Socioeconomic Characteristics

Blood donors tend to have more education and higher incomes than the general population. Piliavin[2] cites a study showing that donor's incomes were 30% higher than those of nondonors. In her own studies, she found those with some college education to be the most overrepresented group compared to nondonors. Lightman[10] found that 60% of blood donors in Toronto, Canada, had some post–high school education, compared to 20% for the entire city. Bowman et al.[9] found that 77% of their donors had some post–high school education, with a range of 60% to 80% in the different blood

centers participating in the study. In a separate study, 69% of all donors and 79% of multi-gallon donors had more than a high school education.[8]

Employment

In Bowman's study,[9] 80% of donors were employed full time and another 9% part time. Seven percent were retired, which is consistent with the 10% of donors who were 60 years old or older.

MOTIVATION OF WHOLE BLOOD DONORS

Psychosocial Theories Applicable to Blood Donation

Piliavin[2] discusses five psychosocial theories that might apply to blood donor motivation. These are (a) Becker's model of commitment, (b) the opponent process theory, (c) the attribution/self-perception framework, (d) the identity theory, and (e) the theory of reasoned action. These can be described briefly as summarized from Piliavin.[2]

In Becker's theory of commitment, the action or decision is based on background factors or preconceptions. These factors influence whether the person takes the initial action; the person is subsequently influenced by the first few experiences. In the opponent process theory, the stronger the negative feelings before the action, the stronger the positive feelings after successfully completing the action. Thus, despite initial fears or negative feelings, a good experience with donation could lead to a strongly positive attitude about continued donation despite very negative feelings before donation. The opponent process theory was developed to explain an involvement in various negative or potentially unpleasant activities. It attempts to account for the continuation of activities that were initially associated with negative feelings. The attribution theory postulates that if an individual believes that there is an external reason for the action, the action is attributed to that external force. In the identity theory, the sense of self is developed from the variety of social roles in which the individual engages. In the theory of reasoned action, the critical factor leading to an act is the development of an intention to carry out the act.

Integrated Model

Piliavin[2] believes that all five of the theories outlined above have some relevance to blood donation. The identity theory is thought to be "overarching" and that the "sense of self as donor is clearly the central factor among the personal determinants of donation." Becker's model applies to making the commitment to donate; the opponent-process and attribution theories relate to the development of a sense of the individual as a blood donor; and the theory of reasoned action is involved in translating the person's idea of himself or herself as a blood donor into action to donate. In integrating these theories, Piliavin[2] believes that the decision to donate is based on "childhood experience factors" negatively influenced by "pain and inconvenience" and positively influenced by "social pressures."

Giving and Not Giving

The reasons for donating are summarized generally[2] as (a) extrinsic rewards and incentives, (b) intrinsic rewards and incentives, (c) perceived community needs, (d) perceived community support, (e) social pressure, and (f) addiction to donation. The reasons for not donating include (a) medical ineligibility, (b) fear, (c) reactions and deferral (poor experiences), and (d) inconvenience and time requirements. Oswalt,[5] in reviewing 60 English-language reports regarding motivation for blood donation, concluded that the following factors were motivations to donate: (a) altruism and humanitarianism, (b) personal or family credit, (c) social pressure, (d) replacement, and (e) reward. Reasons for not donating included (a) fear, (b) medical excuses, (c) reactions, (d) apathy, and (e) inconvenience. Rados[11] also found that fear, inconvenience, and never being asked were the most common reasons given for not donating. In general, the issues described above have seemed to appear rather consistently in these and other studies[12] of donor motivation or nondonation. Because they have been consistent over time, most recruitment strategies attempt to take these factors into consideration.

THE DONATION EXPERIENCE AND FACTORS INFLUENCING CONTINUED DONATION

Although the first blood donation is anxiety producing, it is usually accompanied by good interactions with the donor staff and good feelings about the donation and oneself. Thus, most donors realize that they are reasonably able to give and plan to do so again.[2] With continued donation, the experience becomes easier and the reasons for continuing to donate become more "internal."[2]

Over time a "blood donor role" develops in repeat donors, and this strengthens self-commitment to blood donation, including "friendships contingent on donating, a self-description as a regular donor, an increase in the ranking of the blood donor role, greater expectations from others, and even more donations."[2]

Donors who are deferred are less likely to return to donate after the reason for the temporary deferral has passed.[2] This is not surprising, since deferral breaks the good feelings that might have developed about donation and makes future donation more difficult. Experiencing a reaction also reduces the likelihood of a donor returning.[2] This is because the donor begins to see himself or herself as someone who has trouble donating, and the reaction experience modifies any previous positive feelings about donation. Surprisingly, most multi-gallon donors report that they do not receive recognition for their donation, and the knowledge that a friend or relative was a blood donor did not make them more likely to donate.[8] These observations are consistent with the general view that the initial donation is motivated primarily by external factors and continued donation primarily by internal factors.[13]

Social Influences on Blood Donation

Because blood donation is not done in private, it is by definition a "social" act.[2] It is not surprising that social factors and issues have a strong influence on blood donation.

Social norms of the community affect donation behavior. For example, general publicity about blood donation in the community creates the perception that blood donation is an active part of the community, thus setting the stage for positive decisions by individuals to donate. This, along with "intrinsic" motivational appeals, builds a community norm for blood donation.

Family History of Donation or Blood Use

Blood donors are more likely to have had family members who were blood donors.[2] It is not clear whether blood use by a relative or close friend influences the likelihood that one will be a blood donor.[5]

The Donation Situation

Blood is collected in both fixed and mobile sites. Fixed sites are facilities that are permanently outfitted to serve as a blood donation center. These sites are usually within the blood center or hospital but may be in freestanding locations such as office buildings or shopping malls. The proportion of blood that is collected in fixed sites is not known. A very large portion of the U.S. blood supply is collected in mobile sites. A mobile site is a location that usually serves a purpose other than blood donation. At the mobile site, or "bloodmobile," all of the equipment and supplies necessary for blood collection are portable and are brought in for a few hours or days for the blood collection activity. These mobile sites are in many other kinds of settings, including offices, high schools, social clubs, churches, colleges, manufacturing companies, public buildings, or shopping malls. Donors at mobile sites are more likely to be first-time donors, giving under social pressure, and thus with less internal motivation to donate, and they are more likely to experience a reaction or less-than-optimal experience.[2] However, the influence that these settings have on the likelihood that an individual will donate or will have a good experience and be willing to donate again is not well understood. There are differences between those who donate at fixed sites and those who donate at mobile locations.[2] Donors at fixed sites report more internal motivation, whereas those at mobile sites report more external motivation. This would be consistent with the structure of mobile sites, which are usually arranged around a blood "drive" of some sort involving a community group or a particular need, thus providing the "external" motivation. At fixed sites, the donor is usually called by blood center staff and the donation scheduled as part of the general ongoing blood collection activity, but there is no relation to a particular community or social group or patient.

WHOLE BLOOD DONOR RECRUITMENT STRATEGIES

It is generally believed that the most effective way to get someone to donate blood is to ask directly and personally.[6,14] For instance, in one study comparing two recruitment techniques, the direct "foot in the door" approach was found to be superior to a general request to participate in a donor program.[15] When people were asked their reasons for not donating, the most common response was "no one ever asked."[6] The wide variety

of settings in which blood is collected may also affect an individual's willingness to donate. Different motivations may apply to donation in different settings, or the setting may influence an individual's willingness to donate. However, for either the fixed or mobile site, substantial efforts are made to specifically ask the individual to donate and, if possible, schedule the donation. This request may be made by paid staff of the donor organization or by volunteers. It is not clear whether either type of individual is more effective. Many blood centers with large donor programs have implemented computerized calling systems that integrate the donor files with the donor's history along with automated dialing systems to maximize the efficiency of the telephoning process.

Usually blood donors are asked to give to the general community blood supply. Sometimes donors are asked to donate blood for one or more specific patients. Newman et al.[16] found that these patient-related blood drives were easier to organize, produced more blood, and left the donors and staff with a stronger sense of satisfaction because of the more personal nature of the experience.

Very little structured social science research has been directed to the issue of minority involvement in the blood donation process. Some success in increasing blood donation by minorities has been achieved by involving more minority staff in the recruitment and blood donation process (Wingard M, quoted in reference 2). Compared to Hispanic nondonors, Hispanic donors were found to be better educated, to be more likely to speak English, to have higher job status, and to be more likely to have parents who were donors.[17] The study concluded that there is a need for improved education for Hispanic donors about the safety of blood donation. It was mentioned previously that the age of blood donors is probably increasing, not only because of the general aging of the population but also because of the extending of age limits for blood donation. As donation has been found to be safe and more older persons are donating, no unique recruitment strategies targeted to older donors have been implemented for that group.

Another issue in donor recruitment is whether to devote more effort to recruitment of new donors or to maintaining existing donors. New donors add to the overall files and replace donors inevitably lost due to attrition or disqualification. Thus, it is essential to replenish the donor pool. However, once people are in the donation habit, strategies to encourage them to continue result in the collection of substantial amounts of blood for less effort than is required to recruit new donors. Therefore, the dilemma is not in choosing only one of these strategies but in balancing the effort between them to maintain an adequate donor file but also to produce new donors with a reasonable amount of effort. A recent American Association of Blood Banks (AABB) Think Tank report[1] recommended that new strategies be developed for donor motivation to attract qualified new donors and retain previous donors, all of which could be facilitated if the major blood banking organizations could collaborate in blood donor recruitment campaigns.

ORGANIZATIONAL INFLUENCES

There are different types of organizations involved in collecting blood and providing the nation's blood supply (see Chapter 2). The different types of organizations may influence people's willingness to donate. This may be because different people prefer to

donate to particular organizations. Such preferences could be due to the nature of the organization or the individual donor's motivation. One major difference among organizations is hospital-based donor programs versus community-based freestanding blood centers. Because the community-based blood center serves multiple hospitals, the organization (and, by extension, a donation made to it) carries an image of service to the general medical community along with a feeling of community pride and allegiance. The nature of the community organization may also influence the individual's willingness to donate. About half of the blood collection in community centers is carried out by the American Red Cross. The other half of blood collection is performed by freestanding organizations whose mission is the provision of blood services. People's attitudes about the American Red Cross or the particular community blood organization could influence their willingness to donate. In contrast, a hospital-based program is associated with a specific medical center and can take advantage of the image of that center and its physicians, programs, and patients. Although there are no definitive studies, it seems likely that these factors influence the types of donors and their motivation for donating to different organizations. The differences between organizations involved may also affect the setting in which the blood is collected and thus may indirectly influence the donors or their motivation. For instance, hospital-based donor programs are more likely to use fixed sites for blood collection. While community-based blood centers use some fixed sites, they use mobile sites more extensively than hospital programs.

APHERESIS DONORS

During early phases of the development of cytapheresis, donors were usually friends or relatives of the patients or else they were staff members of the hospital or blood bank. For instance, in one of the first platelet donor programs (established at M.D. Anderson Hospital in 1963), there was no organized donor recruitment program.[18] Instead, the donors themselves as well as blood bank staff served as informal recruiters. Important factors motivating people to become donors in this program were the relationship with the donor center staff, knowledge of the specific patient's progress, and blood "credits" used to decrease the cost of blood components. As it became clear that cytapheresis would become a more widely used method of producing blood components and the procedures began to take a place in the more routine operation of blood centers and hospitals, attention was directed to more formal and structured donor recruitment programs. This raised considerations in addition to those for whole blood donors. The cytapheresis procedure is longer and thus requires more of a time commitment. In addition, the side effects, the nature of adverse reactions to donation, and the donor medical assessment were all different from whole blood donation. One of the important uses for cytapheresis is to provide HLA-matched platelets. This placed an additional responsibility on the donors and added the cost of HLA typing of the donors. Blood centers wished to have some assurance that the donors would actually donate before the blood center incurred the cost of HLA typing. Thus, the types of people to be approached about donation, the information they would be given, and the strategy to be used to obtain the best decision from the donor and potentially the highest acceptance rate became topics of great interest.

A key step in the development of cytapheresis donor programs was a conference that was held to address the scientific, legal, and ethical issues.[19] Issues such as the cost-effectiveness of platelet transfusion, individual rights, informed consent, donor decision-making mechanisms, and personal autonomy were discussed in the context of plateletpheresis donation. The results of this conference formed a sound basis for the development of cytapheresis donor programs. Because of the additional burden of cytapheresis donation, frequent whole blood donors were selected as possible cytapheresis donors. A number of efforts developed simultaneously. In Seattle, recruitment efforts were targeted to repeat whole blood donors; the provision of informational materials was often sufficient to attract them into cytapheresis donation.[20] These early cytapheresis donors were predominantly female and older than whole blood donors. Most remained dedicated to the program; those who dropped out did so primarily because of logistical issues.[20] In a detailed psychosocial evaluation of 20 donors in an active program, Szymanski et al.[21] found that the donors had a strong drive to achieve but also had low self-esteem and that donation strengthened their self-esteem and made them feel more worthy. Thus, the platelet donation was not only an altruistic act of giving, but it also filled some personal needs of the individual. Recently the recruitment of cytapheresis donors has come full circle: initially, plateletpheresis donors were recruited for marrow donation, but now individuals who have agreed to be marrow donors for transplantation are being recruited as new cytapheresis donors.[22]

BONE MARROW DONORS

With increasing use of bone marrow transplantation to treat a wider variety of diseases and with the success of the treatment improving, the lack of a suitable family donor for most patients became a major limitation in the availability of this treatment. Until the late 1970s, it was believed that the requirement for histocompatibility between the donor and recipient precluded the use of volunteer donors not related to the patient. Then in dramatic fashion, a successful transplant was carried out using marrow donated by a volunteer not related to the patient.[23] This opened the urgent need for large numbers of HLA-typed individuals who would be willing to donate marrow. A remarkable story unfolded, resulting in the establishment of the National Marrow Donor Program.[24]

Initially it was believed that it might be improper or even unethical to ask volunteers unrelated to the patient to donate marrow. The risks of donation, the discomfort, the nature of the patient's preparation for the transplant, and lethal consequences of withdrawal by the donor all contributed to an atmosphere in which this kind of donation seemed unlikely. However, the possibility was pursued in a small number of centers—primarily the University of Iowa, the American Red Cross Blood Center in St. Paul, Minnesota (in collaboration with the University of Minnesota), and the Blood Center of Southeastern Wisconsin. One of the major first steps was a conference sponsored by the University of Minnesota at which the legal, ethical, social, financial, and practical issues in unrelated volunteer marrow donation were discussed.[25] The involvement of the two community blood centers added strength at this early stage because they were separate from the transplant centers and also because of the involvement of representa-

tives of the general community as part of their governing boards. As these organizations began to consider establishing a marrow donor program, the results of the conference strengthened the belief that there were proper ways to inform people of the opportunity and the consequences of donation and to provide the opportunity to become a donor if desired.[25] The initial ethical principles involved respect for life, promotion of good, prevention of harm, justice, fairness, truth-telling, and individual freedom.[25]

Because of the extensive commitment required of donors it was decided to approach multi-gallon blood donors and apheresis donors.[26] This had the added benefit that most were already apheresis donors who had been HLA typed, and this avoided the cost of additional HLA typing. The "recruitment" involved providing an extensive description of marrow transplantation, the situations in which it was used, the results of transplantation including actual survival statistics, the marrow donation process, and the steps that would lead up to marrow donation. A donor advocate was made available to each donor, and the potential donor received a physical examination by a physician uninvolved with the transplant program or the donor center. That physician then served as the medical advisor to the potential donor. The recruitment process drew heavily on the considerable experience of sociological studies of families making the decision to donate an organ either to a relative or for cadaver transplantation.[27,28] The informed consent process was given very heavy weight in the recruitment process.[26] Remarkably, almost three-fourths of the Minnesota donors who were provided an extensive description of the marrow donor program elected to participate.[26] Similar experience emerged from the Blood Center of Southeastern Wisconsin, where 81% of 763 previously HLA-typed donors agreed to participate in a marrow donor program.[29] In the Minnesota study, the demographics of those who elected to participate were not different from those who declined. Important factors in the donor's decision whether or not to participate in the program were religion, experience with the medical system, and the spouse's attitude regarding marrow donation.[26]

At about this time, marrow registries were being established in Europe and by families of patients who were unable to obtain a transplant because of the lack of a family donor. Pressure grew to expand the small U.S. registries that had established the practicality of this kind of donation and to develop some method to integrate the search process among the operating registries. To evaluate this situation, a consensus conference was sponsored by the National Institutes of Health. The key recommendations were to continue to evaluate the effectiveness of small registries but that no large-scale national effort was appropriate.[30] In a remarkable political turn of events, Dr. Robert Graves, a Colorado rancher and veterinarian whose daughter received the first unrelated-donor transplant, convinced the Congress to provide funds for the U.S. Navy to establish contract marrow donor centers and a coordinating center. This became the National Marrow Donor Program.[24]

As experience with marrow donation by unrelated volunteers increased, it became apparent that although there are complications of marrow donation, the donation process and its consequences were well tolerated and accepted by donors.[31] The limitations of cytapheresis donors as marrow donors soon became evident, as the need for donors mushroomed far beyond the number of available cytapheresis donors. Thus, donor recruitment efforts were expanded to the general public. Initially, there was con-

cern that people who had never donated blood would not be sufficiently well informed or willing to make the necessary commitment. These fears were rapidly proven to be unfounded. General community appeals for donors resulted in the recruitment of donors who became as committed to the program as the cytapheresis donors.[32,33] The national marrow donor file has now grown to more than 2 million volunteers in the United States and many more worldwide. The extensive experience with marrow donation establishes the effectiveness of the recruitment process and the lifesaving impact of the therapy on patients.[34]

REFERENCES

1. Malloy D, McDonough B, Fuller M. A look to the future of blood banking and transfusion medicine: report from an American Association of Blood Banks Foundation Managerial Think Tank. Transfusion 1991;31:450–463.
2. Piliavin JA, Callero PL, eds. Giving Blood. The development of an altruistic identity. Baltimore, MD: Johns Hopkins University Press, 1991.
3. Communications strategy for public education for the National Blood Resource Education Program, National Institutes of Health. Washington, DC: US Department of Health and Human Services, 1990.
4. Linden JV, Gregorio DI, Kalish RI. An estimate of blood donor eligibility in the general population. Vox Sang 1988;54:96–100.
5. Oswalt RM. A review of blood donor motivation and recruitment. Transfusion 1977;17:123–135.
6. Drake AW, Finkelstein SN, Sopolsky HM. The American Blood Supply. Cambridge, MA: MIT Press, 1982.
7. Burnett JJ. Examining the profiles of the donor and nondonor through a multiple discriminant approach. Transfusion 1982;22:138–142.
8. Royse D, Doochin KE. Multi-gallon blood donors: who are they? Transfusion 1995;35:826–831.
9. Bowman R, Clay M, Therkelsen D, et al. Donor attitudes about exporting and importing blood. Transfusion. In press.
10. Lightman ES. Continuity in social policy behaviors: the voluntary blood donorship. J Soc Policy 1982;10:53–70.
11. Rados DL. How donors and nondonors view people who do not give blood. Transfusion 1977;17:221–224.
12. Boe GP, Ponder LD. Blood donors and non-donors: a review of the research. Am J Med Tech 1981;47:248–253.
13. Gardner WL, Cacioppo JT. Multi-gallon blood donors: why do they give? Transfusion 1995;35:795–798.
14. Jason LA, Rose T, Ferrari JR, Barone R. Personal versus impersonal methods for recruiting blood donations. J Soc Psychol 1984;123:139–140.
15. Hayes TJ, Dwyer FR, Greenwalt TJ. Coe NA. A comparison of two behavioral influence techniques for improving blood donor recruitment. Transfusion 1984;24:399–403.
16. Newman BH, Burak FQ, McKay-Peters E, Pothiawala MA. Patient-related blood drives. Transfusion 1988;28:142–144.
17. Thompson WW. Blood donation behavior of Hispanics in the lower Rio Grande Valley. Transfusion 1993;33:333–335.
18. Wendlandt GM, Lichtiger B. A highly specialized and motivated volunteer population: platelet donors. Transfusion 1977;17:218–220.
19. Wieckowicz M. Single donor platelet transfusions: scientific, legal, and ethical considerations. Transfusion 1976;16:193–199.
20. Meyer DM, Hillman RS, Slichter SJ. Plateletapheresis program. I. Donor recruitment and commitment. Transfusion 1984;24:287–291.

21. Szymanski LS, Cushna B, Jackson BCH, Szymanski IO. Motivation of plateletpheresis donors. Transfusion 1978;18:64–68.
22. Bolgiano DC, Smith S, Slichter SJ. Strategies to recruit plateletpheresis donors from a registry of HLA-typed, unrelated, bone marrow donors. Transfusion 1993;33:675–678.
23. Hansen JA, Clift RA, Thomas ED, Buckner CD, Storb R, Giblett ER. Transplantation of marrow from an unrelated donor to a patient with acute leukemia. N Engl J Med 1980;303:565–567.
24. Stroncek D, Bartsch G, Perkins HA, et al. The National Marrow Donor Program. Transfusion 1993;33:567–577.
25. McCullough J, Bach FH, Coccia P, et al. Bone marrow transplantation from unrelated volunteer donors: summary of a conference on scientific, ethical, legal, financial, and other practical issues. Transfusion 1982;22:78–81.
26. McCullough J, Rogers G, Dahl R, et al. Development and operation of a program to obtain volunteer bone marrow donors unrelated to the patient. Transfusion 1986;26:315–323.
27. Simmons RG. Related donors: costs and gains. Transplant Proc 1977;9:143–145.
28. Kamstra-Hennen L, Beebe J, Stumm S, Simmons RG. Ethical evaluation of related donation: the donor after five years. Transplant Proc 1981;13:60–61.
29. McElligott MC, Menitove JE, Aster RH. Recruitment of unrelated persons as bone marrow donors—a preliminary experience. Transfusion 1986;26:309–314.
30. Leventhal BG, chairman. Should a national bone marrow donor registry be established? In: Technology Assessment Meeting Statement: Donor registries for bone marrow transplantation, May 13–15, 1985. Bethesda, MD: National Institutes of Health, 1985:6–8.
31. Stroncek D, Strand R, Scott E, et al. Attitudes and physical condition of unrelated bone marrow donors immediately after donation. Transfusion 1989;29:317–322.
32. Stroncek D, Strand R, Hofkes C, McCullough J. The changing activities of a regional marrow donor program. Transfusion 1994;34:58–62.
33. Stroncek DF, Strand RD, Hofkes CL, McCullough J. Comparison of the effectiveness of potential marrow donors recruited from apheresis donors or whole blood donors and through appeals to the general public. Transfusion 1991;31:138–141.
34. Stroncek DF, Holland PV, Bartch G, et al. Experiences of the first 493 unrelated marrow donors in the National Marrow Donor Program. Blood 1993;81:1940–1946.

FOUR

BLOOD DONOR MEDICAL ASSESSMENT AND BLOOD COLLECTION

A crucial feature of the recruitment of blood donors to make subsequent donations is the experience donors have at each donation. Thus, it is important that the blood collection staff provide a warm, friendly, professional, and efficient environment in which the medical assessment and blood donation can take place. This experience involves the facilities, the professionalism of the staff, and the social interaction between the donor and the staff.

Because blood is considered to be a drug and is regulated under U.S. Food and Drug Administration (FDA) law, most aspects of the selection of potential donors and the collection of blood are carried out under requirements established by the FDA. This chapter attempts to provide concepts and rationale for blood donor assessment and blood collection and does not refer to every specific FDA requirement. It should be understood, however, that all of these activities must conform to FDA requirements, which can be found in the Code of Federal Regulations and various FDA guidelines. For blood banks that desire accreditation by the American Association of Blood Banks, the standards of that organization must also be followed. The Technical Manual of the American Association of Blood Banks[1] is an excellent reference that provides details for much of the content of this chapter.

MEDICAL ASSESSMENT OF WHOLE BLOOD DONORS

The approach to the selection of blood donors is designed around two themes: to ensure the safety of the donor and to obtain a high-quality blood component that is as safe as possible for the recipient. Some particular steps that are taken to ensure that blood is as safe as possible are (*a*) using only volunteer blood donors, (*b*) questioning donors about

their general health before their donation is scheduled, (c) obtaining a medical history before donation, (d) conducting a physical examination before donation, (e) conducting laboratory testing of donated blood, (f) checking the donor's identity against a donor deferral registry, and (g) providing a method by which after donation the donor can confidentially designate the unit as unsuitable for transfusion.

Registration

When the donor initially presents at the donation site, identifying information is obtained for the permanent record. This includes name, address, telephone number, birth date, social security number (if allowed in that state), and previous donation history including any names under which previous donations might have been made. Individuals may donate no more often than every 56 days to prevent iron depletion. At the time of registration, the prospective donor is given information about blood donation, transmissible disease testing, and factors or behavior that would preclude blood donation. Information may also describe the agencies that are notified in the event of a positive test result for a transmissible disease. While obtaining the medical history, a staff member asks the donor questions about these factors and describes the risk behavior for HIV infection. It is required that the identity of each donor be checked against a registry of individuals known to be unacceptable as blood donors.[2] It is assumed that people have no reason to donate blood under false names, and so this questioning is done primarily to identify women whose name may have changed due to marriage. Some blood banks do this "donor deferral registry" check at the time of registration to avoid collecting blood from anyone on the registry, and other blood banks carry out this check at the blood center later before the unit of collected blood is made available for distribution. Either a paper or computerized deferral registry may be used depending on the preference of the particular blood bank. Although this process is required by the FDA and is widely used throughout the United States, there has never been a thorough study to establish its value. During the registration, the use of the "confidential unit exclusion" (CUE) is also described (see below).

For many years people were deferred from donating blood after 65 years of age. However, as the population has aged, with many more people living active, healthy lives well beyond their 65th year, the arbitrary use of an age limit for blood donation has been reexamined. In one study of 244 healthy volunteers age 63 or older, the donors were found to have more medical conditions and medications than younger donors but did not experience more adverse reactions to donation.[3] In a separate study of more than 600 donors between ages 66 and 78, the incidence of adverse reactions was no greater in the elderly donors than in donors under age 66.[4] Elderly donors have slightly decreased iron stores,[5] but these donors can safely contribute to the nation's blood supply but should do so no more often than four times per year. In an accompanying editorial, Schmidt[6] points out that "blood donation by the healthy adult is remarkably safe and data show that this is true well into old age." Thus, most blood centers do not have a specific upper age limit for blood donors but evaluate donors on an individual basis. The lower age limit for blood donation is usually 17 years. Most states have passed laws that allow donation at this age even though it is below the age of 18 at which individu-

als can take legal responsibility for their actions. These special laws dealing with blood donation are intended to enable high school students to donate without obtaining parental consent.

Medical History

The medical history is an extremely important part of the selection of donors because it can reveal reasons why donation might not be wise for the donor or reasons why the donor's blood might constitute an increased risk for the patient. The interview usually takes about 10 minutes. In addition to specific questions, the interviewer attempts to establish some rapport with the potential donor and to make an assessment of the donor's general condition. This is important to establish that the donor is in good general health, is not under the influence of drugs, and is able to give informed consent for the donation. The interview must be conducted in a setting that provides privacy for the donor. While complete visual privacy is not always possible, visual distractions must be minimized and the donor's answers must not be audible to others. The interview consists of some questions that the donor answers in writing and some verbal responses to questions asked by the interviewer. Several different ways of seeking information from the donor have been used. These include different kinds of brochures, videos, and direct questioning. In studies comparing these approaches, direct questioning elicits the most accurate information.[7,8] The nature of these sex-related questions is very specific, and the act of directly questioning the donor about these behaviors has certainly changed the interaction and relationship between the donor and the blood bank.[9]

During the past few years, the medical history has increased in length and complexity, and certain questions have been added that deal with very sensitive issues. A complete list of the questions is provided in Table 4.1. The questions designed to protect the safety of the donor include those regarding age and medications and whether the donor is under the care of a physician or has a history of cardiovascular or lung disease, seizures, present or recent pregnancy, recent donation of blood or plasma, recent major illness or surgery, unexplained weight loss, or unusual bleeding. Questions designed to protect the safety of the recipient include those related to the donor's general health; the presence of a bleeding disorder; receipt of growth hormone; exposure to or history of jaundice, liver disease, hepatitis, AIDS (or symptoms of AIDS), Chagas' disease, or babesiosis; the injection of drugs; receipt of coagulation factor concentrates, blood transfusion, a tattoo, acupuncture, ear piercing, or an organ or tissue transplant; travel to areas endemic for malaria; recent immunizations; contact with persons with hepatitis or other transmissible diseases; ingestion of medications especially aspirin; presence of a major illness or surgery; or previous notice of a positive test for a transmissible disease. In addition, there are several questions related to AIDS risk behavior. These include whether the potential donor has had sex with anyone with AIDS, given or received money or drugs for sex, had sex with another male (for males), or had sex with a male who has had sex with another male (for females).

The medical history is an extremely effective part of ensuring the safety of the blood supply. For instance, the implementation of questions about behavior that would put potential donors at risk for HIV infection decreased the HIV infectivity of blood in

Table 4.1 Blood donor medical history questions

HAVE YOU EVER:

1. Given blood under a different name?
2. Been refused as a blood donor or told not to donate blood?
3. Had chest pain, heart disease, or lung disease?
4. Had cancer, convulsions, a blood disease, or a bleeding problem?
5. Been given growth hormone or taken Tegison for psoriasis?
6. Had Chagas' disease or babesiosis?
7. Had yellow jaundice, liver disease, hepatitis, or a positive test for hepatitis?
8. Had AIDS or a positive test for the AIDS virus; had sex, even once, with anyone who has?
9. Used a needle, even once, to take any drug (including steroids)?
10. Taken clotting factor concentrates for a bleeding problem, such as hemophilia?
11. At any time since 1977 taken money or drugs for sex?
12. MALE DONORS: Had sex with another male, even once, since 1977?

IN THE LAST 3 YEARS, HAVE YOU:

1. Had malaria or been outside the United States or Canada?

IN THE LAST 12 MONTHS, HAVE YOU:

1. Received blood or had an organ or tissue transplant?
2. Had a tattoo, ear or skin piercing, acupuncture, or an accidental needle stick?
3. Had close contact with a person with yellow jaundice or hepatitis, or have you been given hepatitis B immune globulin (HBIG)?
4. Had or been treated for syphilis or gonorrhea or had a positive test for syphilis?
5. Given money or drugs to anyone to have sex with you?
6. Had sex with anyone who has ever taken money or drugs for sex?
7. Had sex with anyone who used a needle, even once, to take any drug (including steroids)?
8. Had sex with anyone who has taken clotting factor concentrates for a bleeding problem, such as hemophilia?
9. Been in jail for more than 72 consecutive hours?
10. Been under a doctor's care, had a chronic or major illness, or had surgery?
11. Had any shots or vaccinations?
12. FEMALE DONORS: Had sex with a male who has had sex even once since 1977 with another male?

HAVE YOU:

1. Given blood, plasma, or platelets in the last 8 weeks?
2. FEMALE DONORS: Been pregnant in the last 6 weeks, or are you pregnant now?
3. Taken any pills, medications, Accutane, or Proscar in the last 30 days?
4. Taken piroxicam (Feldene), aspirin, or anything that has aspirin in it in the last 3 days?
5. Do you understand that if you have the AIDS virus, you can give it to someone else even though you may feel well and have a negative AIDS test?
6. Do you have a blood relative who has Creutzfeldt-Jakob disease (CJD), or have you ever had a dura mater transplant?
7. Are you giving blood because you want to be tested for AIDS?
8. Are you feeling well and healthy today?
9. Have you had a recent weight loss of 10 pounds or more that you can't explain?
10. My present weight is _____ lb.

the San Francisco Bay area by 90% even before the use of the HIV screening test.[10] One concern has been that people who have engaged in high-risk behavior might seek to donate blood to obtain a test for HIV. In some situations this seems to be true. Of 30 HIV-positive blood donors in Paris, 47% had known risk behaviors and 50% admitted to having donated to obtain a test for HIV.[11] In a larger study of HIV-seropositive blood donors, the reasons for donation in spite of having participated in behavior that placed them at risk of HIV infection were failure to read carefully or comprehend the deferral information, group pressure, a desire to be tested, and belief that the testing would identify any infected blood.[12]

Occasionally, situations arise in which the donor's physician believes that donation would be safe, but the blood bank does not accept the donor. For instance, because the genesis of malignant disease is not known, donors with a history of cancer (other than minor skin cancer or carcinoma in situ of the cervix) are usually deferred, even though it is not expected that transfusion of blood from these donors would transmit cancer. Some medications may make the individual unsuitable as a blood donor because of the condition requiring the medication, while other medications may be potentially harmful to the recipient. Often the potential donor's physician is not aware of the impact some medications may have on donated blood and thus advises the individual that he or she could donate blood. Many other conditions must be evaluated individually by the blood bank physician, whose assessment of conformance with FDA regulations— which consider blood a pharmaceutical—may not always coincide with another physician's view of the health of the potential donor.

Physical Examination of the Blood Donor

The physical examination of a potential donor does not involve disrobing and a general physical examination as might occur in a physician's office. The blood donor physical examination includes determination of the potential donor's temperature, pulse, blood pressure, weight, and hemoglobin. Each of these has FDA-mandated limits. In addition, the donor's general appearance and behavior are assessed for any signs of illness or the influence of drugs or alcohol. The skin at the venipuncture site is examined for signs of intravenous drug abuse, lesions suggestive of Kaposi's sarcoma, and local lesions that might make it difficult to cleanse the skin and thus lead to contamination of the blood unit during venipuncture.

There are weight requirements for donors because it is necessary to balance the amount of blood collected in relation to the donor's estimated blood volume and also the amount of blood in relation to the volume of anticoagulant in the collection container. It is preferable to collect no more than 15% of the donor's estimated blood volume. In addition, the volume of blood in the container should be between 405 and 495 mL (that is, 450 mL $\pm 10\%$). Thus, including specimens for testing, the amount of blood drawn could total 525 mL. Units containing 300 to 404 mL can be used for transfusion but must be labeled as low-volume units. If the volume is less than 300 mL, some of the anticoagulant must be removed to maintain the proper ratio of blood to anticoagulant and avoid hemolysis. To integrate the volumes of blood needed in the container

with the weight ranges of donors, an arbitrary lower weight limit of 110 lb has been established. There is no upper weight limit, although extremely obese potential donors may have other health problems or inadequate venous access precluding donation. The pulse should be regular and between 50 and 100 per minute, although potential donors who have a slower pulse due to involvement in an active exercise program may donate with approval of the transfusion medicine physician.

The hemoglobin is usually tested by a screening method in which a drop of blood is placed in a copper sulfate solution of a known specific gravity so that the falling of the blood drop within the solution indicates an adequate hemoglobin content. The blood drop can be obtained from the finger, but many blood banks obtain the blood from an earlobe puncture. There has been some debate about the use of the earlobe site but it is generally accepted. If the hemoglobin screening test indicates a hemoglobin level below that required for donation, usually a microhematocrit is performed. The minimum acceptable hemoglobin for women is lower (12.5 g/dL) than that for men (13.5 g/dL) because of the normally lower hemoglobin values in women. Apparently the hemoglobin fluctuates with temperature, being lower in hot weather. This may lead to an increase in deferrals due to low hemoglobin during the summer months.[13]

Special Blood Donations

There are several situations involving blood donation in which the blood may be collected by the donor center but will not be used as part of the community's general blood supply. Examples of these include autologous donation, directed donation, patient-specific donation, and therapeutic bleeding. In some of these situations the FDA requirements for blood donation may not apply. These situations are described in Chapter 6.

COLLECTION OF WHOLE BLOOD

The time during blood collection provides another opportunity for the blood center staff to interact with the donor to reinforce the professionalism and set the stage for the donor's willingness to return for subsequent donations. In a way this becomes the first step in the recruitment of the donor for the next donation (see Chapter 3).

Labeling

The first step in the collection process is labeling of all containers, tubes, and related materials. This is an extremely important step because it relates all tubes, specimens, documents, and components to the identity of the donor. Virtually all blood banks use bar-coded labels, and much of the subsequent tracking of specimens, test results, and individual components is done by computers using these labels. Computer systems are generally used to accumulate all data relevant to the individual donation to determine whether the components are suitable for transfusion and can be released into usable inventory. Thus, there are detailed and specific steps in the process at the donor bedside to ensure the accuracy of all materials.

Blood Containers

Blood must be collected into FDA-licensed containers, each of which is sterile and can be used only once. The containers are made of plasticized material that is biocompatible with blood cells and allows diffusion of gases to provide optimal cell preservation (see Chapter 5). These blood containers are combinations of multiple bags connected by tubing so that components can be transferred between bags without being exposed to air. This is referred to as a "closed system." This system of separation of the whole blood into its components in a closed system thus minimizes the chance of bacterial contamination while making it possible to store each component under the conditions and length of time that are optimum for that component. Whole blood is almost never used today; essentially all blood is separated within 6 hours of collection into red cells, platelets, plasma, and sometimes cryoprecipitate (see Chapter 5). This separation of blood into its components maximizes the use of the whole blood by making specific components available for specific clinical situations and enabling each component to be stored under the conditions optimal for that component (see Chapters 5, 11, and 12).

Anticoagulant Preservative Solutions

Several anticoagulant preservative solutions are available. The anticoagulants are various formulas of citrate solutions. The blood may be stored in these solutions and used for transfusion, or most of the supernatant may be removed and the cells stored in other "additive" solutions. The composition and effects of these anticoagulant and preservative solutions are discussed more completely in Chapter 5.

Selection of the Vein and Preparation of the Venipuncture Site

Blood is drawn from a vein in the antecubital fossa. The vein selected should be large enough to accommodate a 16 gauge needle. Careful selection of the vein makes the venipuncture quick and easy, thus providing good blood flow and a quality component but also minimizing the discomfort to the donor and making the donation experience as pleasant as possible. The choice of the vein will also minimize the likelihood of inadvertently damaging a nerve or puncturing an artery (see section on Adverse Reactions to Donation). A blood pressure cuff is usually used to impede venous return and distend the vein.

To minimize the chance of bacterial contamination, the blood must be drawn from an area free of skin lesions, and the phlebotomy site must be properly cleansed. It is not possible to sterilize the skin, but steps are taken to greatly reduce the level of skin flora. This essentially involves scrubbing with a soap solution, followed by tincture of iodine or iodophor complex solution. The selection of the venipuncture site and its sterilization are very important steps since bacterial contamination of blood can be a serious, even fatal complication of transfusion.[14,15]

Venipuncture

Most blood collection equipment uses 16 gauge needles, and the entire set is closed and connected so that the needle is integral. The venipuncture is done with a needle that can

be used only once so as to avoid contamination. Most phlebotomists use a two-step process in which the needle first penetrates the skin, then after a brief pause the needle is inserted into the vein. The pause is so brief that it may not be noticeable to the donor. The phlebotomist must be aware of the needle placement to minimize the likelihood of puncturing a nerve or artery.

Blood Collection

Usually the blood container is placed on a scale, which may have a device to cut off the flow when the container reaches a set weight indicating that the desired volume of blood has been collected. The blood must flow freely and be mixed with anticoagulant frequently as it fills the container to avoid the development of small clots. The actual time for phlebotomy and bleeding is usually about 7 minutes and almost always less than 10 minutes. If the blood flow is slow, clots may form in the tubing before the blood mixes with the anticoagulant in the container. Although there is no FDA-defined maximum allowable time for the collection of a unit of blood, most blood banks establish a maximum. This is usually no more than about 15 minutes. There is no difference in factor VIII or platelet recovery between units collected in less than 8 minutes versus those collected in 8 to 12 minutes.[16] Extremely rapid blood flow or the appearance of bright red blood may indicate an arterial puncture. This can be confirmed by feeling the pressure building in the blood container. An arterial puncture is nearly unmistakable because of the very rapid filling and pressure that develops in the blood container.

During blood donation, there is a slight decrease in systolic and a rise in diastolic blood pressure and peripheral resistance along with a slight fall in cardiac output but little change in heart rate.[17] FDA regulations allow withdrawal of 450 mL ± 10% of whole blood. This is mixed with 63 mL of anticoagulant composed of citrate, phosphate, and dextrose (CPD). The amount of blood withdrawn must be within prescribed limits to be in the proper ratio with the anticoagulant, otherwise the blood cells may be damaged or anticoagulation may not be satisfactory (see Chapter 5).

At the conclusion of blood collection, the needle is removed and the donor is asked to apply pressure to the vein in the antecubital fossa for at least 1 or 2 minutes. Many blood centers have a policy of asking the donor to raise his or her arm to minimize the venous pressure while pressure is applied to the vein. When there is no bleeding, discoloration, or evidence of a hematoma at the venipuncture site, the donor should be evaluated for other symptoms of a reaction to donation. If none are present, the donor can move off the donor table to the refreshment area. The donor should be observed during this time, as the movement into an upright posture may bring on lightheadedness or even fainting. Donors should also be observed while having a postdonation refreshment, because some lightheadedness may develop during that time.

CONFIDENTIAL UNIT EXCLUSION (CUE)

The medical history is designed to identify potential donors who have engaged in behavior that places them at risk of HIV infection. However, some donors may be unwilling to admit to these behaviors when questioned directly by the interviewer, or

the donor may be under peer pressure to donate and be unable or unwilling to explain the reason for deferral if the questions are answered truthfully. Thus, a system was developed to enable donors to complete the donation process but ensure that their blood would not be used for transfusion. While transfusion medicine professionals would prefer that potential donors answer the questions honestly, it is recognized that this may not always occur. The system was established not to encourage dishonesty but to respond to situations in which donors may not provide all of the desired information to the donor center.

The confidential unit exclusion is a process in which the donor is provided an opportunity after completing the blood donation to indicate that the blood should not be used for transfusion. All donors must make a designation of whether their blood is to be used for transfusion. These designations are done using a bar code that is readable only by computer, so it is impossible for anyone to know the designation that has been made. Since everyone makes a designation and the choice is legible only to the computer, the donor can confidentially ensure that the unit will not be used for transfusion if the donor has reason to believe that he or she might be at risk for HIV infection. When the unit is designated not for transfusion, it still undergoes the same testing as units intended for transfusion. This has made it possible to determine the incidence of HIV seropositivity in blood designated not for transfusion compared to the general donor population.

POSTDONATION CARE AND ADVERSE REACTIONS TO BLOOD DONATION

Postdonation Care

Donors are advised to drink extra fluids to replace lost blood volume. The nature of the fluid is not as important as consuming some fluid, except that alcoholic beverages are not recommended. The consumption of fluids helps to restore stamina and minimize the postural hypotension that may occur for several hours after donation. Alcohol is a vasodilator and may cause a shift of blood flow to the periphery, resulting in reduced cerebral blood flow and hypotension or fainting. Even after the loss of a few hundred milliliters of blood, some donors are subject to lightheadedness or even fainting if they change position quickly. Therefore, donors are also advised not to return to work for the remainder of the day in an occupation where fainting would be hazardous to themselves or others. Donors are also advised to avoid strenuous exercise for the remainder of the day of donation. This minimizes the chance of development of a hematoma at the venipuncture site and the chance of fainting due to diversion of blood from the central nervous system into peripheral vasculature.

Adverse Reactions

A reaction occurs following approximately 4% of blood donations, but fortunately most reactions are not serious.[18,19] Minimizing donor reactions begins with the selection of the site for blood collection, the staff training, the general treatment the donor receives

Table 4.2 Adverse reactions to whole blood donation

Hypovolemia	Syncope
	Lightheadedness
	Diaphoresis
	Nausea
	Vomiting
Vasovagal effects	Syncope
	Bradycardia
	Diaphoresis
	Pallor
Venipuncture	Hematoma
	Nerve injury
	Local infection
	Thrombophlebitis

from the staff, and the ambiance of the blood collection situation. These factors are important, because reactions increase when the blood collection situation is crowded, noisy, or hot or when the donor endures a long wait.[20] Donors who have reactions are more likely to be younger, to be unmarried, to have a higher pre-donation heart rate and lower diastolic blood pressure, and to be first-time donors or to have donated fewer times than donors who do not experience reactions.[21]

Adverse reactions to blood donation can be categorized generally as those due to (a) hypovolemia, (b) vasovagal effects, and (c) complications of the venipuncture (Table 4.2). The most common symptoms of reaction to blood donation are weakness, cool skin, diaphoresis, and pallor. A more extensive but still moderate reaction may involve dizziness, pallor, hypertension, hypotension, and/or bradycardia. Bradycardia is usually taken as a sign of a vasovagal reaction rather than hypotensive or cardiovascular shock, in which tachycardia would be expected. In a more severe form, the reaction may progress to loss of consciousness, convulsions, and involuntary passage of urine or stool. The most common cause of these symptoms is thought to be a vasovagal reaction to the psychological stress of the situation or to neurologic factors rather than hypovolemia due to loss of blood volume. In the past a common response to a donor reaction was to have the donor rebreathe into a paper bag. This is effective only if the lightheadedness is due to hyperventilation and reduced bicarbonate levels. Actually, most reactions do not have this basis and the paper bag may only add to the tension of the situation. This is not recommended as routine practice but should be reserved for situations in which it seems clear that hyperventilation is a major part of the reaction. Other systemic reactions may include nausea, vomiting, and hyperventilation, sometimes leading to twitching or muscle spasms, convulsions, or serious cardiac difficulties. These kinds of serious reactions are very rare (see below).

No clinically significant effects have been reported for long-term multi-gallon donations of whole blood. However, some studies have reported immunologic abnormalities, including decreases in natural killer cells, total lymphocyte levels, and proliferative

response to mitogens.[22] The most comprehensive study did not identify differences between donors and nondonors in lymphocyte levels or function.[22] At present it is not considered that long-term blood donation adversely affects immunologic function.

Severe Reactions to Blood Donation

Although most reactions are mild, severe reactions can occur. These include seizures, myocardial infarction, tetany, and death. Popovsky[19] recently reviewed 4,100,000 blood donations and found very severe reactions in 0.0005% or one per 198,110 allogeneic blood donations. These were defined as severe reactions because they required hospitalization. The kinds of reactions included severe vasovagal reaction, angina, tetany, and problems related to the venipuncture site. Most reactions occurred during donation while the donor was at the donor site, although 6% occurred more than 3 days later. Reactions were more likely in first-time donors. If this incidence is generalized to the national blood collection activity of 12 to 14 million donations per year, approximately 60 to 70 such reactions may occur.

Seizures

Because seizures may occur following blood donation, a history of seizures has disqualified donors in the past. In a recent study,[23] donors with a history of seizures that were well controlled at the time of donation had no greater likelihood of experiencing a reaction to donation than donors who had never had seizures. Thus, blood banks may begin to modify their requirements regarding a history of seizures.

Nerve Injuries

During venipuncture, the needle may accidentally strike a nerve. Newman and Waxman[24] reviewed 66 blood donation-related nerve injuries that occurred in 419,000 donations (one per 21,000 donations). The injuries caused numbness or tingling, pain, and/or loss of arm or hand strength. Some of the donors developed a hematoma following donation, but it could not be determined whether the nerve damage was related to the hematoma or direct injury by the needle. One-third of the injuries resolved in less than 3 days, but 2% lasted longer than 6 months and 6% resulted in residual mild localized numbness. This incidence of nerve injuries is similar to the one in 26,700 donations reported by Berry et al.[25] and implies that approximately 500 to 600 such injuries may occur annually from the 12 to 14 million blood donations in the United States.

Hematoma and Arterial Puncture

A hematoma occurs commonly after blood donation even though the arm is inspected and donors are advised to apply pressure to the area. Usually these hematomas are not serious but cause some local discoloration of the antecubital fossa. There may be some leakage of blood, which may soil the donor's clothes resulting in the donor asking the blood center to pay for cleaning of the garment. A more serious but rare complication

is the development of a large hematoma due to venous leakage from an arterial puncture. This can cause pressure on vessels or nerves in the antecubital fossa, and serious injury may result. Reports of symptoms suggesting this type of complication should be dealt with urgently by the blood center so that the donor can receive rapid attention and drainage of the fossa if necessary to prevent more serious injury.

ADVERSE REACTIONS IN APHERESIS DONORS

Apheresis

Rather than being prepared from a standard unit (pint) of whole blood, components can also be obtained by apheresis. In apheresis, the donor's anticoagulated whole blood is passed through an instrument in which the blood is separated into red cells, plasma, and a leukocyte/platelet fraction. Then the desired fraction or component can be removed and the remainder of the blood returned to the donor. Several liters of donor blood can be processed through the instrument, and therefore a larger amount of the desired component can be obtained than from one unit (pint) of whole blood. Apheresis can be used for collection of platelets, lymphocytes, granulocytes, plasma, or hematopoietic stem cells. The use of apheresis for the production of blood components is discussed more fully in Chapter 7. In this chapter the focus is on the medical assessment of apheresis donors. The medical assessment and physical examination of potential cytapheresis donors is based on the effects of the procedure and potential complications. Thus, these factors will be discussed first to provide a basis for the description of the medical assessment and physical examination of these donors.

Adverse Reactions

Adverse reactions in apheresis donors (Table 4.3) are similar in character to those encountered in whole blood donation except that there is a lower incidence of vasovagal reactions and a higher incidence of paresthesias during apheresis. This is probably due to the infusion of the citrate used to anticoagulate the donor's blood while it is in

Table 4.3 Potential complications and adverse reactions to cytapheresis donation

Reactions similar to whole blood donation
Citrate toxicity
Hematoma
Mechanical hemolysis
Air embolus
Platelet depletion
Lymphocyte depletion
Plasma protein depletion

the cell separator. In leukapheresis, donors may be given corticosteroids to elevate the granulocyte count, and the sedimenting agent hydroxyethyl starch is used in the cell separator to improve the granulocyte yield. Each of these agents can cause specific kinds of reactions or complications in the donors. The additional donor selection and monitoring requirements for apheresis are designed to prevent the development of reactions or complications due to excess removal of blood cells or plasma.

Citrate Toxicity

In a careful study relating the dose of citrate, symptoms, electrocardiographic changes, and ionized calcium, Olson et al.[26] showed that when citrate infusion rates were maintained below 65 mg/kg/hr, donors did not experience symptoms nor demonstrate electrocardiographic abnormalities. Donors with similar levels of hypocalcemia may demonstrate wide variability in symptoms.[27] Komatsu and Shikata[28] observed a remarkable number of electrocardiographic abnormalities in platelet and leukapheresis donors. These abnormalities involved bradycardia, sometimes severe (less than 45); supraventricular and ventricular premature contractions; right bundle-branch block; ST segment elevation or depression; and tall, flattened, or inverted T waves. Some of the donors experienced nausea, vomiting, hypotension, fainting, or convulsions. The donors received ACD formula A at a ratio of 1:8 with whole blood. This high level of citrate infusion may have accounted for the large number of electrocardiographic abnormalities. Citrate reactions are managed by slowing the flow rate of the instrument and thus slowing the rate of citrate infusion. This is quite effective in eliminating these reactions, and most apheresis personnel are very aware of this process. Citrate toxicity can also occur if tubing is not properly placed in the pumps and the citrate solution is allowed to flow freely into the donor.[29]

Circulatory Effects

Because the extracorporeal volume of the cytapheresis instruments is small (usually less than 200 mL), hypovolemia is rare and these donors do not experience circulatory problems. Also, since they are usually experienced whole blood donors, they rarely experience vasovagal reactions.

Air Embolus

Because the blood is actively pumped into the donor's veins, there is the theoretical possibility that air could be pumped into the donor if air entered the system. Some of the early models of apheresis instruments contained bubble chambers connected to a device that stopped the pumps if the chamber became filled with air. Air emboli have occurred but no serious consequences have been reported. Contemporary instruments do not contain safety devices to prevent air embolus and so this complication remains a remote possibility. Staff members must be aware of this possibility and ensure that containers and tubing sets do not develop leaks that would allow air to enter the system.

Hematoma

Hematomas may develop after removal of the needles used for apheresis just as after whole blood donation. There is no reason that this should be a more or less frequent complication than following whole blood donation. However, because blood is returned to the donor by active pumping, if the needle becomes dislodged, the blood will continue to be injected into the antecubital fossa under pressure, and a substantial hematoma may develop quickly. Usually the donor will complain of pain and, if so, the pumps should be stopped quickly to minimize the amount of blood injected into the antecubital fossa.

Mechanical Hemolysis

Because blood is pumped through tubing and centrifuges of various configurations, hemolysis is a theoretical complication due to constricted tubing or the geometry of the flow pathways. Although these complications are rare, they have been reported to occur about 0.07% or once per about 1,500 procedures.[30] This means that a busy apheresis program would experience one or two incidents each year. This is a bit more frequently than these problems seem to occur in practice.

Platelet Depletion or Damage

Plateletpheresis does not damage the donor's remaining platelets, and the donor's platelet function is normal following donation.

Red Cell Loss

Collection of platelets, granulocytes, lymphocytes, or stem cells by cytapheresis results in very little red cell loss. Thus, red cell depletion is not considered a possible complication. Red cell loss can occur due to instrument failure whereby the blood in the instrument is lost. If this occurs, it is treated as if the donor had donated a unit of blood and must then undergo the usual waiting period before another donation can be scheduled.

Potential Complications of Serial Donations

Because cytapheresis donors can donate more often than whole blood donors, there are some complications that could result from multiple frequent donations. These involve depletion of cells or plasma proteins. Platelet depletion is of course a primary concern if donors undergo frequent plateletpheresis during a short period. In one study[31] of 2,069 plateletphereses in 352 donors, or an average of six procedures per donor, the following important observations were made that formed the basis of subsequent FDA regulations for the selection and monitoring of cytapheresis donors: (a) among women, platelet counts averaged 12% higher than those of males, (b) about 3% of all donors had platelet counts less than 150,000/μL before their first platelet donation, c) the preapheresis platelet count was the best predictor of the postapheresis platelet count, (d) if

donors with a preapheresis count of less than 150,000 were excluded, only 13% of donations resulted in a postapheresis count of less than 100,000, (*e*) the platelet count decreased about 30% immediately following apheresis, (*f*) the platelet count returned to normal about 4 to 6 days after apheresis, and (*g*) there was a slight rebound in platelet count above the initial count about 8 to 11 days after apheresis.[31] In another rather dramatic example, a female donor underwent 101 donations during a 33-month period, with donation frequencies ranging from once to three times weekly.[32] Her platelet count remained in the range of 135,000 to 430,000 during this time. Lymphocyte studies were not reported. There was no decrease in immunoglobulins.

Lymphocyte depletion could result from frequent multiple donations because of the substantial lymphocyte content of the plateletpheresis component. Senhauser et al.[33] found a 23% decrease in total lymphocyte count, a 25% decrease in T cells, and a 47% decrease in B cells in donors who underwent nine plateletphereses in 1 year compared to those who gave 1 to 4 units of whole blood in the same time. Koepke et al.[34] also found a 20% decrease in total lymphocyte count and a substantial decrease in B cells in frequent cytapheresis donors. In another study of 25 volunteers who underwent an average of 72 platelet donations during about 8 years, there was a decrease in total lymphocytes, T4 cells, T4/T8 ratio, and response to mitogen stimulation.[35] Thus, it seems clear that frequent plateletpheresis over short periods can deplete the lymphocyte pool and alter immune function, although this has not proved to be a practical problem.

There are only a few studies of frequent granulocyte donors. Strauss et al.[36] reported 13 donors who gave between 12 and 29 times on consecutive days. Platelet and hemoglobin levels remained unchanged, but leukocyte levels decreased. Some donors had skin rashes, probably due to the hydroxyethyl starch (HES). Hypertension and peripheral edema are potential complications from fluid accumulation caused by the HES.

MEDICAL ASSESSMENT OF APHERESIS DONORS

The selection of donors for plateletpheresis, leukapheresis, and plasmapheresis uses the same general criteria used for whole blood donors.[1] Because of the unique nature of apheresis, there are some additional donor requirements. These additional requirements are based on the unique complications that may occur from apheresis, the nature of the procedures, and the fact that because few red cells are removed, donors can undergo cytapheresis more often than whole blood donation. The amount of blood components removed from apheresis donors must be monitored. To be consistent with whole blood donation, not more than 200 mL of red cells may be removed in 2 months.[1] If for some reason, such as instrument failure, it is not possible to return the red cells to the donor, then the donation is treated as if it were a whole blood donation, and the donor cannot donate again for 8 weeks. For consistency with plasma donation, not more than 1,000 to 1,200 mL of plasma per week may be retained.[1] When donors undergo apheresis more often than every 8 weeks, this is referred to as "serial" donation, and cumulative records must be maintained of the details of these donations and the records must be reviewed

periodically by a physician. The laboratory testing of donors and apheresis components is the same as for whole blood donation. Thus, the likelihood of disease transmission from apheresis components is the same as for a component from whole blood.

Plateletpheresis Donors

Plateletpheresis donors must meet the same medical requirements as whole blood donors, but a platelet count is not necessary before the initial donation because the decrease in platelet count following donation is not so extensive as to create a risk for the donor. Following plateletpheresis, the donor's platelet count declines by about 30% and does not return to preplateletpheresis levels for about 4 days.[31] At least 48 hours must elapse between platelet donations. If donors are to donate more frequently than every 4 weeks, a platelet count must be done to ensure that it is at least 150,000 per microliter before a subsequent donation.[1] Either the platelet count can be obtained before the donation or a count obtained at the end of the previous donation can be used. Platelet donors should not have taken aspirin or drugs that interfere with platelet function within 3 days of donation.

Leukapheresis Donors

Because the HES used in granulocyte collection is a blood volume expander, some blood banks use lower blood pressure levels than those used for whole blood donors when selecting granulocyte donors. This is not a requirement, however. Donors also may receive corticosteroids to increase their granulocyte count and the granulocyte yield (see Chapter 7). Thus, donors should be questioned about conditions that might be exacerbated by corticosteroids. These include hypertension, peptic ulcers, and diabetes. Because corticosteroids are given to granulocyte donors, these donors usually do not donate frequently at short intervals. If this were to be done, it would need to be under the close supervision of a physician with written plans for monitoring the donor for side effects of accumulation of HES.

Plasmapheresis Donors

If plasma is donated no more than every 8 weeks, the donor assessment procedures are the same as for whole blood. The FDA limitations for plasma removal are no more than 1,000 to 1,200 mL of plasma at one donation depending on the donor's weight.[1] These volumes may be slightly different when semiautomated instruments are used. Donors may give plasma more often than every 8 weeks, and this is called "serial" plasmapheresis. Donors may give again in 48 hours as for platelets but not more than twice within a 7-day period. For donors undergoing plasmapheresis more often than once every 4 weeks, the serum protein must be monitored and found to be within normal limits.[1]

Physical Examination of Apheresis Donors

The physical examination of cytapheresis donors is the same as for whole blood donation.

THERAPEUTIC BLEEDING

Blood may be collected as part of the therapy of diseases such as polycythemia vera or hemochromatosis. Because the procedure is being performed as a therapy, these individuals are patients, not donors. Their medical assessment then is focused on determining that the phlebotomy is safe for the patient. The patients may meet all of the criteria for whole blood donation except for the presence of the disease for which they are undergoing phlebotomy. Often the patient or his or her physician asks that the blood be used for transfusion as a way of comforting the patient. However, usually blood collected as therapeutic bleeding is not used for transfusion, since the cause of the disease is not known, and because of this the donors do not meet the FDA requirements.

REFERENCES

1. Vengelen-Tyler V, ed. Technical Manual. Standards for blood banks and transfusion services, 12th ed. Arlington, VA: American Association of Blood Banks, 1996.
2. Grossman BJ, Springer KM, Zuck TF. Blood donor deferral registries: highlights of a conference. Transfusion 1992;32:868–872.
3. Simon TL, Rhyne RL, Wayne SJ, Garry PJ. Characteristics of elderly blood donors. Transfusion 1991;31:693–697.
4. Pindyck J, Avorn J, Kuriyan M, et al. Blood donation by the elderly—clinical and policy considerations. JAMA 1987;257:1186–1188.
5. Garry PJ, VanderJagt DJ, Wayne SJ, et al. A prospective study of blood donations in healthy elderly persons. Transfusion 1991;31:686–692.
6. Schmidt PJ. Blood donation by the healthy elderly. Transfusion 1991;31:681–683.
7. Mayo DJ, Rose AM, Matchett SE, et al. Screening potential blood donors at risk for human immunodeficiency virus. Transfusion 1991;31:466–474.
8. Gimble JG, Friedman LI. Effects of oral donor questioning about high-risk behaviors for human immunodeficiency virus infection. Transfusion 1992;32:446–449.
9. Sayers MH. Duties to donors. Transfusion 1992;32:465–466.
10. Busch MP, Young MJ, Samson SJ, et al. Risk of human immunodeficiency virus (HIV) transmission by blood transfusions before the implementation of HIV-1 antibody screening. Transfusion 1991;31:4.
11. Lefrere JJ, Elghouzzi MH, Salpetrier J, Duc A, Dupuy-Montbrun MC. Interviews of individuals diagnosed as anti-human immunodeficiency virus-positive through the screening of blood donations in the Paris area from 1991 to 1994: reflections on the selection of blood donors. Transfusion 1996;36:124–127.
12. Doll LS, Petersen LR, White CR. Human immunodeficiency virus type 1-infected blood donors: behavioral characteristics and reasons for donation. Transfusion 1991;31:704–709.
13. Lau P, Hansen M, Sererat M. Influence of climate on donor deferrals. Transfusion 1989;28:559–562.
14. Sazama K. Reports of 355 transfusion-associated deaths: 1976 through 1985. Transfusion 1990;30:583–590.
15. Morduchowicz G, Pitlik SD, Huminer D, Alkan M, Drucker M, Rosenfeld JB, Block CS. Transfusion reactions due to bacterial contamination of blood and blood products. Rev Infect Dis 1991;13:307–314.
16. Reiss RF, Katz AJ. Platelets and factor VIII as functions of blood collection time. Transfusion 1976;16:229–231.
17. Logic JR, Johnson SA, Smith JJ. Cardiovascular and hematologic responses to phlebotomy in blood donors. Transfusion 1963;3:83–93.
18. Tomasulo PA, Anderson AJ, Paluso MB, Gutschenritter MA, Aster RH. A study of criteria for blood donor deferral. Transfusion 1980;20:511–518.
19. Popovsky MA, Whitaker B, Arnold NL. Severe outcomes of allogeneic and autologous blood donation: frequency and characterization. Transfusion 1995;35:734–737.

20. Ogata H, Iinuma N, Nagashima K, Akabane T. Vasovagal reactions in blood donors. Transfusion 1980;679–683.

21. Kasprisin DO, Glynn SH, Taylor F, Miller KA. Moderate and severe reactions in blood donors. Transfusion 1992;32:23–26.

22. Lewis SL, Kutvirt SG, Simon TL. Investigation of the effect of long-term whole blood donation on immunologic parameters. Transfusion 1992;32:51–56.

23. Krumholz A, Ness PM, Hauser WA, Douglas DK, Gibble JW. Adverse reactions in blood donors with a history of seizures or epilepsy. Transfusion 1995;35:470–474.

24. Newman BH, Waxman DA. Blood donation-related neurologic needle injury: evaluation of 2 years' worth of data from a large blood center. Transfusion 1996;36:213–215.

25. Berry PR, Wallis WE. Venipuncture nerve injuries. Lancet 1977;1:1236–1237.

26. Olson PR, Cox C, McCullough J. Laboratory and clinical effects on the infusion of ACD solution during plateletpheresis. Vox Sang 1977;33:79–87.

27. Ladenson JH, Miller WV, Sherman LA. Relationship of physical symptoms, ECG, free calcium, and other blood chemistries in reinfusion with citrated blood. Transfusion 1978;18:670–679.

28. Komatsu F, Shikata M. Abnormal electrocardiographic findings in apheresis donors. Transfusion 1988;28:371–374.

29. Uhl L, Maillet S, King S, Kruskall MS. Unexpected citrate toxicity and severe hypocalcemia during apheresis. Transfusion. In press. (October issue)

30. Robinson A. Untoward reactions and incidents in machine donor apheresis. Transfusion Today 1990;7:7–8.

31. Lasky LC, Lin A, Kahn RA, McCullough J. Donor platelet response and product quality assurance in plateletpheresis. Transfusion 1981;21:247.

32. Bongiovanni MB, Katz RS, Wurzel HA. Long-term plateletpheresis of a donor. Transfusion 1980;20:465–466.

33. Senhauser DA, Westphal RG, Bohman JE, Neff JC. Immune system changes in cytapheresis donors. Transfusion 1982;22:302–304.

34. Koepke JA, Parks WM, Goeken JA, Klee GG, Strauss RG. The safety of weekly plateletpheresis: effect on the donor's lymphocyte population. Transfusion 1981;21:59–63.

35. Matsui Y, Martin-Alosco S, Doenges E, et al. Effects of frequent and sustained plateletapheresis on peripheral blood mononuclear cell populations and lymphocyte functions of normal volunteer donors. Transfusion 1986;26:446–452.

36. Strauss RG, Goeken JA, Eckermann I, McEntegart CM, Hulse JD. Effects of intensive granulocyte donation on donors and yields. Transfusion 1986;26:441–445.

PREPARATION, STORAGE, AND CHARACTERISTICS OF BLOOD COMPONENTS AND PLASMA DERIVATIVES

This chapter describes the preparation, storage conditions, and characteristics of blood components. The clinical uses of the components are described in Chapters 11 and 12.

WHOLE BLOOD

In the United States, whole blood is rarely used. Within a few hours or days, some coagulation factors, especially V and VIII, and platelets decrease in quantity or lose viability in stored whole blood. Therefore, virtually all whole blood collected in the United States is separated into its components, and each component is stored under conditions optimal for that component. This results in a large number of different components being available for transfusion therapy (Tables 5.1 and 5.2). The separation of whole blood into its components makes it possible to retain all of the activities of the original unit of whole blood. Some physicians continue to use whole blood for selected indications such as cardiovascular surgery and exchange transfusion of the neonate. There is a general difference of opinion between transfusion medicine physicians and some clinicians, who believe that whole blood is necessary for certain indications. It is difficult to resolve these differences by clinical trials, and the blood banking system in the United States is so structured to produce components that there is little interest on the part of transfusion medicine physicians to change. Technically, it is possible to provide, through a combination of blood components, everything that can be provided in fresh whole blood. However, there may be a few limited situations in which relatively fresh whole blood might be preferable to a mixture of components.

Table 5.1 Components produced by blood banks and the medical use of these components

Component	Medical use
Red blood cells	Oxygenation of tissues
Platelets	Prevention or cessation of bleeding
Fresh frozen plasma	Cessation of bleeding
Cryoprecipitate	Cessation of bleeding
Cryoprecipitate-poor plasma	Plasma exchange
Granulocytes	Treatment of infection
Frozen red blood cells	Storage of rare blood
Leukocyte-depleted red cells	Prevention of reactions and certain diseases

PREPARATION OF BLOOD COMPONENTS FROM WHOLE BLOOD

Anticoagulant Preservative Solutions

The development of preservatives along with the discovery of blood groups were the two key advances that made transfusion possible (see Chapter 1). The beginning of red cell preservation can be traced to Peyton Rous, who later was awarded the Nobel Prize for his work with viruses. Rous and Turner[1] showed that glucose delayed in vitro hemolysis. During the period between World Wars I and II, Mollison[2] in England developed an acidified citrate and glucose solution for red cell preservation, variants of which are the mainstay of present-day preservatives. These solutions are composed of citrate for anticoagulation, dextrose for cell maintenance, and phosphate buffers (Table 5.3). Whole blood or red blood cells can be stored in these solutions for periods ranging from 21 to 35 days.

Experience with red cell preservation then established that adenosine triphosphate loss correlates with poor viability, and addition of adenine at the beginning of preservation increases ATP and improves red cell viability.[3] It was also known that 2,3-diphosphoglycerate (2,3-DPG) declined in stored red cells, but the significance of this was not appreciated until it was shown that decreased 2,3-DPG was associated with increased affinity of hemoglobin for oxygen.[4-6] Thus, there was considerable interest in developing solutions that would maintain both ATP and 2,3-DPG while allowing removal of the maximum volume of plasma for production of derivatives. These interests led to an overall assessment of the changes that occur during red cell storage, referred to as the storage lesion (Table 5.4). This information has formed the basis of the development of artificial storage media for red cells. During the past few years, it has been possible to extend the duration of red cell storage by placing the red cells in special "additive" solutions. Several solutions are available containing various combinations of saline, adenine, phosphate, bicarbonate, glucose, and mannitol using the names Adsol, Nutricell, and SAGM[7-10] (Table 5.5). These solutions provide better nutrients that maintain red cell viability longer during storage and also maintain red cell enzymes and red cell function. Using the additive solutions allows red cell preservation for 42 days.

Table 5.2 Licensable products produced from whole blood

Red cell components	Red blood cells
	Red blood cells deglycerolized
	Red blood cells deglycerolized irradiated
	Red blood cells frozen
	Red blood cells frozen irradiated
	Red blood cells frozen rejuvenated
	Red blood cells frozen rejuvenated irradiated
	Red blood cells irradiated
	Red blood cells leukocytes removed
	Red blood cells leukocytes removed irradiated
	Red blood cells rejuvenated
	Red blood cells rejuvenated deglycerolized
	Red blood cells rejuvenated deglycerolized irradiated
	Red blood cells rejuvenated irradiated
	Red blood cells washed
	Whole blood CPD irradiated
	Whole blood cryoprecipitate removed
	Whole blood leukocytes removed
	Whole blood modified—platelets removed
	Whole blood platelets removed irradiated
Plasma components	Cryoprecipitate AHF
	Cryoprecipitate AHF irradiated
	Cryoprecipitate AHF pooled
	Fresh frozen plasma
	Fresh frozen plasma irradiated
	Liquid plasma
	Plasma
	Plasma irradiated
Platelets	Platelet-rich plasma
	Platelets
	Platelets irradiated
	Platelets pheresis
	Platelets pheresis irradiated

Abbreviations: AHF, antihemophilic factor; CPD, citrate-phosphate-dextrose.

Blood Processing for the Preparation of Components

The techniques for collection of whole blood are described in Chapter 4. Because most blood is separated into its components, the whole blood is collected into sets involving multiple bags (Fig. 5.1). The blood first enters the primary bag, where it is mixed with anticoagulant-preservative solution. After collection, the manner in which the blood is handled depends on the intended use of the unit (Fig. 5.2). The whole blood is kept at a temperature either between 1°C and 6°C or between 20°C and 24°C. If red blood cells and plasma are to be produced, the blood is kept between 1°C and 6°C. When the blood is collected in a fixed site, the blood can be placed in a regular blood storage refrigera-

Table 5.3 Content of anticoagulant-preservative solutions (g/L)

	ACD-A	CPD	CP2D	CPDA-1
Trisodium citrate	22.00	26.30	26.30	26.30
Citric acid	8.00	3.27	3.27	3.27
Dextrose	24.50	25.50	51.10	31.90
Monobasic sodium phosphate		2.22	2.22	2.22
Adenine				0.275

Source: Vengelen-Tyler V, ed. Technical Manual, 12th ed. Arlington, VA: American Association of Blood Banks, 1996:136.

tor. If the collection is on a mobile unit, special insulated containers are used that contain ice and maintain a temperature between 1°C and 6°C. If platelets are to be prepared from the whole blood, the blood must be maintained at room temperature (20°C to 24°C), because exposure to cold damages the platelets. Maintenance of the blood at room temperature is done by placing the units in containers specially designed to maintain the temperature between 20°C and 24°C. It is recognized that the blood will not

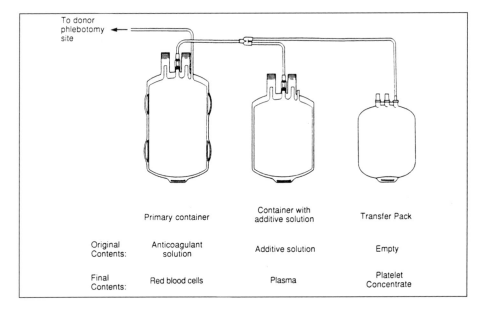

Figure 5.1 Diagram showing unit of whole blood and integral plastic bag system used for preparing blood components.

**Table 5.4 Changes occurring during
red cell storage: the storage lesion**

Increase	Decrease
Lactate	ATP
Pyruvate	2,3-DPG
Ammonia	Intracellular potassium
Intracellular sodium	pH
Membrane vesicles	
Plasma hemoglobin	

attain the temperatures of the storage containers (1°C to 6°C or 20°C to 24°C) for several hours, but the blood must be placed in the environment that will begin to bring the temperature of the blood to the desired storage temperature.

To prepare the components, large high-speed centrifuges that accommodate four or six units of whole blood are used. Important factors in the centrifuge techniques include the rotor size, centrifuge speed, time at maximum speed, and braking mechanism or

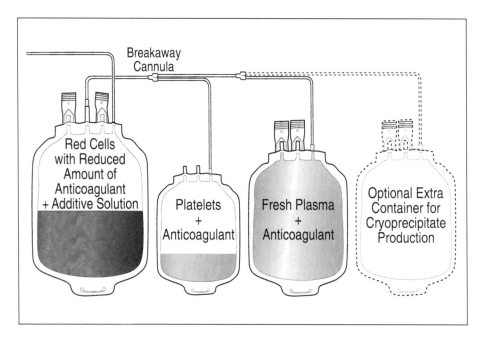

Figure 5.2 Diagrammatic illustration of the separation of whole blood into red cells, plasma, and platelet concentrate.

deceleration phase. The whole blood is manipulated differently depending upon the components desired. If platelets are to be prepared, the whole blood is centrifuged using one set of conditions; if platelets are not to be prepared, a different set of conditions is used (see below). After removal of the platelet-rich plasma, the additive solution is added to the concentrated red cells for optimum red cell preservation.

RED BLOOD CELLS

Description of Component

Red blood cells are the cells remaining after most of the plasma has been removed from whole blood. This blood component is often called "packed red cells" or "packed cells." If platelets or fresh frozen plasma are not being produced from the original unit of whole blood, the red cells can be separated from the plasma at any time during the storage period of the blood. Usually the red cells and plasma are separated within 8 hours of collection, because for the plasma to be used as a source of factor VIII it must be placed in the freezer before 8 hours after collection. This separation can be done by centrifugation or sedimentation. Centrifugation is used when the red cells are being prepared within a few hours after collection, because usually this is done as part of a large-scale operation, and speed is important. Usually the unit of whole blood is centrifuged to produce a platelet concentrate and/or to recover plasma. Therefore, the centrifugation conditions (time and speed) are determined by the method being used to prepare the platelets or plasma. If the unit of whole blood is allowed to remain undisturbed for several hours, the red cells sediment and the plasma can be removed. When sedimentation is used, the red cells are not as concentrated; as a result, the red cell unit has a lower hematocrit and less plasma is recovered than when centrifugation techniques are used. Because the plasma is valuable as a source for production of plasma derivatives, it is desirable to recover the maximum amount of plasma, and therefore sedimentation currently is not often used to separate whole blood into its components.

The unit of red cells has a volume of about 350 mL and will contain a minimum of 154 mL of red cells (405 mL × 38% hematocrit). Usually the red cell unit contains about 190 mL of red cells (450 × 42% hematocrit) and has a hematocrit of about 60%. The fluid portion of the unit (approximately 130 mL) is primarily the additive preservative solution, although about 20 mL of plasma remains from the original unit of whole blood. The characteristics of a unit of red cells stored in an additive are illustrated in Table 5.6. One unit of red cells will increase the hemoglobin concentration and hematocrit in an average-sized adult (70 kg) by about 1 g/dL and 3%, respectively.

Storage Conditions and Duration

Red cells are stored at 1°C to 6°C for different times depending on the anticoagulant preservative used. The storage period may range from 21 to 42 days. The end of the storage period is referred to as the expiration date or the "outdate." The cells must be

Table 5.5 Content of additive solutions (mM)

	AS-1 (Adsol)	AS-3 (Nutricell)	AS-5 (Optisol)
Dextrose	111.00	55.50	45.40
Adenine	2.00	2.22	2.22
Monobasic sodium phosphate	0	23.00	0
Mannitol	41.20	0	45.40
Sodium chloride	154.00	70.00	150.00

Source: Vengelen-Tyler V, ed. Technical Manual, 12th ed. Arlington, VA: American Association of Blood Banks, 1996:136.

stored in refrigerators with good air circulation and that are designed for blood storage. Household refrigerators are not suitable. The temperature in the refrigerator must be monitored and should be recorded periodically, e.g., every 4 hours. There should be an alarm system to warn staff if the temperature moves outside the acceptable limits. When blood is transported to the patient care area for transfusion, it may be allowed to warm to 10°C and still be suitable for return to the blood bank and reissue to other patients.

Clinical Uses

Red cells are transfused to treat symptomatic anemia or to replace clinically significant blood loss. The specific indications are discussed more fully in Chapters 11 and 12.

Table 5.6 Characteristics of red cells in AS-1 (Adsol) for 42 days of storage*

	Days of Storage						
Indices	0	7	14	21	28	35	42
pH (at 37°C)	7.00	6.86	6.69	6.55	—	6.43	3.34
RBC ATP (mmol/g Hgb)	4.69	4.97	4.83	4.50	3.75	3.47	3.24
RBC DPG (mmol/g Hgb)	10.88	8.16	1.96	0.87	0.65	0.54	0.65
Supernatant sodium (mEq/L)	152	135	131	124	—	126	123
Supernatant potassium (mEq/L)	1.6	17	27	34	—	44	46
Supernatant glucose (mg/dL)	909	780	724	697	660	617	604
Hemolysis (%)	0.02	0.06	0.11	0.14	0.20	0.16	0.24

Source: McCullough J. Transfusion medicine. In: Handin RI, Lux SE, Stossel TP, eds. Blood: Principles and practice of hematology. Philadelphia: J.B. Lippincott Company, 1995:1956.

*AS-1 cells: N = 13; volume = 325 + 29 mL; hematocrit = 58 + 4%; mean red cell mass = 188 mL; mean supernatant volume = 136 mL; mean total hemoglobin = 19.3 g%.

FROZEN OR DEGLYCEROLIZED RED BLOOD CELLS

Description of Component

Red blood cells, frozen or deglycerolized, are the cells that have been stored in the frozen state at optimal temperatures in the presence of a cryoprotective agent, which is removed by washing before transfusion. The red cells must be frozen within 6 days after collection, and they can be stored for up to 10 years. The cryoprotectant commonly used is glycerol, which must be removed before transfusion. The method of freezing and storage must preserve at least 80% of the original red cells, and at least 70% of those cells must survive 24 hours after transfusion.

Freezing of red cells is based on work from almost 50 years ago showing that glycerol protected human red cells from freezing injury.[11] During the next few years following this discovery, several reports established that red cells preserved with glycerol were clinically effective.[12–14] From this work, two basic methods were developed.[15,16] These were referred to as the "high-" and "low-" concentration glycerol methods. The glycerol concentration is related to the rate of freezing, which determines the nature of the freezing injury to the cells. When freezing is slow, extracellular ice forms, which increases the extracellular osmolarity, causing intracellular water to diffuse out of the cell and resulting in intracellular dehydration and damage.[15] This type of injury is prevented by solutes such as glycerol that penetrate the cell and minimize the dehydration.[15] Because the freezing process is slower, higher concentrations of cryoprotectant are required. Usually glycerol at about 40% concentration is used. Red cells preserved with this high concentration of glycerol can be stored at about $-85°C$, a temperature that is achievable by mechanical freezers. Rapid freezing causes intracellular ice crystals and resulting cell damage.[15] However, because the freezing is faster, lower concentrations of cryoprotectant are effective.[17] Usually about 20% glycerol is used.[17] This lower concentration of glycerol necessitates storage of red cells at a temperature of about $-196°C$, achievable only by using liquid nitrogen.

These two methods—with different freezing rates, concentrations of glycerol, storage conditions, and processes for removing the glycerol—involve different technologies.[15,16] Technology development played a major role in making red cell freezing clinically available. During the 1970s, a disposable plastic bowl and semiautomated washing system were developed that greatly facilitated glycerol removal from high-concentration red cells.[18–20] A separate system using sugars to agglomerate red cells and allow washing to remove glycerol was used for a time,[21] but it was replaced by more simple semiautomated techniques. In the rapid-freeze method, the concentration of glycerol is low enough that its removal is more simple. Glycerol removal can be done in ordinary blood bags; complex instruments are not required. To summarize, the high-concentration glycerol method involves more simple freezing and storage but complex deglycerolizing procedures. The low-concentration glycerol method involves complex freezing and storage but simple deglycerolizing procedures.[15] Both of these methods are used today.

Red cells must be frozen within 6 days of collection to provide acceptable post-transfusion survival. Red cells that have been stored longer than 6 days can be frozen if they are "rejuvenated."[20] Rejuvenation restores metabolic functions after the red cells

are incubated with solutions containing pyruvate, inosine, glucose, phosphate, and adenine followed by freezing.[22] This is a helpful strategy to freeze red cells in several limited situations, such as (*a*) red cells found after 6 days of storage to be very rare, (*b*) red cells donated for autologous transfusion but the surgery is postponed, and (*c*) rare red cells thawed but not used. The rejuvenation and subsequent freezing process is complex and expensive. It is available but not widely used.

Clinical Uses

In the 1970s, frozen red cells gained popularity as a form of leukocyte-depleted red cells. Initial studies suggested that frozen red cells might have a reduced risk of transmitting hepatitis.[23,24] A third reason for interest in frozen red cells was that the almost complete absence of plasma prevented allergic reactions or anaphylactic reactions in IgA-deficient patients. It was even thought that if the instruments, costs, and technology could be simplified, depots of frozen red cells could be used to supplement the general blood supply in times of shortage. However, the trend to increased use of frozen red cells changed, and at present this component has a very limited role. Subsequent studies established that frozen red cells can transmit hepatitis,[25,26] and so this application did not materialize. New filtration systems were developed that provided much more effective leukodepletion at lower cost. The technology was never simplified to the point that it became a practical way to provide blood for the general inventory in times of shortage.[27] More simple systems for washing red cells became available. Thus, today the use of frozen red cells is for the storage of red cells from donors with very rare antigen composition. This usually means donors who lack a very high-frequency antigen or in whom the combined absence of several antigens makes the red cells extremely rare. These individuals may donate for general allogeneic use or for their own use. Although its use is much more limited than was anticipated by advocates of frozen red cells during the 1970s, this is an extremely valuable strategy for blood banks and transfusion medicine. Substantial stockpiles of very rare red cells can be established. Individual blood banks may maintain some rare red cells, but large stockpiles of rare red cells are available through the American Association of Blood Banks and the American Red Cross Rare Donor Registries. These rare donor registries can be accessed through any AABB-accredited immunohematology reference laboratory or American Red Cross regional blood center.

WASHED RED CELLS

The definition of washed red cells is rather vague. These are the red cells remaining after washing with a solution that will remove almost all of the plasma.[28] Thus, the requirements for this component do not specify the nature of the washing solution or the exact composition of the final component. Red cells can be washed by adding saline to the red cells in an ordinary bag, centrifuging them and removing the supernatant, or by using semiautomated washing devices such as those used for deglycerolization.[29–31] Depending on the solution and technique used, the washed red cells may have a variable

content of leukocytes and platelets. There is usually some red cell loss during the washing step, and the resulting red cell unit may contain a smaller dose of red cells than a standard unit. In general, the characteristics of washed red cells are the removal of approximately 85% of the leukocytes, loss of about 15% of the red cells, and loss of more than 99% of the original plasma.[29–31] Because the washing usually involves entering the storage container, the washed red cells have a storage period of 24 hours.

Clinical Uses

Because washing removes virtually all of the plasma and some of the leukocytes, washed red cells have been used to prevent febrile transfusion reactions, allergic reactions, hives, and urticaria and to prevent reactions to plasma in patients who are IgA deficient. There are more effective methods for leukodepletion, and washed red cells are not recommended for prevention of febrile reactions. They should be reserved for patients who have problems related to plasma. Thus, patients who have allergic reactions to plasma or are IgA deficient benefit from receiving washed red cells.

FRESH FROZEN PLASMA

Description of Component

Fresh frozen plasma (FFP) is plasma separated from whole blood and placed at $-18°C$ or lower within 8 hours of collection. Fresh plasma may be frozen by placing it in a liquid freezing bath composed of ethanol and dry ice, or between blocks of dry ice, or in a mechanical or a blast freezer. The unit of FFP has a volume of about 200 to 250 mL and contains all of the coagulation factors present in fresh blood. Occasionally FFP is produced as a byproduct of plateletpheresis, and this results in a unit of FFP with a volume of about 500 mL. The electrolyte composition of FFP is that of freshly collected blood and the anticoagulant solution. FFP is not considered to contain red cells, and so is usually administered without regard to Rh type. However, there have been occasional rare reports suggesting that units of FFP contain a small amount of red cell stroma that can cause immunization to red cells.[32] Because it contains ABO antibodies, the plasma must be compatible with the recipient's red cells.

Storage Conditions and Duration

Fresh frozen plasma is stored at $-18°C$ or below and can be stored for up to 1 year after the unit of blood was collected. Although there is no defined temperature below which FFP can be stored, freezers capable of maintaining very low temperatures such as $-65°C$ are not usually used for storage of FFP, because these freezers are expensive to operate and there is no reason to keep the FFP that cold. FFP is usually thawed in a 37°C water bath. However, it takes about 15 to 20 minutes to thaw one or two units and someone must occasionally manipulate the unit to speed thawing by breaking up the pieces of ice. This time requirement is a substantial difficulty when FFP is needed for actively bleeding patients. Several approaches have been used, including larger water

Table 5.7 Indications for the use of fresh frozen plasma

Replacement of isolated coagulation factor deficiencies
Reversal of warfarin effect
Massive blood transfusion
Antithrombin III deficiency
Immunodeficiency
Thrombotic thrombocytopenic purpura

Source: Consensus Conference. Fresh frozen plasma: indications and risks. JAMA 1985;253:551–553.

baths and water baths with agitating trays so that staff members do not need to manipulate the units. Another more promising approach is the use of microwave ovens for thawing FFP.[33,34] The concern with microwave thawing has been the uneven energy distribution within the unit of FFP and resulting "hot spots" and damage to proteins. As microwave devices have improved, it appears that these problems have been overcome, and use of microwaves for this purpose is increasing.

Clinical Uses

There are six generally accepted indications for use of FFP[35] (Table 5.7). These are documented coagulation factor deficiencies, multiple factor deficiencies, and massive transfusion in selected patients. FFP can be used for the treatment of deficiencies of factors II, V, VII, IX, X, or XI, because specific component therapy is usually not available for these factors. FFP can also be used to reverse the warfarin effect if this must be done more quickly than could be accomplished by the administration of vitamin K. In addition, FFP can be used to treat deficiencies of protein C and protein S. Fresh frozen plasma may be helpful in patients experiencing massive transfusion, but this is not recommended on a prophylactic basis or according to some formula (see also Chapter 12). FFP can be used as a source of antithrombin III, although concentrates of antithrombin III are now available. FFP is also useful in patients with secondary immunodeficiency associated with severe protein-losing enteropathy, although at present parenteral nutrition is often effective in preventing this immunodeficiency. FFP is also used regularly as replacement solution for plasma exchange in patients with thrombotic thrombocytopenic purpura. These uses are described more completely in Chapters 11 and 12. FFP is not indicated for use as a volume expander or a nutritional source.[35] There has been concern that FFP is overused, and despite the consensus conference this overuse may be continuing.

PLASMA

Description of Component

Plasma from a unit of whole blood can be removed at any time during the storage period of the whole blood unit or up to 5 days after the unit outdates. This plasma can be stored for up to 5 years at $-18°C$ or lower. If the plasma is not frozen but instead is

stored at 1°C to 6°C, it can be stored no longer than 5 days after the expiration of the original unit of whole blood from which it was prepared. Because it was not frozen within 8 hours after the whole blood was collected, plasma is not a satisfactory source of coagulation factors V and VIII. Other coagulation factors are present, however. Because the plasma is removed from the whole blood after several days of storage, the electrolyte concentrations of the plasma will reflect those of stored whole blood. Thus, plasma may have elevated levels of ammonia and potassium (Table 5.6).

Clinical Uses

There are few indications for the use of plasma. It may be used to treat deficiencies of coagulation factors other than V and VIII if concentrates of those factors are not available. Examples are factors II, V, VII, and XI. Plasma could also be used instead of FFP for replacement therapy in liver disease or for reversal of warfarin effect. Some transfusion medicine physicians believe that plasma can be used in patients with disseminated intravascular coagulation or hemodilution due to massive transfusion. The need for factors V and VIII make FFP preferable. Cryoprecipitate-poor plasma has been used as replacement solution when thrombotic thrombocytopenic purpura is treated with plasma exchange (see Chapter 19). This plasma may also be provided to manufacturers for production of albumin, immunoglobulins, or laboratory reagents.

CRYOPRECIPITATE

Description of Component

Coagulation factor VIII is a cold insoluble protein. Pool and Shannon[36] took advantage of this characteristic to develop a method to recover most of the factor VIII from a unit of whole blood in a concentrated form. Cryoprecipitate is the cold insoluble portion of fresh frozen plasma (FFP) that has been thawed between 1°C and 6°C. The cold insoluble material is separated from the thawed plasma immediately and refrozen within 1 hour. Although there are no specific requirements for the volume of a unit of cryoprecipitate, it is usually 5 mL or more, but less than 10 mL. At least 75% of the cryoprecipitate units must contain at least 80 units of factor VIII. Cryoprecipitate is not a suitable source of coagulation factors II, V, VII, IX, X, XI, and XII.[37] Several factors influence the content of factor VIII in cryoprecipitate, including the blood group of the donor (group A higher than group O), the anticoagulant (citrate-phosphate-dextrose [CPD] higher than acid-citrate-dextrose [ACD]), the age of the plasma when frozen, and the speed of thawing the FFP.[38] Cryoprecipitate also contains fibrinogen and von Willebrand factor. Each bag of cryoprecipitate contains about 250 mg of fibrinogen.[37]

Cryoprecipitate can be produced from large volumes of plasma obtained from a limited number of donors by stimulating them with desmopressin acetate and collecting plasma by exchange transfusion.[39] While this makes it possible to provide most of the factor VIII for a patient from a limited number of donors, the process is very complex logistically and has not gained widespread acceptance.

Cryoprecipitate is stored at −18°C or below and can be kept for up to 1 year.

Thawing

Cryoprecipitate is thawed at 37°C, usually in a water bath. Care must be taken to ensure that the water bath is not contaminated and that the bags of cryoprecipitate are placed inside another bag (overwrap) to minimize the chance of contamination. When using cryoprecipitate, it is customary to pool several bags so that only one container is sent to the patient care area for transfusion. Some blood centers pool several bags of cryoprecipitate before freezing them; this is more convenient for the transfusion service because it eliminates the need to pool individual bags of cryoprecipitate after they are thawed. After thawing, the cryoprecipitate is usually maintained between 1°C and 6°C.

Clinical Uses

Soon after the development of cryoprecipitate, it became the mainstay of treatment for hemophilia A because it was the first concentrated form of factor VIII.[40,41] This remained the product of choice until commercial coagulation factor concentrates became available in the mid- to late 1970s. When commercial concentrates of fibrinogen were removed from use because of the high risk of hepatitis, interest developed in using cryoprecipitate as a source of fibrinogen.[37] This has become the major use of cryoprecipitate, and occurs in massive transfusion or activation of the coagulation system. Another use of the fibrinogen in cryoprecipitate is as fibrin sealant or glue (see Chapter 11). Because cryoprecipitate is the only source of concentrated von Willebrand factor, it is used to treat active hemorrhage or to prepare for invasive procedures in patients with severe forms of the disease.

PLATELET CONCENTRATES—WHOLE BLOOD

Description of Component

The official term for this component is platelets. These are platelets suspended in plasma prepared by centrifugation of whole blood. They are also often referred to as "random-donor" platelet concentrates. Platelets may also be produced by cytapheresis, and this is discussed in Chapter 7. At least 75% of the units of random-donor platelets must contain at least 5.5×10^{10} platelets.[28] Although there is no required volume of the random-donor platelet concentrate, these units usually have a volume of about 50 mL to maintain viability and function during the storage period.

There are two methods for preparing platelets: the platelet-rich plasma (PRP) method and the buffy coat method.[42] In the United States, platelets are prepared using the PRP method; in Europe, the buffy coat method is used.[42] The PRP method uses low G forces ("soft" spin), and the platelet-rich plasma easily separates from the red cells. Studies defining the optimum centrifuge time and speed have reported times ranging from 2.7 to 20 minutes and G forces from 2,160 to 3,731.[43–46] The PRP is transferred into a satellite bag to separate it from the red cells (Fig. 5.2). This must be done within 8 hours after the blood is collected. The platelet-rich plasma is then centrifuged at higher G forces ("hard" spin) and the platelet-poor plasma is removed, leaving a

platelet concentrate and the plasma (Fig. 5.3). After the plasma is removed, the platelet concentrate is left undisturbed or, preferably, placed on the platelet storage rotating device for 1 hour to minimize platelet damage and allow for spontaneous resuspension.[47] In the PRP method the first step is a soft spin and the second step a hard spin. Because of the soft spin, about 20% of the plasma and 20% to 30% of the platelets remain with the red cells.[42] Another 5% to 10% of platelets are lost during the second centrifugation step when the PRP is converted to a platelet concentrate. Thus, the PRP method yields about 60% to 75% of the original platelets, a red cell unit containing about 40 mL of plasma, and about 50% or more of the leukocytes in the original unit of whole blood. The disadvantages of this method are the loss of some plasma that could be used for fractionation and the high leukocyte content of the platelets.

When platelets are produced by the buffy coat method, the whole blood is centrifuged at a higher G force (hard spin) to create a buffy coat that also contains the platelets. Most of the platelets (85%) and leukocytes are contained in this buffy coat and can be separated from the red cells. Because the whole blood centrifugation step involves higher G forces, the red cells are more tightly packed and more plasma is obtained along with the buffy coat. However, to obtain most of the buffy coat, it is necessary to remove some of the red cells, and so there is a loss of about 20 to 25 mL

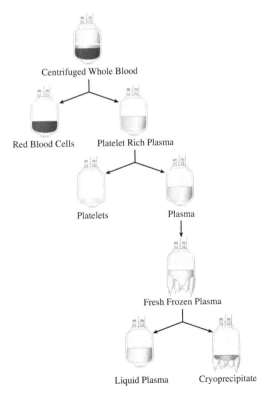

Figure 5.3 Illustration of components produced from a unit of whole blood.

of red cells.[42] To obtain a platelet concentrate, the buffy coat is centrifuged using low G forces, and the platelets are separated from the leukocytes and red cells. Thus, in this method, the first step is a hard spin and the second step a soft spin. It is thought that the use of the soft spin in the second centrifugation may result in platelets that function better than those obtained by the PRP method, in which the second centrifugation is a hard spin when there is less whole blood to "cushion" the platelets.[48] The effectiveness of the second centrifugation step is improved if several units of buffy coat are pooled, usually in groups of six.[42] When units of buffy coat are pooled for the second centrifugation, they may be suspended in an artificial platelet preservation solution (platelet additive solution) that improves the separation and the quality of platelets during storage.[49,50] Also during the second centrifugation step, the platelets are passed through a filter as they are separated, thus removing most of the leukocytes and producing a leukocyte-depleted platelet component.

Storage Conditions and Duration

During the 1960s, platelet transfusion was limited not only by undeveloped methods for platelet collection but also by the inability to store platelets and the resulting necessity to transfuse them shortly after they were produced.[51] A landmark study[52] in the late 1960s established that if platelets were maintained at room temperature, they were effective clinically for up to 96 hours. Further studies confirmed that platelets stored at 20°C to 24°C maintained functional effectiveness for several days.[53–56] Subsequent studies have established that many variables affect the quality of platelets during storage.[43,57] In addition to temperature, these other variables include the anticoagulant preservative solution, storage container, type of agitation, and volume of plasma. With the shift away from the ACD anticoagulant used when platelet preparation was developed, it was established that CPD and CPD-adenine solutions are satisfactory platelet preservatives.[43,58] Storage undisturbed was found to be inferior to gentle agitation, and horizontal agitation preferable to end-over-end agitation.[59] The composition, surface area, and size of the storage container influence the ability for carbon dioxide to diffuse out and oxygen to enter the platelet concentrate, and storage containers specifically designed to optimize platelet quality are now used routinely.[60,61]

The aggregate experience indicated that maintenance of the pH above 6.0 is the crucial factor indicating satisfactory platelet preservation. This combination of storage container, agitation, preservative solution, temperature, and the use of about 50 mL of plasma provide satisfactory preservation of platelets for up to 7 days.[60,62] However, several instances of bacterial contamination of platelet concentrates stored for this period were reported,[63,64] and the storage time was reduced to the 5 days currently used.[65]

Optimal platelet preservation requires about 50 mL of plasma to maintain the pH above 6.0. Several platelet concentrates are usually pooled to provide an adequate dose for most patients (see Chapter 11). For some patients, the volume of plasma in the final pooled component is too large, and plasma must be removed prior to transfusion. This involves another centrifugation step after the platelets have been pooled, and there has been concern that this would damage the platelets and result in an unsatisfactory transfusion. The loss of platelets during this concentration step has been reported to be from

15% to as much as 55%.[66,67] Several centrifugation procedures have been recommended.[66,67] Concentration or volume reduction of pooled platelets can be carried out successfully and is often done for small patients or those receiving large volumes of blood components or intravenous fluids.

The leukocyte content of the platelet concentrates is an important issue. Leukocytes are involved in febrile nonhemolytic transfusion reactions (see Chapter 14) and in alloimmunization leading to platelet refractoriness (see Chapters 11 and 12). The conditions used to centrifuge whole blood influence the leukocyte content of the platelet concentrate, but most platelet concentrates contain 10^8 or more leukocytes. This is a dose adequate to cause transfusion reactions and to alloimmunize patients. During the past few years, filters have become available that remove most of the leukocytes in the platelet concentrate (see below).

GRANULOCYTES

Granulocytes for transfusion are prepared by cytapheresis (see Chapter 7). However, it is not always possible to obtain granulocyte concentrates by cytapheresis in time to respond to the patient's critical condition. Some investigators and blood banks have prepared granulocytes from units of whole blood.[68,69] Granulocytes can be isolated from units of fresh whole blood by sedimentation with hydroxyethyl starch or by centrifugation,[68,69] but the dose of cells obtained by these methods is inconsistent and may not be adequate even for a neonate.[70] Doses of 0.25×10^9 are reported from units sedimented with hydroxyethyl starch, and this is below the 1×10^9 desired for transfusion to a neonate.[70] The possibility of obtaining granulocytes from units of whole blood is usually raised in a crisis; the blood bank often does not have procedures to prepare the cells, and it may not be possible logistically to test the blood for transmissible disease. These conditions add to the difficulty of obtaining a suitable component. Thus, although preparation of granulocytes from units of fresh whole blood may occasionally be helpful, usually the dose is inadequate and this is not a recommended approach.

HEMATOPOIETIC STEM AND PROGENITOR CELLS

Hematopoietic stem cells are being obtained from several sources, including marrow, peripheral blood, and cord blood (see Chapters 17 and 18). Stem cells from these different sources are undergoing an increasing variety of processing methods. Methods for the short-term liquid preservation of stem cells are not well developed. Many cell processing methods (see Chapter 18) lead to a suspension of hematopoietic stem and progenitor cells of varying composition for which frozen preservation is desired. Despite the variety of manipulations of the source or starting material, the freezing and storage methods themselves are rather standard.

The usual method for freezing stem cells uses liquid nitrogen as the freezing system, dimethyl sulfoxide (DMSO) as the cryoprotectant, and controlled-rate freezing.[71,72] The most critical stages in the process are freezing and thawing. If the cooling rate is too slow, extracellular ice crystals form and damage the cells due to the increased

osmolarity of the external solution. If the cooling rate is too fast, intracellular ice crystals form and damage the cells, leading to lysis. The cryoprotective agent, DMSO, binds to water and slows the formation of ice crystals both internally and externally, thus protecting the cell. A particularly important stage in the freezing process is the transition from liquid to solid. The heat of fusion is released then, and the time required to pass through this phase is important. To control the entire freezing process, a programmed freezing apparatus has been used to control the rate of temperature change.[71] The best cooling rate is $-1°C$ to $-3°C$ per minute.[71–73] When freezing is complete, the cells are stored in liquid nitrogen at about $-196°C$. This provides better preservation than higher temperatures,[72,74] and these conditions preserve stem cells for up to 11 years.[75]

There are toxicities associated with marrow transfusion, and these seem to be related to the amount of DMSO the patient receives.[76] In an effort to minimize the amount of DMSO administered and also to simplify the freezing procedure, recent studies have used a combination of lower concentrations of DMSO along with hydroxyethyl starch and albumin.[77–79] In this system, the stem cells suspended in the cryoprotectant are placed in special containers and frozen in a mechanical freezer at about $-80°C$. In this system, the freezing rates are apparently about the same as in the controlled-rate liquid nitrogen system,[79] and the cells are protected satisfactorily.[77,78] The cells are also stored at $-80°C$ in a mechanical freezer, reducing the cost and complexity of the system. The maximum duration of storage in this system is not established. More work is needed to establish that this freezing and preservation method is as satisfactory as the traditional liquid nitrogen method.

Thawing is another important step in the use of hematopoietic stem cells. It has been believed for many years that thawing must be rapid[72] to avoid formation of free water as the ice crystals melt. In addition, DMSO has been thought to be toxic to stem cells upon prolonged exposure, and thus transfusion should be accomplished as soon as possible after thawing.[80] Traditionally, the stem cells have been thawed in a 37°C water bath in the patient's room and transfused immediately. However, a recent study found no toxicity when stem cells were incubated with 10% DMSO for up to 1 hour.[81] Thus, it may become possible to modify the thawing procedure to wash away the DMSO and reduce the reactions associated with DMSO transfusion.[76]

IRRADIATION OF BLOOD COMPONENTS

The techniques and clinical indications for irradiating blood components are described in Chapter 11.

LEUKODEPLETION OF BLOOD COMPONENTS

Definition of Component

Leukocyte-depleted red cells are cells prepared by a method known to retain at least 80% of the original red cells. When these cells are intended for use as a component to prevent febrile transfusion reactions, the final leukocyte content must be less than

5×10^8, and when intended for other purposes (see Chapters 11 and 12), the leukocyte content must be less than 5×10^6.[28]

History of Leukodepletion

During the 1960s and 1970s, it was recognized that leukocytes were important in the pathogenesis of febrile nonhemolytic transfusion reactions and could cause alloimmunization that would later interfere with organ transplantation or platelet transfusion (see Chapters 14 and 15). Thus, considerable interest developed in removing leukocytes before transfusion. Early methods involved centrifuging the red cells (either upright or inverted); sedimenting red cells with dextran or hydroxyethyl starch; filtration with nylon or cotton wool; or washing, freezing, and deglycerolizing[31]. These methods removed from 65% to 99% of the original leukocytes and 5% to 20% of the original red cells. A huge body of literature developed describing the advantages and disadvantages of the different methods and some of the clinical effects of their use. Although they are of historical interest, these studies are not described extensively here because the methods are not used today. Leukodepletion continues to be a very major issue in transfusion medicine, because even more adverse effects of leukocytes contained in blood components have been identified (Table 5.8). The consequences of these effects are described in more detail in Chapter 14 and in many review articles.[82–84] The exact role leukocytes play in some of these situations is not resolved, and thus the optimum strategies for the preparation and use of leukodepleted red cells are still evolving. As these adverse effects of leukocytes have been more extensively described, the technology for producing leukodepleted red cells has evolved to provide more extensive leukocyte depletion than was possible using the methods mentioned above.

The blood filters routinely used for many years and today for routine transfusions have a pore size of 170 to 260 μm and serve to filter out clots and fibrin strands. They do not effectively remove leukocytes and are sometimes referred to as first-generation filters. In the late 1970s, adult respiratory distress syndrome was recognized and microaggregates that form in stored blood were thought to be at least partly responsible (see Chapters 12 and 14). Filters with a pore size of 20 to 40 μm were developed to remove these microaggregates. These filters, composed of polyester or plastic screens or depth filters of foam or fibers,[85] effectively remove about 90% of the original leukocytes. They are referred to as second-generation filters. As ideas developed about the role of leukocytes in the consequences described above, there was interest in removing even more leukocytes (see Chapter 14). Clinical and animal studies suggested that red cells intended to prevent febrile nonhemolytic transfusion reactions must contain fewer than 5×10^8 leukocytes, and those intended to prevent alloimmunization fewer than 5×10^6 leukocytes.[28] The latter requires removal of about 99.9% of the leukocytes. More sophisticated filters have been developed to accomplish this. These are sometimes referred to as 3 log 10, 3 log, or third-generation filters and are manufactured by Pall Corporation and Baxter Healthcare, Inc. With the development of these new very effective filters, several procedural issues have surfaced. The remainder of this discussion deals with the technique of preparing leukodepleted red cells using these new highly effective filters.

Table 5.8 Adverse effects of leukocytes in blood components

Immunologic effects	Alloimmunization
	Febrile nonhemolytic transfusion reactions
	Refractoriness to platelet transfusion
	Rejection of transplanted organs
	Graft versus host disease
	Transfusion-related acute lung injury
Immunomodulation	Increased bacterial infections
	Increased recurrence of malignancy
Infectious disease transmission	Cytomegalovirus infection
	HTLV-I infection
	Epstein-Barr virus infection

Leukodepletion Filters

The filters currently in use are composed of synthetic microfibers in a nonwoven web.[86] The filter material may be modified to alter the surface charge and improve the effectiveness. The mechanism of leukocyte removal is probably a combination of physical or barrier retention and also biological processes involving cell adhesion to the filter material.[86] Because leukocytes are contained in red cell and platelet components, filters have been developed for both of these components. Filters are available as part of multiple-bag systems including additive solutions so that leukocytes can be removed soon after collection and the unit of whole blood converted into the usual components. Filtration removes 99.9% of the leukocytes along with a loss of 15% to 23% of the red cells.[83,87] There are some failures of filtration to achieve the desired leukodepletion. This failure rate ranges from 0.3% to 2.7%.[83,87]

The availability of these filters and the different degrees of leukocyte removal necessary for the prevention alloimmunization compared with transfusion reactions has raised several practical operational matters. These include (*a*) the timing of filtration during the usable life of the component, (*b*) whether filtration in the laboratory is preferable to filtration at the bedside, (*c*) the laboratory techniques suitable for quality control testing of these components, and (*d*) the consistency of the leukodepletion procedure under different conditions.

It appears that febrile nonhemolytic transfusion reactions are caused not only by leukocyte antigen-antibody reactions but also by the cytokines produced by leukocytes in the transfused blood component (see Chapter 14). This would be more effectively prevented if the leukocytes were removed immediately after the blood is collected, avoiding the formation of cytokines. This is referred to as "prestorage" leukodepletion. Since most patients do not receive leukodepleted red cells, this prestorage leukodepletion creates a separate inventory that must be managed. The usage of leukodepleted red cells is still small enough that the separate inventory is limited and may be difficult to manage in such a way that the cells are always available but not wasted. The leukodepletion can be performed by filtering the red cells at the bedside at the time of transfu-

sion. This bedside filtration has the advantage of not requiring a separate inventory but the disadvantage of allowing cytokines to accumulate during blood storage, and thus being less effective in preventing febrile transfusion reactions. Another concern is that the techniques of bedside filtration may not be as effective in removing leukocytes as filtration in the laboratory under standardized conditions and with a good quality control program. Despite these concerns, there are no data to indicate that bedside filtration is less effective.

Another issue is the methods for quality control testing of red cells leukodepleted by these new high-efficiency filters. Because the leukocyte content of the depleted units is very low, the usual methods for leukocyte counting are not accurate.[82,83,87] It has been necessary to develop new or modify existing methods for this purpose. These include the Nageotte chamber and flow cytometry.[82,84]

Leukodepletion of Platelets

Filters are available for leukodepletion of platelets as well as red cells. This is necessary if it is hoped to prevent alloimmunization or disease transmission in patients receiving platelet transfusion. The platelet filters result in a loss of about 20% to 25% of the platelets and have a rate of failure in achieving fewer than 5×10^5 leukocytes of about 5% to 7%.[83,87]

Clinical Uses of Leukodepleted Components

There is considerable debate about the indications for leukodepleted red cells and platelets for some situations (Table 5.9). Prevention of febrile transfusion reactions and alloimmunization of leukocyte antigens have been accepted for some time. More recent studies have established the value of leukodepleted blood components in preventing the development of platelet refractoriness[88] and transmission of cytomegalovirus (CMV).[89] Preventing CMV transmission by the removal of the leukocytes (where the cytomegalovirus is thought to reside) would be an ideal strategy because of the difficulty in finding an adequate supply of CMV-negative blood components, especially in some parts of the United States. Several small studies suggested that leukocyte depletion might be effective in preventing CMV transmission.[90,91] The largest study comparing components leukocyte depleted by filtration with CMV antibody-negative components establishes that filtered leukocyte-depleted components are effective in preventing CMV transmission.[89] There has been some debate about whether this study provides adequate data on which to base the practice of using leukodepleted blood components for prevention of CMV. In the filtration arm, three of 250 patients demonstrated CMV seroconversion, and in the antibody-screened arm, two of 252 demonstrated CMV seroconversion. This difference was not significant. However, of the patients receiving filtered components, all developed CMV disease, whereas of the patients receiving CMV antibody-negative components, none developed disease but only seroconversion. These differences are not significant. It has become the practice in the institutions where this study was done to use components leukodepleted by filtration interchangeably with CMV antibody-negative components, thus confirming the belief of the investigators in the conclusions of the study.

Table 5.9 Indications and nonindications for leukocyte-reduced blood components*

Established indications	Prevention of recurrent nonhemolytic febrile transfusion reactions to red blood cell transfusions
	Prevention or delay of alloimmunization to leukocyte antigens in selected patients who are candidates for transfusion on a long-term basis
Nonindications	Prevention of transfusion-associated graft versus host disease
	Prevention of transfusion-related acute lung injury due to the passive administration of antileukocyte antibody
	Patients who are expected to have only limited transfusion exposure Acellular blood components (for example, fresh frozen plasma, cryoprecipitate)

Source: Lane TA, Anderson KC, Goodnough LT, et al. Leukocyte reduction in blood component therapy. Ann Intern Med 1992;117:151–162.

*Unless otherwise stated in the text, a third-generation filter or an equivalent technique should be used to reduce the leukocyte content of blood components.

Another currently debated issue is whether leukodepleted blood components avoid alloimmunization and platelet refractoriness. Several studies have supported this concept.[85,92–95] In the most recent and largest study, leukodepletion prevented the development of alloimmunization and platelet refractoriness in newly diagnosed patients with acute myelogenous leukemia[88]. It seems that use of leukodepleted components is the optimum therapy for patients who may receive many transfusions and in whom platelet refractoriness should be avoided.

The use of leukodepleted components is currently one of the most actively discussed issues in transfusion medicine. The indications for leukodepleted components are increasing but still constitute a relatively small portion of total component use. As a result, it is difficult for blood suppliers to develop efficient and economical systems to produce leukodepleted components on a large scale. A very major consideration in this discussion and the future of leukodepleted components is whether it can be established that there is an immunomodulatory effect of transfusion that can be alleviated by leukodepletion (see Chapter 14). If so, then there will probably be a shift to almost if not complete use of leukodepleted components. Apart from the scientific data, it seems as if an evolution to the most pure form possible of each component is desirable.

PLASMA DERIVATIVES

General

Procedures for the fractionation of plasma were developed during the 1940s in response to World War II (see Chapter 1). A large pool of plasma, often up to 10,000 L or 50,000 donor units, is processed using cold ethanol fractionation. In cold ethanol, different plasma proteins have different solubilities, which allows their separation. This large-

scale separation and manufacturing process results in the isolation of several proteins from plasma that are prepared for therapeutic use. These are called plasma derivatives (Table 5.10). For the past 50 years, the major derivatives have been albumin, immune serum, γ-globulin, and, during the past 20 years, coagulation factor VIII concentrate. Until the past few years, techniques were not available to sterilize some blood derivatives after manufacture. Thus, because of the large number of units of donor plasma in each pool, the chance of contamination of the pool with viruses (i.e., hepatitis, HIV, etc.) was high and the risk of disease transmission from these nonsterilized blood derivatives was high.[96,97] This risk was accentuated because much of the plasma that serves as the raw material for the manufacture of blood derivatives is obtained from paid donors, a group known to provide blood with an increased likelihood of transmitting disease.[98] Until recently, only albumin and immune globulin carried no risk of disease transmission; albumin because it was sterilized by heating and immune globulin because none of the known infectious agents were contained in that fraction prepared from the plasma. Because of the recognition of the high risk of disease transmission by coagulation factor concentrates, methods were developed to sterilize them.[99,100]

Coagulation Factor Concentrates

Coagulation factor concentrates have evolved rapidly and extensively during the past 15 years.[101] Although these concentrates have been known to transmit hepatitis since they first became available, the risk has been reduced over the years by improvements to the donor history, the addition of laboratory tests for transmissible agents, and the introduction in the mid-1980s of methods to treat the concentrates to separate and inactivate viruses. Currently, the major methods of viral inactivation for plasma-derived concentrates are (a) dry heating, in which the sealed final vial is heated between 80°C and 100°C, (b) pasteurization, in which the concentrate is heated to 60°C while still in solution before lyophilization, (c) vapor heating, in which the lyophilized powder is exposed to steam before bottling, and (d) solvent-detergent treatment, in which the organic solvent tri-n-butyl-phosphate (TNBP) and the detergent Tween 80 or Triton X100 are added at intermediate processing steps. At present, the solvent-detergent method is most commonly used. The pasteurization and vapor heating methods result in substantial loss of factor VIII activity.[99,100]

Each of these methods uses a different strategy of viral inactivation. There are differing amounts of data about the effectiveness of these viral inactivation methods, since not all of their products have been subjected to randomized controlled trials. In general, it appears that the methods are effective in inactivating virus with a lipid envelope, but infections with non-lipid envelope viruses such as parvovirus B19[102] and hepatitis A[103] have been reported.

The first recombinant-produced coagulation factor VIII concentrates became available in late 1992 and 1993. Thus, experience with these products is rather limited, but it appears that these products transmit no diseases. The factor VIII is produced in murine cell lines, and both fetal calf serum and murine monoclonal antibodies are used in the production process. The products are subjected to viral inactivation steps, even though there should be no way that human viruses could contaminate the products.

Table 5.10 Plasma-derivative products

Albumin	Restoration of plasma volume subsequent to shock, trauma, surgery, and burns
Alpha$_1$ proteinase inhibitor	Used in the treatment of emphysema caused by a genetic deficiency
Antihemophilic factor	Treatment or prevention of bleeding in patients with hemophilia A
Anti-inhibitor coagulant complex	Treatment of bleeding episodes in the presence of factor VIII inhibitor
Antithrombin III	Treatment of bleeding episodes associated with liver disease, antithrombin III deficiency, and thromboembolism
Cytomegalovirus immune globulin	Passive immunization subsequent to exposure to cytomegalovirus
Factor IX complex	Prophylaxis and treatment of hemophilia B bleeding episodes and other bleeding disorders
Factor XIII	Treatment of bleeding and disorders of wound healing due to factor XIII deficiency
Fibrinogen	Treatment of hemorrhagic diathesis in hypofibrinogenemia, dysfibrinogenemia, and afibrinogenemia
Fibrinolysin	Dissolution of intravascular clots
Haptoglobin	Supportive therapy in viral hepatitis and pernicious anemia
Hepatitis B immune globulin	Passive immunization subsequent to exposure to hepatitis B
IgM-enriched immune globulin	Treatment and prevention of septicemia and septic shock due to toxin liberation in the course of antibiotic treatment
Immune globulin (intravenous and intramuscular)	Treatment of agammaglobulinemia and hypogammaglobulinemia; passive immunization for hepatitis A and measles
Plasma protein fraction	Restoration of plasma volume subsequent to shock, trauma, surgery, and burns
Rabies immune globulin	Passive immunization subsequent to exposure to rabies
Rh$_O$(D) immune globulin	Treatment and prevention of hemolytic disease of fetus and newborn resulting from Rh incompatibility and incompatible blood transfusions
Rubella immune globulin	Passive immunization subsequent to exposure to German measles
Serum cholinesterase	Treatment of prolonged apnea after administration of succinylcholine chloride
Tetanus immune globulin	Passive immunization subsequent to exposure to tetanus
Vaccinia immune globulin	Passive immunization subsequent to exposure to smallpox
Varicella-zoster immune globulin	Passive immunization subsequent to exposure to chicken pox

Source: From information provided by the American Blood Resources Association.

Experience with these recombinant products is limited but very encouraging.[104,105] Factor VIII is a very antigenic protein. A major concern is whether there will be an increased incidence of factor VIII inhibitors as a result of the transfusion of recombinant-produced factor VIII. At present, it is not clear whether recombinant factor VIII is more likely than plasma-derived factor VIII to cause development of factor VIII inhibitors. Infusion of factor VIII reduces immune function, and this effect is more pronounced the less pure the factor VIII product.[106]

Coagulation factor VIII concentrates produced by recombinant DNA techniques are much more expensive than those produced from plasma. It is estimated that plasma-derived factor VIII may be produced by a direct cost as low as $0.05 per factor VIII unit, although the material typically sells for approximately $0.85 per unit.[107] Recombinant-produced factor VIII concentrates typically sell for more than $1.00 per unit. Despite these price differences, the high-purity (high-cost) plasma-derived and the recombinant products are the most widely used.

Factor IX concentrates did not become free of transmission of most viruses until 1991.[107] Factor IX concentrates vary in purity. The less pure concentrates contain other coagulation factors and cause some degree of hypercoagulability.[108]

Immune Serum Globulins

Immune serum globulin (Ig or γ-globulin) prepared by the traditional plasma fractionation technique has been very effective in preventing bacterial infections in patients with agammaglobulinemia and in preventing certain viral infections in immunologically normal persons (Table 5.10). This immune globulin is administered intramuscularly because it contains aggregated or oligomeric molecules of Ig which, when injected intravenously, activate complement, resulting in severe reactions.[109] However, several important limitations were created by the necessity of intramuscular administration. These include dose limitations, painful injections because of the volume required, and difficulty maintaining plasma levels of IgG due to dose limitations. Immune globulin suitable for intravenous administration became available in the United States in about 1985. Four brands are currently available. These are prepared from the plasma of normal donors and thus can be expected to have an antibody content reflective of normal healthy individuals in a large population. There are some differences in the IgA content, the relative proportions of IgG subclasses, and in vitro activity against some viruses. The differences in IgA content are clinically important, as brands that contain much IgA may cause a reaction if given to an IgA-deficient patient with anti-IgA. The importance of the other differences among the brands has not been established.

Intravenous immune globulin (IVIG) is approved for use by the U.S. Food and Drug Administration for treatment of individuals with impaired humoral immunity, specifically for primary (congenital) immune deficiency, and for (idiopathic) autoimmune thrombocytopenia. The availability of intravenous immunoglobulin makes it possible to maintain the serum IgG level near normal in immunodeficient patients. The amount required varies with the size of the patient and the indication. Usually 100 to 200 mg/kg per month is used as a starting dose for patients with primary immunodefi-

ciencies. Larger doses are usually used for patients with autoimmune thrombocytopenic purpura. The intravenous half-life of the intravenous immunoglobulin is 21 to 25 days, which is similar to native IgG.

The value of intravenous immunoglobulin in other immune deficiency states such as in acquired immune deficiency syndrome (AIDS) or autoimmune diseases has not been established. As with immune globulin preparations used intramuscularly, intravenous immunoglobulin with especially high activity against a particular virus can be prepared from plasma that has a high level of antibody to that virus. One example is cytomegalovirus-intravenous immunoglobulin, which showed promise in early clinical trials.[110,111] However, this material is not widely available, and the effectiveness of leukodepletion in preventing CMV infection makes it unlikely that CMV immune globulin will be developed for clinical use. A large use of IVIG is developing in patients undergoing marrow transplantation in an effort to reduce infections and possibly ameliorate graft versus host disease. No formal structured studies are available to establish the value of IVIG in this situation.

Adverse reactions to intravenous immunoglobulin occur with 2% to 10% of injections. These are local, such as erythremia, pain, phlebitis, or eczema. Systemic symptoms include fever, chills, myalgias, back pain, nausea, and vomiting. Some reactions in some patients are dose related and can be reduced or eliminated by slowing the rate of infusion. The nature and frequency of adverse reactions may differ among the different products, but this is not clear and is beyond the scope of this chapter.

Since intravenous immunoglobulin is made from large pools of human plasma, it contains a variety of antibodies, including those against blood groups and possibly anti-HBs, anti-HBc, anti-cytomegalovirus, etc. Donor screening should eliminate some of these (i.e., anti-HIV), but patients may have transiently positive tests for certain antibodies that are passively acquired from the intravenous immunoglobulin. For instance, marrow transplant patients being treated with intravenous immunoglobulin had a 49% incidence of positive direct antiglobulin test and a 25% incidence of positive red cell antibody detection.[112] Transient hemolysis has been reported in patients with autoimmune thrombocytopenic purpura being treated with intravenous immune globulin. Thus, although hemolysis is unusual, a large proportion of patients receiving intravenous immune globulin will develop circulating or cell-bound blood group antibodies. This should be considered if unexplained hemolysis occurs in patients being treated with intravenous immune globulin.

BLOOD SUBSTITUTES

The functions of blood can be grouped generally as maintenance of intravascular volume, delivery of oxygen to tissues, provision of coagulation factors, provision of some defense mechanisms, and transportation of metabolic waste products. This discussion of blood substitute, or artificial blood, deals only with the oxygen-delivery function. Thus, more appropriate terms are hemoglobin or red cell substitute. Platelet substitutes or artificial platelets are under development but will not be covered here.

History

For years there has been considerable interest in the use of a red cell substitute that would effectively transport oxygen from the lungs to the tissues. The ideal acellular red cell substitute would not require crossmatching or blood typing, could be stored preferably at room temperature for a long period, have a reasonable intravascular life span and thereafter be excreted promptly, and be free of toxicity or disease transmission. The two compounds that have undergone the most study are hemoglobin and perfluorocarbons. Hemoglobin chemically binds oxygen, whereas perfluorocarbons have a solubility for oxygen 20 times greater than water.

Perfluorocarbon Compounds

The physiologic benefit of this high solubility for oxygen has been demonstrated dramatically by the survival of mice completely immersed in a solution of well-oxygenated perfluorocarbons. During the 1980s, a specific perfluorocarbon product underwent clinical trials in patients who required urgent medical care and who refused to receive blood components. The amount of oxygen that can be delivered is based on the oxygen content of inspired air. At ambient oxygen tension, the perfluorocarbon product was not effective, but when patients breathed 100% oxygen, perfluorocarbon provided increased oxygen consumption, an increased mixed venous oxygen tension, and an increased mixed venous hemoglobin saturation.[113]

A study of 186 patients revealed no important adverse effects of the perfluorocarbon on hemodynamics, blood gases, hematologic parameters, coagulation tests, electrolytes, renal function, and liver enzymes.[114] However, the perfluorocarbon product was toxic to macrophages[115] and in some patients caused bronchospasm, leukopenia, thrombocytopenia, and complement activation.[116] In a careful study, eight severely anemic patients (hemoglobin levels of 1.2 to 4.5 g/dL) who received the perfluorocarbon product were compared with 15 who did not.[117] All patients refused blood transfusion. The amount of perfluorocarbon that could be given to patients and the oxygen tension, even when 100% oxygen was inspired, were such that the perfluorocarbon contributed only about half the oxygen-carrying capacity of the patient's plasma. The amount of oxygen delivered by the perfluorocarbon was not clinically significant and the patients did not benefit. The major observation in this study was the ability of all the patients to tolerate remarkably low hemoglobin levels and the lack of the need for increased arterial oxygen content in the 15 control patients who had hemoglobin levels of approximately 7 g/dL.

Hemoglobin-Based Blood Substitutes

Work with hemoglobin solutions has progressed steadily. Hemoglobin can be prepared in solution by lysis of red cells. If the remaining cell stroma is removed, the stroma-free hemoglobin is relatively nontoxic and nonantigenic. However, stroma-free hemoglobin in solution has a short intravascular life span and has a low P_{50} (the point at which 50% is saturated). Thus, research has focused on modifying the structure of the hemoglobin

molecule or binding hemoglobin to other molecules to overcome these two problems. Much of this work is proprietary, and thus little information is available in the scientific literature. However, at least one stroma-free hemoglobin product has undergone extensive in vitro study, animal trials,[118] and substantial experience in humans. The company has constructed a plant to manufacture the blood substitute and is currently arranging for a supply of red cells for further manufacture into this product. It seems likely that in the not-too-distant future a hemoglobin substitute will become available.

Potential Clinical Uses and Impact of Hemoglobin Substitutes

It has been presumed, especially by financial analysts interested in the potential of companies developing blood substitutes, that these would extensively replace present red cell transfusion. It is likely that hemoglobin substitutes will supplement, not replace, most red cell transfusions. The short intravascular half-life of these substitutes make them impractical for long-term red cell replacement (for instance, in chronically anemic patients). The substitutes can be used for immediate restoration of oxygen delivery such as in trauma, or in other urgent situations involving massive blood loss where red cells are not available quickly. Since blood typing and crossmatching would not be necessary, hemoglobin substitutes might be stocked in ambulances and used by paramedics outside of health care facilities. Thus, the substitutes might be carried in emergency vehicles, stocked in emergency departments, or used by the military or civilians in situations where access to blood is limited. In addition, the availability of hemoglobin substitutes will probably create new therapeutic strategies. Other potential uses of hemoglobin substitutes include organ perfusion and preservation prior to transplantation, and improving oxygen delivery to tissues that have an impaired blood supply. If it is true that the blood substitutes are hemoglobin based and are used primarily for situations in which red cells are not now used, then there would be an expanded need for red cells to serve as the basic material for further manufacture of the blood substitute. If the use of hemoglobin solutions follows this course, the need for donated blood might increase instead of decline, as might have been expected.

REFERENCES

1. Rous P, Turner JR. The preservation of living red blood cells in vitro. I. Methods of preservation. II. The transfusion of kept cells. J. Exp Med 1916;23:219–248.
2. Loutit JF, Mollison PL. Advantages of disodium-citrate-glucose mixture as a blood preservative. Br Med J 1943;2:744.
3. Simon ER. Red cell preservation: further studies with adenine. Blood 1962;20:485–491.
4. Benesh R, Benesh RE. The influence of organic phosphates on the oxygenation of hemoglobin. Fed Proc 1967;26:673.
5. Chanutin A, Curnish RR. Effect of organic and inorganic phosphates on the oxygen equilibrium of human erythrocytes. Arch Biochem 1967;121:96–102.
6. Benesch R, Benesch RE. Intracellular organic phosphates as regulators of oxygen release by haemoglobin. Nature 1969;221:618–622.
7. Hogman CF, Hedlund K, Zetterstrom H. Clinical usefulness of red cells preserved in protein-poor media. N Engl J Med 1978;299:1377.

8. Hogman CF. Additive system approach in blood transfusion: birth of the SAG and Sagman systems. Vox Sang 1986;51:339–340.

9. Moroff G, Holme S, Keegan T, Heaton A. Storage of Adsold-preserved red cells at 2.5 and 5.5°C: comparable retention of in vitro properties. Vox Sang 1990;59:136–139.

10. Simon TL, Marcus CS, Myhre BA, Nelson EJ. Effects of AS-3 nutrient-additive solution on 42 and 49 days of storage of red cells. Transfusion 1987;27:178–182.

11. Smith AU. Prevention of hemolysis during freezing and thawing of red blood cells. Lancet 1950;2:910.

12. Sloviter HA. Recovery of human red blood-cells after freezing. Lancet 1951;1:823–824.

13. Chaplin H, Mollison PL. Improved storage of red cells at −20°C. Lancet 1953;1:215–218.

14. Tullis JL, Ketchel MM, Pyle HM, et al. Studies on the in vivo survival of glycerolized and frozen human red blood cells. JAMA 1958;168:399–404.

15. Meryman HT. The cryopreservative of blood cells for clinical use. In: Brown EB, ed. Progress in Hematology, vol. 11. New York: Grune & Stratton, 1979:193–227.

16. Valeri CR. Frozen blood. N Engl J Med 1966;275:365–431.

17. Rowe AW, Eyster E, Kellner A. Liquid nitrogen preservation of red blood cells for transfusion: a low glycerol-rapid freeze procedure. Cryobiology 1968;5:119–128.

18. Latham A, Steimen LE. Development of an expendable liner and automated solution system for red cell glycerolization. Vox Sang 1962;7:102–103.

19. Meryman HT, Hornblower M. A method for freezing and washing red blood cells using a high glycerol concentration. Transfusion 1972;12:145–156.

20. Valeri CR. Simplification of the methods for adding and removing glycerol during freeze-preservation of human red blood cells with the high or low glycerol methods: biochemical modification prior to freezing. Transfusion 1975;15:195–218.

21. Huggins CE. Preservation of blood by freezing with dimethylsulfoxide and its removal by dilution and erythrocyte agglomeration. Vox Sang 1963;8:99–100.

22. Valeri CR, Zaroulis CG. Rejuvenation and freezing of outdated stored human red cells. N Engl J Med 1972;287:1307–1312.

23. Tullis JL, Hinman J, Sproul MT, Nickerson RJ. Incidence of posttransfusion hepatitis in previously frozen blood. JAMA 1970;214:719–723.

24. Carr JB, de Quesada AM, Shires DL. Decreased incidence of transfusion hepatitis after exclusive transfusion with reconstituted frozen erythrocytes. Ann Intern Med 1973;78:693–695.

25. Haugen RK. Hepatitis after the transfusion of frozen red cells and washed red cells. N Engl J Med 1979;301:393–395.

26. Alter HJ, Tabor E, Meryman HT. Transmission of hepatitis B virus infection by transfusion of frozen-deglycerolized red blood cells. N Engl J Med 1978;298:637–642.

27. Telischi M, Hoiberg R, Rao KRP, et al. The use of frozen, thawed erythrocytes in blood banking—a report of 28 months' experience in a large transfusion service. Am J Clin Pathol 1977;68:250–257.

28. Standards for Blood Banks and Transfusion Services, 16th ed. Bethesda, MD: American Association of Blood Banks, 1994.

29. Buchholz DH, Charette JR, Bove JR. Preparation of leukocyte-poor red blood cells using the IBM 2991 blood cell processing. Transfusion 1978;18:653–662.

30. Tenczar FJ. Comparison of inverted centrifugation, saline washing, and dextran sedimentation in the preparation of leukocyte-poor red cells. Transfusion 1973;13:183–188.

31. Polesky HF, McCullough J, Helgeson MA, Nelson C. Evaluation of methods for the preparation of HL-A antigen-poor blood. Transfusion 1973;13:383–387.

32. Ching EP, Poon MC, Neurath D, et al. Red blood cell alloimmunization complicating plasma transfusion. Am J Clin Pathol 1991;96:201–202.

33. Churchill WH, Schmidt B, Lindsey J, et al. Thawing fresh frozen plasma in a microwave oven. Am J Clin Pathol 1992;97:227–232.

34. Thompson KS, O'Kell RT. Comparison of fresh-frozen plasmas thawed in a microwave oven and in a 37°C water bath. Am J Clin Pathol 1981;75:851–853.

35. National Institutes of Health Consensus Conference. Fresh frozen plasma: indications and risks. JAMA 1985;253:551–553.

36. Pool JG, Shannon AE. Simple production of high potency anti-hemophilic globulin (AHG) concentrates in a closed bag system. Transfusion 1965;5:372.

37. Ness PM, Perkins HA. Cryoprecipitate as a reliable source of fibrinogen replacement. JAMA 1979;241:1690–1691.
38. Gunson HH, Bidwell E, Lane RS, Wensley RT, Snape TJ. Variables involved in cryoprecipitate production and their effect on factor VIII activity. Br J Haematol 1978;43:287–295.
39. McLeod BC, Scott JP. Use of "singe donor" factor VIII from plasma exchange donation. JAMA 1984;252:2726–2729.
40. Hattersley PG. The treatment of classical hemophilia with cryoprecipitates. JAMA 1966;198:243–247.
41. Simson LR, Oberman HA, Penner JA. Clinical evaluation of cryoprecipitated factor VIII. JAMA 1967;199:122–126.
42. Murphy S, Heaton WA, Rebulla P. Platelet production in the old world—and the new. Transfusion 1996;36:751–754.
43. Slichter SJ, Harker LA. Preparation and storage of platelet concentrates. II. Storage and variables influence platelet viability and function. Br J Haematol 1976;34:403–419.
44. Kahn RA, Cossette I, Friedman LI. Optimum centrifugation conditions for the preparation of platelet and plasma products. Transfusion 1976;16:162–165.
45. Reiss RF, Katz AJ. Optimizing recovery of platelets in platelet rich plasma by the simplex strategy. Transfusion 1976;16:370–374.
46. Slichter SJ, Harker LA. Preparation and storage of platelet concentrates. I. Factors influencing the harvest of viable platelets from whole blood. Br J Haematol 1976;34:395–402.
47. Mourad N. Studies on release of certain enzymes from human platelets. Transfusion 1968;8:363–367.
48. Fijnheer R, Pietersz RN, de Korte D, et al. Platelet activation during preparation of platelet concentrates: a comparison of the platelet-rich plasma and the buffy coat methods. Transfusion 1990;30:634–638.
49. Eriksson L, Hogman CF. Platelet concentrates in an additive solution prepared from pooled buffy coats. I. in vitro studies. Vox Sang 1990;59:140–145.
50. Bertolini F, Rebulla P, Riccardi D, et al. Evaluation of platelet concentrates prepared from buffy coats and stored in a glucose-free crystalloid medium. Transfusion 1989;29:605–609.
51. Levin RH, Freireich EJ. Effect of storage up to 48 hours on response to transfusions of platelet rich plasma. Transfusion 1964;4:251–256.
52. Murphy S, Gardner FH. Platelet preservation—effect of storage temperature on maintenance of platelet viability—deleterious effect of refrigerated storage. N Engl J Med 1969;380:1094–1098.
53. Murphy S, Sayer SN, Gardner FH. Storage of platelet concentrates at 22°C. Blood 1970;35:549–557.
54. Handin RI, Valeri CR. Hemostatic effectiveness of platelets stored at 22°C. N Engl J Med 1971;285:538–543.
55. Becker GA, Tuccelli MT, Kunicki T, Chalos MK, Aster RH. Studies of platelet concentrates stored at 22 C and 4 C. Transfusion 1973;13:61–68.
56. Filip DJ, Aster RH. Relative hemostatic effectiveness of human platelets stored at 4°C and 22°C. J Lab Clin Med 1978;91:618–624.
57. Kunicki TJ, Tuccelli M, Becker GA, Aster RH. A study of variables affecting the quality of platelets stored at "room temperature." Transfusion 1975;15:414–421.
58. Scott EP, Slichter SJ. Viability and function of platelet concentrates stored in CPD- adenine (CPDA-1). Transfusion 1980;20:489–497.
59. Holme S, Vaidja K, Murphy S. Platelet storage at 22°C: effect of type of agitation on morphology, viability, and function in vitro. Blood 1978;52:425–435.
60. Murphy S, Kahn RA, Holme S, et al. Improved storage of platelets for transfusion in a new container. Blood 1982;60:194–200.
61. Simon TL, Nelson EJ, Murphy S. Extension of platelet concentrate storage to 7 days in second-generation bags. Transfusion 1987;27:6–9.
62. Heal JM, Blumberg N, Masel D. An evaluation of crossmatching, HLA, and ABO matching for platelet transfusions to refractory patients. Blood 1987;70:23.
63. Heal JM, Singal S, Sardisco E, Mayer T. Bacterial proliferation in platelet concentrates. Transfusion 1986;26:388–390.
64. Braine HG, Kickler TS, Charache P, et al. Bacterial sepsis secondary to platelet transfusion: an adverse effect of extended storage at room temperature. Transfusion 1986;26:391.
65. Schiffer CA, Lee EJ, Ness PM, Reilly J. Clinical evaluation of platelet concentrates stored for one to five days. Blood 1986;67:1591–1594.

66. Simon TL, Sierra ER. Concentration of platelet units into small volumes. Transfusion 1984;24:173–175.

67. Moroff G, Friedman A, Robkin-Kline L, et al. Reduction of the volume of stored platelet concentrates for use in neonatal patients. Transfusion 1984;24:144–146.

68. Rock G, Zurakowski S, Baxter A, Adams G. Simple and rapid preparation of granulocytes for the treatment of neonatal septicemia. Transfusion 1984;24:510–512.

69. Wheeler JG, Abramson JS, Ekstrand K. Function of irradiated polymorphonuclear leukocytes obtained by buffy-coat centrifugation. Transfusion 1984;24:238–239.

70. Strauss R. Current issues in neonatal transfusions. Vox Sang 1986;51:1–9.

71. Rowe AW, Rinfret AP. Controlled rate freezing of bone marrow. Blood 1962;20:636–637.

72. Pegg DE. Freezing of bone marrow for clinical use. Cryobiology 1964;1:64–71.

73. Lewis JP, Passovoy M, Conti SA, et al. The effect of cooling regimens on the transplantation potential of marrow. Transfusion 1967;7:17–32.

74. Malinin TI, Pegg DE, Perry VP, et al. Long-term storage of bone marrow cells at liquid nitrogen and dry ice temperature. Cryobiology 1970;7:65–69.

75. O'Grady LF, Lewis JP. The long-term preservation of bone marrow. Transfusion 1972;12:312–316.

76. Stroncek DF, Fautsch SK, Lasky LC, Hurd DD, Ramsay NKC, McCullough J. Adverse reactions in patients transfused with cryopreserved marrow. Transfusion 1991;31:521–527.

77. Rosenfeld CS, Gremba C, Shadduck RK, Zeigler ZR, Nemunaitis J. Engraftment with peripheral blood stem cells using noncontrolled-rate cryopreservation: comparison with autologous bone marrow transplantation. Exp Hematol 1994;22:290–294.

78. Preti RA, Razis E, Ciavarella D, et al. Clinical and laboratory comparison study of refrigerated and cryopreserved bone marrow for transplantation. Bone Marrow Transplant 1994;13:253–260.

79. Makino S, Harada M, Akashi K, et al. A simplified method for cryopreservation of peripheral blood stem cells at −80 degrees C without rate-controlled freezing. Bone Marrow Transplant 1991;8:239–244.

80. Douay L, Gorin NC, David R, et al. Study of granulocyte-macrophage progenitor (CFUc) preservation after slow freezing of bone marrow in the gas phase of liquid nitrogen. Exp Hematol 1982;10:360–366.

81. Rowley SD, Anderson GL. Effect of DMSO exposure without cryopreservation on hematopoietic progenitor cells. Bone Marrow Transplant 1993;11:389–393.

82. Bordin JO, Heddle NM, Blajchman MA. Biologic effects of leukocytes present in transfused cellular blood products. Blood 1994;84:1703–1721.

83. Lane TA, Anderson KC, Goodnough LT, et al. Leukocyte reduction in blood component therapy. Ann Intern Med 1992;117:151–162.

84. Freedman JJ, Blajchman MA, McCombie N. Canadian Red Cross Society symposium on leukodepletion: report of proceedings. Transfus Med Rev 1994;8:1–14.

85. Snyder EL. Clinical use of white cell-poor blood components. Transfusion 1989;29:568.

86. Dzik S. Leukodepletion blood filters: filter design and mechanisms of leukocyte removal. Transfus Med Rev 1993;7:65–77.

87. Kao KH, Mickel M, Braine HG, et al. White cell reduction in platelet concentrates and packed red cells by filtration: a multicenter clinical trial. Transfusion 1995;35:13–19.

88. TRAP Trial Study Group. A randomized trial evaluating leukocyte-reduction and UV-B irradiation of platelets to prevent alloimmune platelet refractoriness. N Engl J Med 1997. In press.

89. Bowden RA, Slichter SJ, Sayers M, et al. W. A comparison of filtered leukocyte-reduced and cytomegalovirus (CMV) seronegative blood products for the prevention of transfusion-associated CMV infection after marrow transplant. Blood 1995;86:3598–3603.

90. van Prooijen HC, Visser JJ, van Oostendorp WR, de Gast GC, Verdonck LF. Prevention of primary transfusion-associated cytomegalovirus infection in bone marrow transplant recipients by the removal of white cells from blood components with high-affinity filters. Br J Haematol 1994;87:144–147

91. Gilbert GL, Hudson IL, Hayes KL, et al. Prevention of transfusion-acquired cytomegalovirus infection in infants by blood filtration to remove leucocytes. Lancet 1989;1228–1231.

92. Class FHJ, Smeenk RJT, Schmidt R, et al. Alloimmunization against the MHC antigens after platelet transfusions is due to contaminating leukocytes in the platelet suspension. Exp Hematol 1981;9:84.

93. Eernisse JG, Brand A. Prevention of platelet refractoriness due to HLA antibodies by administration of leukocyte-poor blood components. Exp Hematol 1981;9:77.

94. Schiffer CA, Dutcher JP, Aisner J, et al. A randomized trial of leukocyte depleted platelet transfusion to modify alloimmunization in patients with leukemia. Blood 1980;56:182a. Abstract.
95. Sniecinski I, O'Donnell MR, Nowicki B, Hill LR. Prevention of refractoriness and HLA-alloimmunization using filtered blood products. Blood 1988;71:1402.
96. Factor IX complex and hepatitis. Food Drug Admin Drug Bull 1976;6:22.
97. Evatt B, Gompaerts E, McDougal J, Ramsey R. Coincidental appearance of LAV/HTLV antibodies in hemophiliacs and the onset of the AIDS epidemic. N Engl J Med 1985;312:483.
98. Walsh JH, Purcell RH, Morrow AG, et al. Post-transfusion hepatitis after open-heart operations: incidence after administration of blood from commercial and volunteer donor populations. JAMA 1970;211:261.
99. Prince AM, Horowitz B, Brotman B. Sterilization of hepatitis and HTLV-III viruses by exposure to try (n-butyl) phosphate and sodium cholate. Lancet 1986;1:706.
100. Aronson, DL. The development of the technology and capacity for the production of factor VIII for the treatment of hemophilia A. Transfusion 1990;30:748.
101. Kasper CK, Lusher JM. Transfusion Practices Committee: Recent evolution of clotting factor concentrates for hemophilia A and B. Transfusion 1993;33:422–434.
102. Azzi A, Ciappi S, Zakvrezeska K, et al. Human parvovirus B19 infection in hemophiliacs first infused with two high-purity virally attenuated factor VIII concentrates. Am J Hematol 1992;39:228–230.
103. An outbreak of hepatitis A related to a solvent/detergent treated factor VIII concentrate (Alphanate). MMWR 1996;45:29–32.
104. Lusher JM, Arkin S, Abildgaard CF, et al. Recombinant factor VIII for the treatment of previously untreated patients with hemophilia A. N Engl J Med 1993; 328:453–457.
105. Bray GL, Gomperts ED, Courter S, et al. A multicenter study of recombinant factor VIII (recombinate): safety, efficacy, and inhibitor risk in previously untreated patients with hemophilia A. Blood 1994;83:2428–2437.
106. deBiasi R, Rocino A, Miraglia E, et al. The impact of a very high purity factor VIII concentrate on the immune system of human immunodeficiency virus-infected hemophiliacs: a randomized prospective, two year comparison with an intermediate purity concentrate. Blood 1991;78:1919–1922.
107. Kasper CK. Plasma-derived versus recombinant factor VIII for the treatment of hemophilia A. Vox Sang 1996;70:17–20.
108. Mannucci PM, Bauer KA, Gringeri A, et al. Thrombin is not increased in the blood of hemophilia B patients after the infusion of a purified factor IX concentrate. Blood 1991;76:2540–2545.
109. Barundun S, Kistler P, Jeunet F, et al. Intravenous administration of human gamma globulin. Vox Sang 1962;7:157.
110. Condie RM, O'Reilly RJ. Prevention of cytomegalovirus infection by prophylaxis with an intravenous, hyperimmune, native, unmodified cytomegalovirus globulin. Am J Med 1984;76:134.
111. Meyers JD, Leszczynski J, Zaia JA, et al. Prevention of cytomegalovirus infection by cytomegalovirus immune globulin after marrow transplantation. Ann Intern Med 1983;98:442.
112. Sacher RA. Intravenous gammaglobulin products: development, pharmacology, and precautions. In: Garner RJ, Sacher RA, eds. Intravenous Gammaglobulin Therapy. Arlington, VA: American Association of Blood Banks, 1988:1.
113. Tremper KK, Friedman AE, Levine EM. The preoperative treatment of severely anemic patients with a perfluorochemical oxygen-transport fluid, fluosol-DA. N Engl J Med 1982;307:277.
114. Mitsuno T, Ohyanagi H, Naito R. Clinical studies of a perfluorochemical whole blood substitute (Fluosol-DA). Ann Surg 1982;195:60.
115. Bucala R. Cytotoxicity of a perfluorocarbon blood substitute to macrophages in vitro. Science 1983;220:965.
116. Vercellotti GM, Hammerschmidt DE, Craddock PR, Jacob HS. Activation of plasma complement by perfluorocarbon artificial blood: probable mechanism of adverse pulmonary reactions in treated patients and rationale for corticosteroid prophylaxis. Blood 1982;59:1299.
117. Gould SA, Rosen AL, Sehgal R, et al. Fluosol-DA as a red-cell substitute in acute anemia. N Engl J Med 1986;314:1653.
118. Winslow RM. Blood substitutes: current status. Transfusion 1989;29:753.

AUTOLOGOUS BLOOD DONATION
AND TRANSFUSION

Autologous blood donation is an old concept but was little used until the AIDS epidemic raised patients' and physicians' fears of blood transfusion. Autologous blood is widely believed to be the safest blood[1] and, as a result, interest in and the use of autologous blood increased dramatically during the latter part of the 1980s and the 1990s. The most common form of autologous blood is that deposited in anticipation of elective surgery, also called preoperative autologous blood donation. Other forms of autologous blood are perioperative hemodilution, intraoperative salvage of shed blood, and postoperative salvage of shed blood (Table 6.1). In addition, concerns about blood safety have increased interest in using other methods to avoid the need for transfusion; some of these will be mentioned here. Finally, another approach to minimizing the likelihood of transmission of disease is the development of "limited" donor programs. All of these techniques and strategies are described below.

STRATEGIES TO REDUCE OR AVOID ALLOGENEIC TRANSFUSION

There are several actions that can be used in a combined approach to minimize the use of allogeneic blood (Table 6.2).[2] An excellent example of an overall approach to the specific situation of cardiovascular surgery is provided by one of the pioneers of cardiovascular surgery, Dr. Denton Cooley, who recently described a wonderful, comprehensive program for minimizing the necessity of transfusion of allogeneic blood during cardiovascular surgery.[3] This program involves preoperative considerations such as review of the medical history to identify factors that may predispose patients to

Table 6.1 Types of autologous blood donation and transfusion

Preoperative deposit/donation
Acute normovolemic hemodilution
Intraoperative salvage
Postoperative salvage

excessive blood loss, review of medications that might increase blood loss, use of erythropoietin, and preoperative autologous blood donation, as well as intraoperative considerations such as the use of acute normovolemic hemodilution (ANH), close attention to heparin levels, use of antifibrinolytic agents, use of hypothermia, attention to hemostasis, and intraoperative and postoperative salvage of shed blood (Table 6.3).

The program described by Dr. Cooley illustrates the importance of paying careful attention to factors in the medical history or present medications that might predispose the patient to excessive bleeding and taking steps to deal with any correctable problems in advance of surgery. Once into the transfusion situation, the indications for transfusion become a factor. Recently transfusion practices have become much more conservative. In comparison to common practice a few years ago, patients' hemoglobin levels or platelet counts are now allowed to fall much lower before transfusion, and the use of plasma has been curtailed (see Chapters 11 and 12). These changes in transfusion practice have resulted in fewer transfusions and thus fewer donor exposures. Pharmacologic agents may be used to reduce blood loss.[2] Examples are more careful use of anticoagulants, administration of desmopressin acetate to enhance coagulation (particularly in cardiovascular surgery), and use of protease inhibitors such as epsilon aminocaproic acid (EACA) in fibrinolytic situations or to enhance platelet function (aprotinin). A different approach using pharmacologic agents involves stimulation of hematopoiesis. This can be done for red cells using erythropoietin either to enhance red cell production in the patient in anticipation of blood loss or to increase the number of autologous units that can be donated (see below). Pharmacologic strategies can also be used for granulocytes using either granulocyte colony-stimulating factor (G-CSF) or granulocyte-macrophage colony-stimulating factor (GM-CSF), and possibly for platelets using thrombopoietin or megakaryocyte growth and development factor

Table 6.2 Strategies to reduce or avoid allogeneic transfusion

Change indications for transfusion
Use special surgical and anesthetic techniques
Use pharmacologic agents to:
    Reduce blood loss
    Stimulate marrow
    Increase capability for autologous donations
Use limited-donor programs
Use single-donor components

Table 6.3 Blood management considerations for cardiovascular surgery patients

	Consideration	Comments
Preoperative	Antithrombolytic drugs	Whenever possible, discontinue several days before surgery
	Epoetin alfa	Appropriate for patients at high risk of bleeding complications
	Iron supplementation	Appropriate for patients with low Hb levels or clinical or laboratory signs of anemia
	Preoperative autologous donation of blood	Limited by cost, logistics, and time; recommended only for patients at high risk of bleeding
Intraoperative	Hemodilution	Extreme hemodilution (HCT <20%) may adversely affect platelet function
	Heparinization	Adequate anticoagulation can usually be achieved with a loading dose of 3 mg/kg
	Aprotinin	Reduces blood loss and transfusion requirements; most useful in patients at high risk of bleeding
	Aminocaproic acid	Antiplasminogenic effects
	Desmopressin	Useful in some patients with coagulopathies such as uremic thrombopathy, platelet defects, von Willebrand's disease
	Hypothermia	Moderate levels (22–28%C) should be used; expeditious rewarming reverses adverse effects
	Topical hemostatic agents	Used to create drier operative field and reduce blood loss
	Blood salvage and autotransfusion	Although considered fairly standard practice, unwashed blood collected without systemic anticoagulation could increase clotting products and activated clotting factor proteins
Postoperative	Shed mediastinal blood salvage	Can reduce the need for allogeneic RBC transfusion by 50%; generally ineffective if the volume to be reinfused is <400 mL or 4 h
	Allogeneic transfusion	Should be used only when absolutely necessary
	RBC transfusion	May be needed when Hb <8 g/dL
	Platelet therapy	Consider when platelet level <50,000 cells/mm^3
	Fresh frozen plasma	May be needed when PT >15 s, PTT >40 s, or postoperative chest tube output >300 mL/h for 2 h or >900 mL total in 3 h
	Hypertension	Must be controlled to avoid potential for increased bleeding; plasma expanders can cause or exacerbate hypertension

Source: Cooley DA. Conservation of blood during cardiovascular surgery. Am J Surg 1995;170:53S–59S.
Abbreviations: Hb, hemoglobin; HCT, hematocrit; PT, prothrombin time; PTT, partial thromboplastin time; RBC, red blood cell.

(MGDF) (see Chapter 17). Another strategy that can reduce but not eliminate allogeneic donor exposure is the use of single-donor components when possible. The most common example of this is the use of single-donor platelets obtained by apheresis instead of pooling several units obtained from whole blood to provide one therapeutic dose (see Chapters 5 and 11). Some blood centers make available fresh frozen plasma in large-volume units, thus reducing by about half the number of donor exposures from plasma

transfusions. Finally, limited-donor programs are operated by some centers (see below). This is usually practical only for pediatric patients. While all of these strategies are available, it would be rare to find them all used extensively in one center. Each hospital has its own unique mix of activities designed around these specific steps, but the central theme that pervades transfusion practice today is the more conservative use of blood transfusion and structuring the provision of blood components to take into account the public's concern about transfusion-transmitted diseases.

TRENDS IN THE COLLECTION AND TRANSFUSION OF AUTOLO-GOUS BLOOD

National Trends in Autologous Blood Donation

In one study[4] the amount of predeposit autologous blood increased 23% annually between 1988 and 1992 and the proportion of all blood collected that was autologous more than doubled from 2.5% to 5.7%. In another study,[5] autologous blood increased from 655,000 units in 1989 to 1,117,000 units in 1992 for a 70.5% increase, while total blood collections decreased 3.1%. This represented nearly a doubling of the proportion of the total blood supply provided by autologous donations during this 5-year period. Interestingly, most of this increase in autologous blood collection occurred in blood centers, not hospitals,[5] where it might have been expected because of the close interaction between the hospital blood bank and the clinicians planning to use the autologous blood. There is also a regional difference in autologous blood collection.[5] Autologous blood represented an average of 9.9% of the blood collected by blood centers in the Pacific region compared to 3.2% by blood centers in the New England region. Despite the large increase in autologous donations, this is far short of predictions that autologous blood could provide 20% of all blood used. It now seems unlikely that such extensive use of autologous blood will ever occur.

National Trends in Autologous Blood Transfusion

From 1989 to 1992, there was a 6.2% decrease in the total number of units of red cells transfused in the United States.[5] During the same period, the number of units of autologous red cells used increased 59%.[5] However, this increased usage of autologous blood was not as great as the increase in autologous donations, and the result was that 49.1% of autologous units were not used.[5] This poor utilization rate was attributed to donation for procedures with a low probability of use, donation beyond the expected need, lack of clear criteria for transfusing autologous blood, and hesitancy to use suitable autologous blood as part of the general community blood supply.[5] Thus, although use of autologous blood is quite popular and is seen by many patients as a valuable way to reduce the possibility of disease transmission, the policies and procedures for its use in an operationally efficient and cost-effective way are not yet well developed. These issues are discussed in more detail below.

PREOPERATIVE AUTOLOGOUS BLOOD DONATION

Autologous Donor Blood

An individual may donate blood for his or her own use if the need for blood can be anticipated and a donation plan developed. Most commonly, this occurs with elective surgery. It is important to thoughtfully plan the autologous blood donation schedule so that blood is collected only for procedures for which there is substantial likelihood that the blood will be used. Without this type of planning, there is a very high rate of wastage of autologous blood, and the costs are quite high. The procedures for which some form of autologous blood is recommended have been summarized by the National Heart, Lung, and Blood Institute Expert Panel on the Use of Autologous Blood (Table 6.4).[6] In general, autologous blood is recommended only for procedures for which blood would be crossmatched and that involve at least a 10% chance of blood use. Examples are major orthopedic procedures, radical prostatectomy, vascular surgery, and open heart surgery. Examples of situations in which autologous donation is not recommended include cholecystectomy, herniorrhaphy, and normal delivery. It is essential

Table 6.4 Autologous blood collection techniques in selected surgical procedures

Surgical procedure	Autologous blood collection technique*			
	PABD	IBS	PBS	ANH
Coronary artery bypass graft	+	+	+	+
Major vascular surgery	+	+	−	+
Primary hip replacement	+	+	+	+
Revision hip replacement	+	+	+	+
Total knee replacement	+	−	+	−
Major spine surgery with instrumentation	+	+	+	+
Selected neurologic procedures (e.g., resection of arteriovenous formation)	+	+	−	+
Hepatic resections	+	+	−	+
Radical prostatectomy	+	+	−	+
Cervical spine fusion	−	−	−	−
Intervertebral discectomy	−	−	−	−
Mastectomy	−	−	−	−
Hysterectomy	−	−	−	−
Reduction mammoplasty	−	−	−	−
Cholecystectomy	−	−	−	−
Tonsillectomy	−	−	−	−
Vaginal and cesarean deliveries	−	−	−	−
Transurethral resection of the prostate	−	−	−	−

Source: National Heart, Lung, and Blood Institute Expert Panel on the Use of Autologous Blood. Transfusion alert: use of autologous blood. Transfusion 1995;35:703–711.
Abbreviations: ANH, acute normovolemic hemodilution; IBS, intraoperative blood salvage; PABD, preoperative autologous blood donation; PBS, postoperative blood salvage.
*+ Indicates use of the technique is considered appropriate; − indicates use of the technique is considered inappropriate.

to define the specific situations in which autologous blood is indicated and then define the amount of blood desired for each of those situations. The hospital's standard surgical blood order system can be used to estimate the amount of blood likely to be used, and a plan for autologous donation can be developed based on that schedule. One specific suggested plan has been published.[7] A practical approach to the implementation and operation of a hospital-based autologous donation and transfusion program has also been published,[8] and an excellent review of autologous blood utilization shows relationships between estimated blood loss, hematocrit changes during hospitalization, cost-effectiveness of autologous blood, and programs for collecting the blood.[9] An example of strategies combining all of the different autologous blood collection and transfusion methods is illustrated in Table 6.3.

If patient candidates for autologous blood donation meet the usual FDA criteria for blood donation, their blood may be "crossed over"—that is, used for other patients—if the original autologous donor has no need for the blood. If the autologous donor does not meet the FDA criteria for blood donation, the blood must be specially labeled, segregated during storage, and discarded if not used by that specific patient. There is no general agreement about the desirability of the practice of crossing over autologous units. Some studies show similar rates of transmissible disease markers in autologous and allogeneic donors,[10] and others show increased rates among autologous donors.[11] AuBuchon and Dodd[12] described the structure of the data that should be obtained to define the relative risk of autologous blood and to form the basis of practice. Unfortunately, almost a decade later the data are not available. Because of the concern about the possible inadvertent transfusion of an infectious unit to someone other than the autologous donor, most blood banks do not cross over autologous blood to patients other than the donor-patient.

Occasionally a healthy person wishes to donate blood for long-term storage for himself or herself in the event of a future unforeseen need. This is not recommended because of the low possibility that the blood will be available where and when needed and the high cost of the long-term storage.

Medical Requirements and Evaluation for Autologous Blood Donation

The medical history for autologous donation is the same as for allogeneic donation except that since the donor is actually a patient, additional emphasis should be placed on questions about medications and medical conditions or illnesses. There are no age or weight restrictions for autologous donation.[13] However, because severe reactions are more likely in older donors,[14] this should be taken into account when evaluating potential donors. One of the types of severe reactions in allogeneic donors who are in good health is cardiovascular events,[14] and deaths have occurred following blood donation by individuals who met all the FDA criteria for blood donation.[15] Therefore, there is some difference of opinion regarding the safety of donation by patients with cardiovascular risk factors.[8,16,17] Several specific cardiovascular conditions have been proposed as contraindications for autologous blood donation (Table 6.5).

Pregnant women may donate, although this is not recommended routinely since these patients rarely require transfusion.[6] Donors with known or suspected bacteremia

Table 6.5 Cardiovascular conditions proposed as contraindications to autologous blood donation

Idiopathic subaortic stenosis
Aortic stenosis
Left main coronary artery disease
Unstable angina
Cardiac failure
Recent myocardial infarction
Ventricular arrhythmia
Atrioventricular block
Symptoms of disease on the day of donation

Source: Yomtovian R. Practical aspects of pre-operative autologous transfusion. Am J Clin Pathol 1997;107:S28–S35.

should not donate autologous blood because of the possibility of transfusion of contaminated blood (see Chapter 15). Examples of such situations are patients with ulcers that might be associated with bacteremia or patients with recent gastroenteritis that might be due to *Yersinia enterocolitica.*

The autologous donor's hemoglobin may be lower (11 g/dL) than that required for allogeneic donors (12.5 g/dL), and autologous donors may donate as often as every 72 hours up to 72 hours prior to the planned surgery. Usually it is only possible to obtain 2 to 4 units of blood before the hemoglobin falls below 11 g/dL. The planned donations ideally should begin 4 to 6 weeks before the anticipated blood use. Although blood can be donated up to 72 hours before surgery, a mathematical model[18] has suggested that donations closer to surgery than 15 days are not effective because the patient's hemoglobin does not have time to recover, resulting in the patient receiving the blood back due to the iatrogenic anemia induced by the blood donations. This was confirmed in a large study showing that blood use increased when the last autologous unit was donated less than 15 days before elective surgery.[19] Oral iron therapy is usually recommended to facilitate erythropoiesis in response to blood donation. However, many patients experience gastrointestinal side effects that limit the iron therapy.

The final decision on whether to withdraw blood from an autologous donor rests with the medical director of the blood bank. Often consultation between the donor's (patient's) physician and the blood bank physician is necessary to arrive at a wise course of action.

Collection Processing and Storage of Autologous Blood

Procedures for the selection of veins for phlebotomy, cleaning the venipuncture site, use of containers and other equipment for blood collection, and the actual collection are similar to the procedures used for collection of allogeneic blood (see Chapter 4). If desired, the amount of anticoagulant in the primary container can be reduced by transferring some anticoagulant to a satellite bag. This makes it possible for autologous

blood to be collected from children or small adults.[20] All autologous units must be labeled "for autologous use only." Components can be made from autologous units, but if so, each component must be labeled as autologous and recording systems must ensure that these components are used only for the donor-patient.

Usually autologous blood is collected within a few weeks of its intended use and is stored in the liquid state as is done for the ordinary blood supply. The red cells can be frozen for longer-term storage if it is desired to allow the donor's red cell mass to replenish itself. However, this adds substantially to the cost of the blood and is rarely done. Another reason to consider freezing the red cells is if the planned use is delayed. For instance, if the donor-patient develops a cold or other transient reason to postpone elective surgery, it may be desirable to freeze the red cells for later use. Alternatively, the red cells can be returned to the donor-patient, but this is not recommended because transfusion will suppress the donor's red cell production.

Adverse Reactions to Autologous Blood Donation

There is some disagreement regarding whether adverse reactions are more common in autologous than allogeneic donors. This comparison is complicated by the fact that autologous donors tend to be older than allogeneic donors and to have medical conditions that would preclude many of them from allogeneic donation. Two reports show no increase in adverse reactions in autologous donors,[12,21] but another found that first-time autologous donors, females, and those taking cardiac glycosides had a higher risk of reaction than nonautologous donors.[22] Very severe reactions resulting in hospitalization were found to occur 12 times more often in autologous donors than in allogeneic donors and may occur as often as once in 17,000 donations.[14] Thus, although it is not clear whether the overall incidence of adverse reactions is greater in autologous than allogeneic donors, this form of blood donation is not without risk. Autologous donation should be used only after careful consideration of the particular patient's medical condition and potential transfusion needs.

Laboratory Testing of Autologous Blood

Autologous blood must be typed for ABO and Rh antigens, just as with allogeneic blood. If the blood is to be kept in the institution where it is collected and used only for the autologous donor, no infectious disease testing is required. If the blood is to be shipped to another institution for transfusion, at least the first unit must be tested for transmissible diseases.[13] Subsequent units donated within 30 days need not be tested. If any of the transmissible disease tests are positive, the unit must be labeled with a biohazard label. This is sometimes confusing or disconcerting to physicians and patients. The biohazard label implies to them that the blood is unsafe, but it is an FDA requirement intended to alert health care personnel to the potential hazard presented by the blood, which has a positive test for a transmissible disease.

At the time of admission to the hospital for the planned blood use, a blood specimen should be obtained from the patient and compatibility testing carried out with the autologous unit. The nature of the compatibility can be established by the hospital but

should consist of at least confirming the ABO compatibility between the patient's sample and the unit of blood. It is preferable to use the hospital's routine compatibility testing system for autologous units as well as allogeneic units to minimize the chance of error caused by special handling of the autologous units.

Donation of Autologous Blood by Patients Known to Be Infectious

Autologous blood is thought to be the safest blood available, but it may be of even greater benefit to human immunodeficiency virus (HIV)-infected than noninfected patients.[23] A debate has developed over whether patients known to be infectious, particularly with HIV, should be allowed to donate autologous blood.[23] The concerns are mainly twofold: that medical personnel might accidentally become infected with the blood (via needle puncture, etc.) and that the blood might be inadvertently transfused to someone other than the patient-donor. Ethical principles that have been applied to this situation include the principle of autonomy, whereby the patient has a right to decide what should and should not be done to him or her, and the principle of justice, whereby equity is ensured to all involved or potentially affected by the decision.[24] The denial of treatment to any specific group of patients is considered unethical,[23] which seems to indicate that it would be unethical to deny the opportunity to donate autologous blood to a patient solely on the basis of HIV status.[23] A detailed analysis of the risks and benefits indicated that these are in balance only when donation is by a patient with hepatitis C.[25] Any other kinds of infections carry greater risks of harm to others than benefits to the patient. However, in the absence of more extensive data, a national policy has not yet been developed. Such a policy must depend on the "interplay of the medical utility of such blood and the public health implications of an accident or error resulting in the inadvertent transmission of virus to an innocent party."[23] Each institution must establish its own local policy on this issue.

Use of Erythropoietin to Increase Autologous Blood Donation

Erythropoietin (EPO) acts on receptors primarily found on erythroid cells to increase proliferation and differentiation of immature erythroid cells in the marrow (see Chapter 17). Thus, it is possible that administration of EPO might be of benefit to potential donors of autologous blood. The increased red cell production could benefit the patient-donor in at least three ways: (1) make it possible to donate more blood, (2) make it possible to donate when he or she might not have been able to do so at all because of anemia, and (3) provide faster recovery of hemoglobin after autologous donation, resulting in a higher hemoglobin at the time of surgery. Based on analysis of 13 reports, Spivak concluded that the administration of EPO to autologous blood donors increases the number of units of blood they can donate.[26] However, the value of EPO administration remains a bit unclear, since this strategy usually has not been shown to reduce the need for allogeneic donor blood.[26] In one study of orthopedic surgery in rheumatoid arthritis patients, the use of EPO did increase the amount of blood donated preoperatively but also the amount of allogeneic blood the patients received.[27] Another example of a specific situation in which EPO administration was helpful is a patient with anemia of

chronic disease who had multiple red cell antibodies and in whom EPO made possible autologous donation for elective surgery.[28] In general, the main advantage of EPO administration may be in patients who are anemic prior to considering autologous donation. These studies also established that the increased red cell production that is under way at the time of surgery can reduce the need for allogeneic blood use even in the absence of autologous blood.[26]

UTILIZATION OF PREOPERATIVE AUTOLOGOUS DONATED BLOOD

Utilization

A substantial amount of literature has been published describing the use of autologous blood in various specific clinical situations (Table 6.4). The major issue of interest in this regard is whether the donation of autologous blood causes changes in the patient on admission to the hospital that would alter the transfusion therapy. That is, if the patient is admitted with a lower hemoglobin level, he or she may ultimately receive more blood than comparable patients who have not donated autologous blood. There are no extensive, convincing data to settle this issue. In one study,[29] patients who donated autologous blood prior to elective hysterectomy had lower hematocrits upon admission and received more transfusions during their hospitalization. In general, it seems quite likely that patients who have donated autologous blood will have lower hemoglobins at the time of elective surgery. This raises the question of whether the indications for transfusion of autologous units should be the same as for allogeneic units. Because there are risks associated with autologous units, many transfusion medicine physicians have suggested that indications should be the same. Others contend that since the risk-benefit relationship for autologous transfusion is different than for allogeneic transfusion, the indications should be different. There are some data suggesting that those who donate autologous blood have a different transfusion experience from patients who do not. Patients undergoing hip and knee arthroplasty who had donated autologous blood received less blood that nonautologous donors.[30] In another study of orthopedic surgery patients, those who had donated autologous blood received fewer transfusions than nondonors.[31] Thus, although the availability of autologous blood might lead physicians to transfuse it more liberally, some data such as the previous examples suggest that physicians might be more conservative when autologous blood is available. Each hospital must establish its own guidelines regarding the indications for autologous blood. Suggested transfusion audit criteria have been published.[32,33]

Cost-Effectiveness

The cost of autologous blood is greater than that of allogeneic blood. Additional time is required for scheduling, for the donor interview, for labeling and making decisions regarding transmissible disease testing, and for record keeping. Other costs of autologous blood are for special shipping if the unit is not collected in the hospital where it will be used and for additional handling and quarantine within the hospital blood bank. Most blood banks apply a surcharge or extra handling fee to cover these additional

costs. Ironically, although autologous blood is considered the safest blood for the patient, governmental agencies and health care providers may refuse to pay the extra costs of autologous blood, thus placing a financial disincentive on its use.

Because approximately 50% of autologous blood donated preoperatively is not used,[5] this results in other additional costs. Recently, a study of the cost-effectiveness of preoperative autologous blood[34] demonstrated that the expected health benefit was only approximately 2 to 4 hours of additional life span. This translates to a cost ranging from $235,000 to more than $23 million per quality-adjusted life year resulting from the use of autologous blood. Separate studies have estimated that the cost per life year saved ranged from $40,000 to more than $1 million when autologous blood was used, depending on the likelihood of transfusion during the surgical procedures.[35,36] Thus, autologous blood is considerably more costly than allogeneic blood for the benefits received and does not fit within the usual range of medical procedures thought to be cost-effective. However, the widespread use of autologous blood is another example of the lack of impact of cost-effectiveness on the specific practices used within transfusion medicine. The cost-effectiveness of autologous blood could be improved by developing and operating better systems to determine when autologous donation should be used.

COMPLICATIONS OF TRANSFUSION OF AUTOLOGOUS BLOOD

Although it is widely accepted that autologous blood is the safest blood for a particular patient, complications of autologous transfusion can occur (Table 6.6). These include problems in handling the autologous blood such as allowing units to outdate, units being misplaced by the blood bank, or transfusing allogeneic units out of sequence instead of available autologous units. If the donor has bacteremia, the unit may be contaminated and the patient then receives contaminated blood. If the donor has unsuspected hemolytic syndrome, hemolysis can occur at the time of transfusion.[37] Occasionally blood is improperly handled or the transfusion techniques are not satisfactory (see Chapters 13, 14, and 15). This can result in the transfusion of hemolyzed blood. These same problems can occur with autologous blood. The most serious problem is transfusing the unit to the wrong patient. In one study of 251,228 autologous units, it was determined that transfusion errors occurred once for every 15,600 units or once in 14,800 patients.[38] A separate study estimated that the likelihood that a unit of autologous blood will be given to the wrong patient is 1 in 30,000 to 50,000 units.[6] In a questionnaire to American Association of Blood Banks (AABB) institutions, 1.2% reported erroneously transfusing a unit to the wrong patient.[8] The overall estimate of the risks of autologous transfusion then can be estimated as 1 per 15,000 to 50,000 units.

ACUTE NORMOVOLEMIC HEMODILUTION

As experience has been gained with the successful use of colloid and crystalloid to manage acute blood loss, this approach has been applied in a controlled setting to collect blood from patients for autologous transfusion. This has been called acute normovolemic hemodilution (ANH). In acute ANH, whole blood is withdrawn immediately

Table 6.6 Complications of autologous transfusion

Donor-related	Bacterial contamination of unit
Clerical	Allogeneic units used out of sequence when autologous units available
	Autologous units not available when needed
	Autologous unit transfused to wrong patient—hemolysis; disease transmission
	Autologous unit allowed to outdate
Mechanical	Hemolysis due to improper collection, handling, or storage of unit
	Hemolysis due to improper transfusion technique

before or after induction of anesthesia. As the blood is removed, blood volume is maintained with infusion of large volumes of crystalloid (3:1 ratio with volume of blood removed) or colloid (1:1 ratio with volume of blood removed). ANH involves removal of the amount of blood projected to reduce the hematocrit level to approximately 28%, although more extreme reductions of hematocrit are sometimes attempted. The advantages of ANH are (a) production of autologous blood, (b) availability of fresh blood containing platelets and coagulation factors, (c) reduction in the amount of red cell loss during surgery because intraoperative bleeding occurs at a lower hematocrit after blood donation, and (d) hemodynamics and oxygen availability may actually be increased due to the lower hematocrit and there may be decreased operating time and possibly postoperative improvements in pulmonary, renal, and myocardial function.[39]

During hemodilution, there are several compensatory mechanisms to maintain oxygen delivery. These include increased cardiac output,[40,41] decreased blood viscosity with resulting decreased peripheral vascular resistance, thus enhancing cardiac output. Peripheral vascular resistance is maximally reduced at a hematocrit level of approximately 30%,[42] and maximum oxygen transport capacity occurs at a hematocrit level of approximately 30%.[43] Thus, it is thought that the patient may have better hemodynamics at the lower hematocrit that results from the blood donation just prior to surgery.

In ANH, the blood is collected from large-bore catheters placed into the central vein or even an artery (usually the radial artery). The blood is collected into standard plastic blood bank containers containing CPD anticoagulant and stored at room temperature, usually right in the operating room.[43–45] Special containers and tubing sets are available for this purpose.[45] It is essential that the personnel collecting the blood be familiar with important steps such as mixing the blood during collection, proper labeling, and storage conditions. Specific procedures should be available and the staff should be familiar with them. Formulas are available to calculate the volume of blood that can be removed from patients with different starting hematocrits and different weights to achieve a final hematocrit of 30%.[45] Criteria for patient selection should be determined in advance by written protocol (Table 6.7). Usually ANH is reserved for patients in whom the expected blood loss is 1 liter or more or 20% or more of the patient's estimated blood volume.

ANH has been used to provide autologous red cells in orthopedic surgery, major general surgery, liver resection, and cardiovascular surgery.[40,43,44,46–53] There are reports of a 15% to 90% decrease in the use of allogeneic red cells (multiple studies

Table 6.7 Criteria for acute normovolemic
hemodilution

Expected blood loss > 1 liter or 20% blood volume
Hemoglobin > 12 g/dL
Absence of coronary heart disease
Absence of coagulopathy
Absence of liver disease
Absence of severe hypertension
Absence of severe pulmonary disease
Absence of severe renal disease

Source: Adapted from Vengelen-Tyler V, ed. Technical
Manual. Standards for blood banks and transfusion services, 12th ed. Arlington, VA: American Association of
Blood Banks, 1996; and Stehling L, Zauder HL. Acute
normovolemic hemodilution. Transfusion 1991;31:
857–868.

reviewed).[45] This would seem to indicate that ANH is very effective, and from this one would expect that it is widely used. However, there is not universal agreement about the value, safety, and cost-effectiveness of ANH. Despite the references listed above, there are only a few structured studies of ANH and most involve small numbers of patients and few or no controls. However, it seems unlikely that large, properly structured, controlled studies will be done. Thus, the data on safety and the effectiveness of ANH in avoiding allogeneic red cell transfusion are not as compelling as it might seem from the references cited. Regarding safety, in any large number of surgical patients, there will be many who have silent coronary vascular disease, in whom ANH might be dangerous. Thus, it seems that the best setting for ANH is in young, otherwise healthy patients undergoing elective surgery with a large expected blood loss and where the surgical and anesthesia team is experienced in techniques of ANH.

INTRAOPERATIVE BLOOD SALVAGE

Development of Blood Salvage

There are a number of situations in which blood can be collected from the operative site or extracorporeal circuits and returned to the patient. This process is known as intraoperative salvage. With the development of cardiovascular surgery, it became apparent that the blood lost during surgery and in the pump oxygenator could be recovered and returned to the patient. Pump devices were improved, extracorporeal anticoagulation techniques refined, and safety systems such as bubble traps introduced to minimize the likelihood of complications when blood was salvaged from the operative site. This practice became more routine, and it also became apparent that the approach could be used to salvage blood in other types of surgical procedures.[54] At about the same time, it was recognized clinically that blood shed from sources such as the chest was defib-

rinated and could be returned to the patient after being washed. Further stimulating interest in blood salvage was the dramatic growth in coronary artery bypass surgery during the 1970s and 1980s. Thus, gradually, an incentive developed for manufacturers to develop devices specifically designed for salvage of blood shed during surgery.

Devices Used for Intraoperative Blood Salvage

There are three types of blood salvage devices: (1) canisters, (2) cell processing units, and (3) single-use reservoirs.[55,56] The canisters use a sterile plastic liner in a rigid container attached to a suction device. Anticoagulant is added as the shed blood is aspirated into the canister. When the container is full, it can be connected to a cell-washing device or removed and taken to the laboratory for washing and concentration of the red cells. These units are less expensive than the other devices and are used when the amount of blood loss is expected to be small. Cell-processing devices are similar to instruments used for apheresis. They are semicontinuous-flow systems in which the blood is aspirated, anticoagulated with heparin or citrate,[55] and washed to remove the anticoagulants as well as platelets, plasma, and most debris if present. These devices are more complex and use more expensive software than the canisters and so the semicontinuous devices are used when blood loss is expected to be substantial, usually greater than 1 liter. The single-use reservoir is a simple device that allows salvage of blood with immediate return to the patient but no washing or cell concentration steps. Because of the lack of a washing step, this approach is used only for procedures that are expected to generate minimal debris.

In the operation of a blood salvage program, collaboration among surgeons, anesthesiologists, and transfusion medicine professionals is important because of the technical considerations as well as the selection of patients and equipment.[54,56,57] For instance, when blood is salvaged from noncardiovascular surgery in which the patients are not anticoagulated, the washing is particularly important, since the shed blood will usually contain activated coagulation factor proteins.[58,59] The transfusion of these activated coagulation factor proteins can cause severe reactions. It is also essential to ensure that hemolysis does not occur from improper use of the device, since transfusion of red cells with high levels of free hemoglobin can also cause severe reactions. Since the recovered shed blood will be primarily red cells when transfused, patients who receive large amounts of salvaged blood may develop a "depletion" coagulopathy even though they will have received little allogeneic blood. Blood replacement strategies should account for this possibility. Intraoperative salvage is contraindicated in patients with bacteremia or for salvaging blood from a surgical field thought to be contaminated. Intraoperative salvage is also not used for surgeries involving malignancies because of the theoretical possibility of dissemination of tumor cells. Tumor cells have been found in the cell salvage devices.[60] The potential complications of intraoperative blood salvage can be summarized as[54] coagulopathy, air embolus, infection, fat embolus, drug effects due to aspiration of drugs into salvage devices, and microaggregate effects. Because of the complexities of blood collection, storage, and transfusion and the patient selection necessary to operate a safe and effective program, thorough procedures and documentation are important. Often blood bank personnel can work in col-

laboration with surgery personnel to develop and monitor the program and carry out ongoing quality control.

Intraoperative blood salvage has been used in cardiovascular, vascular, orthopedic, gynecologic, urologic, transplant (especially liver), and occasionally trauma patients.[54] In one study of cardiovascular surgery patients, blood salvage resulted in an overall reduction of 62% of the mean number of red cells transfused.[61] There are fewer studies of intraoperative blood salvage than for ANH, and those that are available are small and not well controlled. However, blood salvage is used more extensively than ANH, but the optimum conditions, the expected blood loss, and the devices used for each situation are not well defined.

POSTOPERATIVE BLOOD SALVAGE

Following surgery, it may be possible to collect shed blood and return it to the patient in some circumstances. The most extensive experience with this is in cardiovascular surgery, although in the past few years interest has developed in salvaging blood from joints following joint replacement surgery. Several devices are available for collection of blood, and these usually involve a chest tube drainage system with integral blood bag and filter. Blood salvaged from postoperative drainage is usually not anticoagulated The obvious advantage is to obtain the patient's own shed blood for autologous transfusion. However, there are several concerns with postoperative salvage: (*a*) the wound drainage is usually dilute, and so the volume of red cells actually obtained may not be large; (*b*) the red cells in the drainage are usually partially hemolyzed; (*c*) there is activation of the coagulation system and the drainage contains activated coagulation proteins; and (*d*) the drainage may contain cytokines and drainage may occur over a prolonged time, resulting in red cells that are damaged by exposure to room temperature. Because the postoperative salvaged blood is not washed before transfusion, the quality of the red cells being transfused may be poor or even dangerous for the patient. Thus, as for ANH, it is valuable for these procedures to be developed in collaboration with the blood bank and for personnel to be knowledgeable and follow procedures so as to ensure the transfusion of a safe and effective red cell component.

DIRECTED-DONOR BLOOD

Directed donors are friends or relatives who wish to give blood for a specific patient. It is estimated that in 1992, a total of 436,000 units of blood were donated as directed-donor units.[5] This represented 3.2% of the total available blood supply, which was an increase of 24.6% since 1989. The appeal of directed-donor blood is that the patient hopes those donors will be safer than the regular blood supply. Before much experience had been gained with directed-donor blood, some transfusion medicine professionals feared that this blood would be less safe than the general community supply because the donors would be under considerable pressure to donate and might not be candid about their medical and risk-behavior history. In general, the data do not indicate that

directed donors are either more or less safe than regular donors. Directed donors do not have a lower incidence of transmissible disease markers,[62–64] and directed-donor blood is no more safe than allogeneic blood donated for the general blood supply. Conversely, there is no evidence that the incidence of positive transmissible disease tests is increased in directed donors, which would cause directed-donor blood to be less safe. Thus, the transmissible disease testing data do not provide a factual rationale for directed donations. Despite this, directed-donor blood has considerable appeal to many patients, and it continues to be a meaningful part of the blood supply for some hospitals. A few blood banks refuse directed donations, but most accept these donors as a service to the patients. Each hospital must also decide whether to sequester the blood and use it only for the intended patient or to allow the directed-donor blood to become part of the community's general blood supply if it is not used for the originally intended patient. If directed-donor units are to be "crossed over" into the general supply, the donors must meet all the usual FDA requirements for routine blood donation. In either situation, directed-donor blood requires additional attention and record systems for the blood center and hospital, thus increasing the cost and creating the possibility for errors to occur and the blood to be unavailable when desired for the particular patient.

PATIENT-SPECIFIC DONATION

There are a few situations in which appropriate transfusion therapy involves collecting blood from a particular donor for a particular patient. Examples are donor-specific transfusions prior to kidney transplantation, maternal platelets for a fetus projected to have neonatal thrombocytopenia, or family members of a patient with a rare blood type. In these situations, the donors must meet all the usual FDA requirements, except that they may donate as often as every 3 days so long as their hemoglobin remains above the normal donor minimum of 12.5 g/dL.[65] The units donated must undergo all routine laboratory testing.[65]

MINIMAL DONOR EXPOSURE PROGRAMS

Programs that attempt to limit the number of donors to which a patient is exposed usually involve pediatric patients, because their size makes their blood requirements smaller than for most adults. Limiting the donor exposures can be accomplished by some laboratory techniques, by selected-donor programs, and by the use of single-donor components.

Laboratory Techniques

Sterile connector devices can be used to allow multiple entry into a unit of red cells so that a patient can receive multiple transfusions of cells from the same donor.[66–68] The advantage of reducing donor exposures must be balanced against the use of blood that ages while being stored. Many pediatricians and neonatologists prefer to use blood less

than 7 to 10 days old, especially for seriously ill neonates. This may limit the number of transfusions that can be provided from one unit of red cells even though the technology is available to enter the container under sterile conditions multiple times.

Donor Programs

One approach is the use of a model to predict the patient's blood needs.[66] This allows the use of either one unit of blood designated for that specific patient or the use of one unit to supply several patients. This approach improves the efficiency of blood use but does not necessarily reduce the number of donor exposures. The Mayo Clinic physicians reported a unique program for children undergoing cardiovascular surgery, in which the parents donated platelets by apheresis before surgery; during surgery, blood salvage was used along with blood from one dedicated donor.[67] This reduced donor exposures by 80%. Strauss et al.[68] were able to obtain all of the blood needed by pediatric patients undergoing elective surgery from an individual donor dedicated to each patient by lowering the hematocrit necessary for donation. Thus, programs like these can result in reduction of donor exposures for some pediatric patients. The cost is probably higher than those of allogeneic donor programs, and the usual FDA donor requirements cannot be applied to donor selection. Very few such programs are in operation.

REFERENCES

1. Surgenor DM. The patient's blood is the safest blood. N Engl J Med 1987;316:542–544.
2. AuBuchon JP. Minimizing donor exposure in hemotherapy. Arch Pathol Lab Med 1994;118:380–391.
3. Cooley DA. Conservation of blood during cardiovascular surgery. Am J Surg 1995;170:53S–59S.
4. Forbes JM, Laurie ML. The Northfield Blood Collection Report. Community Blood Center Collections, 1988–1992. Evanston, IL: Northfield Laboratories, Inc., 1993.
5. Wallace EL, Surgenor DM, Hao HS, An J, Chapman RH, Churchill WH. Collection and transfusion of blood and blood components in the United States, 1989. Transfusion 1993;33:139.
6. National Heart, Lung, and Blood Institute Expert Panel on the Use of Autologous Blood. Transfusion alert: use of autologous blood. Transfusion 1995;35:703–711.
7. Axelrod FB, Pepkowitz SH, Goldfinger D. Establishment of a schedule of optimal preoperative collection of autologous blood. Transfusion 1989;29:677–680.
8. Yomtovian R. Practical aspects of preoperative autologous transfusion. Am J Clin Pathol 1997;107:S28–S35.
9. Goodnough LT, Monk TG, Brecher ME. Autologous blood procurement in the surgical setting: lessons learned in the last 10 years. Vox Sang 1996;71:133–141.
10. Kruskall MS, Popovsky MA, Pacini DG, Donovan LM, Ransil BJ. Autologous versus homologous donors—evaluation of markers for infectious disease. Transfusion 1988;28:286–288.
11. Grossman BJ, Stewart NC, Grindon AJ. Increased risk of a positive test for antibody to hepatitis B core antigen (anti-HBC) in autologous blood donors. Transfusion 1988;28:283–285.
12. AuBuchon JP, Dodd RY. Analysis of the relative safety of autologous blood units available for transfusion to homologous recipients. Transfusion 1988;28:403–405.
13. Vengelen-Tyler V, ed. Technical Manual. Standards for blood banks and transfusion services, 12th ed. Arlington, VA: American Association of Blood Banks, 1996.
14. Popovsky MA, Whitaker B, Arnold NL. Severe outcomes of allogeneic and autologous blood donation: frequency and characterization. Transfusion 1995;35:734–737.
15. Sazama K. 355 reports of transfusion-associated deaths. Transfusion 1990;30:583.

16. Kruskall MS. Controversies in transfusion medicine: the safety and utility of autologous donations by pregnant patients—pro. Transfusion 1990;30:168.
17. Kruskall MS, Leonard S, Klapholz H. Autologous blood donation during pregnancy: analysis of safety and blood use. Obstet Gynecol 1987;70:938.
18. Cohen JA, Brecher ME. Preoperative autologous blood donation: benefit or detriment? a mathematical analysis. Transfusion 1995;35:640–644.
19. Larson N, Foyt M, Marengo-Rowe A. Late donation of autologous units increases allogeneic transfusion requirements. Transfusion 1995;35:24S.
20. Mayer MN, de Montalembert M, Audat F, et al. Autologous blood donation for elective surgery in children weighing 8–25 kg. Vox Sang 1996;70:224–228.
21. McVay PA, Andrews A, Kaplan EB, et al. Donation reactions among autologous donors. Transfusion 1990;30:249.
22. Hillyer CD, Hart KK, Lackey DA III, Lin LS, Bryan JA. Comparable safety of blood collection in "high-risk" autologous donors versus non-high-risk autologous and directed donors in a hospital setting. Am J Clin Pathol 1994;102:275–277.
23. Yomtovian R, Kelly C, Bracey AW, et al. Procurement and transfusion of human immunodeficiency virus-positive or untested autologous blood units: issues and concerns: a report prepared by the Autologous Transfusion Committee of the American Association of Blood Banks. Transfusion 1995;35:353–361.
24. Macpherson CR, Grindon AJ. Ethical issues in autologous transfusion. Transfusion 1995;35:281–283.
25. Vanston V, Smith D, Eisenstaedt R. Should patients with human immunodeficiency virus infection or chronic hepatitis donate blood for autologous use? Transfusion 1995;35:324–330.
26. Spivak JL. Recombinant human erythropoietin and its role in transfusion medicine. Transfusion 1994;34:1–4.
27. Mercuriali F, Gualtieri G, Sinigaglia L, et al. Use of recombinant human erythropoietin to assist autologous blood donation by anemic rheumatoid arthritis patients undergoing major orthopedic surgery. Transfusion 1994;34:501–506.
28. Thompson FL, Powers JS, Graber SE, Krantz SB. Use of recombinant human erythropoietin to enhance autologous blood donation in a patient with multiple red cell allo-antibodies and the anemia of chronic disease. Am J Med 1991;90:398–400.
29. Kanter MH, van Maanen D, Anders KH, et al. Preoperative autologous blood donations before elective hysterectomy. JAMA 1996;276:798–801.
30. Churchill WH, Chapman RH, Rutherford CJ, et al. Blood product utilization in hip and knee arthroplasty: effect of gender and autologous blood on transfusion practice. Vox Sang 1994;66:182–187.
31. Julius CJ, Purchase KS, Isham BE, Howard PL. Patterns of autologous blood use in elective orthopedic surgery: does the availability of autologous blood change transfusion behavior? Vox Sang 1994;66:171–175.
32. Silberstein LE, Kruskall MS, Stehling LC, et al. Strategies for the review of transfusion practices. JAMA 1989;262:1993–1997.
33. Stehling L, Luban NLC, Anderson KC, et al. Guidelines for blood utilization review. Transfusion 1994;34:438–448.
34. Etchason J, Potz L, Keeler E, et al. The cost-effectiveness of preoperative autologous blood donations. N Engl J Med 1995;332:719–724.
35. Birkmeyer JD, Goodnough LT, AuBuchon JP, Noordsy PG, Littenberg B. The cost-effectiveness of preoperative autologous blood donation for total hip and knee replacement. Transfusion 1993;33:544–550.
36. Birkmeyer JD, AuBuchon JP, Littenberg B, et al. Cost-effectiveness of preoperative autologous donation in coronary artery bypass grafting. Ann Thorac Surg 1994;57:161–169.
37. Baussaud V, Mentec H, Fourcade C. Hemolysis after autologous transfusion. Ann Intern Med 1996;124:931–932.
38. Linden JV. Autologous blood errors and incidents. Transfusion 1994;34:28S. Abstract.
39. Utley JR, Moores WY, Stephens DB. Blood conservation techniques. Ann Thorac Surg 1981;31:482–490.
40. Laks H, Pilon RN, Klovekorn WB, et al. Acute hemodilution: its effects on hemodynamics and oxygen transport in anesthetized man. Ann Surg 1974;180:103–109.

41. Fowler NO, Holmes JC. Blood viscosity and cardiac output in acute experimental anemia. J Appl Physiol 1975;39:453–456.
42. Messmer K, Sunder-Plassman L, Klovekorn WP, et al. Circulatory significance of hemodilution: rheological changes and limitations. Adv Microcirc 1972;4:1–77.
43. Martin E, Hansen E, Peter K. Acute limited normovolemic hemodilution: a method for avoiding homologous transfusion. World J Surg 1987;11:53–59.
44. Kramer AH, Hertzer NR, Beven EG. Intraoperative hemodilution during elective vascular reconstruction. Surg Gynecol Obstet 1979;149:831–836.
45. Stehling L, Zauder HL. Acute normovolemic hemodilution. Transfusion 1991;31:857–868.
46. Cutler BS. Avoidance of homologous transfusion in aortic operations; the role of autotransfusion, hemodilution, and surgical technique. Surgery 1984;95:717–723.
47. Sejourne P, Poirier A, Meakins JL, et al. Effect of haemodilution on transfusion requirements in liver resection. Lancet 1989;2:1380–1382.
48. Bowens C, Spahn DR, Frasco PE, et al. Hemodilution induces stable changes in cardiovascular and regional myocardial function. Anesth Analg 1993;76:1027–1032.
49. Lilleaasen P, Stokke O. Moderate and extreme hemodilution in open-heart surgery: fluid balance and acid-base studies. Ann Thorac Surg 1978;25:127–133.
50. Zubiate P, Kay JH, Mendez AM, et al. Coronary artery surgery—a new technique with use of little blood, if any. J Thorac Cardiovasc Surg 1974;68:263–267.
51. Rosberg B, Wulff K. Hemodynamics following normovolemic hemodilution in elderly patients. Acta Anaesthesiol Scand 1981;25:402–406.
52. Buckley MJ, Austen WG, Goldblatt A, Laver MB. Severe hemodilution and autotransfusion for surgery of congenital heart disease. Surg Forum 1971;22:160–162.
53. Dale J, Lilleaasen P, Erikssen J. Hemostasis after open-heart surgery with extreme or moderate hemodilution. Eur Surg Res 1987;19:339–347.
54. Williamson KR, Taswell HF. Intraoperative blood salvage: a review. Transfusion 1991;31:662–675.
55. Zauder HL. Intraoperative and postoperative blood salvage devices. In: Stehling L, ed. Perioperative Autologous Transfusion. Arlington, VA: American Association of Blood Banks, 1991:25–37.
56. Popovsky MA, Devine PA, Taswell HF. Intraoperative autologous transfusion. Mayo Clin Proc 1985;60:125.
57. Glover JL, Broadie TA. Intraoperative autotransfusion. World J Surg 1987;11:60–64.
58. Griffith LD, Billman GF, Daily PO, Lane TA. Apparent coagulopathy caused by infusion of shed mediastinal blood and its prevention by washing of the infusate. Ann Thorac Surg 1989;47:400–406.
59. Sieunarine K, Lawrence-Brown MMD, Brennan D, et al. The quality of blood used for transfusion. J Cardiovasc Surg 1992;33:98–105.
60. Yaw PB, Sentany M, Link WJ, Wahle WM, Glover JL. Tumor cells carried through autotransfusion—contraindication to intraoperative blood recovery? JAMA 1975;231:490–492.
61. McCarthy PM, Popovsky MA, Schaff HV, et al. Effect of blood conservation efforts in cardiac operations at the Mayo Clinic. Mayo Clin Proc 1988;63:225–229.
62. Grindon AJ. Infectious disease markers in directed donors in the Atlanta region. Transfusion 1991;31:872–873. Letter to the Editor.
63. Starkey NM, MacPherson JL, Bolgiano DC, Simon ER, Zuck T, Sayers MH. Markers for transfusion-transmitted disease in different groups of blood donors. JAMA 1989;262:3452–3454.
64. Cordell RR, Yalon VA, Cigahn-Haskell C, McDonough B, Perkins HA. Experience with 11,916 designated donors. Transfusion 1986;26:484–486.
65. Standards for Blood Banks and Transfusion Services, 16th ed. Bethesda, MD: American Association of Blood Banks, 1994.
66. Wang-Rodriguez J, Mannino FL, Liu E, Lane TA. A novel strategy to limit blood donor exposure and blood waste in multiply transfused premature infants. Transfusion 1996;36:64–70.
67. Brecher ME, Taswell HF, Clare DE, Swenke PK, Pineda AA, Moore SB. Minimal-exposure transfusion and the committed donor. Transfusion 1990;30:599–604.
68. Strauss RG, Wieland MR, Randels MJ, Koerner TAW. Feasibility and success of a single-donor red cell program for pediatric elective surgery patients. Transfusion 1992;32:747–749.

PRODUCTION OF COMPONENTS BY APHERESIS

Blood component therapy developed because of the use of plastic bag systems to allow separation of whole blood into some of its parts (see Chapters 1, 5, and 11). This led to important advances in hemotherapy and made possible many of the medical and surgical therapies used today. Rather than being limited to the acquisition of blood components in the number and ratio present in one unit of whole blood, the situation described above created considerable interest in developing techniques to selectively remove only the desired component and return the remainder to the donor, thus making it possible to process large volumes of donor blood and obtain a larger dose of the desired component from one donor. Pioneering work by Abel in 1914[1] demonstrated that this could be done. He removed whole blood, retained the plasma, and returned the red cells to the donor. During the 1950s and 1960s, these procedures were developed using combinations of the plastic bags and tubing sets used for whole blood collection. A standard unit of blood was removed, the desired component (either plasma or platelets) separated, and the remainder of the blood returned to the donor; the process was repeated several times, thus producing a larger amount of the desired component than would have been obtained from one unit of whole blood.[2] Although this method worked, it was time consuming, cumbersome, and expensive. Therefore, more automated methods were sought. There was particular motivation to develop these techniques for platelet collection. As platelet transfusions began to be used more extensively, it became apparent that some transfusions did not result in the expected increase in platelet count. In some situations, the poor response was due to alloimmunization with the formation of either HLA or platelet-specific antibodies. Platelets from certain HLA-identical siblings provided an excellent response in some patients.[3,4] The need for single-donor platelet collection methods was strengthened when it was established that transfusion of HLA-matched platelets from donors unrelated to the patients was successful,[5–7] and that platelets only partially HLA matched with the patient could provide a good response.[8] This general

establishment of the clinical effectiveness of transfusions in which all of the platelets were obtained from one donor added momentum to the development of plateletpheresis procedures.

Semiautomated apheresis methods were developed generally by two separate research groups.[9] In Boston, the centrifuge apparatus developed for plasma fractionation by Edwin Cohen was modified to process whole blood from normal donors,[10] and at the National Institutes of Health a blood cell separator was developed to aid in the treatment of leukemia.[11] Both of these approaches ultimately led to the sophisticated blood cell separators available today for the processing of large volumes of donor blood and the selective removal of the desired blood component. Thus, a major advance in the production of blood components and component therapy was the development and large-scale implementation of apheresis.

PRINCIPLES OF APHERESIS

Apheresis, meaning to take away, refers to the process of selectively removing one component of whole blood and returning the remainder to the donor. The term plasmapheresis was used by Abel in 1914 to describe his initial work.[1] Apheresis can be done on standard units of whole blood with plastic bag systems to isolate platelets (plateletpheresis) or plasma (plasmapheresis). However, this procedure is time consuming and is no longer widely used. Today most apheresis is done using semiautomated instruments sometimes called blood cell separators. In apheresis, the donor's whole blood is anticoagulated and passed through the instrument in which the blood is separated into red cells, plasma, and a leukocyte-platelet fraction. Then the desired fraction or component can be removed and the remainder of the blood recombined and returned to the donor. Several liters of donor blood can be processed through the instrument, and therefore a larger amount of the desired component can be obtained than from one unit (450 mL) of whole blood. Several blood cell separator instruments are available. Some operate in a continuous flow and others with intermittent flow; some require two venipunctures (an outflow and return) and others only one venipuncture.

Apheresis Instruments

There are several different instruments available for the collection of platelets, granulocytes, lymphocytes, peripheral blood stem cells, or plasma by apheresis. All of the instruments used for normal-donor apheresis use centrifugation to separate the blood components. The instrument operation is controlled by a microprocessor. This operation includes the blood flow rate, the anticoagulant added to the whole blood entering the system, the centrifuge conditions, the component separation, and the recombination of the remaining components and returning them to the donor.

Instruments available for plateletpheresis were recently summarized by the U.S. Food and Drug Administration (FDA) (Table 7.1). Granulocytes can be collected by at least three instruments. These instruments also can be used to collect lymphocytes. Specific procedures have been described only for the collection of peripheral blood stem

Table 7.1 Instruments available in the United States for collection of blood components by apheresis

Instrument	Manufacturer	Component produced				
		Platelets	Granulocytes	MNCs	PBSCs	Plasma
CS-3000	Fenwal	X	X	X	X	
Amicus	Baxter	X				
Autopheresis C	Baxter					X
Spectra	COBE	X	X	X	X	
V50	Haemonetics	X	X			
PCS	Haemonetics	X				X
MCS*	Haemonetics	X				X

*The MCS also collects red cells.

cells. Pertinent comments about collection of each component are given below. For details of the operation of the instrument and collection procedure, the manufacturer's instructions and references should be consulted.

CURRENT APHERESIS ACTIVITY IN THE UNITED STATES

Apheresis can be used for collection of platelets, leukocytes, or plasma but in the past has not been used for red cell collection because the maximum volume of red cells that can be removed according to FDA regulations can be obtained in a standard unit of 450 mL of whole blood. Recent protocols involving the collection of the equivalent of two units of red cells have been initiated, but considerable work remains to be done before this becomes an FDA-licensed procedure. The medical uses of the components produced by apheresis are discussed in Chapters 11 and 12. In the early years of platelet transfusion therapy, platelet concentrates were produced from whole blood. The use of apheresis, particularly for platelet production, is increasing substantially. Between 1982 and 1984 the number of plateletpheresis procedures performed in the United States was estimated to have increased from 80,000 to 120,000 annually, or 50% in 2 years. More recently, it has been estimated that 638,000 plateletpheresis procedures were done during 1992, representing about 46% of the total platelet production in the United States and an increase in plateletpheresis of 74% since 1989.[12] This change is even more remarkable if one considers that one apheresis procedure can produce the number of platelets usually obtained from six different units of whole blood. This suggests that the number of plateletpheresis procedures done in 1992 substitutes for the platelets from 3,828,000 units of whole blood and represents a decreased need for 1,638,000 units of whole-blood platelets just since 1989. The advantages and uses of platelets obtained by apheresis are discussed in Chapter 11.

The plasma collection and fractionation industry in the United States developed during the 1960s using manual plastic bag methods for plasma collection by plasmapheresis. Today, virtually all plasma collected in the United States for fractionation into

coagulation factor concentrates, albumin, and immune globulin is obtained by semiautomated instrument plasmapheresis. It has been estimated that 13 million plasmapheresis procedures are carried out annually in the United States, resulting in an average of 700 mL of plasma each or a total of 9 million liters of plasma (see Chapter 2).

Ten to fifteen years ago, leukapheresis was used to produce granulocyte concentrates for transfusion therapy of infections unresponsive to antibiotics.[13] However, leukapheresis provides only a marginally adequate dose of granulocytes for therapeutic benefit, and its use has declined to very low levels (see Chapter 11). There may be a resurgence in leukapheresis now that cytokines can be used to elevate the donor's granulocyte count and increase the yield of granulocytes (see Chapter 17).

Leukapheresis can also be used for the collection of mononuclear cell concentrates containing peripheral blood stem cells, which are used for autologous and more recently allogeneic stem cell (marrow) transplantation[14–18] (also see Chapter 17). This is a rapidly expanding and exciting new role for apheresis, but the number of these procedures is small and not likely to become very large because of the specialized use of the stem cell component.

PLATELETPHERESIS FOR THE PRODUCTION OF SINGLE-DONOR PLATELET CONCENTRATES

The official name of this component is platelets, pheresis. In daily practice, this component is usually called single-donor platelets or plateletpheresis concentrates. They are a suspension of platelets in plasma prepared by cytapheresis. A unit or bag of plateletpheresis concentrate must contain at least 3×10^{11} platelets in at least 75% of the units tested. Plateletpheresis usually requires about 1½ hours and involves processing 4,000 to 5,000 mL of the donor's blood through the instrument. Platelets obtained by plateletpheresis are processed, tested, and labeled similar to whole blood (see Chapter 8). This includes ABO and Rh typing and testing for all required transfusion-transmitted diseases. The plateletpheresis concentrate may be stored for 5 days at 20°C to 24°C if it is collected in a closed system. The number of platelets contained in each concentrate is determined, although this information may not necessarily be recorded on the label. Each platelet concentrate has a volume of approximately 200 mL and contains very few red cells (less than 0.5 mL), and so red cell crossmatching is not necessary. Quality control tests must show that at least 75% of the apheresis platelet concentrates produced by each facility contain 3×10^{11} platelets or more. The white blood cell content varies depending on the instrument and technique used for collection.

The effects of plateletpheresis on donors are discussed in Chapter 4.

Development of Centrifugation Instruments for Cytapheresis

Intermittent-flow centrifugation   With the development of plasma fractionation during the 1940s, it was necessary to carry out continuous-flow washing of blood inside a bacteriologically closed centrifuge with no limitation of the volumes that could be processed. The special centrifuge system developed by Edwin Cohn (a professor of bio-

chemistry at Harvard who originated the plasma fractionation procedure) was modified for use as a blood processor in collaboration with the Arthur D. Little Corporation (ADL) and one of its engineers, Allan Latham, and later James Tullis, M.D., a Harvard hematologist.[19] The original motivation to modify the Cohn ADL bowl was for washing and deglycerolizing previously frozen red cells. However, because of the difficulty in obtaining an adequate supply of platelets, it soon became apparent that the Latham bowl could be used to separate whole blood and collect platelets.[20,21] Soon a freestanding device, the Model 10, containing the centrifuge bowl was produced by Abbott Laboratories, but they did not choose to go into the business of manufacturing medical devices. The procedure was cumbersome because the bowl was made of stainless steel and had many parts, all of which had to be cleaned and sterilized between uses, and although it was a major innovation, it was not practical for routine or large-scale use. A new company called Haemonetics was formed and soon produced a more sophisticated instrument, the Model 30. The centrifuge bowl system was later made from Lucite and adapted to a special centrifuge[10] that became the Haemonetics system. This system was sterile, more self-contained, and included anticoagulant solutions, storage bags, and ancillary materials. In the operation of the Haemonetics system using the Cohn ADL bowl, donor blood was pumped into the spinning centrifuge bowl and underwent separation, and the plasma was pumped out of the bowl until the operator observed the concentrated platelets at the exit port. The platelet-rich plasma was then diverted into a separate collection container, and after collection of approximately 50 mL of platelet-rich plasma the blood flow was reversed and the platelet-poor whole blood returned to the donor. Several of these cycles were carried out until the desired amount of platelets had been collected or the donation time caused donor fatigue. The operator monitored the development of a buffy coat layer and diverted the platelets into the collection container at the desired time. This system represented a major improvement because of the sterile containers and convenient package.[22] A large and a small bowl were developed so that the maximum volume of blood could be processed in as short a time as possible. An amount of platelets equal to approximately 8 units of whole blood was obtained and no serious or unexpected side effects were seen in the donors. Experience with this disposable plateletpheresis system was gained rapidly in many centers, and it became clear that a large number of platelets could be collected safely from volunteer donors.[23–26]

Continuous-flow centrifugation   In the early 1960s, the need for a blood cell separator type of instrument became apparent to an engineer from IBM Corporation whose child was being treated for leukemia at the National Cancer Institute (NCI). Because of this, IBM Corporation collaborated with the NCI to develop an instrument that could be used to separate the cellular elements of blood in a continuous flow in vivo and return the plasma and red cells to the donor.[27,28] Although the instrument was originally designed for granulocyte collection, it was also suitable for plateletpheresis.[11] The instrument was cumbersome and had many parts that had to be cleaned and sterilized before each use. The collection system was modified, however, to become the IBM 2997, which functioned quite well for platelet collection. Later, when IBM left the medical device field, the instrument became the COBE plateletpheresis system, which evolved into the current COBE Spectra. Later, a third instrument, the Fenwal CS-3000,

which used a disposable flow pathway and no rotating seal, was developed for platelet-pheresis.[29,30]

These three basic instruments—the Haemonetics models, the COBE blood cell separator models, and the Fenwal CS-3000—are the mainstay of platelet production in the United States. In one study[31] directly comparing three instruments and another[32] comparing two of them, none was found to be superior overall to the others. Each instrument has certain strengths that make it advantageous based on the desires of the particular blood center.

COBE Spectra

The original IBM blood cell separators evolved to the Model 2997, which forms the basis of the Spectra instrument. The Model 2997 used a disposable plastic system shaped somewhat like a belt but with one or two integral separation chambers (Fig. 7.1). Various versions of the blood separation chamber made it possible for the instrument to be used for plateletpheresis, leukapheresis, or plasma exchange. The current version of this system is the Spectra. This system is closed (to allow for storage of the platelets for several days) and has an integral needle for blood withdrawal, isolated pressure monitoring, and sterile barrier filters for solution attachment.[33] The blood flows into the sealless disposable plastic loop, where the first portion of the loop serves as the first separation chamber. Blood is separated into red cells and platelet-rich buffy coat layers. During passage through the second portion of the loop, the platelets are separated, resulting in platelets, plasma, and red cells exiting the system separately. The red cells and plasma are recombined and returned to the donor via either a separate venipuncture site or the withdrawal site.[34] In earlier versions of the instrument the operator adjusted the flow rates of the different channels to obtain optimum yields. In the present Spectra version of this instrument, the blood separation interface is maintained automatically by the microprocessor controls, thus reducing operator time and increasing reproducibility. Prior to starting the procedure, the operator enters the donor's height, weight, gender, hematocrit, and platelet count into the microprocessor. The microprocessor then controls the procedure to obtain the desired platelet yield. Usually 3 to 4 × 10^{11} platelets are obtained in about 90 minutes.[33–35]

Fenwal CS-3000

The CS-3000 is controlled by a microprocessor and uses disposable plastic tubing and flexible separation chamber set for the entire blood flow pathway.[29,36] The instrument is primed automatically using saline and acid-citrate-dextrose (ACD) anticoagulant. After the venipuncture is completed and the donor connected to the instrument, the plateletpheresis procedure is initiated by selecting the start/resume mode on the instrument. The donor's platelet count (from this visit or a previous donation) is entered and the instrument's microprocessor calculates the volume of blood that should be processed to obtain a platelet yield of 3.9 × 10^{11}. The collection procedure is automated, and so the instrument begins the procedure. Blood is pumped out of the donor's vein at a rate of 35 to 55 mL/minute, is mixed with citrate anticoagulant, and then enters

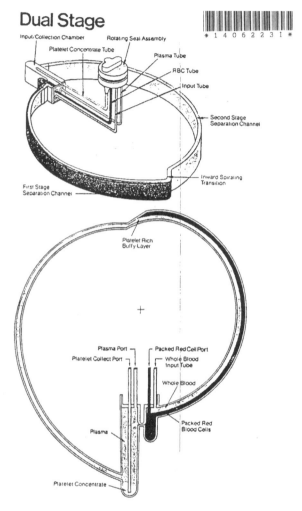

Figure 7.1. IBM 2997 blood separation channel: dual stage. *(Reprinted with permission of COBE Laboratories, Inc., Lakewood, CO.)*

the first of two blood separation chambers. In the first chamber whole blood is separated into platelet-rich plasma and red cells. The platelet-rich plasma then enters a second chamber, where it is separated into platelet concentrate and platelet-poor plasma. The platelet-poor plasma is combined with the red cells and returned to the donor via either a second venipuncture or via the single venipuncture in a modification of the original CS-3000.[29] The length of the collection procedure is determined by the automated calculations within the instrument. Usually about 90 to 120 minutes is required to obtain the desired yield of platelets. The flow rate can be increased to about 65 mL/minute to shorten the donation time while maintaining satisfactory platelet

yields.[37] A unique feature of the CS-3000 is the lack of a rotating seal connecting the fixed tubing (attached to the donor) to the rotating separation chamber.

Fenwal Amicus

This instrument was just released for use in Europe, and little information about its operation or the components it produces was available at the time of this writing. It is intended by Fenwal to be the successor to the CS-3000.

Haemonetics

The Haemonetics system uses a disposable, transparent Lucite centrifuge bowl for blood separation.[10,22,38–40] After venipuncture is performed and the donor is connected to the instrument, the operator activates the instrument and blood is pumped from the donor into the centrifuge bowl. ACD anticoagulant is added to the blood as it leaves the donor. The centrifuge bowl spins at approximately 4,800 rpm and continuously separates the blood as it enters the bowl. When the volume of blood removed from the donor exceeds the capacity of the bowl, plasma begins to exit the bowl and is collected in a bag. The platelet/buffy coat layer accumulates at the top of the red cells, and as the bowl continues to fill, this layer moves toward the exit port. When the platelets—visible as a white band between the red cells and plasma—reach the exit port, a valve is activated, diverting the flow pathway into a separate bag where the platelets are collected. When the platelets have been collected, the blood flow is stopped, the pumps reversed, and the plasma and red cells recombined and returned to the donor. This cycle of filling the centrifuge bowl is repeated several times to obtain the desired platelet yield. In early versions of this system, the operator determined when to alter the flow pathways to collect platelets, but in later versions this has become more automated.

Recently an enhanced version of the Haemonetics system called the Multiple Component System (MCS) has become available. The MCS has the flexibility to collect various combinations of platelets, plasma, and red cells. In an early study, the equivalent of one single-donor platelet concentrate (3×10^{11} platelets) and one unit (220 mL) of red cells were collected in about 87 minutes using this system.[41] The MCS was used in a separate study to collect the equivalent of one half unit of single-donor platelets (1.98×10^{11}) and one to two units of plasma.[42] This exciting approach may finally be the first step to providing flexibility in the donor center to determine on a daily basis or for individual donors the particular mix of components to collect.

Function and Storage of Platelets Obtained by Apheresis

Another important issue in the development and widespread implementation of plateletpheresis was the quality of the platelets. Several studies[23,24,29,43–47] established that platelets collected using these plateletpheresis systems had in vitro function and in vivo survival characteristics equal to platelets prepared from whole blood. The platelets survived normally when autologous transfusions of radiolabeled platelets were given to normal research donors, and platelets collected by apheresis caused the expected

increase in platelet count in thrombocytopenic patients.[48] Because of the large number of platelets obtained by apheresis, the preservation medium, the size and composition of the storage container, and the acceptable length of storage were issues.[29,49] Subsequently, as platelet storage containers were produced from newer plastics that allowed better gas diffusion, it became possible to store platelet concentrates produced by apheresis in a smaller volume.

Reducing the Volume of the Platelet Concentrate

The dose of platelets necessary in some situations may result in a volume of plasma in the platelet concentrate that is too large for the patient to safely tolerate. Examples of these situations are transfusions to small children or the need for large doses of platelets to average-sized adults. In this situation, the platelet concentrate can be centrifuged and excess plasma removed safely anytime during the 5-day storage period.[50] It is important that the centrifugation technique be gentle and that the laboratory gain some experience with the technique to ensure that there is not excessive damage to platelets before attempting this for patient therapy.

LEUKAPHERESIS FOR THE PRODUCTION OF GRANULOCYTE CONCENTRATES

This blood component is called granulocytes, pheresis. The component is a suspension of granulocytes in plasma prepared by cytapheresis.[51] A granulocyte concentrate must contain at least 1×10^{10} granulocytes in at least 75% of the units tested. Neither the American Association of Blood Banks (AABB) Standards nor FDA regulations specify the number of units that must be tested for quality control purposes. However, since only a few granulocyte concentrates are prepared by most blood banks, it is customary to test all concentrates.

Development of Leukapheresis Instruments

As mentioned above, investigators at the National Cancer Institute (NCI) entered into collaboration with IBM Corporation to develop a device that could separate the cellular elements of blood on a continuous flow in vivo and return the plasma and red cells to the donor.[27,28] This relationship developed because of the personal involvement of Mr. George Judson, an IBM engineer whose child was being treated at the NCI. The child was being treated by leukodepletion rather than chemotherapy, and collaborative efforts were made to develop an instrument for more efficient leukocyte removal. Supposedly, the first blood cell separator was constructed primarily of material obtained at a Bethesda, Maryland, hardware store.[52] Because the instrument was developed at the NCI, the plans were in the public domain. The American Instrument Company obtained these plans and developed their version of the device.

During leukapheresis with these instruments, the donor would undergo venipuncture in each arm. Blood was pumped out of one vein and through the blood

cell separator, where the granulocytes were removed, and the remaining blood was returned to the other arm.[53] Blood flowed to the bottom of the centrifuge bowl by a central channel, flowed outward along the bottom, and up the sides where the red cells were packed against the walls.[54] Blood separation occurred in a polycarbonate bowl with a clear plastic cover through which the operator could view the separation of plasma, buffy coat, and platelets. Each of these components was drawn off by a separate peristaltic flow pump adjusted by the operator to maintain optimum cell separation. The key to these instruments was the rotating seal, one section of which was attached to the rotating centrifuge bowl and the other fixed to the blood inflow and outflow lines.[54] The NCI-IBM Blood Cell Separator contained a blood reservoir so that the donor could be bled intermittently but blood flow into the centrifuge was continuous. The Aminco Celltrifuge was a more simple instrument without the reservoir system, but this necessitated continuous bleeding of the donor. These systems, like the original Latham bowl for plateletpheresis, were very cumbersome because they were made of multiple reusable parts that had to be cleaned, sterilized, and reassembled between procedures. To simplify the procedure and to use more disposable equipment, IBM developed the Model 2997 blood cell separator. In this instrument, the centrifuge bowl was replaced with a disposable hollow plastic blood separation channel attached at both ends to the input and output blood flow ports to form a closed loop.[55] This instrument then formed the basis for the development of the IBM, and later COBE, plateletpheresis instruments.

As the Latham bowl and the Haemonetics system were being developed for plateletpheresis, attempts were made to use this also for granulocyte collection. The IFC was operated in much the same way as for plateletpheresis, but the operator then adjusted the blood flow rates and time of component collection to remove the buffy coat rather than the platelet layer.[56–58]

Subsequently a new generation of apheresis instrument technology was developed, including a microprocessor to control the operation of the instrument combined with a system that lacked the rotating seal present on the IBM, Celltrifuge, and Haemonetics devices. This system, the Fenwal CS-3000, made possible different types of blood separation because different unique separation chambers were developed for the particular component desired. This system had the additional advantage of being completely closed and enabling sterile collection and thus storage of products for longer than the 24-hour limitation.

These instruments extracted approximately 20% to 40% of the granulocytes that passed through them, but because of the relatively low level of circulating granulocytes in normal donors, it was necessary to process a large volume of blood to obtain a usable dose of granulocytes. Initial development of the instruments and experience with granulocyte transfusions involved collecting cells from patients with chronic myelogenous leukemia (CML). However, there were the obvious problems of the use of abnormal or malignant cells and the limited number of CML patients available to donate. Additional strategies were needed to increase the granulocyte yield. The two major approaches used were the addition of blood sedimenting agents to improve granulocyte separation within the centrifuge and the treatment of donors with corticosteroids to increase the level of circulating granulocytes.

Hydroxyethyl Starch in Leukapheresis

The separation between granulocytes from the upper layer of red cells is poor because the density of granulocytes is similar to that of some red cells. Although several agents can be used to sediment red cells in vitro, hydroxyethyl starch (HES) is used because it is licensed in the United States and is not associated with unacceptable reactions or alteration of coagulation tests. The granulocyte yield is doubled when HES is added to the leukapheresis system by constant infusion.[59–61] Several studies of the effects of HES established that the nature and incidence of reactions are acceptable for use on normal donors, the potential for blood volume overload when administered to normal donors can be easily managed during the procedure, there is no adverse affect on laboratory values or platelet or granulocyte function, and there are no adverse long-term effects.[53]

Corticosteroid Stimulation of Donors Prior to Leukapheresis

The second approach to increase the granulocyte yield was to increase the donor's circulating granulocyte count. Corticosteroids seemed to be the drug of choice, and dexamethasone was selected because it could be given either orally several hours before leukapheresis or parenterally at the beginning of the procedure. This is a very effective method to increase the granulocyte yield even further than is accomplished by adding HES to the separation system.[56,62,63]

Leukapheresis

Leukapheresis procedures are usually more complex and lengthy than plateletpheresis. The donor receives up to 500 mL of HES to improve the efficiency of granulocyte extraction and may receive corticosteroids to increase the yield by elevating the level of circulating granulocytes. Dexamethasone 60 mg can be given orally the evening before or hydrocortisone 4 mg/m^2 intravenously 6 to 12 hours before leukapheresis. Much of the initial work with granulocyte collection was done with the IBM Blood Cell Separator or the Haemonetics Model 30 instruments. The leukapheresis procedure takes 2 to 3 hours, a longer time than plateletpheresis, to process more blood and improve the granulocyte yield. Usually 6,500 to 8,000 mL of the donor's blood is processed through the instrument, with removal of about 50% of the granulocyte, resulting in a yield of 1 to 2 $\times$ 10^{10} granulocytes in a volume of about 200 mL. Later the centrifuge bowl of the Blood Cell Separator was replaced with a blood separation channel composed of a disposable hollow plastic tube attached at both ends to the input and output blood flow ports to form a closed loop. Within the plastic tubing channel a barrier was placed, against which the buffy coat containing leukocytes accumulated. Red cells moved around one side of the barrier and plasma around the other side, thus making it possible to separate these three components.[55] This device became the Model 2997.

When the Haemonetics system is used for granulocyte collection, HES is added to the inflow line, causing both a platelet and a granulocyte layer to become visible at the outlet port. The operator then adjusts the blood flow rates and time of complete collec-

tion to obtain primarily the buffy coat rather than the platelet layer.[56–58] Using this technique, an average of 1 to 1.4 × 10^{10} granulocytes from normal donors using HES and 1.7 × 10^{10} using both HES and dexamethasone were obtained.[56–58]

Because granulocytes do not completely separate from the red cells, granulocyte concentrates usually contain a substantial amount of red cells (hematocrit 10% or about 20 mL of red cells), and therefore crossmatching is necessary. The granulocyte content of each concentrate is determined but not necessarily indicated on the label. There are no FDA minimum requirements defining the composition of granulocyte concentrates; American Association of Blood Banks Standards require that 75% of units contain at least 1 × 10^{10} granulocytes.

Filtration Leukapheresis

This method of granulocyte collection is described because of historical interest, but it is not used today. A nylon fiber filter system was developed to collect granulocytes.[64] This was a very effective method of procuring granulocytes for transfusion, and soon a small, free-standing filtration leukapheresis (FL) set using a peristaltic pump to pass the blood over the filters was manufactured.[65,66] This system yielded a larger number of cells than the centrifuge procedures, but one drawback was that heparin anticoagulation of the donor was necessary. Another even more difficult problem was that some damage to the granulocytes resulted from their adhesion to the fibers. Granulocytes obtained by FL were more vacuolated and morphologically altered, had slightly reduced phagocytosis,[67–70] normal oxygen consumption and chemotaxis,[70] and reduced intravascular circulation in rats[69] and humans.[70] Incubation of normal granulocytes with nylon fibers caused release of intracellular enzymes indicative of degranulation.[67] Thus, it became clear that granulocytes obtained by FL had a mild to moderate impairment in bacterial killing and decreased intravascular recovery and survival. Also, a severe transient neutropenia occurred a few minutes after the donor's blood came in contact with the nylon fibers.[68,71,72] Some donors, predominantly women, experienced severe abdominal or perineal pain,[73] and some male donors experienced severe priapism. Activation of the complement system in blood being returned to the donor was suspected to be the cause of the neutropenia in FL.[74,75] With these reports of donor complications and the establishment of the pathophysiologic mechanism, use of FL for granulocyte collection was rapidly discontinued, and FL is no longer used.

Function of Granulocytes Obtained by Leukapheresis

There is no evidence that the collection procedure damages the granulocytes. Granulocytes collected by centrifuge leukapheresis techniques demonstrate normal bacterial killing, phagocytosis NBT dye reduction (an indication of granulocyte metabolism), chemiluminescence, superoxide production, and chemotaxis.[76–79] Studies of granulocytes in vivo using isotope-labeled cells showed that granulocytes obtained by leukapheresis, isotope labeled, and transfused to the cell donor (autologous) had a normal intravascular recovery and survival and migrated to sites of inflammation.[76,80–82] The

use of corticosteroids in donors to improve the granulocyte yield does not adversely affect the function of the cells in vitro or in vivo.[77,78,80]

Storage of Granulocytes for Transfusion

Granulocytes have a life span in the circulation of only a few hours, and so storage of granulocytes as part of a routine blood bank operation is difficult. Granulocytes retain bactericidal capacity and metabolic activity related to phagocytosis and bacterial killing for 1 to 3 days of storage at refrigerator temperatures, although chemotactic response declines by 30% to 50% after 24 hours.[83,84] The loss of chemotaxis is only about 30% after the first day of storage if the cells are maintained at room temperature.[80,84] Studies using ^{111}In-labeled granulocytes showed that storage of granulocytes between 1°C and 6°C for 24 hours was associated with a reduction in the percentage of transfused cells that circulated and about a 75% reduction in migration into a skin window,[81] but storage at room temperature for 8 hours did not reduce the intravascular recovery, survival, or migration into a skin chamber.[81] In vivo recovery, survival, or migration was reduced further when granulocytes were stored longer than 8 hours at room temperature or for even 8 hours between 1°C and 6°C. Thus, it appears that granulocytes can be stored for up to 8 hours at room temperature before transfusion. Even so, this results in some deterioration of in vitro and in vivo function. It is recommended that granulocytes be transfused within a very few hours. AABB standards allow storage for up to 24 hours at 20°C to 24°C.

Donor-Recipient Matching for Granulocyte Transfusion

Granulocyte concentrates must be ABO-compatible with the recipient because of the substantial volume of red cells in the concentrates. ABO antigens are probably not present on granulocytes (see Chapter 9). The clinical impact of ABO incompatibility on granulocyte transfusion was evaluated in one study.[85] A small number of ^{111}In-labeled granulocytes free of red blood cells were injected into ABO-incompatible recipients. The intravascular recovery, survival, and tissue localization of the cells were not different from those seen when similar injections were given to ABO-compatible subjects. This study was not intended to encourage the use of ABO-incompatible granulocyte transfusions, but this could be considered if granulocyte concentrates that are depleted of red blood cells could be prepared.

Studies using CML cells showed that incompatibility by leukoagglutination or lymphocytotoxicity (LC) was associated with the failure of transfused cells to circulate or localize at sites of inflammation.[86,87] Studies in dogs also showed that immunization to granulocytes interfered with the outcome of transfusion. However, most animals' sera reacted in several different leukocyte antibody assays, so the optimum laboratory testing technique could not be specified. Studies using ^{111}In-labeled granulocytes in humans established that granulocyte-agglutinating (GA) antibodies were associated with decreased intravascular recovery and survival, failure of the cells to localize at known sites of inflammation,[88] and excess sequestration of transfused granulocytes in the pulmonary vasculature.[88, 89] However, applying these research data to the practical

operation of a blood bank and granulocyte transfusion service is difficult. Granulocytes can be stored for only a few hours, and cells are not usually available for crossmatching to allow selection of compatible donors. The only practical approach has been to screen the patients' serum against a panel of cells periodically (i.e., two or three times weekly) to determine whether the patient is alloimmunized. If so, HLA-matched unrelated donors or family members can be selected for leukapheresis. However, the problem of donor-recipient matching and compatibility testing for granulocyte transfusion has never been solved in the practical operational sense.

LYMPHOCYTAPHERESIS FOR THE COLLECTION OF MONONUCLEAR CELLS

Lymphocytes have not usually been collected as a blood component for transfusion. Recently, lymphocytapheresis has been used to obtain mononuclear cell concentrates for several purposes. These include serving as starting material for the production of cells for adoptive immunotherapy or as a concentrate enriched in peripheral blood stem cells. Lymphocytapheresis also may be done as a therapeutic procedure to treat immune diseases by the physical removal of lymphocytes (see Chapter 19).

Lymphokine-Activated Killer Cells and Natural Killer Cells

Lymphokine-activated killer (LAK) cells are peripheral blood lymphocytes that are collected by apheresis and then cultured with interleukin-2 and other additives, resulting in cells that are cytotoxic to tumor cells but not to nonmalignant cells (see Chapter 18). LAK cells generated from the patient's own lymphocytes have been used as experimental therapy for several forms of malignancy. Although the ultimate role of this adoptive immunotherapy is not known, the approach of collecting autologous lymphocytes by apheresis, then modifying the lymphocytes in vitro for later autologous use seems likely to undergo continued clinical investigation during the next few years.

Mononuclear Cells for Graft versus Leukemia Effect

Following stem cell transplantation for chronic myelogenous leukemia, mononuclear cells from the marrow donor have been transfused to reduce the likelihood of recurrent malignancy by taking advantage of the graft versus leukemia effect (see Chapter 18). The cells are collected using standard lymphocytapheresis techniques.

Mononuclear Cells for Antiviral Effect

Peripheral blood mononuclear cells can be cultured to generate clones of cells with specific activity against Epstein-Barr virus or cytomegalovirus. These cloned cells, expanded in vitro, have been transfused to restore patients' immunity to cytomegalo-

virus and to treat posttransplant lymphoproliferative disease due to Epstein-Barr virus (see Chapter 18). The cells that are cloned for production of these experimental therapeutic materials are collected using standard lymphocytapheresis procedures.

Lymphocytapheresis

Lymphocytes can be collected using any of the three systems—COBE Spectra, Fenwal CS-3000, or Haemonetics. Each system has a mononuclear cell collection procedure that very efficiently yields 1 to 3 × 10^{10} mononuclear cells.

CYTAPHERESIS FOR THE PRODUCTION OF PERIPHERAL BLOOD STEM CELLS

Hematopoietic stem cells are present not only in the marrow but also in the peripheral circulation. These hematopoietic stem cells can be collected from the peripheral blood by cytapheresis and are called peripheral blood stem cells (PBSCs). Normally the number of circulating PBSCs is small—much less than in the marrow. However, after the marrow suppression of chemotherapy, there is a rebound and the number of PBSCs increases substantially. This made it possible to collect PBSCs from patients undergoing chemotherapy, especially for malignancies in which there was suspected marrow involvement. The PBSCs—expected to contain few, if any, malignant cells—were then used as marrow rescue following the chemotherapy. These autologous transplants of PBSCs made new chemotherapy regimens possible and also established that PBSCs could be used successfully for autologous marrow transplantation.[90-95]

For several years, use of PBSCs was limited to autologous transplants. It was feared that the large number of T lymphocytes contained in the PBSC concentrates would cause severe graft versus host disease and that T-depletion would result in an unacceptably large loss of PBSCs. These concerns have now been overcome by the rapidly expanding successful experience with allogeneic stem cell transplants using PBSCs.[15-18,95-99] The advantages of donating for a stem cell transplant by apheresis instead of under general anesthesia in the operating room are substantial. As a result, there is great interest in developing policies and procedures for the collection of PBSCs from normal donors.[100-103]

Because the number of PBSCs circulating in normal individuals is low, methods have been sought to increase the level of circulating PBSCs. Several cytokines or hematopoietic growth factors will accomplish this, but most have unacceptable side effects or donor risks. Granulocyte colony-stimulating factor (G-CSF) has its primary effect on granulocyte development and maturation but also increases the level of circulating PBSCs. Although G-CSF causes some side effects, they are modest and are not considered to present major risks to normal donors. Thus, G-CSF has been used in experimental protocols to mobilize PBSCs from normal donors to establish the expected side effects, to develop the collection procedures, and for experimental allogeneic transplantation.

Collection Procedures

Either the COBE Spectra or the Fenwal CS-3000 can be used for the collection of PBSCs. The CS-3000 procedure uses the TNX upgrade and unique program settings and modified interface detection settings and centrifuge speeds.[104,105] The granulocyte separation chamber and the small-volume collection chamber are used.[104,105] In the COBE Spectra, the mononuclear cell procedure is used for PBSC collection. The operator enters the donor's hematocrit, height, weight, and gender and a microprocessor controls the addition of anticoagulant and the separation process. Because the cell separation depends on centrifugal force and dwell time in the gravitational field, the microprocessor varies the centrifuge speed if the blood flow rate varies. The operator can customize the procedure if desired, and the separation and actual collection of the PBSC component are determined by the operator observing the interface between red cells and buffy coat. During collection, the operator monitors the collection interface and the color of the collection material to optimize the resulting PBSC concentrate. PBSCs can be collected from small children, but adjustments are necessary in priming the system and managing the donors.

For normal donors, the usual skin preparation, venous access, needles or catheters, solutions, and software are used. Blood flow rates of 40 to 80 mL/minute are used depending on the donor's venous access and blood flow tolerance. Ideas are not fixed regarding the volume of blood that should be processed. The traditional mononuclear cell collection procedures involve processing 10 to 15 L of blood over 2 or 3 hours, although it has been recommended that a large volume of blood be processed in order to increase the PBSC yield.[104] This observation[104] that there may be recruitment of CD34+ cells during extended apheresis has led to the use of procedures of up to 40 L over 5 hours or more to increase the number of CD34+ cells obtained during one procedure. However, many patients or donors do not have vascular access that accommodates these long procedures. In addition, it is not clear that the CD34+ cell levels remain stable or increase (recruitment) during apheresis of normal donors, and so the length of the procedure is still under evolution.

Effects of PBSC Collection on Normal Donors

The major clinical effects of PBSC collection on donors are caused by the G-CSF the donors receive to mobilize the PBSCs. Almost all donors experience some side effect.[103] The most common of these is bone pain, but headache, fatigue, and flu-like symptoms also occur. The donor's leukocyte count increases to 30,000 to 40,000 per microliter and the platelet count decreases by about 40%.[106] The leukocyte and platelet counts return to normal by about day 16, or about 10 days after the apheresis donation and discontinuing the G-CSF. There is an increase in alkaline phosphatase, alanine aminotransferase, lactate dehydrogenase, and sodium and a decrease in glucose, potassium, bilirubin, and blood urea nitrogen.[103] Thus, although most donors experience some side effects, these are mild and should interfere with PBSC donation only rarely.[101,103]

Table 7.2 Effects of G-CSF dose on the quantity of cells collected by one apheresis procedure from healthy people treated with G-CSF for 5 days (number of cells collected)

Cell type	All components ($n = 150$)		
	Mean ± SD	Median	Range
WBCs ($\times 10^9$)	35.0 ± 16.4	32.4	11.9–163.3
MNCs ($\times 10^9$)	33.3 ± 14.4	31.4	11.9–139.6
CD34+ cells ($\times 10^8$)	4.1 ± 2.9	3.3	0.70–16.6
CD34+ cells ($\times 10^6$ per L processed)	48.4 ± 33.7	39.9	7.7–193.5
RBC (mL)	7.2 ± 4.0	7.6	0–22.1
Neutrophils ($\times 10^9$)	1.71 ± 3.59	0.64	0–27.6
Platelets ($\times 10^{11}$)	4.8 ± 11.0	4.7	2.5–9.2

Source: Stroncek DF, Clay ME, Smith J, et al. Composition of peripheral blood progenitor cell components collected from healthy donors. Transfusion 1997; 37:411–417.

Characteristics of the PBSC Concentrates

Large quantities of CD34+ cells can be collected from normal donors given G-CSF for 5 days. G-CSF doses of 7.5 or 10 mg per day provide a greater yield than 5 mg per day,[102] but it is not clear whether there are statistically significant differences in the CD34+ cell yield between 7.5 and 10 mg per day.[102] Because the donor side effects increase with increasing doses of G-CSF, we recommend that donors be given 7.5 mg of G-CSF per kilogram per day to mobilize peripheral blood CD34+ cells.[102] The composition of the PBSC component is shown in Tables 7.2 and 7.3. Most PBSC components

Table 7.3 Effects of G-CSF dose on composition of WBCs collected by apheresis from healthy donors given 5 days of G-CSF (percentage of cells collected)

Cell type	All components ($n = 150$)		
	Mean ± SD	Median	Range
Lymphocytes	65.6 ± 13.7	67.5	27.0–93.0
Monocytes	22.5 ± 8.8	22.3	3.0–49.0
Neutrophils	3.6 ± 5.2	2.0	0.37
Bands	0.3 ± 0.9	0	0–8
Metamyelocytes	0.4 ± 1.0	0	0–5
Myelocytes	6.0 ± 5.8	5	0–39
Promyelocytes	0.5 ± 1.1	0	0–5
Blasts	0.4 ± 1.0	0	0–4
Basophils	0.7 ± 0.9	0.5	0–4

Source: Stroncek DF, Clay ME, Smith J, et al. Composition of peripheral blood progenitor cell components collected from healthy donors. Transfusion 1997; 37:411–417.

contain only a small volume of red cells (mean, 7 mL) but a rather large total number of neutrophils (1.7×10^9) and platelets (4.8×10^{11}).[102] This number of platelets is similar to the number of platelets ordinarily provided in a platelet transfusion, and this may provide an additional benefit from the PBSC transfusion. The concentrate usually has a volume of about 200 mL and contains approximately 3×10^{10} mononuclear cells and 4×10^8 CD34+ cells.

The total number of CD34+ cells collected is similar for the COBE Spectra and the Fenwal CS-3000, but the composition of the components is slightly different (Table 7.4). PBSCs collected using the Fenwal CS-3000 contained more mononuclear cells, and those collected using the COBE Spectra contained more granulocytes. The PBSC concentrates collected with both instruments contained a similar number of CD34+ cells and platelets. The instruments seem to perform similarly, and local operator or institutional preferences may make one or the other more desirable.

Quality Control of PBSC Concentrates

Since there is no definitive test for the primordial hematopoietic stem cell, quality control of these peripheral blood stem cell concentrates is not standardized. Cell culture techniques can be used to determine CFU-GM, BFU-E, and CFU-MIX colonies and the number of CD34+ cells. In practice, the dose for transplantation is usually based on cell counting to obtain at least 3×10^8 mononuclear or 5×10^6 CD34+ cells per kilogram of the recipient's body weight. The results of progenitor assays are not available for about 2 weeks and thus can be used only in retrospect for research purposes.

There is considerable variation in the number of CD34+ cells collected (Fig. 7.2). In our experience,[102] a single cytapheresis procedure yields a median dose of 780 to $1,658 \times 10^6$ CD34+ cells. In approximately 42% of the procedures, this would be an adequate cell dose to transplant 5×10^6 CD34+ cells per kilogram to a 75-kg recipient. In 86% of donors, two cytapheresis procedures would yield an adequate cell dose for transplanting the 75-kg recipient. These numbers were obtained by processing approximately 10 L of whole blood. Other reports involving processing of 15 to 20 L of blood for each cytapheresis procedure suggest that larger numbers of CD34+ cells could be obtained.[104] Thus, a higher proportion of procedures could result in a dose of cells suitable for transplantation.

Storage of PBSCs

Because of the variability in the number of cells that may be obtained, the strategy for using the cells for transplantation cannot always be the same. If the dose needed for transplantation can be obtained with one procedure, the cells can be transfused immediately. However, if two or three apheresis procedures are necessary, it may be desirable to freeze the concentrates and transfuse them all at once. However, the freezing and thawing may alter the composition of the PBSC concentrates, and so some transplant physicians give the cells fresh each day until the desired dose is obtained. Alternatively, the concentrate collected on the first day is stored in the liquid state and transfused with the concentrate collected on the second day. The use of PBSCs is so new that issues such

Table 7.4 Quantity of cells in the PBSC components

Cell type	CS-3000 ($n = 15$)	Spectra ($n = 14$)	p
WBCs ($\times 10^9$)	40.9 ± 21.7	33.1 ± 10.7	0.24
Neutrophils ($\times 10^9$)	1.38 ± 1.88	5.53 ± 8.71	0.001
Mononuclear cells ($\times 10^9$)	39.6 ± 21.9	26.9 ± 5.6	0.02
Platelets ($\times 10^9$)	507 ± 98	531 ± 116	0.54
CD34+ cells ($\times 10^9$)	470 ± 353	419 ± 351	0.69

Source: Stroncek DF, Clay ME, Smith J, Jaszcz WB, Herr G, McCullough J. Comparison of two blood cell separators in collecting peripheral blood stem cell components. Transfus Med 1997;7:95–99.

as these are still being evaluated and new strategies being developed. Studies performed some years ago suggested that bone marrow progenitors were best preserved at 4°C.[107] However, little research has focused on the optimum conditions for preservation of stem cells. Since the optimum conditions for storage of hematopoietic stem cells are not well established, it is preferable either to transfuse the cells soon after collection or to freeze them within a few hours of collection.

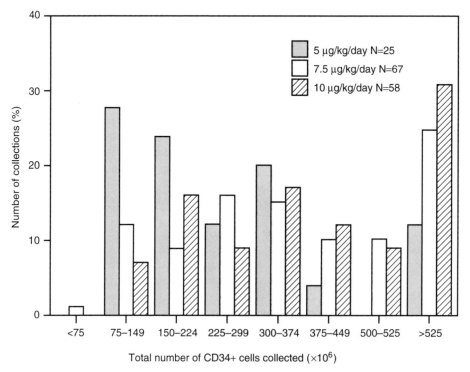

Figure 7.2 CD34+ cell yield in peripheral blood concentrates collected from normal donors. *(Reproduced with permission from Stroncek DF, Clay ME, Smith J, et al. Composition of peripheral blood progenitor cell components collected from healthy donors. Transfusion 1997;37:414.)*

COMPLICATIONS OF CYTAPHERESIS IN NORMAL DONORS

Some potential complications of apheresis apply to all types of procedures because they have to do with the instrument or activities that are common to all types of procedures. These are vasovagal reactions, anticoagulation, citrate toxicity, and hematoma. Other potential complications are unique to certain apheresis procedures. These will be considered separately.

Vasovagal Reactions

These reactions are similar to those associated with whole blood donation. The symptoms include weakness, pallor, diaphoresis, bradycardia, cold clammy skin, lightheadedness or fainting, and, if severe, convulsions. The treatment is as described for whole blood donors (see Chapter 4).

Anticoagulation

The anticoagulant used for plateletpheresis is citrate. The toxicity due to calcium binding is a much more sensitive problem than in vivo anticoagulation. Thus, bleeding due to citrate anticoagulation is not an issue. In the distant past, the Celltrifuge device used for leukapheresis involved administration of heparin to the donors. With the Celltrifuge the heparin was combined with citrate so that usually 2,000 to 4,000 units of heparin were administered. Although this was a modest dose, it did cause the partial thromboplastin time (PTT) to increase to about 1.5 times normal. For filtration leukapheresis, heparin doses of 10,000 units or more were used, causing very substantial prolongation of PTT and an anticoagulated state that lasted for several hours after donation. Although no reports of severe hemorrhage appeared in the literature, this degree of anticoagulation was of concern, and the development of apheresis systems that did not require heparin was a substantial improvement. Today, anticoagulation is done only with citrate solutions, and so the adverse effects are related to binding of calcium by the citrate.

Citrate Toxicity

Elevations of blood citrate can cause paresthesias, muscle cramping, tetany, cardiac arrhythmia, and other symptoms. The plateletpheresis procedure involves the administration of citrate solutions to donors, almost as a form of massive autologous transfusion, because 4 to 6 L of their blood is withdrawn, passed through the instrument, citrated, and returned to them during the 2- to 3-hour procedure. During the development of apheresis techniques, there was a considerable interest in determining the particular citrate solution that would be optimal, the acceptable dose of citrate, and the nature and incidence of side effects. Acid-citrate-dextrose (ACD), citrate-phosphate-dextrose (CPD), and sodium citrate were tried by different investigators at different times. The concentration of citrate in the anticoagulant, the amount of citrate administered, and the rate of administration were important issues in projecting the potential citrate toxicity.[108,109] The greatest concern was the potential of cardiac arrhythmia. Infusion of full-strength ACD

solution caused a decrease in ionized calcium of 22% to 32%, serum citrate levels of 22 to 26 mg/dL, and a QT interval prolongation of 0.08 second.[108,109] Half-strength ACD solution, or formula B, resulted in a decrease in ionized calcium of 16%, a serum citrate concentration of 12 mg/dL, and a 0.04-second QT interval prolongation.[108] It was established that citrate doses of 1 mg/kg/minute that maintained ionized calcium levels at 3 mg/dL or greater were well tolerated. Symptoms of hypocalcemia, primarily paresthesias and muscle cramping, were rather common[108,109] and remain so today. They can be managed easily by slowing the rate of blood flow and administering milk. However, despite years of experience with plateletpheresis and the safeguards built into instruments, errors can still occur that result in citrate toxicity.[110]

Hematoma

Blood is returned to the donor under pressure by pumps within the apheresis instrument. Thus, if the return needle becomes dislodged, a rather extensive hematoma can develop quickly. The signs of this are pain, discoloration, or oozing at the venipuncture site. If this occurs, the blood flow is discontinued immediately, pressure is applied, and the hematoma is managed as described for whole blood donation.

Instrument-caused hemolysis   Determinations of haptoglobin[10] and red cell survival[10] established that the Latham bowl used in the Haemonetics system did not cause sufficient red cell damage to interfere with normal red cell survival. Other studies established that instrument-caused hemolysis was not a problem with continuous-flow centrifugation systems.[111] Thus, it was established that hemolysis was not a complication of the passage of large volumes of donor blood through the apheresis instruments.

Platelet depletion and thrombocytopenia   Initially it was necessary to establish the extent of decrease in platelet count that would occur following removal of platelets equivalent to several units of the donor's blood and to determine the period required for the platelet count to return to pre-apheresis levels. As experience with plateletpheresis increased, it became clear that the platelet yield was related to the donor's platelet count and that the platelet count decreased less than expected based on the number of platelets collected.[22,23,25,26,29,112] For instance, in one study[22] the average number of platelets collected was 4.16×10^{11} and the average decrease in total circulating platelets was 2.19×10^{11}. In another study, the mean decrease in total circulating platelets was 3.4×10^{11} and the mean number of platelets collected was 4.2×10^{11}.[29] Thus, it appeared that platelets were mobilized during the apheresis procedure. This was documented using indium[111] labeled platelets[113] that showed that as platelets were removed from the circulation, they were replaced with platelets mobilized from the splenic pool.

To ensure that donors would not be at risk of bleeding after donating, there was renewed interest in the distribution and variation in platelet counts in normal, healthy people. It was found that the average platelet count in females was about 12% higher than that in males.[26,114] Although the decrease in platelet count varied somewhat with the procedure used, a decrease of 20% to 35% generally occurred. The platelet count returned to baseline levels about 4 days after donation.[26,112] In donors who underwent

repeated plateletpheresis, the platelet count decreased somewhat more but then stabilized. Thus, it appeared that platelets could be donated safely approximately every 4 days.

Blood volume shifts Because of the administration of HES during leukapheresis, there was concern that a net increase in blood volume might occur because HES is used as a blood volume expander. This could lead to hypertension or acute heart failure. The volume of HES administered ranged from 200 to 400 mL and, combined with the removal of approximately 50 to 200 mL of granulocyte concentrate, did not result in complications due to excess blood volume.

Air embolus Because the first instruments used—particularly the Aminco Celltrifuge—involved a rotating two-part seal, there was a possibility of air entering the system and being pumped into the donor's veins. Thus, it was necessary to insert into the flow pathway and tubing systems of these instruments a chamber in which air that might enter the system could be accumulated. The chamber was attached to a sensing device that would automatically stop the pumps if air accumulated, thus avoiding creating an air embolus in the donor. Monitoring these air sensors was an important part of quality control of these instruments. There were several anecdotal, unpublished reports of donors who did receive an air embolus. Apparently none of these caused serious problems.

Lymphocyte depletion Because a relatively large number of lymphocytes were removed during plateletpheresis, concern developed about the possibility of lymphocyte depletion and altered immunologic status in normal donors undergoing frequent plateletpheresis.[115] It has been estimated that at least 10^{11} lymphocytes must be removed over a short time and/or the individual's lymphocyte count must be less than 500 per microliter for clinical immunosuppression to occur.[116] Wright et al.[117] provided some of the first very complete data addressing this issue when they carried out lymphapheresis using the Aminco Celltrifuge. Patients (not normal donors) underwent a 4-hour lymphapheresis two to three times per week for 5 to 7 weeks (for a total of 13 to 18 procedures). Each apheresis procedure involved removal of approximately 3.5×10^9 lymphocytes, or up to 2.5×10^{10} lymphocytes per week. A fall in lymphocyte count of about 25% occurred after the first three procedures, and the count remained stable for approximately the second week. The study established that at least 10^9 lymphocytes must be removed daily for several days for a measurable decline in lymphocyte count to occur. Although lymphocyte depletion can occur with repeated lymphapheresis, the number of lymphocytes removed during ordinary plateletpheresis, even on multiple occasions during a relatively short period of time, was established not to be a clinical risk for normal donors.

The present concern about the leukocyte content of blood components has led to alterations in apheresis procedures to minimize the leukocyte content. As a result, most plateletpheresis procedures today remove about 1×10^6 to 5×10^7 leukocytes. Loss of this number of leukocytes is very unlikely to lead to leukocyte depletion or any clinical effects on the donor's immune function.[116]

Complications Unique to Plateletpheresis

Virtually all of the cytapheresis procedures carried out in normal donors are plateletpheresis. Normal donors undergoing plateletpheresis may report an adverse reaction following up to 50% of procedures when asked; however, such reactions cause the procedure to be discontinued in only 0.1% to 1.0% of the time.[118] These reactions are almost entirely due to citrate toxicity and can be alleviated by slowing the rate of blood return and thus the rate of citrate infusion.

Complications Unique to Leukapheresis

The complications related to leukapheresis are usually not different from those in plateletpheresis except that donors receive hydroxyethyl starch, which may cause headache due to blood volume expansion. A few cases of a lichen planus-like skin rash—apparently caused by HES—have been reported.

Complications Unique to Mononuclear Cell Apheresis for Collection of PBSCs

Because of the low level of circulating PBSCs in normal donors, donors receive the hematopoietic growth factor G-CSF to mobilize PBSCs and increase the yield (see Chapter 17). G-CSF is associated with a rather high frequency of side effects. Thus, virtually all of the complications and side effects of the donation of mononuclear cells as a source of PBSCs are related to the administration of the G-CSF.

PLASMAPHERESIS AND SOURCE PLASMA

Plasma is the starting material for the further manufacture of some diagnostics and plasma "derivatives." Derivatives are described in more detail in Chapter 2, and the selection and medical evaluation of plasma donors is described in Chapter 4. Some plasma is that removed from units of whole blood, but during the past few years there has been an almost complete shift so that today most plasma, especially that used for the manufacture of derivatives, is obtained by plasmapheresis. Approximately 13 million plasmapheresis procedures, producing approximately 9 million liters of plasma, are carried out in the United States annually (see Chapter 2). In the past, plasmapheresis was done using sets of multiple plastic bags and involved separation of the blood from the donor such that there was a chance for erroneous return of red cells to the incorrect donor. During the past few years, new instruments have become available that are semiautomated and require less operator involvement while producing larger amounts of plasma at a reasonable cost. The instruments in use in the United States are the Baxter Autopheresis C, the Haemonetics V50, and the Haemonetics PCS. This section focuses on the techniques used for plasmapheresis.

The Haemonetics PCS can be used to collect platelet-poor or platelet-rich plasma. Usually one venipuncture is used and the system can be set up in about 5 minutes. This

includes loading the disposable plastic set into the instrument, connecting the anticoagulant and solution bags, recording appropriate data, and placing the collection bags. The venipuncture area is prepared as for whole blood collection (see Chapter 4) and the venipuncture is done using the needle integral with the disposable plastic set used for the procedure. The operator then activates the instrument, and blood flow is initiated by the pumps in the instrument. Anticoagulant is metered into the blood flowing into the instrument in the proper ratio, and the centrifuge bowl is filled until the optical sensor detects the red cell interface and stops the inflow of blood. During this filling phase of the cycle, the plasma has been diverted into the collection bag. After the plasma-cell interface has reached the detector, the blood flow is reversed and the red cells are pumped from the bowl back to the donor. The cycle is then repeated until the desired amount of plasma is obtained. Usually about 500 mL of plasma can be obtained in about 30 minutes.[119] The Haemonetics V50 can be used to collect platelets, granulocytes, plasma, or combinations of these. Thus, the operation of the V50 instrument is less automated and the operator must determine which component is to be collected and make manual adjustments during the collection procedure to obtain the desired component.

The Baxter Autopheresis C plasmapheresis instrument operates on a different principle from the Haemonetics devices. The Autopheresis C combines filtration and centrifugation to separate blood in a smaller chamber (and possibly more efficiently). The instrument setup and donor preparation are the same as described for the Haemonetics systems and for whole blood collection. For the Autopheresis C, blood is withdrawn from the donor into a closed, disposable plastic set with a total extracorporeal volume of about 165 mL. Blood separation occurs in a small (7-mL) cylinder that is part of the system. A magnet causes rotation of the cylinder inside a larger compartment. The cylinder is composed of a membrane, and as the cylinder rotates, plasma moves peripherally through the membrane, thus providing the filtration part of the separation system. The system does not operate in a continuous-flow manner; blood is returned intermittently to the donor through the single venipuncture and the process is repeated. This system, like the Haemonetics systems, collects about 500 mL of plasma in about 30 minutes.[120,121]

REFERENCES

1. Abel JJ, Rowntree LC, Turner BB. Plasma removal with return of corpuscles. J Pharmacol Exp Ther 1914;5:625–641.
2. Kliman A, Gaydos LA, Schroeder LR, Freireich EJ. Repeated plasmapheresis of blood donors as a source of platelets. Blood 1961;18:303–309.
3. Yankee RA, Grumet FC, Rogentine GN. The selection of compatible platelet donors for refractory patients by lymphocyte HL-A typing. N Engl J Med 1969;27:1208–1212.
4. Grumet FC, Yankee RA. Long-term platelet support of patients with aplastic anemia—effect of splenectomy and steroid therapy. Ann Intern Med 1970;73:1–7.
5. Thorsby E, Helgesen A, Gjemdal T. Repeated platelet transfusions from HL-A compatible unrelated and sibling donors. Tissue Antigens 1972;2:397–404.
6. Yankee RA, Graff KS, Dowling R, Henderson ES. Selection of unrelated compatible platelet donors by lymphocyte HL-A matching. N Engl J Med 1973;288:760–764.
7. Lohrmann HP, Bull MI, Decter JA, et al. Platelet transfusions from HL-A compatible unrelated donors to alloimmunized patients. Ann Intern Med 1974;80:9–14.

8. Duquesnoy RJ, Filip DJ, Rodey GE, Aster RH. Transfusion therapy of refractory thrombocytopenic patients with platelets from donors selectively mismatched for cross-reactive HLA antigens. Transplant Proc 1977;9:221–224.

9. McCullough J. Introduction to apheresis donations including history and general principles. In: McLeod BC, Price TH, Drew MJ, eds. Apheresis: Principles and practice. Bethesda, MD: AABB Press, 1997:19–36.

10. Tullis JL, Tinch RJ, Baudanza P, et al. Plateletpheresis in a disposable system. Transfusion 1971;11:368–377.

11. Graw RG, Herzig GP, Eisel RJ, Perry S. Leukocyte and platelet collection from normal donors with the continuous flow blood cell separator. Transfusion 1971;11:94–101.

12. Wallace EL, Surgenor DM, Hao HS, An J, Chapman RH, Churchill WH. Collection and transfusion of blood and blood components in the United States, 1989. Transfusion 1993;33:139–144.

13. McCullough J. Leukapheresis and granulocyte transfusion. Clinical reviews in clinical laboratory science. Boca Raton, FL: CRC Press, 1979:275.

14. Korbling M, Huh YO, Durett A, et al. Allogeneic blood stem cell transplantation: peripheralization and yield of donor-derived primitive hematopoietic progenitor cells (CD34+ Th-1dim) and lymphoid subsets, and possible predictors of engraftment and graft-versus-host disease. Blood 1995;86:2842–2848.

15. Weaver CH, Buckner CD, Longin K. Syngeneic transplantation with peripheral blood mononuclear cells collected after the administration of recombinant human granulocyte colony-stimulating factor. Blood 1993;82:1981–1984.

16. Bensinger WI, Clift RA, Anasetti C, et al. Transplantation of allogeneic peripheral blood stem cells mobilized by recombinant human granulocyte colony stimulating factor. Stem Cells 1996;14:90–105.

17. Bensinger WI, Buckner CD, Shannon-Dorcy K, et al. Transplantation of allogeneic CD34+ peripheral blood stem cells in patients with advanced hematologic malignancy. Blood 1996;88:4132–4138.

18. Bensinger WI, Weaver CH, Appelbaum FR. Transplantation of allogeneic peripheral blood stem cells mobilized by recombinant human granulocyte colony-stimulating factor. Blood 1995;85:1655–1658.

19. Tullis JL, Tinch RJ, Gibson JG, Baudanza P. A simplified centrifuge for the separation and processing of blood cells. Transfusion 1967;7:232–242

20. Tullis JL, Eberle WG, Baudanza, Tinch R. Platelet-pheresis description of a new technique. Transfusion 1968;8:154–164.

21. Miller WV, Gillem HG, Yankee RA, Schmidt PJ. Pooled platelet concentrates prepared in a new blood bank centrifuge. Transfusion 1969;9:251–254.

22. Szymanski IO, Patti K, Kliman A. Efficacy of the Latham blood processor to perform plateletpheresis. Transfusion 1973;13:405–411.

23. Nusbacher J, Scher ML, MacPherson JL. Plateletpheresis using the Haemonetics Model 30 cell separator. Vox Sang 1977;33:9–15.

24. Chao FC, Tullis JL, Tinch J, et al. Plateletpheresis by discontinuous centrifugation: effect of collecting methods on the in vitro function of platelets. Br J Haematol 1979;39:177–187.

25. Glowitz RJ, Slichter SJ. Frequent multiunit plateletpheresis from single donors: effects on donors' blood and the platelet yield. Transfusion 1980;20:199–205.

26. Lasky LC, Lin A, Kahn RA, McCullough J. Donor platelet response and product quality assurance in plateletpheresis. Transfusion 1981;21:247–260.

27. Freireich EJ, Judson G, Levin RH. Separation and collection of leukocytes. Cancer Res 1965;25:1517–1520.

28. Buckner D, Eisel R, Perry S. Blood cell separation in the dog by continuous flow centrifugation. Blood 1968;31:653–672.

29. Katz AJ, Genco PV, Blumberg N, et al. Platelet collection and transfusion using the Fenwal CS-3000 cell separator. Transfusion 1981;21:560–563.

30. Ito Y, Suaudeau J, Bowman RL. New flow-through centrifuge without rotating seals applied to plasmapheresis. Science 1975;189:999–1000.

31. Mintz PD, Coletta U. Prospective comparison of plateletpheresis with three cell separators using identical donors. Lab Med 1987;18:537–539.

32. Kalmin ND, Grindon AJ. Comparison of two continuous-flow cell separators. Transfusion 1983;23:197–200.

33. Simon TL, Sierra ER, Ferdinando B, Moore R. Collection of platelets with a new cell separator and their storage in a citrate-plasticized container. Transfusion 1991;31:335–339.

34. McLeod BC, McKenna R, Viernes A, et al. Plateletpheresis with the COBE Spectra single needle access option. J Clin Apheresis 1991;6:24–27.

35. Kuriyan M, Opalka A. Leukoreduced platelet apheresis production with a modified COBE spectra collection protocol. J Clin Apheresis 1995;10:85–86.

36. Buchholz DH, Porten JH, Menitove JE, et al. Description and use of the CS-3000 blood cell separator for single-donor platelet collection. Transfusion 1983;23:190–196.

37. Strauss RG, Ludwig GA, Randels MJ, Winegarden DC. Efficacy and safety of Fenwal CS-3000 plateletpheresis performed at a rapid donor blood flow rate: rapid plateletpheresis with Fenwal CS-3000. J Clin Apheresis 1991;6:21–23.

38. Aisner J, Schiffer CA, Wolff JH, Wiernik PH. A standardization technique for efficient platelet and leukocyte collection using the Model 30 blood processor. Transfusion 1976;16:45.

39. Hogge DE, Schiffer CA. Collection of platelets depleted of red and white cells with the "surge pump" adaptation of a blood cell separator. Transfusion 1983;23:177–181.

40. Schoendorfer DW, Hansen LE, Kenney DM. The surge technique: a method to increase purity of platelet concentrates obtained by centrifugal apheresis. Transfusion 1983;23:182–189.

41. Valbonesi M, Frisoni R, Florio G, et al. Single-donor platelet concentrates produced along with packed red blood cells with the Haemonetics MCS 3p: preliminary results. J Clin Apheresis 1994;9:195–199.

42. Szymanski IO, Ciavarella D, Rososhansky S, Napychank PA, Snyder EM. Evaluation of platelets collected by a new portable apheresis device. J Clin Apheresis 1993;8:66–71.

43. Slichter SJ. Efficacy of platelets collected by semi-continuous flow centrifugation (Haemonetics Model 30). Br J Haematol 1978;38:131–140.

44. Katz A, Houx J, Ewald L. Storage of platelets prepared by discontinuous flow centrifugation. Transfusion 1978; 18:220–223.

45. Patel IP, Ambinder E, Holland JF, Aledort LM. In vitro and in vivo comparison of single-donor platelets and multiple-donor pooled platelets transfusions in leukemic patients. Transfusion 1978;18:116–119.

46. Turner VS, Hawker RJ, Mitchell SG, Seymour Mead AM. Paired in vivo and in vitro comparison of apheresis and "recovered" platelet concentrates stored for five days. J Clin Apheresis 1994;9:189–194.

47. Maguire LC, Henriksen RA, Strauss RG. Function and morphology of platelets produced for transfusion by intermittent-flow centrifugation plateletpheresis or combined platelet-leukapheresis. Transfusion 1981;21:118–123.

48. Daly PA, Schiffer CA, Aisner J, Wiernik PH. A comparison of platelets prepared by the Haemonetics Model 30 and multiunit bag plateletpheresis. Transfusion 1979;19:778–781.

49. Rock GA, Blanchette VS, Wong SC. Storage of platelets collected by apheresis. Transfusion 1983;23:99–105.

50. Moroff G, Friedman A, Robkin-Kline L, Gautier G, Luban NLC. Reduction of the volume of stored platelet concentrates for use in neonatal patients. Transfusion 1984;24:144–146.

51. Standards for Blood Banks and Transfusion Services, 16th ed. Bethesda, MD: American Association of Blood Banks, 1994.

52. Millward BL, Hoeltge GA. The historical development of automated hemapheresis. J Clin Apheresis 1982;1:25–32.

53. McCullough J. Leukapheresis and granulocyte transfusion. CRC Crit Rev Clin Lab Sci 1979;10:275.

54. Jones AL. Continuous-flow blood cell separation. Transfusion 1968;8:94–103.

55. Hester JP, Kellogg RM, Mulzet AP, et al. Principles of blood separation and component extraction in a disposable continuous-flow single-stage channel. Blood 1979;54:254–268.

56. Huestis DW, White RF, Price MJ, Inman M. Use of hydroxyethyl starch to improve granulocyte collection in the Latham blood processor. Transfusion 1975;15:559–564.

57. Sussman LN, Coli W, Pichetshote C. Harvesting of granulocytes using a hydroxyethyl starch solution. Transfusion 1975;15:461–465.

58. Aisner J, Schiffer CA, Wiernik PH. Granulocyte transfusions: evaluation of factors influencing results and a comparison of filtration and intermittent centrifugation leukapheresis. Br J Haematol 1978;38:121.

59. Mishler JM, Hadlock DC, Fortuny IE, et al. Increased efficiency of leukocyte collection by the addition of hydroxyethyl starch to the continuous flow centrifuge. Blood 1974;44:571–581.

60. McCredie KB, Freireich EJ, Hester JP, Vallejos C. Increased granulocyte collection with the blood cell separator and the addition of etiocholanolone and hydroxyethyl starch. Transfusion 1974;14:357–364.

61. Mishler JM, Higby DJ, Rhomberg W. Hydroxyethyl starch and dexamethasone as an adjunct to leukocyte separation with the IBM blood cell separator. Transfusion 1974;14:352–356.

62. Price TH, Glasser L. Neutrophil collection using modified fluid gelatin—effect on in vitro and in vivo neutrophil function. Transfusion 1985;25:238–241.

63. Lowenthal RM, Park DS. The use of Dextran as an adjunct to granulocyte collection with the continuous-flow blood cell separator. Transfusion 1975;15:23–27.

64. Djerassi I, Kim JS, Suvansri U, Mitrakul C, Ciesielka W. Continuous flow filtration—leukopheresis. Transfusion 1972;12:75–83.

65. Buchholz DH, Schiffer CA, Wiernick PH, Betts SW, Reilly JA. Granulocyte harvest for transfusion: donor response to repeated leukapheresis. Transfusion 1975;15:96–106.

66. Katz AJ, Houx J, Morse EE. Factors affecting the efficiency of filtration leukapheresis. Transfusion 1977;17:67–70.

67. Klock JC, Bainton DF. Degranulation and abnormal bactericidal function of granulocytes procured by reversible adhesion to nylon wool. Blood 1976;48:149–161.

68. Wright DG, Kauffmann JC, Chusid MJ, Herzig GP, Gallin JI. Functional abnormalities of human neutrophils collected by continuous flow filtration leukopheresis. Blood 1975;46:901–911.

69. Roy AJ, Yankee RA, Brivkalns A, Fitch M. Viability of granulocytes obtained by filtration leukapheresis. Transfusion 1975;15:539–547.

70. McCullough J, Weiblen BJ, Deinard AR, et al. In vitro function and post-transfusion survival of granulocytes collected by continuous-flow centrifugation and by filtration leukapheresis. Blood 1976;48:315–326.

71. Schiffer CA, Aisner J, Wiernik PH. Transient neutropenia induced by transfusion of blood exposed to nylon fiber filters. Blood 1975;45:141–146.

72. Rubins JL, MacPherson JL, Nusbacher J, Wiltbank T. Granulocyte kinetics in donors undergoing filtration leukapheresis. Transfusion 1976;16:56–62.

73. Wiltbank TB, Nusbacher J, Higby DJ, MacPherson JL. Abdominal pain in donors during filtration leukapheresis. Transfusion 1977;17:159–162.

74. Hammerschmidt DE, Craddock PR, McCullough J, et al. Complement activation and pulmonary leukostasis during nylon fiber filtration leukapheresis. Blood 1978;51:721–730.

75. Nusbacher J, Rosenfeld SI, MacPherson JL, Thiem PA, Leddy JP. Nylon fiber leukapheresis: associated complement component changes and granulocytopenia. Blood 1978;51:359–365.

76. McCullough J, Weiblen BJ, Deinard AS, et al. In vitro function and post-transfusion survival of granulocytes collected by continuous-flow centrifugation and by filtration leukapheresis. Blood 1976;48:315.

77. Glasser L, Huestis DW, Jones JF. Functional capabilities of steroid-recruited neutrophils harvested for clinical transfusion. N Engl J Med 1977;297:1033.

78. Glasser L. Functional considerations of granulocyte concentrates used for clinical transfusions. Transfusion 1979;19:1.

79. Strauss RG, Maguire LC, Koepke JA, Thompson JS. Properties of neutrophils collected by discontinuous-flow centrifugation leukapheresis employing hydroxyethyl starch. Transfusion 1979;19:192.

80. Price TH, Dale DC. Blood kinetics and in vivo chemotaxis of transfused neutrophils: effect of collection method, donor corticosteroid treatment, and short term storage. Blood 1979;54:977.

81. McCullough J, Weiblen BJ, Fine D. Effects of storage of granulocytes on their fate in vivo. Transfusion 1983;23:20.

82. Dutcher JP, Schiller CA, Johston GS, et al. The effect of histocompatibility factors on the migration of transfused 111indium-labeled granulocytes (abstract). Blood 1984;58:181.

83. Glasser L. Effect of storage on normal neutrophils collected by discontinuous-flow centrifugation leukapheresis. Blood 1977;50:1145.

84. McCullough J. Liquid preservation of granulocytes. Transfusion 1980;20:129.

85. McCullough J, Clay ME, Loken MK, Hurd JJ. Effect of ABO incompatibility on fate in vivo of 111indium granulocytes. Transfusion 1988;28:358.

86. Eyre HJ, Goldstein IM, Perry S, Graw RG Jr. Leukocyte transfusions: function of transfused granulocytes from donors with chronic myelocytic leukemia. Blood 1970;36:432.

87. Applebaum FR, Trapani RJ, Graw RG. Consequences of prior alloimmunization during granulocyte transfusion. Transfusion 1977;17:460.

88. McCullough J, Clay M, Hurd D, et al. Effect of leukocyte antibodies and HLA matching on the intravascular recovery, survival, and tissue localization of 111indium granulocytes. Blood 1986;67:522.

89. Dutcher JP, Fox JJ, Riggs C, et al. Pulmonary retention of indium-111-labeled granulocytes in alloimmunized patients (abstract). Blood 1982;58:171.

90. Pettengell R, Gurney H, Radford JA, et al. Granulocyte colony-stimulating factor to prevent dose-limiting neutropenia in non-Hodgkin's lymphoma: a randomized controlled trial. Blood 1992;80:1430–1436.

91. Welte K, Gabrilove J, Bronchud MH, Platzer E, Morstyn G. Filgrastim (r-metHuG-CSF): the first 10 years. Blood 1996;88:1907–1929.

92. Brandt SJ, Peters WP, Atwater SK, et al. Effect of recombinant human granulocyte-macrophage colony-stimulating factor on hematopoietic reconstitution after high-dose chemotherapy and autologous bone marrow transplantation. N Engl J Med 1988;318:869–876.

93. Bishop MR, Anderson JR, Jackson JD, et al. High-dose therapy and peripheral blood progenitor cell transplantation: effects of recombinant human granulocyte-macrophage colony-stimulating factor on the autograft. Blood 1994;83:610–616.

94. Nemunaitis J, Rabinowe SN, Singer JW, et al. Recombinant granulocyte-macrophage colony-stimulating factor after autologous bone marrow transplantation for lymphoid cancer. N Engl J Med 1991;324:1773–1778.

95. Bensinger W, Singer J, Appelbaum F, et al. Autologous transplantation with peripheral blood mononuclear cells collected after administration of recombinant granulocyte stimulating factor. Blood 1993;81:3158–3163.

96. Nemunaitis J, Anasetti C, Storb R, et al. Phase II trial of recombinant human granulocyte-macrophage colony-stimulating factor in patients undergoing allogeneic bone marrow transplantation from unrelated donors. Blood 1992;79:2572–2577.

97. Korbling M, Przepiorka D, Huh YO. Allogeneic blood stem cell transplantation for refractory leukemia and lymphoma: potential advantage of blood over marrow allografts. Blood 1995;85:1659–1665.

98. Kessinger A, Smith DM, Strandjord SE, et al. Allogeneic transplantation of blood-derived, T cell-depleted hemopoietic stem cells after myeloablative treatment in a patient with acute lymphoblastic leukemia. Bone Marrow Transplant 1989;4:643–646.

99. Schmitz N, Dreger P, Suttorp M, et al. Primary transplantation of allogeneic peripheral blood progenitor cells mobilized by filgrastim (granulocyte colony-stimulating factor). Blood 1995;85:1666–1672.

100. Goldman J. Peripheral blood stem cells for allografting. Blood 1995;85:1413–1415.

101. Korbling M, Przepiorka D, Gajewski J, et al. With first successful allogeneic transplantations of apheresis-derived hematopoietic progenitor cells reported, can the recruitment of volunteer matched, unrelated stem cell donors be expanded substantially? Blood 1995;86:1235–1239.

102. Stroncek DF, Clay ME, Smith J, et al. Composition of peripheral blood progenitor cell components collected from healthy donors. Transfusion 1997;37:411–417.

103. Stroncek DF, Clay ME, Petzoldt ML, et al. Treatment of normal individuals with granulocyte-colony-stimulating factor: donor experiences and the effects on peripheral blood CD34+ cell counts and on the collection of peripheral blood stem cells. Transfusion 1996;36:601–610.

104. Hillyer CE, Lackey DA, Hart KK, Stempora LL, Bray RA, Bender JG, Donnenberg AD. CD34+ progenitors and colony-forming units—granulocyte macrophage are recruited during large-volume leukapheresis and concentrated by counterflow centrifugal elutriation. Transfusion 1993;33:316–321.

105. Rosenfeld CS, Cullis H, Tarosky T, Nemunaitis J. Peripheral blood stem cell collection using the small volume collection chamber in the Fenwal CS-3000 Plus blood cell separator. Bone Marrow Transplant 1994;13:131–134.

106. Stroncek DF, Clay ME, Smith J, et al. Changes in blood counts after the administration of granulocyte-colony-stimulating factor and the collection of peripheral blood stem cells from healthy donors. Transfusion 1996;36:596–600.

107. Lasky LC, McCullough J, Zanjani ED. Liquid storage of unseparated human bone marrow: evaluation of hematopoietic progenitors by clonal assay. Transfusion 1986;26:331.

108. Olson PR, Cox C, McCullough J. Laboratory and clinical effects of the infusion of ACD solution during plateletpheresis. Vox Sang 1977;33:79–87.

109. Szymanski IO. Ionized calcium during plateletpheresis. Transfusion 1978;18:701–708.

110. Uhl L, Maillet S, King S, Kruskall MS. Unexpected citrate toxicity and severe hypocalcemia during apheresis. Transfusion 1977;37:1063–1065.

111. McCullough J, Fortuny IE. Laboratory evaluation of normal donors undergoing leukapheresis on the continuous flow centrifuge. Transfusion 1973;13:394–398.

112. Schiffer CA, Aisner J, Schmukler M, Whitaker CL, Wolff JH. The effect of hydroxyethyl starch on in vitro platelet and granulocyte function. Transfusion 1975;14:473–475.

113. Heyns AP, Badenhorst PN, Lotter MG, Pieters H, Wessels P. Kinetics and mobilization from the spleen of indium-111-labeled platelets during platelet apheresis. Transfusion 1985;25:215–218.

114. Stevens RF, Alexander MK. A sex difference in the platelet count. Br J Haematol 1977;37:295–300.

115. Senhauser DA, Westphal RG, Bohman JE, Neff JC. Immune system changes in cytapheresis donors. Transfusion 1982;22:302–304.

116. Strauss RG. Effects on donors of repeated leukocyte losses during plateletpheresis. J Clin Apheresis 1994;9:130–134.

117. Wright DG, Karsh J, Fauci AS, et al. Lymphocyte depletion and immunosuppression with repeated leukapheresis by continuous flow centrifugation. Blood 1981;58:451–458.

118. Strauss RG. Mechanism of adverse effects during hemapheresis. J Clin Apheresis 1996;11:160–164.

119. Gilcher RO, Gardner JC. Haemonetics V50 and plasma collection system: common concerns and troubleshooting. J Clin Apheresis 1990;5:106–109.

120. McCombie N, Rock G. Logistics of automated plasma collection. J Clin Apheresis 1988;4:104–107.

121. Rock G, Tittley P, McCombie N. Plasma collection using an automated membrane device. Transfusion 1986;26:269–271.

EIGHT

LABORATORY TESTING OF DONATED BLOOD

Each unit of whole blood or each apheresis component undergoes a standard battery of tests (Table 8.1). These tests include determining the blood type and the presence of red cell antibodies and tests for transmissible diseases. Additional tests for cytomegalovirus or HLA antibodies may be performed as an option. Seven tests are done for transmissible diseases, five of which have been introduced since 1985. The total number of test results for each unit of donated blood is about 15, depending on the specific methodology used. This dramatic increase in transmissible disease testing has quickly and fundamentally altered the nature of blood donor centers and has presented a huge increase in workload. For instance, during the last 5 years of the 1980s, the American Red Cross Blood Service carried out about 95 million more transmissible disease tests than during the first half of that decade.[1] In addition, since each unit of whole blood is separated into several components and there is a donor history record and two or three tubes of blood for tests, each donation generates up to 30 different data elements. Each of these must be properly identified and all data amalgamated to ensure that all testing and donor-related information is complete and the results are satisfactory before the blood or components can be released into the transfusion inventory. Since busy blood collection centers deal with hundreds of donors each day, this virtual explosion of data has led to the development and implementation of sophisticated new computer systems; where possible, automated laboratory testing equipment is integrated into these systems. Thus, the modern blood center uses pharmaceutical-type manufacturing processes to ensure accuracy[2] and cost-effectiveness.

Table 8.1 Tests of donor blood

Blood grouping tests
    ABO typing
    Rh typing

Red cell antibody detection

Transmissible disease testing
    Treponemal antigen
    Hepatitis BS antigen
    Hepatitis BC antibody
    Hepatitis C antibody
    HIV 1 and 2 antibody
    HIV antigen
    HTLV I and II antibody

Optional tests
    Cytomegalovirus
    Platelet antigen typing
    Rare red cell antigens
    IgA levels

SAFETY OF THE BLOOD SUPPLY

During the past decade, fear of transfusion has increased among the public, and physicians have become more cautious in the use of blood components. However, the nation's blood supply is safer than ever (see Chapter 15). Changes in donor selection and laboratory testing have been added, and new approaches to quality have led to better process control.[2] Although this chapter focuses on laboratory testing of donated blood, each step in the overall process of donor evaluation and testing adds to blood safety in important ways; laboratory testing of donated blood is only one of these (Table 8.2). For instance, in San Francisco, changes in the medical history and donor selection criteria caused a 90% decrease in the HIV infectivity of the blood supply even before the introduction of a test for HIV.[3] The introduction of new tests for transmissible diseases has further reduced the proportion of infectious donors. Screening of the donor's identity against donor deferral registries detects individuals who have been previously deferred as blood donors but who for various reasons attempt to donate again. These and many other changes have resulted in the improvement in blood safety.

The incidence of infectious units of blood after all screening tests are negative ranges from 1 per 63,000 units for hepatitis C, to 1 per 493,000 for HIV, and 1 per 641,000 for HTLV[4] (see Chapter 15). The aggregate risk is estimated to be 1 per 34,000 units.[4] Since the average transfused patient receives 3.8 units of blood,[5] the average overall risk of acquiring a transmissible disease is about 0.01% per patient transfused. Thus, although the blood supply is safer than ever, transfusion is not risk-free and should be undertaken only after careful consideration of the patient's clinical situation and specific blood component needs.

Table 8.2 Methods of reducing the infectivity of the blood supply

Recruitment health criteria
Medical history
Physical examination
Donor deferral registry
Laboratory testing
Donor callback
Confidential unit exclusion

RED CELL BLOOD GROUP TESTING

Testing of donated blood is carried out on blood specimens obtained for this purpose at the time of donation. The blood is collected in separate tubes or a pouch in the tubing through which the blood passes. The maximum volume of blood that can be retained for testing is about 30 mL.

ABO Typing

The most common cause of a fatal transfusion reaction is the administration of ABO-incompatible red cells (see Chapter 14). Therefore, the ABO and Rh typing of the donor units is of critical importance. Usually ABO and Rh typing are carried out together along with red cell antibody detection testing, since all of these tests involve red cell antibody-antigen interaction. The ABO and Rh typing can be done in a variety of systems, including slides, tubes, solid-phase microplates, gel systems, or affinity columns. Complex semiautomated instruments are available for typing large numbers of blood samples. These instruments handle the specimen from start to finish adding reagents, carrying out the incubation, reading the reaction, and providing the result, which can be interpreted by the computer in the instrument or provided for manual interpretation. The choice of the particular method and instrument will depend on the specific circumstances at the donor center. Processing several hundred blood specimens manually or in tubes is cumbersome and probably not very efficient. Automation is usually used. However, it is not feasible to purchase an expensive instrument to type only a few samples. Manufacturers are making efforts to develop semiautomated instruments based on the solid-phase or gel technology so that the benefits of automation can be brought to smaller donor centers. There are some similarities in methodology among all of the test system configurations. Antisera or reagent red cells are added, and tests of both red cells and serum are carried out at room temperature. The cell suspension is usually centrifuged or manipulated in some way to foster agglutination. An effort is made to disperse the cell suspension, and the resulting mixture is observed either visually or by an instrument.

For ABO typing, both the red cells and the serum are always typed. The red cells are tested with anti-A, anti-B, and anti-A, B (group O) sera. The A, B (group O) serum is used to detect weak subgroups of A (see Chapter 9), because the anti-A or anti-B in

Table 8.3 Common causes of ABO typing discrepancies

Technical causes	Incorrect matching of red cell and serum test results
	Incorrect recording of results
	Failure to add serum or red cells to test
	Failure to recognize hemolysis as a positive test result
	Improper warming of test system
	Incorrect ratio of red cells to serum
	Improper centrifugation
	Bacteriologic contamination of reagents
	Weak antigen on test red cells
	Fibrin clots
Patient and donor-related causes	Cold agglutinins
	Abnormal serum protein values
	Infusion of rouleaux-inducing agent
	Antibody against dye in test serum
	Antibody against ingredient in medium
	Antibody active at room temperature
	Weak or absent antibody due to age or disease
	Non-ABO antibodies
	Recent transfusion
	Previous stem cell transplant
	Polyagglutinable state
	Neonatal patient
	Immunodeficient patient

serum from type O individuals reacts more strongly with some weak subgroups than anti-A or anti-B sera. Some of the weak subgroups of A require incubation before a reaction can be seen, and they may be missed in routine testing. During the past few years, blood typing reagents have been increasingly produced using monoclonal antibody techniques. These reagents have much greater specificity and strength of reactivity than older reagents that were human allosera. In addition to testing the red cells with antisera, the serum of each donor is tested against A and B red cells to determine which, if any, ABO antibodies are present. The group A test red cells should be A1 to provide the strongest reactions. Commercial reagent A and B cells are almost, if not always, Rh negative. This is to avoid apparent false-positive reactions in the ABO typing tests if anti-Rh antibodies are present in the donor and react with the A or B Rh positive reagent red cells. The ABO typing is done using both red cells and serum to take advantage of the known relationship of ABO antigens and antibodies to strengthen the validity of the test result. Any discrepant test result must be resolved before the donor unit can be labeled and released from quarantine into the usable inventory. The common causes of ABO typing problems are listed in Table 8.3.

Rh Typing

There are many antigen specificities in the Rh system, but the D antigen is highly immunogenic, and alloantibodies to the D antigen can cause severe or fatal hemolytic disease of the newborn or transfusion reactions (see Chapter 9). Individuals who pos-

sess the D antigen are said to be Rh positive, and those who lack it are Rh negative. Because of the clinical importance of alloantibodies to the Rh(D) antigen, all donated blood is typed for this antigen but not others within the Rh system. This makes it possible to select Rh-negative red cell components for patients who are Rh negative. Most Rh-negative individuals do not have circulating anti-D, and so the combination of cell and serum typing done for ABO is not done for Rh. Rh typing reagents have been more complex than ABO reagents. Because ABO antibodies are usually a combination of IgG and IgM and cause direct agglutination at room temperature, it was possible to carry out ABO typing tests without extensive incubation or the need for agents to potentiate the antigen-antibody reaction. However, anti-D is usually an IgG-type antibody that does not cause direct agglutination at room temperature. Thus, potentiating agents such as antihuman globulin (AHG) were necessary to demonstrate the reaction. However, this requires incubation at 37°C, washing, and addition of the AHG. To simplify the typing procedure and to make it similar to ABO typing, reagents called high protein or rapid tube have been used for Rh typing because they promoted rapid agglutination of red cells coated with anti-D without incubation and the use of AHG. The production of an ideal high-protein or rapid tube reagent for Rh typing was unique to different companies, and sera from different companies sometimes gave different reactions with a few individuals' red cells. Red cells from some individuals would react with some antisera but not others. These individuals were said to have a Du or weak D antigen (see Chapter 9). Since their red cells contain some D antigen, it is important to detect these individuals. This is done by testing all donors who are initially found to be Rh negative for the weak D. Weak D antigen tests use Rh antisera specially designed for this purpose. These antisera are polyclonal high-protein, chemically modified low-protein, or a combination polyclonal-monoclonal low-protein reagents. The test involves incubating the donor's red cells with the Rh typing sera, washing the cells, adding AHG, centrifuging the mixture, and observing it for agglutination. If no agglutination occurs, the donor is considered to be Rh negative; if agglutination occurs, the donor has a weak D and the unit of red cells is labeled as Rh positive. Even though the donor's red cells tested negative in the original Rh typing test, the presence of the weak D antigen makes the red cells possibly immunogenic and they must be considered Rh positive.

It is not customary to type donor blood for other antigens of the Rh system, because either they are less antigenic than D, the phenotype frequencies are such that incompatibility between donor and recipient are less common, and/or the antibodies are less clinically dangerous.

Red Blood Cell Antibody Detection

Blood donors who have been previously pregnant or transfused may have red cell alloantibodies in their plasma. These antibodies can cause a positive direct antiglobulin test, shortened red cell survival, or hemolysis in the recipient.[6–8] Thus, transfusion of antibody in components containing donor plasma should be avoided. Production of red cells using present methods leaves a small amount of residual plasma compared to the larger amount of plasma that remained with the red cells before the use of additive solutions for red cell storage (see Chapter 5). Thus, with present methods there is probably little chance that an amount of antibody large enough to cause a clinical problem would

be transfused with a unit of red cells. However, plasma or platelets may also be prepared from the donor unit, and these plasma-containing components could provide passive antibody. Other reasons to search for red cell antibodies in donor plasma are (a) the presence of an antibody means that the donor's red cells are negative for the corresponding antigen, and this is a convenient way to identify antigen-negative donors, (b) the donor's plasma may be a useful source of antibody reagent, and (c) the antibody may lead to better understanding of a blood group system. Thus, units of donated blood are screened for red cell antibodies. Plasma containing components from units found to contain antibodies are not used for transfusion. Approximately 0.5% of donor units will test positive in the antibody detection test.

Since the red cell antibodies of concern are formed in response to pregnancy or transfusion, American Association of Blood Banks (AABB) standards require antibody detection testing only of those donors.[9] However, from a practical standpoint it is more convenient for the blood bank to screen all donor units. This avoids the possibility that a unit that should be screened will be missed or that clerical errors will result in release of a unit that contains an antibody. Because the donor antibody is diluted when it is transfused, the donor antibody detection procedure may be different from that used to detect antibodies in patients. In donor antibody detection tests, serum from several donors or several reagent red cell suspensions may be pooled. This reduces the sensitivity of the test but also reduces costs and appears not to reduce safety. Pooling of both donor sera and reagent red cells is not recommended. The antibody detection method must demonstrate clinically significant antibodies, but one of several different techniques can be used to accomplish this. The techniques include incubation at 37°C with reagent red cells in one of the following media: saline, albumin, low ionic strength, polyethylene glycol, or polybrene. The sensitivity of these methods and the particular antibodies they detect varies (see Chapter 10), as does their desirability for donor antibody detection. Tests are not carried out at room temperature because of the large number of nonspecific or non-clinically significant cold antibodies that are detected. Currently the most common donor antibody detection method uses two or occasionally three different reagent red cell suspensions and 37°C incubation of donor serum suspended in albumin for 30 minutes followed by antihuman globulin. This is a reasonable compromise providing a high likelihood of detecting red cell antibodies and yet minimizing the likelihood of obtaining false-positive reactions.

For a time in the 1970s, the autoanalyzer was used, but for the most part, red cell antibody detection has been done using the traditional tube test methods. During the past few years, several new technologies have been developed for the detection of red cell antibody-antigen reactions. These include gel and solid-phase systems and affinity columns. These methods are discussed more fully in Chapter 10. All three test systems can be used for red cell antibody detection. When solid-phase tests are used for red cell antibody screening,[10,11] the microtiter plates are covered with either ghosts of the reagent red cells or antihuman globulin. For plates covered with red cell ghosts, the donor's serum is added and the antibody-antigen reaction occurs on the plate surface. Antibody binding is detected by adding anti-IgG coated red cells. For plates covered with antihuman globulin, the antibody-antigen reaction can occur in the fluid phase and the mixture added to the wells where IgG coated red cells adhere to the AHG coated

plates. In the affinity column system, the antibody antigen reaction can also occur in the fluid phase. Antihuman globulin is added, and the reagent red cells are then added to the microwell plates. If antibody was present, the IgG–anti-IgG complex on the red cell binds to the plate coated with staphylococcal protein A. These solid-phase tests are similar in their ability to detect donor antibodies, although the titers of the antibodies differ in the different methods.[11]

Automated devices using bar code scanners and designed for large-scale screening in donor centers have been developed for the solid-phase system. In addition, specific automated devices for large-scale testing of donor blood have been developed. These methods are usually based on agglutination, which is read by photometers or visually as precipitates on filter paper. The instruments incorporate automated sample and reagent dispensing, have bar code readers for sample identification, and use anticoagulated blood so that both red cells and plasma can be sampled from the same tube and centrifugation with sample separation is not necessary.

Each blood center will establish the method that provides the most satisfactory results for their donor population and technical staff.

Positive Direct Antiglobulin Tests in Normal Donors

A positive direct antiglobulin test (DAT) occurs in about 1 per 7,000 to 14,000 donors.[12,13] Occasionally the positive DAT result is caused by a viral infection or immune disease, but usually there is no explanation for this positive test result when the donors are observed for long periods.[12] At normal ionic strength, about 2×10^3 molecules of IgG are bound to the red cell. The amount of IgG binding can be increased by lowering the ionic strength of the medium or treating the cells with enzymes. Probably the positive DATs in normal donors are due to unknown factors causing increased binding of IgG to the red cells. Some reports of higher incidence of positive DATs in normal donors are probably the result of inclusion of patients with disease. Recently three donors were described in whom a positive DAT was due to antiphospholipid antibodies.[12] The authors speculate that the positive DAT was caused by nonspecific binding of the antibody onto phospholipids of the red cell membrane. These antiphospholipid antibodies are associated with several autoimmune disorders (including systemic lupus erythematosus, infections, or malignancy), and the antibodies may occur in apparently healthy people. These three donors also had false-positive serologic tests for syphilis, although most donors with a positive DAT do not. For instance, the three reported donors accounted for only 10% of the donors found to have a positive DAT. Thus, antiphospholipid antibodies probably do not account for most of the cases of positive DATs in normal donors.

TESTING FOR TRANSMISSIBLE DISEASES

General Concepts of Testing for Transmissible Diseases

The use of laboratory tests to eliminate potentially infectious blood from the blood supply has been in place since the 1950s, when syphilis testing became routine. The use

of testing to improve the safety of transfusion therapy is discussed more fully in Chapter 15. The decision to implement a test and the strategy used in dealing with the test results are complex issues. The quality of the test, the prevalence of the disease in the donor population, and the likelihood of transmission of the disease to blood recipients are some of the important factors to consider. The impact of a test done on millions of individuals must also be considered. Tests that perform very well in a patient population have different ramifications in a normal donor population. For instance, a test with a specificity of 99% might be considered good, but still 1% of positive tests will be false. When such a test is done on 12 million blood donors and has a positive rate of 0.1%, this means that 12,000 individuals will be falsely labeled as having a positive test result. If such a test is an important step in improving the safety of the blood supply, it should be implemented, but along with the implementation, plans must be in place to deal with the donors who will have a false-positive test result. Confirmatory testing should be available to distinguish those who are truly positive from those who are not, and effective systems must be in place to carry out the confirmatory testing and provide this information. For donors who have a true positive test, complete and accurate information must be available describing the significance of the test result. An excellent example of this situation is described below for hepatitis C.

A major issue in testing for transmissible diseases, especially HIV, is that several of the assays detect antibodies, and there is an interval between infection and antibody formation. During this interval, known as the "window phase", the individual is infectious but has a negative test. Test kit manufacturers devote considerable effort to designing their test kits to provide maximum sensitivity and shorten this window phase as much as possible.

The viral serology tests are based on the enzyme-linked immunosorbent assay (EIA) principle. The EIA is considered a screening test. For most of the assays, if the initial test result is positive, it is repeated in duplicate. If both of the subsequent results are negative, the test is considered to be negative and the unit of blood is suitable for use. If one or both of the subsequent results are positive, the result is considered to be "repeat reactive" and the unit of blood cannot be used. The assays are carried out in microtiter plates, and the antigen may be bound to beads or to the wells of the microtiter plates. Automatic pipetters and washers are used, but the plates are moved manually from step to step during the assay; there is not a single large device that carries the assay from start to finish.

The tests for specific transmissible diseases are (a) serologic test for syphilis, (b) hepatitis B surface antigen, (c) anti-hepatitis B core, (d) anti-hepatitis C virus, (e) anti-human immunodeficiency virus types 1 and 2, (f) human immunodeficiency virus antigen, and (g) anti-human T-cell lymphotrophic virus I and II (Table 8.4). The hepatitis B core antibody test has been used as a surrogate test for non-A, non-B hepatitis and until recently was not expected to be of value in detecting hepatitis B.[14] Alanine aminotransferase (ALT) was used as another surrogate test for non-A, non-B hepatitis, but with the discovery of the hepatitis C virus and implementation of hepatitis C testing, the ALT is no longer of value and is no longer required.[14] Some blood banks continue to test blood for ALT if they wish to provide plasma for the production of derivatives

Table 8.4 Present transfusion-transmitted disease screening

Agent	Disease
Treponema	Syphilis
Hepatitis B$_S$ antigen	Hepatitis B
Hepatitis B$_C$ antibody	Hepatitis B
	Hepatitis non-A, non-B
	HIV
Hepatitis C antibody	Hepatitis C
HIV 1 and 2 antibody	AIDS
HIV antigen	AIDS
HTLV I antibody	Leukemia
	Lymphoma
	Tropical paresis
HTLV II antibody	Disease unknown
CMV*	CMV disease

*For immunodeficient patients only

to be sold in Europe, where ALT testing is still required. Donor blood is not tested for hepatitis A because this form of hepatitis is not transmitted by transfusion.

An important aspect of the conduct of testing for transmissible diseases is the method of handling the result data. Transcription errors are known to occur in medical laboratories, and they certainly occur in the management of transmissible disease test results. For instance, in New York, four patients were exposed to anti-HIV-positive blood because of transcription errors[15] during a period in which only four other patients were exposed to anti-HIV-positive blood because of a seronegative donation. Thus, the risk from transcription error was as great as that from a window-period donation.

Human Immunodeficiency Virus Testing

For the HIV antibody test, the antigens may be prepared from materials produced by recombinant DNA or from viral extracts, depending on the manufacturer. The composition of the antigenic material used in the assays is mixed to reflect the antigen regions of HIV strains from around the world in an effort to maximize the sensitivity of the assay. The present HIV assays include antigens from both HIV-1 and HIV-2. Because there is greater than 50% homology between HIV-1 and HIV-2 DNA, the HIV-1 test detects about 90% of HIV-2 strains.[16] However, as HIV-2 began to appear in the United States,[17] the U.S. Food and Drug Administration (FDA) requested that HIV test kits include antigens specific for HIV-2. This strategy has been very effective, because although HIV-2 is not common in the United States, there have been no cases of transfusion-transmitted HIV-2.

Confirmatory tests For all blood samples that test repeat reactive, supplemental or confirmatory testing is done. The methods used for this are Western blot and immuno-

fluorescence assays using viral lysate antigens. FDA-approved confirmatory test kits are available for anti-HIV but not for anti-hepatitis C or anti-HTLV. The confirmatory test for anti-HIV is a Western blot that tests for antibody against the following HIV proteins: p24, the major core (gag) protein; gp41, a transmembrane (env) protein; and gp120/160 external (env) protein and an external (env) precursor protein. The results of the Western blot can be positive, indeterminate, or negative. The criteria for positivity on the Western blot are the presence of antibody against any two of these proteins. Sera that react with only one protein are considered indeterminate. These individuals must be deferred from blood donation, although it appears that they are not infected with HIV,[18,19] and it has been proposed that they be reinstated as blood donors.[20,21] False-positive screening test results for anti-HIV and anti-HTLV (not confirmed by Western blot) have been related to receipt of an influenza vaccine.[22,23]

Antibody assay variability and controls   The controls used in the assays are referred to as internal controls because they are provided by the manufacturer as part of the test kits. It has been suggested that external controls might also be helpful, especially external controls that are weakly reactive;[24] however, the FDA does not believe that these external controls add to the effectiveness of the test systems.[25]

There is some variable sensitivity of the assays currently licensed in the United States.[26] It has been proposed[21] that an ongoing comparison of the sensitivity and effectiveness of the various licensed assays be conducted in the United States, although this is not currently done. Some test reagents are licensed for use in other countries but not in the United States. It has been suggested[21] that some of these reagents may be more effective than some of those licensed in the United States and that collaborative ongoing monitoring systems should be established to ensure that assay systems used in the United States have the maximum possible sensitivity and effectiveness.

Shortening the window-phase detection   The FDA has stated its commitment to shorten the window phase. One approach is to adjust the assays to detect IgM anti-HIV in hopes of detecting antibody earlier in the course of infection. Another approach to shortening the window phase is to shift the test methodology away from antibody detection to detection of the infectious agent. The FDA is committed to this shift.[27] The major difficulty is to find a method sufficiently sensitive to detect the infectious agent in the circulation but with a minimal rate of false positivity and at a level of complexity and cost that would be practical for widespread use for screening millions of blood donors. At an FDA-sponsored conference in 1995, manufacturers estimated that such assays would be available in 3 to 5 years or by late 1998 to 2000.[27]

HIV antigen test   In an effort to detect HIV-infected donors earlier and thus shorten the window phase of infectivity, the FDA required the addition of a test for the HIV antigen. Two studies of several hundred thousand donors had failed to identify any donor who tested positive by the HIV antigen test but negative by the anti-HIV test.[28,29] Thus, it was considered unlikely that HIV antigen screening would be valuable. No test kits were licensed by the FDA for donor screening, and so this was not implemented as a routine part of the donor testing process. However, a few cases of transmission of HIV

from antigen-positive, antibody-negative donors occurred,[30,31] and the FDA reconsidered its position on antigen testing. In late 1995, the FDA recommended that blood banks begin testing for HIV antigen, and soon thereafter test kits were licensed for this purpose. HIV antigen testing is now a standard part of blood donor testing.

Human T-Cell Lymphotrophic Virus

Donors are tested for antibodies to HTLV-I and HTLV-II using an EIA method.[32] The assays from different manufacturers have varying capability to detect HTLV-II. The testing algorithm is the same as that described for HIV. Supplemental confirmatory testing is also done using a Western blot with recombinant DNA–produced and viral lysate antigens.

Hepatitis Tests

Hepatitis B surface antigen Testing for hepatitis B was introduced in 1971 shortly after the discovery of the hepatitis-associated antigen. Test methodology evolved over the years, and at present an EIA system is used. Antibody to hepatitis B surface antigen (HBsAg) is coated onto particles, the donor's serum is added, and any HBsAg binds to the particle and is detected by a second anti-HBs that is linked to an enzyme. The HBsAg test is confirmed using a neutralization step. This is done by adding known anti-HBs and repeating the assay. A substantial reduction in activity signifies a true positive or confirmed positive test.

Hepatitis B core antibody The hepatitis B core antibody (anti-HBc) test was originally introduced in hopes of identifying cases of hepatitis B in a phase with no detectable HBsAg.[33] However, this has not proved to be so, and the anti-HBc test was introduced more as a surrogate marker for non-A, non-B hepatitis.[34–36] More recently, with the introduction of specific testing for hepatitis C, the anti-HBc test is not effective as a surrogate test but has been retained because of the possibility that it does detect a few donors infectious for hepatitis B but with a negative HBsAg test.[14] The anti-HBc test is different than the others in that it is an inhibition-type assay. HBc is bound to the solid phase, and the indicator (enzyme-linked) probe is anti-HBc. The anti-HBc in the probe competes with the donor's serum sample, and if anti-HBc is present in the donor's serum there is less binding of the labeled probe and a reduced assay activity, indicating a positive test. Unfortunately, this type of assay is subject to greater variability than the direct-type assay used for other tests, and this has resulted in a considerable false-positive rate for the anti-HBc test.

Hepatitis C antibody The hepatitis C antibody (anti-HCV) test is also an EIA. Peptides of the HCV are bound to the solid phase, and an enzyme-linked antiglobulin is the detection system. Initially there was no FDA-licensed confirmatory test available, and it appeared that as many as 50% of those who initially tested reactive had false-positive tests.[37–39] The mix of peptides in the assay system has been modified during the past several years, improving the test performance and reducing the proportion of false-positive reactions.[39] A confirmatory test is available using an immunoblot system.[40]

Managing the Results of Transmissible Disease Testing of Donors

Donors must be notified of the results if a screening test is positive. A repeated reactive (positive) screening test result may subsequently be confirmed or not. Thus, the information provided must be tailored to the specific disease and the nature of the test result. For instance, even a nonconfirmed but positive initial screening test for HIV may create serious anxiety.

The information provided should describe the disease, the significance of the test result, and any recommendations or implications this has for the donor's health and future blood donations. The extent to which blood bank personnel should take responsibility for providing this information is an interesting issue. One approach would be to have the donor's physician provide the notification; alternatively, blood bank personnel can take primary responsibility for at least the initial consultation. In general, blood bank organizations have provided the basic information and initial consultation. This is particularly important in notifying people of a positive HIV test. Since the ramifications of this result are so serious, it is important to do this personally and to have information and referral systems to knowledgeable AIDS-treating physicians readily available. Another complicating matter is that the significance of the test result may not be known. For instance, the long-term clinical effect of non-A, non-B hepatitis or hepatitis C has only become clear during the last few years. During the early stages of hepatitis C screening of donors, there was no licensed confirmatory test, and as a result a large portion of the donors who had a positive screening test were not infected but could not be informed of this. Thus, the donors had to be told they had a positive screening test for hepatitis C, but it was not known whether they were infected. Needless to say, this created considerable anxiety and unnecessarily so. Another example is the lack of definitive information on the long-term health impact of an indeterminate Western blot for HIV. While it appears that these donors may not be infected (see above), they are deferred from donating blood and cannot be told definitively that despite a positive screening test they are not infected.

Lookback

When a donor is found to have a positive test for HIV, HTLV, or hepatitis B, records are reviewed to determine whether the individual has donated previously. If so, the hospital to which the blood was provided is notified. They in turn notify the physician of the blood recipient, who is expected to determine whether and how to inform the patient. This process is called lookback. The objectives of lookback are to alert the patient so that he or she can obtain treatment for the disease if indicated and take steps to avoid transmitting the disease to others. Lookback is done for donors with a positive test for HIV, HTLV, and hepatitis B, but not for hepatitis C.

Surrogate Testing Using ALT

Studies during the 1970s and 1980s indicated that blood from donors with an elevated ALT was associated with transmission of non-A, non-B hepatitis (see Chapter 15). In response to these data, many blood banks initiated testing for both anti-HBc and ALT.

Several difficulties were found in using ALT as a donor screening test. The values are influenced by age, gender, race, and weight, and the results are a continuous distribution, making determination of a "cutoff" difficult. Nevertheless, the use of ALT prior to introduction of HCV testing seems to have been helpful in reducing posttransfusion non-A, non-B hepatitis (see Chapter 15). However, with the availability of the specific test for anti-HCV, the ALT no longer contributes to blood safety, and it has been discontinued.[14]

Syphilis Testing of Donated Blood

Syphilis testing has been carried out on donated blood for more than 50 years because of the recognized risk of transfusion-transmitted syphilis[41] (see also Chapter 15). However, very few cases have been reported for years, and in the mid-1980s a move was initiated to discontinue testing. This was because the spirochete is viable in stored blood for only about 96 hours,[14] and the serologic test for syphilis is rarely positive at a time when spirochetes are in the circulation. Thus, the current testing probably does not identify infectious units. However, as the AIDS epidemic began to unfold, the syphilis test was retained as a surrogate marker of risk for sexually transmitted diseases, including HIV. This has not proved to be an effective way to identify HIV-infected donors,[14] and syphilis testing need not be retained for this purpose. At present, many blood components, especially platelets, are stored at room temperature—conditions that will not inactivate the spirochete. Until definitive laboratory studies are available demonstrating its lack of value, syphilis testing continues to be required.

OPTIONAL TESTS OF DONOR BLOOD

Cytomegalovirus

Cytomegalovirus (CMV) infection can be transmitted by blood transfusion, resulting in serious, even fatal, disease (see Chapters 11 and 12). The primary CMV infection can be mild or asymptomatic, and the CMV then remains latent in healthy individuals, whose blood can transmit the disease to susceptible patients.[42,43] It is thought that the virus remains latent in the donor's leukocytes, but efforts to develop a test to detect the virus and thus define true infectivity have not been successful. As a result, the testing strategy has had to identify potentially infectious donors by detecting previous exposure to the virus. This is done using a test for CMV antibody. Alternatively, CMV transmission can be prevented by removing the leukocytes from the blood components (see Chapter 11). This section deals with screening donated blood for anti-CMV to prevent CMV transmission.

Transfusion-transmitted CMV is a risk only for immunosuppressed patients such as neonates or those undergoing marrow transplantation. CMV testing is not done routinely on all donated blood. Several types of CMV antibody detection methods are available, including EIA, latex agglutination, solid-phase immunofluorescence, complement fixation, and indirect hemagglutination. These methods can be used to detect

IgG or IgM antibodies with a specificity of 85% to 98% and a sensitivity of 95% to 99%.[44] The two assay methods used most commonly are the EIA and the latex agglutination test. The EIA is done as described above for other transfusion-transmitted diseases. The microtiter plates are coated with CMV antigen; the patient's serum is added, incubated, and washed away; and any antibody in the patient's serum bound to the plate is detected with the enzyme-linked antibody. The latex agglutination test uses latex particles coated with CMV antigen. Antibodies, if present in the patient's serum, bind to the latex particles and the particles form macroscopically visible agglutinates. The latex test is more convenient to carry out if only a few samples are to be tested, and this test tends to be used in hospitals to screen units of blood in their inventory. The EIA method lends itself better to large-scale testing. Also, since the EIA test is similar to other infectious disease tests, it tends to be the test method of choice in blood centers for screening large numbers of donors. Both tests are done on serum or plasma.

CMV infection is rather common in the general population, with 30% to 80% of blood donors testing positive with the EIA or latex tests; but probably only about 1% to 3% of donors are actually infectious.[44] Unfortunately, these antibody tests do not distinguish those donors who are truly infectious. IgM antibodies may indicate recent infection and suggest that a donor is more likely to be infectious, but this has not proved to be very effective in identifying truly infectious donors. Although polymerase chain reaction is a very sensitive assay to detect viral DNA, this has not yet been developed into a practical screening test for CMV in blood donors. Thus, the donor-screening approach to prevention of transmission of CMV is screening of donors for antibody to CMV and use of only CMV antibody–negative blood components for susceptible patients. An alternative approach involving leukodepleted blood components is described in Chapters 11 and 12.

Other Red Cell Antigens

Donors are not routinely typed for other red cell antigens. Occasionally a blood bank or donor center may wish to screen donors for particular antigens to increase the blood center's rare donor file. The particular antigens being sought depend on local circumstances and the availability of good reagents.

HLA or Granulocyte Antibody Detection in Donors

Because of the possibility that HLA or granulocyte antibodies in donors may be involved in transfusion-related acute lung injury (TRALI) (see Chapter 14), it has been suggested that blood from multiparous donors not be used as whole blood or plasma components unless it has been screened for these antibodies.[45] This practice has not been implemented, possibly because newer information suggests that cytokines or other inciting factors may play an important role in TRALI and screening of donors for these antibodies may not be especially helpful. This remains an important issue, however, and such screening may be implemented in the future so that transfusion of plasma containing these antibodies can be avoided.

Platelet-Specific Antibodies and Antigens

Donors' blood is not routinely tested for platelet-specific antibodies. Occasionally some blood centers may screen donors for a limited time to identify donors negative for the HPA1 (PlA1) platelet-specific antigen. This is the antigen most commonly involved in alloimmune neonatal thrombocytopenia or posttransfusion purpura (see Chapters 10 and 12), and many blood centers like to maintain a file of donors known to lack this antigen. The donors can be called upon to donate platelets if needed for patients with anti-HPA1 antibodies.

Screening Donors for IgA Deficiency

IgA levels are not routinely determined in donated blood. Some blood centers occasionally screen donors for a limited time to establish a file of donors known to be IgA deficient. The donor record can be annotated so that when the individual donates, the plasma from the unit can be frozen and saved for future use for IgA-deficient patients. Also, those donors can be called upon to donate platelets if needed for IgA-deficient patients.

SUMMARY

Laboratory testing of donated blood is composed of both red cell typing and transmissible disease testing. Each of these kinds of tests is under increasing stringency. As electronic systems are used increasingly for data management, repeated laboratory tests are being eliminated, placing increased importance on the accuracy of the original donor type result (see Chapter 10). Transmissible disease tests are an essential part of the strategy to minimize the risks of blood transfusion. The increasing complexity of these tests has led to consolidation of the testing into larger laboratories and the use of computer control systems, making the entire donor testing process much more extensive and intricate than just a decade ago.

REFERENCES

1. McCullough J. The nation's changing blood supply system. JAMA 1993;269:2239-2245.
2. Zuck TF. Current good manufacturing practices. Transfusion 1995;35:955–966.
3. Busch MP, Young MJ, Samson SJ, et al. Risk of human immunodeficiency virus (HIV) transmission by blood transfusions before the implementation of HIV-1 antibody screening. Transfusion 1991;31:4.
4. Schreiber GB, Busch MP, Kleinman SH. The risk of transfusion-transmitted viral infections. N Engl J Med 1996;334:1685–1690.
5. Wallace EL, Churchill WH, Surgenor DM, An J, Cho G, McGurk S, Murphy L. Collection and transfusion of blood and blood components in the United States, 1992. Transfusion 1995;35:802–812.
6. Zoes C, Dube VE, Miller HJ, Vye MV. Anti-A1 in the plasma of platelet concentrates causing a hemolytic reaction. Transfusion 1977;17:29.
7. Franciosi RA, Awer E, Santana M. Interdonor incompatibility resulting in anuria. Transfusion 1967;7:297.

8. Reiner AP, Sayers MH. Hemolytic transfusion reaction due to interdonor Kell incompatibility. Report of two cases and review of the literature. Arch Pathol Lab Med 1990;114:862.

9. Standards for Blood Banks and Transfusion Services. 16th ed. Bethesda, MD: American Association of Blood Banks, 1994:408.

10. Uthemann H, Poschmann A. Solid-phase antiglobulin test for screening and identification of red cell antibodies. Transfusion 1990;30:114–116.

11. Schrem A, Flegel WA. Comparison of solid-phase antibody screening tests with pooled red cells in blood donors. Transfusion 1996;71:37–42.

12. Win N, Islam SIAM, Peterkin MA, Walker ID. Positive direct antiglobulin test due to antiphospholipid antibodies in normal healthy blood donors. Vox Sang 1997;72:182–184.

13. Gorst DW, Rawlinson VI, Merry AH, Stratton F. Positive direct antiglobulin test in normal individuals. Vox Sang 1980;38:99–105.

14. NIH Consensus Development Panel on Infectious Disease Testing for Blood Transfusions. Infectious disease testing for blood transfusion. JAMA 1995;274:1374–1379.

15. Linden JV. Error contributes to the risk of transmissible disease. Transfusion 1994;34:1016. Letter to the Editor.

16. Busch MB, Petersen L, Schable C, Perkins HA. Monitoring blood donors for HIV-2 infection by testing anti-HIV-1 reactive sera. Transfusion 1990;30:184.

17. O'Brian TR, George JR, Holmberg SD. Human immunodeficiency virus type 2 infection in the United States: epidemiology, diagnosis, and public health implications. JAMA 1992;267:2775.

18. Eble BE, Busch MP, Khayam-Bashi H, et al. Resolution of infection status of HIV- seroindeterminate and high-risk seronegative individuals using PCR and virus-culture: absence of persistent silent HIV-1 infection in a high-prevalence area. Transfusion 1992;32:503.

19. Jackson JB. Human immunodeficiency virus (HIV)-indeterminate Western blots and latent HIV infection. Transfusion 1992;32:497.

20. Busch MP, Kleinman SH, Williams AE, et al. Frequency of human immunodeficiency virus (HIV) infection among contemporary anti-HIV-1 and anti-HIV-1/2 supplemental test-indeterminate blood donors. Transfusion 1996;36:37–44.

21. Sayre KR, Dodd RY, Tegtmeier G, Layug L, Alexander SS, Busch MP. False-positive human immunodeficiency virus type 1 Western blot tests in noninfected blood donors. Transfusion 1996;36:45–52.

22. MacKenzie WR, Davis JP, Peterson DE, Hibbard AJ, Becker G, Zarvan BS. Multiple false-positive serologic tests for HIV, HTLV-I, and hepatitis C following influenza vaccination, 1991. JAMA 1992;268:1015–1017.

23. False-positive serologic tests for human T-cell lymphotrophic virus type I among blood donors following influenza vaccination, 1992. MMWR 1993;42:173–175.

24. Linden JV, Wethers J, Dressler KP. Controversy in transfusion medicine: use of external controls in transmissible disease testing: pro. Transfusion 1994;34:550–551.

25. Epstein JS. Controversy in transfusion medicine: use of external controls in transmissible disease testing: con. Transfusion 1994;34:552–553.

26. Busch MP, Courouce AM. Relative sensitivity of United States and European assays for screening blood donors for antibodies to human immunodeficiency viruses. Transfusion 1997;37:352–353.

27. Hewlett IK, Epstein JS. Food and Drug Administration conference on the feasibility of genetic technology to close the HIV window in donor screening. Transfusion 1997;37:346–351.

28. Busch MP, Taylor PE, Lenes BA, et al. Screening of selected male blood donors for p24 antigen of human immunodeficiency type 1. Transfusion Safety Study Group. N Engl J Med 1990;323:1308–1312.

29. Alter HJ, Epstein JS, Swenson SG, et al. Prevalence of human immunodeficiency virus type 1 p24 antigen in US blood donors—an assessment of the efficacy of testing in donor screening. HIV-Antigen Study Group. N Engl J Med 1990;323:1312–1317.

30. Irani MS, Dudley AW, Lucco LJ. Case of HIV-1 transmission by antigen-positive, antibody negative blood. N Engl J Med 1991;325:1174–1175. Letter to the Editor.

31. Roberts CS, Longfield JN, Platte RC, et al. Transfusion-associated human immunodeficiency virus type 1 from screened antibody-negative blood donors. Arch Pathol Lab Med 1994;118:1188–1192.

32. Williams AE, Fang CT, Slamon DJ, et al. Seroprevalence and epidemiologic correlates of HTLV-1 infection in U.S. blood donors. Science 1988;240:643.

33. Chambers LA, Popovsky MA. Decrease in reported posttransfusion hepatitis. Contributions of donor screening for alanine aminotransferase and antibodies to hepatitis B core antigen and changes in the general populations. Arch Intern Med 1991;151:2445.

34. Stevens CE, Aach RD, Hollinger FB. Hepatitis B virus antibody in blood donors and the occurrence of non-A, non-B hepatitis in transfusion recipients: an analysis of the transfusion-transmitted viruses study. Ann Intern Med 1984;101:733.

35. Koziol DE, Holland PV, Alling DW, et al. Antibody to hepatitis B core antigen as a paradoxical marker for non-A, non-B hepatitis agents in donated blood. Ann Intern Med 1986;104:488.

36. Alter HJ, Purcell RH, Holland PV, Alling DW, Koziol DE. Donor transaminase and recipient hepatitis: impact on blood transfusion services. JAMA 1981;246:630.

37. Janot C, Courouce AM, Maniez M. Antibodies to hepatitis C virus in French blood donors. Lancet 1989;2:796.

38. Sirchia G, Bellobuono A, Giovanetti A, Marconi M. Antibodies to hepatitis C virus in Italian blood donors. Lancet 1989;2:797.

39. Kleinman S, Alter H, Busch M, et al. Increased detection of hepatitis C virus (HCV)–infected blood donors by a multiple-antigen HCV enzyme immunoassay. Transfusion 1992;32:805.

40. Evans CS, Tobler L, Polito A, et al. Comparative evaluation of supplemental hepatitis C virus antibody test systems. Transfusion 1992;32:408.

41. Chambers RW, Foley HT, Schmidt PJ. Transmission of syphilis by fresh blood components. Transfusion 1969;9:32.

42. Schrier RD, Nelson JA, Oldstone MBA. Detection of human cytomegalovirus in peripheral blood lymphocytes in a natural infection. Science 1985;230:1048–1051.

43. Diosi P, Moldovan E, Tomescu N. Latent cytomegalovirus infection in blood donors. Br Med J 1969;Dec:660–662.

44. Przepiorka D, LeParc GF, Werch J, Lichtiger B. Prevention of transfusion-associated cytomegalovirus infection—practice parameter. Am J Clin Pathol 1996;106:163–169.

45. Popovsky MA, Chaplin HC, Moore SB. Transfusion-related acute lung injury: a neglected, serious complication of hemotherapy. Transfusion 1992;32:589.

BLOOD GROUPS

RED BLOOD CELL BLOOD GROUPS

New red cell antigen specificities were reported almost monthly during the 1970s and 1980s. Unfortunately, the terminology for these antigens has not been consistent, and this has contributed to the difficulty for nonexperts to understand the blood group systems. Efforts to develop a more consistent and uniform nomenclature system are under way. A working party of the International Society of Blood Transfusion has accepted a total of 255 antigens and classified them as systems, collections, low-frequency antigens, and high-frequency antigens.[1] Of these 255 antigens, 195 are categorized in 23 major discrete systems (Table 9.1). Eleven antigens have sufficiently similar serologic, biochemical, or genetic characteristics that they have been grouped and called "collections." In addition, there are 37 low-incidence and 12 high-incidence antigens thought to be independent of all others. This chapter describes the red cell antigens and systems and the platelet and neutrophil antigens and antibodies that are most commonly involved in the clinical practice of transfusion medicine. For a more comprehensive description of the hundreds of known red cell antigens, the reader is referred to reference texts.[2,3]

The structure of the red cell membrane and the composition of its major components have been studied extensively. Newer techniques for the study of membranes and the ability to identify the genes responsible for individual molecules of the membrane have enabled a virtual explosion in knowledge about the composition of blood group antigens and the genes that control them. The biochemical composition, molecular weight, and number of antigens per red cell have been established for many antigens (Table 9.2). The nature of the molecules and the genes responsible have been identified for all of the 23 blood group systems except Dombrock.

Table 9.1 Major red cell antigen systems containing 195 antigen specificities

Carbohydrate-defined antigens	Protein-defined antigens
ABO	Rh
Lewis	Duffy
P	MNSs
Hh	Kell
	Kidd
	Lutheran
	Gerbich
	Xg
	LW
	Indian
	Knops
	Diego
	Colton
	Kx
	Cartwright
	Cromer
	Dombrock
	Scianna
	Chido/Rogers

Source: Data from Daniels GL, Anstee DJ, Cartron JP, et al. Blood group terminology 1995: from the ISBT Working Party on Terminology for Red Cell Surface Antigens. Vox Sang 1995;69:265–79; Daniels G. Human Blood Groups. Cambridge, MA: Blackwell Science Ltd, 1995; and Reid ME. Molecular basis for blood groups and function of carrier proteins. In: Silbertsein LE, ed. Molecular and Functional Aspects of Blood Group Antigens. Bethesda, MD: American Association of Blood Banks, 1995:75–126.

There are two basic kinds of blood group antigens. One group of antigens is determined by carbohydrates attached to either proteins or lipids. The specificity of these blood group antigens is determined by sugars, and thus the genes responsible for these antigens code for an intermediate molecule, usually an enzyme that creates the antigenic specificity by transferring sugar molecules onto the protein or lipid. Thus, certain proteins exposed on the outer surface of the red cell will express the carbohydrate-determined antigens (Fig. 9.1). The carbohydrate-defined antigens are ABO, Lewis, Hh, P, and the Ii antigens, although the latter are not a true blood group system. The second type of antigen is determined by amino acid sequences of proteins that are directly determined by genes (Table 9.2). It is believed that proteins carrying blood group antigens are inserted into the red cell membrane in one of three ways: single pass, multiple pass, and linked to phosphatidylinositol (Fig. 9.2). The size of the molecule containing the blood group antigens ranges from 25 to 100 kD, and the number of antigen sites from just 1,500 to more than 1,000,000 per red cell (Table 9.2). The following discussion provides a brief synopsis of the major blood group systems.

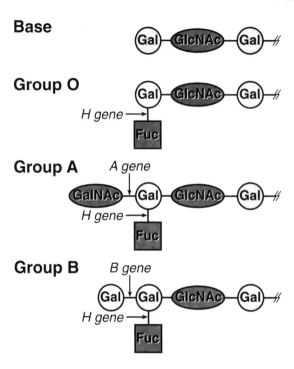

Figure 9.1 Schematic diagram of the site of action of ABH genes. Gal = galactose; Fuc = fucose; GalNAc = N-Acetyl galactosamine

ABO SYSTEM

The ABO system was the first red cell blood group system to be identified, and its discovery led to the Nobel prize for Landsteiner (see Chapter 1).[4] Landsteiner observed the agglutination reactions by mixing various combinations of cells and sera from himself, four doctoral students working in his laboratory, and another subject.[4] This simple set of experiments was the beginning of red cell serology and blood groups. Landsteiner had identified the clinically most important red cell antigen system, because most individuals have circulating A and B antibodies that are usually complement-fixing antibodies and cause intravascular hemolysis. The frequency distribution of the ABO antigens and genes is shown in Table 9.3. The antigenic determinants for A, B, and H are found widely throughout our environment on bacteria, plants, food, dust, etc. Exposure to these antigens causes the normal development of antibodies against whichever ABH antigens are absent in the individual (Table 9.4).

Composition

The ABH antigen activity is determined by sugars that are linked either to polypeptides (forming a glycoprotein) or to lipids (forming a glycolipid). Because the antigenic

Table 9.2 Molecular and biochemical characteristics of some blood group antigens

Blood group antigen	Chromosome of gene location	No. of antigen sites × 10³ red cell	Molecular weight of antigen (kD)	RBC membrane components associated with antigen expression	Antigen composition	cDNA cloned
AB	9	1,000	90–100	Anion transport protein (band 3)	Glycoprotein	Yes
H	19				Glycoprotein	Yes
Ii	Unknown	120	55	Glucose transport protein (band 4.5) Poly-N-acetyl lactosaminyl glycolips	Glycoprotein Glycolipid	Yes —
Lewis	19	Not applicable	Not applicable	Not applicable	Glycosphingolipid	No
P1	22	Unknown	Unknown	Paragloboside plus a terminal D-galactose	Glycosphingolipid	No
P	Unknown	Unknown	Unknown	Globoside I	Glycosphingolipid	No
Pk	Unknown	Unknown	Unknown	Ceramide trihexoside	Glycosphingolipid	Yes
Rh(D)	1	100–200 100–200	30–32 45–100	Polypeptides Polypeptides	Lipoprotein Lipoprotein	Yes —
LW	19	3–5	40	N-Glycans	Glycoprotein	Yes
MN	4	200–1,000	43†	Glycophorin A	Sialoglycoprotein	Yes
Ss	4	50–250	25†	Glycophorin B	Sialoglycoprotein	Yes
Kell	7	3–6	93†	Disulfide bonding required for antigen activity	Glycoprotein	Yes
Kx	X	Unknown	32	Unknown	Unknown	No
Duffy	1	12	40–66	N-Glycans not required for antigen activity	Glycoprotein	Yes
Lutheran	19	1–4	78–85	N-Glycans and disulfide bonding required for antigen activity	Glycoprotein	No

Gerbich	2	60–120 15–20	39* 30*	Glycophorin C Glycophorin D	Sialoglycoprotein Sialoglycoprotein	Yes Yes
Kidd	18	11	50	Unknown	Unknown	No
Xg	X	Unknown	22–29	Unknown	Sialoglycoprotein	No
Colton	7	120–160	40–60	CHIP 28	Glycoprotein	Yes
Complement Rogers (C4A) Chido (C4B)	6 6	Unknown Unknown	96 94	None None	Glycoprotein Glycoprotein	Yes Yes
Diego	17	15	Unknown	Band 3	Glycoprotein	Yes
Yt	7	Unknown	72–160	Acetylcholinesterase	Glycoprotein	Yes
Cromer	1	Unknown	70	Decay accelerating factor	Sialoglycoprotein	Yes
Dombrock	Unknown	Unknown	46–57	Unknown	Glycoprotein	No
Scianna	1	Unknown	60–68	Unknown	Glycoprotein	No
Knops	1	Unknown	200	DR1	Glycoprotein	Yes
Indian	11	6–10	80	CD44	Glycoprotein	Yes

Source: Adapted from McCullough J. Transfusion medicine. In: Handin RI, Lux SE, Stossel TP, eds. Blood: Principles and practice of hematology. Philadelphia: J.B. Lippincott Company, 1995:1958; Daniels GL, Anstee DJ, Cartron JP, et al. Blood group terminology 1995: from the ISBT Working Party on Terminology for Red Cell Surface Antigens. Vox Sang 1995;69:265–79; Daniels G. Human Blood Groups. Cambridge, MA: Blackwell Science Inc, 1995; and Reid ME. Molecular basis for blood groups and function of carrier proteins. In: Silbertsein LE, ed. Molecular and Functional Aspects of Blood Group Antigens. Bethesda, MD: American Association of Blood Banks, 1995:75–126.

*These molecules give anomalous apparent molecular weight on SDS PAGE. Fy antigen activity is observed over a broad range of molecular weights (38–90 kD); the value given corresponds to the region of greatest activity.

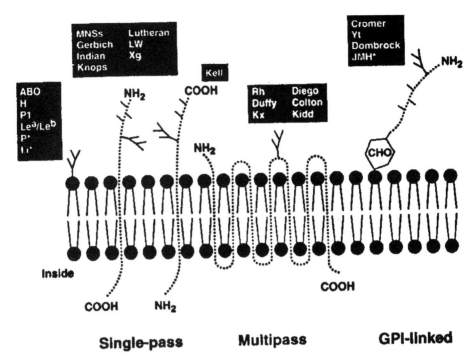

Figure 9.2 Models for insertion of RBC membrane proteins. The blood group systems that are associated with different RBC membrane components are shown in the boxes. An asterisk represents a blood group collection or unassigned high-prevalence antigen. CHO represents carbohydrate moieties. The multipass membrane proteins carrying Rh, Kidd, Diego, Colton, and Kx antigens are oriented with their amino (NH_2) and carboxyl (COOH) termini to the inside of the membrane. The number of membrane passes differs for each protein, as does the glycosylation. *(Reproduced with permission from Reid ME. Molecular basis for blood groups and function of carrier proteins. In: Silbertsein LE, ed. Molecular and Functional Aspects of Blood Group Antigens. Bethesda, MD: American Association of Blood Banks, 1995:75–126.)*

activity is determined by sugars and resides in a carbohydrate structure, the antigens are not directly determined by genes. Instead, the ABH genes determine proteins that are sugar-transferring enzymes collectively called glycosyltransferases. Genes for three different blood group systems (ABO, Hh, and Sese) control the expression of ABO antigens. Each A, B, and H gene codes for a different enzyme (glycosyl transferase), which places a different sugar on the polypeptide or lipid to produce the unique antigen (Table 9.3, Fig. 9.1). The genes for the ABO system are on chromosome 9.[5,6] The O gene is similar to the A gene except for one base deletion that causes a frame shift and premature stop in transcription.[7] The result is lack of production of a functional protein (enzyme), and so there is no product of the O gene. The B gene differs from the A gene in several different ways.[3] Some of the differences have more impact on the resulting

Table 9.3 A_1A_2BO phenotype, gene and genotype frequencies in south England in 1939

Phenotype		Gene		Genotype	
	Frequency		Calculated frequency		Calculated frequency
O	0.43	*O*	0.6602	*O/O*	0.43
A_1	0.35	A^1	0.2090	A^1/A^1	0.04
				A^1/O	0.28
				A^1/A^2	0.03
A_2	0.10	A^2	0.0696	A^2/A^2	0.00
				A^2/O	0.09
B	0.09	*B*	0.0612	*B/B*	0.00
				B/O	0.08
A_1B	0.03			A^1/B	0.03
A_2B	0.01			A^2/B	0.01
	1.00		1.0000		1.00

Source: Adapted from Technical Manual, 12th ed. Bethesda, MD: American Association of Blood Banks, 1996:31.

Table 9.4 Genes and antigens of the ABH system and ABO type of donor red cells suitable for patients of different ABO types

Gene	Glycosyl transferase	Antigen-determining sugar	ABH antigen	ABO type	Antibody present	Preferable donor	Other acceptable donors*
A	*N*-Acetyl galactosamine transferase	*N*-Acetyl galactosamine	A	A	B	A	O
B	D-Galactosyl transferase	D-Galactose	B	B	A	B	O
H	L-Fucosyl transferase	L-Fucose	H	O	A & B	O	None
A & B	All above	All above	A & B	AB	None	AB	A or B or O†

*If blood is used as red blood cells.
†Group A is preferable.

protein,[8] but in general the differences result in the two different enzymes and the different sugar attachments, giving different antigen specificities. Genes for the Hh system are on chromosome 19. The H gene enables the attachment of L-fucose to the polypeptide or lipid chain. If no A or B gene is present, the H specificity remains and the individual is a type O, since the O gene is nonfunctional. These group O red cells do not react with anti-A or anti-B. If an A or B gene or both are present, additional sugars are attached to the L-fucose, giving A, B, or AB specificity. Thus, ABO specificity depends on both the ABO and the Hh genes (Fig. 9.1).

Antigen Distribution and Subgroups

ABH antigens are widely distributed throughout the body. The ABH antigens present on red cells may be in either the glycoprotein or the glycolipid form. ABH glycolipids are also part of most endothelial and epithelial membranes. In addition, the ABH glycolipids are present in a soluble form in plasma. Most other body fluids and secretions contain soluble ABH antigens, but those are in the glycoprotein form. The ability to secrete soluble ABH antigens is controlled by a secretor (Se) gene, which is separate from the ABH system.

In a normal adult, the number of A antigen sites ranges from 1,600,000 (A1 individual) to 800,000 (A2 individual), to 700 (Am individual). The number of B antigen sites is 600,000 to 800,000, and the number of A, B antigen sites about 800,000.[2,3] Normal newborns have approximately one-third the adult numbers of antigen sites. Before the structure and number of A and B antigens was known, it was observed that red cells from some group A individuals react weakly or not at all with anti-A sera. These were called A subgroups and were named intermediate (A int), A3, Ax, Am, Ay, Ael, and Aend. It was thought that different forms of the A antigen might exist and that sera contained mixtures of antibodies to these different A subgroup antigens. Now it appears that these differences in reactivity are caused by variability in the ABO genes, resulting in variations in the A antigens or the number of antigen sites.[3, p. 36] For instance, the A2 gene differs from the A1 gene by one base pair, resulting in a different protein product.[3, p. 28] Some individuals with these weak A subgroups form anti-A antibodies, probably indicating a quantitative difference in their A antigens. However, A2 red cells will absorb anti-A1, suggesting that the differences may be more quantitative. Thus it appears that A subgroups may result from either qualitative or quantitative differences.

The A subgroups are not of major clinical importance but may cause difficulties in the serology laboratory. Approximately 1% to 8% of an A individual's and 20% to 35% of an AB subgroup individual's sera may contain A antibodies. However, these usually do not react at 37°C and are not considered clinically significant. In rare situations where the anti-A reacts at 37°C, donors whose red cells are A2 can be easily identified, and red cells from a compatible donor can be provided. Subgroups of B exist but are rare.[3, p. 43] These individuals may also have anti-B in their serum. Since donors with B subgroup red cells are also rare, group O red cells can be used for transfusion.

Bombay Type

The very rare Bombay phenotype, first recognized in India, lacks the H gene and is homozygous for its allele h (they are hh). The notation Oh is used for the Bombay type. The lack of an H gene does not allow the attachment of L-fucose to the protein or lipid, and thus the individuals express very little H antigen (Fig. 9.1). They type as group O since their red cells do not react with anti-A or anti-B and their serum contains anti-A and anti-B . However, their serum also contains anti-H, which reacts with group O red cells and can cause hemolysis in vivo. It is fortunate that such individuals are rare, because finding compatible red cells is extremely difficult. The only suitable red cells are those from another Bombay individual.

Antibodies of the ABH System

These antibodies begin to appear during the first few months of life, probably from exposure to ABH antigen-like substances in the environment. Because of this, these antibodies are called "naturally occurring," but the implication that they form without antigenic stimulation is incorrect. Anti-A or anti-B antibodies are usually combinations of IgM and IgG. Because of the IgM content, these sera almost always cause agglutination—even at room temperature—of red cells containing the corresponding antigen. The IgM composition makes these antibodies effective in fixing complement, and so they can be very dangerous clinically.

Immunization to A or B antigens can also occur by transfusion of incompatible red cells, inoculation with vaccines containing A or B antigens, transfusion of plasma containing soluble A or B antigens, or pregnancy with an ABO-incompatible fetus. Following these kinds of immunization, the A or B antibody may become more active at 37°C, have a higher IgG component, increase in titer and/or avidity, and become more strongly hemolytic and thus even more clinically dangerous.

Anti-H antibodies can occur in persons with little or no H antigen on their red cells. Thus, Bombay type individuals (who lack the H gene and do not make H antigens) have a very active anti-H, which binds complement and causes hemolysis. A few persons of type A or AB make anti-H, probably because almost all their H antigen has been converted to A or B. These anti-H antibodies usually do not react at body temperatures and do not cause hemolysis.

THE RH SYSTEM

The second most important red cell antigen system is the Rh system. This is because a substantial proportion of the population lacks the major Rh antigen known as D; the likelihood of becoming immunized to the D antigen is very high and anti-D has serious clinical effects, causing hemolytic disease of the newborn and/or transfusion reactions. In addition to the clinical importance of the Rh system, there has been a lively scholarly debate over the years about the genetics of this system.

Discovery

In 1939, Levine and Stetson[9] reported the case of a woman who delivered a fetus affected by hemolytic disease of the newborn and upon receiving a transfusion of her husband's blood experienced a severe transfusion reaction. They hypothesized correctly that the woman had become immunized to a factor that her child had inherited from the husband (father) but that she lacked. In 1940, Landsteiner and Wiener[10] obtained an antibody from guinea pigs and rabbits immunized with rhesus monkey red cells. This serum had a pattern of reactivity similar to that of Levine and Stetson's patient, and so the blood group system was named Rh for rhesus monkey. Later work established that the animal anti-rhesus sera and the human antibody did not detect the same antigen, but by that time the nomenclature was established. The pattern of reactivity and the antigen identified by the animal sera has been named LW in honor of Landsteiner and Wiener. LW is assigned to a different red cell antigen system.

Nomenclature and Genetics

The Rh system contains at least 44 different antigens and many other antigenic specificities that may represent weak versions of these antigens or other antigens not yet established as part of the Rh system. The antigen detected in the original Levine and Stetson patient's serum is the D antigen. This is present in about 85% of North American Caucasians and is the basis for determining Rh positivity or negativity. That is, persons whose red cells contain the D antigen are Rh positive and those whose red cells lack the D antigen are Rh negative.

Four other antigens (C, c, E, and e) were identified that seemed to be inherited in various combinations along with D and became part of the Rh system (Table 9.5). These four antigens, along with D, account for almost all of the Rh-related transfusion problems encountered in practice. Different nomenclature systems have been used to describe the Rh system (Table 9.5). The Wiener system supposed that the gene product was a single entity with multiple serologic specificities.[11] The Fisher-Race system postulated three closely linked loci, each with its own gene and gene product.[12] The terms that each of these nomenclature systems applied to the different patterns of serologic reactivity are shown in Table 9.5. Rosenfield et al.[13] proposed a third nomenclature in which each Rh antigen was assigned a number, and the serologic reactions were used.

Structure and Composition of the D Antigen

A major step forward in understanding the Rh system was the isolation of Rh antigen containing components of the red cell membrane.[14-16] This led to the identification of several nonglycosylated fatty acid acylated polypeptides. The D antigen is a 30-kD protein that is associated with the red cell membrane skeleton. The protein has an external and intramembranous domain but no cytoplasmic domain. The protein probably traverses the membrane several times (Fig. 9.2). There is considerable similarity among the Rh proteins. The C and c antigens differ in only four amino acids, and E and e in only one amino acid. In contrast, the membrane protein in D-positive individuals possess

Table 9.5 Serologic reactions and the Weiner and Fisher-Race nomenclature for the Rh system

Reaction with anti-					Weiner			Fisher-Race[12]		
D	C	E	c	e	Most likely genotype	Phenotype	Antigens	Most likely genotype	Phenotype	Antigens
+	+	O	+	+	R^1r	R_1r	Rh_0 rh' hr' hr"	CDe/cde	CcDee	CDce
+	+	O	O	+	R^1R^1	R_1R_1	Rh_0 rh' hr"	CDe/Cde	CCDee	CDe
+	O	+	+	+	R^2r	R_2r	Rh_0 rh" rh' hr"	cDE/cde	ccDEe	cDEe
+	O	+	+	O	R^2R^2	R_2R_2	Rh_0 rh" hr'	cDE/cDE	ccDEE	cDE
+	+	+	+	+	R^1R^2	R_1R_2	Rh_0 rh' rh" hr' hr"	CDe/cDE	CcDEe	CcDEe
+	O	O	+	+	R^0r	R_0r	Rh_0 hr hr	cDe/cde	ccDee	cDe
O	O	O	+	+	rr	rr	hr' hr"	cde/cde	ccee	ce
O	+	O	+	+	$r'r$	r'r	rh' hr' hr"	Cde/cde	Ccee	Cce
O	O	+	+	+	$r''r$	r"r	rh" hr' hr"	cdE/cde	ccEE	cEe
O	+	+	+	+	$r'r''$	r'r"	rh' rh" hr' hr"	Cde/cdE	CcEe	CcEe

Source: Adapted from McCullough J. Transfusion medicine. In: Handin RI, Lux SE, Stossel TP, eds. Blood: Principles and practice of hematology. Philadelphia: J.B. Lippincott Company, 1995:1961.

36 amino acids lacking in D-negative individuals. The total amount of D protein per red cell is about 60,000 daltons, indicating that the antigen is probably a dimer or trimer of D proteins,[17] because there are approximately 30,000 D antigen sites per cell.[18] These antigens cannot move laterally within the membrane but instead are fixed about 70 nm apart.[19,20] This distance between the D antigen sites probably accounts in part for the lack of complement fixation in D antigen-antibody reactions.

Surprisingly, the D protein has been isolated from Rh(D)-negative red cells.[18] Comparison of the protein isolated from Rh-negative cells with the Rh protein isolated from Rh-positive cells reveals slight differences, probably due to genetic polymorphism.[16,21] It is postulated that the protein molecule isolated from the Rh-negative cells is a mixture of Rh (c) and (e) proteins. The Rh (c) and (E) proteins have recently been isolated,[22] and it appears that D, C, and E have regions of identity and regions of diversity.[23] Thus, it appears that C, D, and E are three distinct proteins.[21] From the amino acid sequences of the Rh polypeptides, genomic studies were carried out.[24,25] This work has identified two genes in the Rh system: RHD and RHCE. There may be one or two copies of the RHD gene. Rh-negative individuals lack the RHD gene and thus that polypeptide. This explains why the d antigen was never found. The RHCE gene codes both the Cc and Ee polypeptides. There are four alleles at this locus: RHCE, RHCe, RHcE, and RHce. The full-length transcript of each gene encodes a polypeptide of 416 amino acids.[26] Thus, it appears that there are two Rh genes, not either one or three. Based on present understanding of the biochemical composition of the Rh antigens and their genetic control, the longstanding debate between Wiener and Race probably ends in a draw[21]—a fitting conclusion.

Weak D, D Variant, Du, and Partial D

Many red cell antigens show different degrees of reactivity, but this is more of a problem with the D antigen because all donors and patients are typed for D and it is important to choose D-negative red cells for D-negative patients. Some individuals who inherit the D antigen have red cells that react weakly or not at all with certain anti-D reagents. Thus, these individuals may appear to be Rh negative. This situation has been called D variant or Du, but the contemporary term is weak D. The term Du will be used here for historical consistency to describe certain situations. The Du phenomenon can be caused by three different mechanisms. First, when a C gene is on the chromosome opposite from the D gene (*trans* position), the D antigen may be weakened. An example of this is *CDe/Cde*. This has been called weak D due to gene interaction. Secondly, a D variant or Du can also occur because of a qualitative difference in the D antigen. Rare individuals lack a portion of the D antigen molecule, and when exposed to the D antigen produce an antibody to that portion of the D antigen they lack. This has been called Du due to D mosaic, but the contemporary term is partial D. Third, the D gene in some individuals codes for an antigen that reacts more weakly. These three forms of Du occur in about 1% of all Rh-positive individuals. The gene interaction and weak D are more common than the D mosaic as causes of Du.

These observations are of intellectual interest but also have clinical impact. Persons who are weak D have the D antigen, although some may lack a part of it. Thus, the rare

recipient who is weak D because of a partial absence of D and receives D-positive red cells could make anti-D. Recipients who are weak D because of gene interaction have all the D antigen and can receive D-positive blood. However, it is not necessary to determine whether recipients who appear to be Rh negative are in fact weak D, because they will receive Rh-negative red cells since they type as Rh (D) negative. Weak D donors are of greater concern. They may type as Rh negative but contain some D antigen that could immunize an Rh-negative recipient. Thus, donor red cells must be tested for Rh (D) using methods that will detect the weak D antigens (see Chapter 7).

Rh Null Type

Rare individuals lack all the Rh antigens. This may be due to the absence of a gene that regulates the expression of Rh antigens or to the presence of an amorphic gene at the Rh locus on chromosome 1. Rh-null individuals have abnormal red cell morphology and hemolytic anemia that is usually sufficiently compensated to result in only mild anemia. If exposed to Rh-positive red cells, these persons make an antibody that reacts with all red cells other than Rh null and is considered to be reactive against the entire Rh molecule.

Rh Antibodies

The most common Rh antibody is anti-D. This is almost always an IgG, does not cause agglutination of red cells in vitro, acts at 37°C, and does not bind complement effectively, but causes hemolytic disease of the newborn or serious transfusion reactions and red cell destruction by accelerated clearance of cells through the mononuclear phagocyte system (Table 9.6).

OTHER RED CELL BLOOD GROUPS

Kell System

The Kell blood group system currently includes 24 alloantigens, which can be grouped into three sets of antithetical antigens, two unpaired high-frequency antigens, and 12 related high-frequency antigens. The primary antigens of this system are Kell (K) and its antithetical antigen Cellano (k). Other antigens of the Kell system are Kp (a, b, and c), and Js (a and b). The antithetical sets are Kk, Kp(a)(b), and Js(a)(b). There is a numerical system for Kell terminology as well. The K gene is an autosomal dominant whose frequency differs considerably in different populations. The Kell system is important clinically because the K antigen is next in immunogenicity after D and because antibodies to Kell system antigens (or anti-K) are usually IgG, react at 37°C, and do not bind complement, but can cause severe hemolytic transfusion reactions and hemolytic disease of the newborn (Table 9.6). It is not customary to type donors or recipients for Kell unless the recipient has a Kell antibody. The Kell gene is located on chromosome 7, has 2,500 base pairs, and encodes for a 732-amino acid protein.[27]

Table 9.6 General laboratory reactions of blood group antibodies

| RBC antigen | Protein | Antibodies | | Binds complement | HDN |
		Optimum temperature	Reaction medium		
ABO	IgM	20°C	Saline	Yes	Yes
Lewis	IgM	20°–37°C	Variable	Yes	No
I	IgM	4°C	Saline	Some	No
P	IgM	4°–20°C	Saline	Only anti-TJA	No
MN	IgM	4°–20°C	Saline	Some anti-Ss	
Lutheran	IgM & IgA	Variable	Saline	Some or AHG	Occas
Rh	IgG	37°C	AHG	No	Yes
Kell	IgG	37°C	AHG	No	Yes
Duffy	IgG	37°C	AHG	No	Rare
Kidd	IgG	37°C	AHG	All	Yes

The Kell molecule is a 93-kD glycoprotein,[27,28] which apparently is associated with a small (20 to 30 kD), poorly characterized second protein.[28] Most, if not all, of the Kell antigens are located on this single 93-kD molecule.[29,30] The antigenicity of Kell antigens is inactivated when the glycoprotein is isolated using reducing conditions that break the disulfide bonds. Thus, the antigen reactivity probably depends on maintenance of the tertiary structure of the surface of the molecule. The Kell molecule glycoprotein molecule is the same size as band 3 of the red cell membrane skeleton; however, these are different molecules.

Another reason that the Kell blood group is interesting is its relationship with chronic granulomatous disease (CGD). In CGD there is a congenital absence of a superoxide-producing cytochrome that interferes with the normal oxidative response of neutrophils so that their bactericidal activity is diminished and patients suffer severe, life-threatening infections. The genetic defect associated with CGD is on the X chromosome near a Kell-related locus, Kx. Trace amounts of Kx antigen are on Kell-positive cells, but cells lacking both K and K (Ko) have elevated levels of Kx. Rare individuals who also lack Kx are said to have the McLeod phenotype. In the McLeod phenotype, the red cells express Kell system antigens weakly and have bizarre shapes, and patients have a chronic compensated hemolytic anemia. The occurrence of the McLeod phenotype in some patients with chronic granulomatous disease led to the discovery that the McLeod syndrome involves a spectrum of abnormalities in addition to those involving the Kell system. Other associated abnormalities occur in red cells (acanthocytosis, compensated hemolysis, increased red cell phosphorylation) the nervous system (areflexia, choreiform movements, mild dysarthria, neurogenic

myopathy, and muscle wasting), the cardiovascular system (cardiomyopathy), and granulocytes (chronic granulomatous disease); other changes such as reduced hapto-globin, elevated creatinine phosphokinase, lactic dehydrogenase, and carbonic anhy-drase may be found.

Duffy System

Duffy was the first blood group locus to be identified on an autosome—chromosome 1. The locus is near the centromere, but it is not clear whether it is on the long or the short arm. The Duffy system is composed of five or possibly six antigens that are not present on other blood cells or body tissues. These are Fy^a, Fy^b, Fy^3, Fy^4, Fy^5, and possibly Fy^6. The composition of the Duffy antigens is not completely understood. It appears that the molecule containing Fy^a and Fy^b is a glycoprotein with a molecular weight between 40,000 and 66,000 daltons.[31] There are approximately 13,000 Fy^a or Fy^b antigen sites on each red cell in persons homozygous for the *Fya* or *Fyb* gene.[32] Red cells from indi-viduals heterozygous for Fy^a or Fy^b contain about 6,000 antigen sites per red cell. These red cells often show a weaker agglutination than homozygous cells in serologic tests—a phenomenon called dosage effect. This can have a practical clinical effect. A patient with a weak anti-Fy^a might have a compatible crossmatch when serum is tested against Fy(a+b+) donor red cells. If an effective antibody screening procedure (see Chapter 7) was not carried out, the patient could receive Fya+ red cells that appeared to be com-patible.

The Duffy system is unusual because the antigen frequency varies substantially in different racial groups. In general, the *Fya* gene has a high incidence in Asians and moderate incidence in Caucasians; *Fya* and *Fyb* have low incidence in Africans. Both antigens are detectable during fetal development and present in normal strength at birth.

Fy^a antibodies may cause severe, even fatal, hemolytic transfusion reactions or severe hemolytic disease of the newborn (HDN); however, transfusion reactions to Fy^a are not frequent and the HDN is usually mild (Table 9.6). Anti-Fy^b is an infrequent cause of transfusion reactions and HDN. Other Duffy system antibodies have not been implicated in clinical problems

One of the most interesting features of the Duffy system is its association with malaria. Fya(a−b−) red cells are resistant to infection by *Plasmodium knowlesi*[33] and probably *Plasmodium vivax*. The malaria parasites are unable to penetrate red cells lacking the Fy^a or Fy^b antigens because they do not establish a junction site.[34] In West Africa most blacks are Fy(a−b−) and are resistant to *P. vivax* malaria; thus, a natural selection process might have been in effect.

Kidd System

The three antigens of the Kidd system (Jk^a, Jk^b, and Jk^3) were discovered during the 1950s; no new antigens in this system have been reported since then. There is a rare null phenotype, Jk(a−b−), and Jk^3 is a high-incidence antigen. Several possible chromo-some locations for the Kidd locus have been reported, but it appears that the most likely of these is chromosome 18.[35] The exact molecule coded by this gene is not yet estab-lished. It may be a 391-amino acid protein with several membrane-spanning domains.[36]

Red cells from individuals homozygous for Jk^a contain about 11,000 antigen sites;[32] Kidd antigens are not present on other blood cells or tissues but are well developed at birth. Kidd antigens may be altered by products of bacteria in infected patients. For instance, *Proteus mirabilis* and *Streptococcus faecalis* can cause Jk(b+) cells to become reactive with anti-Jk^b, and autohemolysis can occur.

Kidd antibodies are usually IgG but can also be a mixture of IgG and IgM. They often bind complement and can cause severe hemolytic transfusion reactions but usually cause only mild HDN (Table 9.6). In vitro Kidd antibodies may react weakly and yet cause severe hemolysis despite being IgG. The relatively low number of Kidd antigen sites (11,000) should mean that the distance between antigen sites is too great for complement activation by an IgG molecule; however, the antigens probably are clustered, thus accounting for weak serologic reactivity, complement activation by IgG, and severe clinical effects.

A unique characteristic of Kidd antibodies is that they often disappear. Thus, they may cause delayed hemolytic transfusion reactions. This occurs when the patient has been immunized previously by pregnancy or transfusion but no longer has circulating antibody, so all the pretransfusion tests are compatible; yet if the patient receives Kidd-positive red cells, the antibody may be resynthesized rapidly, causing hemolysis of the transfused red cells a few hours to days later. An additional feature of Kidd antibodies is their tendency to show "dosage." That is, anti-Jk^a reacts more strongly with red cells homozygous for Jk^a than heterozygous Jk(a+b+) cells. Thus, the antibody can be missed in laboratory tests if proper antibody detection cells are not used (see Chapter 8).

Lutheran System

The Lutheran system has three pairs of antithetical antigens and a seventh antigen that appears to be one involving one of the pairs of antigens. These are Lu^a and Lu^b, Lu^6 and Lu^9, Lu^8 and Lu^{14}, and Lu^{18} and Lu^{19}, also known as Au(a) and (b). In addition, six other antigens have Lutheran system nomenclature because they are phenotypically related to the Lutheran system. However, these "paralutheran" antigens are not genetically related to the Lutheran system. The Lutheran system was known to be linked to the third component of complement and the location of the C3 gene to chromosome 19 led to the localization of the Lutheran gene to that same chromosome.[37] Lutheran antigens are part of a glycoprotein molecule of 78 kD to 85 kD that traverses the red cell membrane. The number of antigen sites has been reported to be 1,000 to 4,000 per cell depending on the zygosity.

The antigens are not well developed at birth, and so antigens and antibodies of the Lutheran system cause only mild hemolytic disease of the newborn. Lutheran antibodies may be IgG or IgM or mixtures of these with IgA (Table 9.6). The most common Lutheran antibodies are anti-Lu^a and anti-Lu^b. Anti-Lu^a is usually not active at body temperatures and thus is not a problem clinically. These antibodies have not been implicated in immediate hemolytic transfusion reactions or in hemolytic disease of the newborn requiring exchange transfusion. Anti-Lu^a is rarely found because the incidence of Lu(a+) red cells is low; thus, patients are rarely exposed to the antigen. Laboratory test

cells often are not Lu(a+), so the antibody is not detected. Fortunately, even if the antibody is missed in the antibody detection test, patients with the antibody would rarely receive a transfusion of Lu(a+) red cells. Anti-Lu^b may cause accelerated destruction of incompatible red cells. However, this antibody is also rarely found because almost all individuals are Lu(b+).

MN System

Long before Rh was known, the M and N antigens were discovered by immunizing rabbits with human red cells. The system has five major antigens: M and N, which are antithetical; S and s, which are antithetical; and U, which is present in all individuals who possess M or N and S or s antigens and in some S− s− individuals. The MN U-negative people are usually blacks. In addition to these five antigens, this system has many variants and includes as many as 37 different antigens.

The composition of antigens of this system is well understood. The antigens of the MNSs system are located on the red cell membrane sialoglycoproteins.[38] The M and N antigens are on the terminal portion of the sialic acid-rich glycoprotein called glycophorin A, of which there are from 200,000 to 1,000,000 copies per red cell. Glycophorin A has a molecular weight of 43,000 and is composed of 131 amino acids. The MN activity is located in approximately 70 external amino acids, the remaining amino acids being intramembranous or intracytoplasmic. The Ss and probably the U antigens are located on the terminal portion of glycophorin B, of which there are 50,000 to 250,000 copies per red cell. The amino acid sequences of these sialic acid-rich glycoproteins and the location of the antigen activity have been described.[2,3] There are two different genes: one each that encodes for glycophorin A and glycophorin B. The genes are located close to each other on chromosome 4.

Antibodies to the MN antigens are usually not clinically active. Although anti-M is often IgG, most MN antibodies have a large IgM component, are usually not active at body temperatures, and only rarely cause hemolysis, transfusion reactions, or hemolytic disease of the newborn (Table 9.6). Unusual examples may be active at 37°C and clinically significant. Anti-N is almost always IgM, not reactive at body temperature, and not clinically significant. Anti-S, anti-s, and anti-U are usually IgG warm active antibodies that may have clinical effects by causing transfusion reactions, hemolysis, or HDN. Anti-S occurs infrequently, anti-s is rare, and anti-U is extremely rare.

P System

Like the MN system, P-system antigens were discovered before the Rh system by injecting animals with human red cells. The three antigens of the P system define five different P-system phenotypes. The antigens are P1, P, and Pk. All but 1 in 100,000 persons have the P antigen. The two most common phenotypes are P1 (P1P) and P2 (PP); each of these phenotypes has trace amounts of Pk. The amount of P1 antigen varies greatly among individuals, is not well developed at birth, and does not reach adult levels until the individual is about 7 years of age. P-negative (pp) individuals lack P1, P, and Pk and are very rare.

The P-system antigenic determinants are carbohydrates that are linked to gly-cosphingolipids in the red cell membrane. P-system antigens, like the I antigens, seem to be formed in a sequence of steps instead of being antithetical and controlled by allelic genes. They seem to originate from a common precursor, and Pk is the precursor of P, but neither Pk nor P is the precursor of P1.[2,3] The biochemistry of P-system antigens is better understood than the genetics. Genetic control of the P-system has been proposed to involve two or three loci. These genes code for enzymes that add the carbohydrates to the lipids in a manner similar to the ABO-system genes.

Antigen structures similar to those of the P-system are found in animal tissue, pigeons, doves, worms, and *Echinococcus* cyst fluid. Thus, many antibodies of the P-system are called "naturally occurring," although as with ABO antibodies this is not technically correct. Because some parasites have antigen structures similar to P-system antigens, anti-P1 is sometimes found in patients with parasitic infections.

Antibodies of the P-system are rather common and can range from cold active and clinically insignificant to those that cause severe hemolysis (Table 9.6). Anti-P1 is common, usually cold active, and not clinically significant unless it reacts at body temperatures. Anti-P1+P+Pk made by people with the rare pp phenotype and anti-P made by people with the rare pk phenotype will cause hemolysis in vitro and in vivo. There is a high incidence of miscarriage in women with the pp phenotype, and it has been suggested that anti-P+P1+Pk may have a pathologic role. Auto anti-P is the specificity of the Donath-Landsteiner antibody found in paroxysmal cold hemoglobinuria. The antibody is often called biphasic because it binds to the red cell at cool temperatures, then causes hemolysis at warmer (body) temperature.

Lewis System

The gene for the Lewis system is linked to the third component of complement and is located on chromosome 19. The Lewis system is not a blood group system. Lewis antigens are soluble in body fluids, and the antigens present in plasma are adsorbed onto red cells. The site of synthesis of Lewis antigens is not known. The Lewis system also differs from most other blood group systems in that the Lewis genes must interact with *Hh* and secretor genes in order for Lewis antigens to be produced. There are two antigens in the Lewis system: Le^a and Le^b. The Lewis antigenic specificity is determined by the carbohydrate fucose. The *Le* gene produces a glycosyltransferase that adds the fucose to a precursor substance (type 1 chain) to produce the Lewis antigen, which is a glycosphingolipid. The exact Lewis antigen produced, however, is determined by the presence or absence of the secretor gene (*Se*). Se determines the location on the precursor substance (type 1 chain) to which the fucose is added by the *Le* gene. If both the Lewis and *Se* genes are present, both Le^a and Le^b are added and the individual is Le(a+b+). However, if only the Lewis gene is present (the individual is sese and lacks the *Se* gene), Le^b is not produced and the individual is Le(a+b−). Thus, two different antigen specificities are produced depending on whether the secretor gene is present. In addition, the ABH makeup of the individual determines the position and linkage of the fucose being added by the Lewis gene, and this creates several variations of the Lewis phenotype. Because of the involvement of the secretor gene, Lewis substance is also

released into the plasma and saliva, which are of primary practical interest in transfusion medicine, but also into milk, gastrointestinal fluids, urine, seminal fluid, ovarian cyst fluid, and amniotic fluid.[3]

Newborns' red cells lack Lewis antigens and there is no Lewis substance in their plasma, although Lewis substance is present in their saliva. The adult Le^a antigen phenotype is attained by about 1 year of age but not until about 7 years for Le^b. Lewis antigens are decreased during pregnancy. During pregnancy there is an increased lipoprotein to red cell mass, which results in a shift of glycolipids from red cells to plasma, reducing the Lewis antigen content on the red cells. Also, the Lewis type of transfused red cells may change. After transfusion, the transfused donor red cells convert to the Lewis type of the recipient. Thus, Lewis antigen may be acquired or lost through the exchange of glycolipids between the plasma and red cell.

Lewis antibodies are common, usually react below body temperature, are mainly or entirely IgM, and are not clinically significant (Table 9.6). These antibodies are usually found in patients who have not been transfused and are thus sometimes called "natural"—a technically incorrect term, since they are probably stimulated by environmental agents. Anti-Le^a is often found in pregnant women, but it is not clear that the antibody is formed after immunization by fetal red cells. Lewis antibodies do not cause HDN. A few examples of anti-Le^a have caused hemolytic transfusion reactions. In these situations usually the antibody reacts at body temperatures, and this can be used as an indication of clinical significance. Other reasons that Lewis antibodies usually do not cause hemolysis are that the patient's antibodies are neutralized by soluble Lewis substance in the plasma of the donor, and the Lewis antigens on the transfused red cells elute into the plasma of the recipient. Lewis antibodies have been implicated in the rejection of transplanted Lewis-positive kidneys.[39] The available information on this subject is conflicting, but Lewis matching of donated kidneys is not done in most transplant programs.

LW System

LW antigen is named for Landsteiner and Wiener because it was the antigen defined on red cells by the original anti-Rh they prepared in rhesus monkeys.[10] Adult D-positive red cells exhibit stronger LW activity than D-negative red cells. Thus, weak examples of anti-LW appear similar to anti-D because they react with D-positive but not with D-negative red cells. This was the situation with the original anti-LW serum, and therefore it reacted similarly to the serum found by Levine and Stetson in their original report of hemolytic disease of the newborn.[9] Thus, the name of the Rh system was from the LW antibody produced in rhesus monkeys but that was in fact an antibody to a different antigen in a different system (LW). The original serum reacted with what is now known as the LW^a antigen. LW^b has been identified and four phenotypes have been observed: LW(a+b−), LW(a+b+), LW(a−b+), and LW(a−b−).

LW antibodies are very rare. Only very rare individuals lack LW^a antigen and can make anti-LW^a. Although LW is a genetically distinct system, this was not recognized for years. Because the expression of LW and Rh is related, LW was thought to be part of the Rh system. LW antibodies may cause accelerated destruction of LW-positive red

cells and thus, when present as an alloantibody, should be considered clinically significant. Anti-LW may also occur as a transient autoantibody in persons who temporarily lose LW antigen activity. This loss may occur during pregnancy or in association with malignancy.[3]

Ii Blood Group Antigens

The Ii blood group system is composed of 16 antigens, the major ones being I and i. The I and i antigens are part of the interior of the oligosaccharide chain that contains the ABH and Lewis antigens. One of the unique things about this system is that the presence of the I and i antigens changes with age. At birth, the i antigen is present and I is almost undetectable. During the first 18 months of life, the i antigen declines and is replaced by I. In most adults, very little i is detectable, except for rare individuals who remain i positive and I negative. At birth the oligosaccharides have the i structure and the action of the I gene causes branching of the linear i oligosaccharide chain to create the I phenotype. I specificity is conferred by the addition of a D- galactose-N-acetyl-D-galactosamine to the i oligosaccharide chain. Thus, it appears that I and i are not alleles but are part of a sequence of steps. The antigen structure is a complex branched chain, and it has been suggested[2,3] that the variety of antibodies that occurs in the I system is due to the formation of antibodies against domains within the antigen molecule. The other I system antigens are rare forms, transitional forms, or a complex with other antigens. The amount of Ii antigen on red cells varies in different individuals, and this also leads to the appearance of different forms of I antigens. I and i antigen are present in a soluble form in serum, saliva, breast milk, urine, amniotic fluid, ovarian cyst fluid, and hydatid cyst fluid.

The major antibodies of this group are anti-I and anti-i. These are usually autoantibodies that are optimally reactive at cold temperatures and not clinically significant. They do not cause HDN, and there is only one report of an anti-I that caused accelerated destruction of I red cells.[40] Almost all normal adults' serum contain anti-I; however, it is also found in cold agglutinin disease and transiently in *Mycoplasma pneumoniae* infection. In cold agglutinin disease, the antibody changes characteristics and is an auto-anti-I, which reacts at body temperature, fixes complement, and causes hemolysis. Anti-i is rare but has been associated with infectious mononucleosis.

Diego (Di)

The Diego system includes two pairs of antithetical antigens: Di^a and Di^b and (Wright) Wr^a and Wr^b. Di^a was the first of these to be discovered and is common in South American Indians but rare in Caucasians. The Diego antigens are part of band 3 of the red cell membrane. Anti-Di^a is not a common antibody because of the rarity of the antigen in the United States; however, the antibody can cause red cell destruction and should be considered clinically significant when present. Anti-Wr^a is common but is often not detected because most red cells used for antibody detection lack the antigen. When present it usually does not cause red cell destruction, and so special efforts are not made to include Wr^a cells on antibody screening panels.

Cartwright (Yt)

The Cartwright system consists of two antigens, one of high incidence and one of low incidence. The antigens are located on red cell acetylcholinesterase. Anti-Yt^a is not common, and anti-Yt^b is very rare. Anti-Yt^a has not caused HDN and usually does not cause hemolysis or transfusion reactions, but occasional examples do cause accelerated red cell destruction.

Xg System

An antibody that reacted more frequently with red cells from females than those from males identified the antigen named Xg^a. The Xg^a gene is carried on the X chromosome, and about 65% of males and 89% of females are Xg^a positive. Anti-Xg^a does not cause HDN nor hemolysis and thus is not considered to be clinically significant.

Dombrock (Do)

The Dombrock system initially included the Do^a and Do^b antigens but has been expanded to include some high-frequency antigens as well. Dombrock antibodies are not common, although anti-Do^a has caused mild HDN or red cell destruction. Anti-Do^b is not considered to be clinically significant.

Scianna (Sc)

Sc1 is a high-incidence antigen, and the antithetical antigen of low incidence is Sc2. An additional antigen, Sc3, is present on the cells of anyone who inherits either Sc1 or Sc2. The low-incidence antigen Radin also belongs to the Sc system. Sc antibodies are rare and have not been reported to cause HDN or accelerated red cell destruction.

Colton (Co)

The Colton system includes a high-incidence antigen (Co^a) and a low-incidence antigen (Co^b). The system also resembles Scianna and Duffy in that there is a third antigen (Co3) that is present whenever there is a functional Co gene. Colton antigens are part of the water transport protein Aquaporin 1, also known as CHIP. Colton antibodies are rare, but anti Co^a has been implicated in HDN and red cell destruction.

Rogers (Rg) and Chido (Ch)

The fourth component of complement (C4) is polymorphic. The Ch and Rg antigens are present on the C4A plasma components that remain attached to the red cell membrane. Thus, these antigens are not integral to the red cell membrane. There are at least six antigens in the Ch group and nine in the Rg group. Individuals who lack all Ch and Rg antigens also therefore lack C4 and have a high incidence of systemic lupus erythematosus. Antibodies to Ch and Rg antigens are not considered clinically significant because they have not been involved in HDN or red cell destruction. They can create problems in laboratory testing (see Chapter 10).

Gerbich (Ge)

The Gerbich system contains seven antigens: three of high incidence and four of low incidence. The antigens are located on glycophorin molecules. Gerbich system antibodies are of variable clinical significance. Some have caused mild HDN or slightly accelerated red cell clearance.

Cromer (Cr)

Ten different antigens have been assigned to the Cromer system. The antigens are located on the decay-accelerating factor, which is a regulatory protein in the complement system. The antibodies have varying clinical significance. None have caused a transfusion reaction or been implicated in HDN, although some Cromer antibodies have caused accelerated red cell destruction.

Knops (Kn)

There are six antigens of the Knops system. These include the Helgeson and McCoy phenotypes. The Knops antigens are located on the CR1 complement receptor, which is the primary complement receptor on red cells. Knops system antigens have different strengths of reactivity, and this is based more on the amount of red cell CR1 than on antigen dosage. Antibodies of the Kn system, like those of Chido and Rogers, have serologic reactivity referred to in the past as "high titer, low avidity." The sera caused weak reactivity, but the reactivity remained even after the serum was extensively diluted. Clinically, the antibodies are not significant because they do not cause transfusion reactions, increased red cell destruction, or HDN. However, they may be clinically significant in the broad sense that they make it difficult to carry out serologic investigations and their reactivity may mask other clinically dangerous antibodies.

Indian (In)

There are two antigens of the Indian system: one of low incidence (In^a) and one of high incidence (In^b). The antigens were discovered in people from the Indian subcontinent, and this was the source of the name of the antigen. The antigens are located on a glycoprotein that is a cellular adhesion molecule and lymphocyte homing receptor. The glycoprotein is present on many tissues, including red cells. Neither anti-In^a nor anti-In^b has been implicated in HDN, but both have caused a transfusion reaction and decreased red cell survival. Thus, they should be considered clinically significant.

HLA

HLA class I antigens are present on red cell membranes in varying amounts ranging from 40 to 550 antigen sites. They are attached to the membrane by β_2-microglobulin. The HLA system is described in more detail in Chapter 16.

ANTIBODIES TO RED CELL ANTIGENS

Antibodies to red blood cell antigens vary widely in their characteristics and in vivo significance. Red blood cell antibodies can be categorized based on their immunoglobulin class, the antigen to which they are directed, the method of stimulation, their optimum temperature of reaction in vitro, whether they fix complement, their action on red cells in vitro, and their in vivo effect (such as whether they cause hemolysis, transfusion reactions, or hemolytic disease of the newborn) (Tables 9.6 and 9.7). A summary of the general characteristics of antibodies of the major red blood cell antigen systems is provided in Table 9.6; however, specific antibodies within each system may exhibit different characteristics, so an appropriate reference text should be consulted before decisions are made regarding the identity or potential clinical effect of a particular antibody.

Almost all red cell antibodies are either IgG or IgM. There are rare examples of IgA red cell antibodies. There are some clinical and laboratory differences between IgM and IgG red cell antibodies (Tables 9.6 and 9.7). The mechanism of action of these antibodies is that the Fab portion of the Ig molecule binds to the antigen combining site on the red cell surface. The avidity and binding constants for this antibody-antigen reaction vary widely for different red cell antibodies. After binding, the heavy chain region of the antibody molecule determines the biologic effect of the antibody by activating complement or reacting with receptors in the fixed macrophages of the liver and spleen to cause accelerated red cell clearance.

The specificities of the most common red cell antibodies found in hospitalized patients, pregnant women, and normal blood donors differ slightly because of the nature of these populations. The incidence of different antibodies depends on the prevalence of the antigen in the population and the immunogenicity of the antigen. Factors that determine immunogenicity are not fully understood. The clinical importance of an antibody depends on whether it is likely to cause red cell destruction and also the incidence of the antibody. For instance, the combination of the 15% incidence of Rh-negative individuals, the 65% likelihood of becoming immunized after exposure to one unit of

Table 9.7 Methods of characterizing red cell antibodies

Physiochemical	IgG, IgM, IgA
Antigen	Iso, auto, hetero
In vitro action	Agglutinating (complete)
	Coating (incomplete, blocking)
	Complement fixing (hemolysin)
Temperature of optimum reaction	Warm, 37°C
	Cold, 20°C to 4°C
Optimum method of detection	Saline medium
	High-protein medium
	Antiglobulin serum required
Method of stimulation	Natural, immune

Rh-positive blood, and the serious clinical effect of anti-D makes the Rh(D) antigen the single most important non-ABO antigen.

FUNCTION OF MOLECULES CONTAINING RED CELL ANTIGENS

The clinical effects of most red cell antigens is because they serve as targets for antibodies, and thus the effects are due to their corresponding antibodies. These effects have been described above with each blood group system. During the past two decades, blood group serologists and transfusion medicine professionals have developed an understanding of the clinical relevance of these different antibodies and the laboratory techniques to identify clinically important red cell incompatibility. Thus, the laboratory detection of these blood group antigens and antibodies have been incorporated into a working system to provide safe and effective red cell transfusions.

Red cell blood group antigens have been of interest to blood bankers because of their role in transfusion therapy but also to geneticists because of their ability to serve as a genetic marker. During the past few years, the chromosomal location of several blood groups has been established (Table 9.2). Linkage between some blood groups and diseases are now known, and this also helps to localize some blood group genes to certain areas of the chromosomes. Studies of the red cell membrane have also begun to yield information about the structure and composition of red cell (blood group) antigens. Thus, the red cell antigens are no longer of interest only to the serologist-blood banker but are recognized increasingly as parts of important structural or functional components of the cell membrane. These antigens are part of molecules involved in many diverse activities. The serologic studies have often provided important links in the investigation of the function of these molecules.

The structural alterations of rare red cell antigens may be associated with hemolytic anemias or abnormal red cell morphology or membrane constituents (Table 9.8). Some clinical conditions such as to malignancies, stress, and pregnancy may alter the expression of blood groups (Table 9.9). Many of a cell's functions are determined by its membrane. Since red cell antigens are contained on molecules of the cell membrane, it is not surprising that certain red cell antigens or alterations in red cell antigens are associated with various functions of the cell. There are several different basic functions provided by red cell blood groups (see below and Table 9.10). Also, in some situations diseases alter the expression of red cell antigens (Table 9.9). Usually the red cell antigen is not directly involved in the function but happens to be located on the same molecule. Thus, the genetic variation that causes serologic problems is not the central function of the molecule but brings the molecules to the attention of transfusion medicine professionals.

Chemokine Receptor

Red cells bind chemokines such as interleukins, and it has been noted that Duffy (a−b−) red cells failed to bind the chemokine IL-8.[41] Thus, the Duffy blood group

serves as a chemokine receptor. The receptor activity is probably on the amino terminal end of the molecule (Fig. 9.2). It appears that the role of the red cell chemokine receptors is to bind and thus inactivate chemokines in the blood.

Transport Protein

Specific (transport) molecules are responsible for transporting nutrients into the cell and washing products out of the cell. Several blood groups are located on these molecules. One major transport molecule is band 3, a transmembrane protein that traverses the membrane multiple times, that is the major anion exchanger. The Diego and Wright blood groups are located on band 3. Because the Wright antigens require expression of glycophorin A, the transport function of band 3 is reduced when red cells are glycophorin deficient. The major water channel protein is the channel-forming integral protein (CHIP). The gene coding for this protein is located on chromosome 7 near the gene for the Colton blood group. It has now been established that the Colton antigens are located on the CHIP molecule.[42] The Kidd antigens are probably part of a molecule that acts as a urea transporter, because Jk(a−b−) cells are resistant to urea lysis. Rh and

Table 9.8 Rare blood types associated with abnormal red cell morphology or membrane constituents

Phenotype	Biochemical modification	Morphologic or functional abnormality
Rh$_{null}$	No Rh or LW antigens	Stomatocytes, spherocytes, partially compensated hemolytic anemia
McLeod	Weak expression of normal Kell antigens; Kx absent	Acanthocytes; partially compensated hemolytic anemia
K$_o$	No normal Kell antigens; Kx present	None observed
P	No normal P antigens; decreased globoside and ceramide trihexoside	None observed
Pk	Normal P1 antigen; CTH increased; globoside decreased	None observed
P1^{pk}	Increased GL3 (NAc galactose transferase deficiency)	None observed
Lu(a−b−)	Not studied	Abnormal scanning electron microscopy: wrinkled, furrowed appearance
En(a−)	Glycophorin A absent; depressed MN antigens; enhanced Rh(D) antigen	None observed
S−s−	Glycophorin B absent or abnormal	None observed
M^{k}M^k	Both glycophorin A and glycophorin B absent	None observed

Source: Adapted from McCullough J. Transfusion Medicine. In: Handin RI, Lux SE, Stossel TP, eds. Blood: Principles and Practice of Hematology. Philadelphia: J.B. Lippincott Company, 1995:1967.

Table 9.9 Clinical conditions with red cell antigen alteration

| Clinical condition | Red cell antigen | | Red cell antibody |
	Depressed	Increased	
Autoimmune hemolytic anemia	Rh-LW	i	Autoanti-D, LW Anti-Kp^b
Leukemia with monosomy 7	ABH Co^a	IiH	
Myelofibrosis	LW Rh ABH		
Hodgkin's disease			Anti-LW
Paroxysmal nocturnal hemoglobinuria		i	
Paroxysmal cold hemoglobinuria			Autoanti-P
Ovalocytosis	Rh, LW Ss, U Kidd Yt^a, Xg^a	H	
Chronic granulomatous disease	Kell		Anti-KL + Kx
Hereditary hemolytic anemia	Rh Kell Colton		
Sickle cell anemia—stress		i	
Pregnancy	LW Lewis Sd^a		Anti-LW Anti-Lewis
Bacterial infections			Acquired B antigen T activation
Chromosomal defects	Rh MN Duffy		

Source: Adapted from McCullough J. Transfusion Medicine. In: Handin RI, Lux SE, Stossel TP, eds. Blood: Principles and Practice of Hematology. Philadelphia: J.B. Lippincott Company, 1995:1966.

Kx may also be involved with membrane transport because portions of the molecules on which they are located span membranes. However, the molecules involved and the function have not been determined.

Complement Pathway

Three blood group systems are part of molecules involved in the complement pathway. The Chido/Rogers antigens are part of the C4 molecule.[43,44] Thus, these antigens are

Table 9.10 Functions of molecules containing red cell blood group antigens

Function	Blood group
Receptor	Duffy, Knops, Indian
Transport protein	Diego, Wright, Colton, Kidd
Complement pathway	Chido, Rogers, Cromer, Knops
Adhesion molecule	Indian, LW, Lutheran
Structural integrity	MN, Ss, Gerbich
Enzymatic activity	Cartwright, Kell ??
Microbial receptor	Duffy, P, Cromer

absorbed onto red cells from the C4 molecules in the circulation. The Cromer antigens are located on the decay accelerating factor (DAF) red cell membrane molecule,[45] and the Knops antigens are part of the C3b complement receptor.[46] The Cromer antigens were helpful in elucidating the cause of paroxysmal nocturnal hemoglobinuria (PNH). The role of DAF is to protect red cells from complement damage, and it was hoped that the rare Cromer-negative individual would establish the key role of the absence of DAF as the cause of PNH. However, Cromer-negative individuals have only a mildly increased sensitivity of complement. This finding led to the discovery that another molecule (CD59) was the key in PNH.

Adhesion Molecule

The Indian blood group antigens are located on the adhesion molecule CD44.[47] CD44 is involved in the adhesion of lymphocytes to endothelium and thus is involved in lymphocyte homing to lymphoid tissues. Also of interest is the possibility that CD44 may be involved in the homing of hematopoietic progenitor cells to marrow extracellular matrix. The LW blood group antigen is located on a membrane protein with a structure similar to intracellular adhesion molecule 2, which is part of a group of molecules that bind leukocytes to endothelium. It is not known whether the LW antigen is actually involved in adhesion. The Lutheran antigen is also part of a membrane-spanning protein and may be active in adhesion, but this has not been established.

Structural Integrity

Glycophorins are major structural proteins on the red cell surface, accounting for most of the negative surface charge that may function to prevent undesirable cell-to-cell interactions. The MN antigens are part of glycophorin A, the Ss antigens are part of glycophorin B, and the Gerbich antigens are part of glycophorins C and D.[48] Rare variants of these blood group antigens are helpful in elucidating the role of glycophorins in red cell structure and function. Red cells that lack glycophorin A (the En(a−) phenotype) or glycophorins A and B (the MkMk phenotype) are apparently normal. However, those that lack glycophorins C and D (Leach phenotype) lead to elliptocytes and decreased deformability.

Enzymatic Activity

The Cartwright blood group antigens are located on the acetylcholinesterase molecule.[49] The role of this enzyme molecule on the surface of red cells is not known. The gene coding for the Kell antigens is quite similar to the gene for zinc-binding peptidases. It is not known whether the Kell protein is enzymatically active.

Microbial Receptor

As a first step in infection, the invading organism must bind to the tissues. The involvement of the Duffy system in malaria is described above. Duffy (a−b−) red cells are resistant to infection by some species of *Plasmodium* because the parasites cannot establish a junction site on the red cell surface in the absence of the Duffy structure.[31,33] *Escherichia coli* has several adhesion molecules. One group of these bind to the DAF glycoprotein, which contains the Cromer blood group. It appears that the Cromer antigen is the receptor for this binding and thus facilitates infection with *E. coli*.[50] The DAF molecule containing Cromer is located on cells other than red cells, and there is a suggestion that binding of *E. coli* to Cromer in the urinary tract facilitates urinary tract infection. This mechanism is more clear with the P blood group system. Some *E. coli* adhesion molecules bind to the glycosphingolipids of the P system, thus increasing the likelihood of urinary tract infection.[51] Some viruses also adhere to molecules containing blood group antigens. The parvovirus B19 adheres to globoside of the P blood group system.[52] Enteroviruses such as coxsackievirus or echovirus use DAF containing the Cromer antigens as receptors. Poliovirus may use the CD44 molecule containing the Indian blood group antigens in its adhesive process.

PLATELETS

The blood group systems of interest on platelets are red cell groups, particularly ABO and Rh, HLA, and platelet-specific antigens.

Platelets contain antigens from several red cell blood group systems, including ABH, Lewis, Ii and P. Platelets do not contain Rh, Duffy, Kell, Kidd, and Lutheran antigens. There is debate as to whether the ABO antigens are integral to the platelet membrane or are adsorbed onto the platelet from their soluble form in plasma. It appears that some ABH antigens are intrinsic to the platelet membrane and some are adsorbed onto the cell surface from the plasma, which contains soluble A and B substance.[53] The density of A antigen sites on platelets is only about 5% of that on red cells.[53] ABO antigens have some importance in platelet transfusion in that it appears that ABO incompatibility reduces the response to transfusion (see Chapter 11).

In contrast to ABH antigens, HLA antigens are integral to the platelet membrane. However, only HLA class I (A and B locus) and not class II (DR) antigens are present.[54] The HLA system is discussed more extensively in Chapter 16, and the clinical impact of the HLA antigens on platelets is discussed in Chapter 12.

Table 9.11 Human platelet alloantigens

System	Antigen	Alternative names	Glyco-protein	Nucleotide change	Amino acid change	Molecular name	Pheno-type*
HPA-1	HPA-1a	Zw^a,Pl^{A1}	GPIIIa	T^{196}	Leu^{33}	GPIIIa-Leu33	97.9
	HPA-1b	Zw^b, Pl^{A2}		C^{196}	Pro^{33}	GPIIIa-Pro33	28.6
HPA-2	HPA-2a	Ko^b	GPIb^a	T^{524}	Thr^{145}	GPIb^a-Thr145	>99.9
	HPA-2b	Ko^a, Sib^a		C^{524}	Met^{145}	GPIb^a-Met145	13.2
HPA-3	HPA-3a	Bak^a, Lek^a	GPIIb	T^{2622}	Ile^{843}	GPIIb-Ile843	80.9
	HPA-3b	Bak^b		G^{2622}	Ser^{a843}	GPIIb-Ser843	69.8
HPA-4	HPA-4a	Yuk^b, Pen^a	GPIIIa	A^{526}	Arg^{143}	GPIIIa-Arg143	>99.9
	HPA-4b	Yuk^a, Pen^b		G^{526}	Gln^{143}	GPIIIa-Gln143	0.0
HPA-5	HPA-5a	Br^b, Zav^b	GPIa	G^{1648}	Glu^{505}	GPIa-Glu505	99.0
	HPA-5b	Br^a, Zav^a, Hc^a		A^{1648}	Lys^{505}	GPIa-Lys505	19.7
HPA-6W	HPA-6bW	Ca^a, Tu^a	GPIIIa	C^{1564}	Gln^{489}	GPIIIa-Gln489	0.7
				G^{1564}	Arg^{489}	(GPIIIa-Arg489)	
HPA-7W	HPA-7bW	Mo^a	GPIIIa	G^{1317}	Ala^{407}	GPIIIa-Ala407	Unkn
				C^{1317}	Pro^{407}	(GPIIIa-Pro407)	
HPA-8W	HPA-8bW	Sr^a	GPIIIa	C^{2004}	Cys^{636}	GPIIIa-Cys636	Unkn
				T^{2004}	Arg^{636}	(GPIIIa-Arg636)	
HPA-9W	HPA-9bW	Max^a	GPIIb	A^{2306}	Met^{837}	GPIIb-Met837	Unkn
				G^{2306}	Val^{837}	(GPIIb-Val837)	
—	—	Gro^a	GPIIIa	A^{1996}	His^{633}	GPIIIa-His633	Unkn
				G^{1996}	Arg^{633}	(GPIIIa-Arg633)	
—	—	Va^a	GPIIIa	—	—	—	—
—	—	Ly^a	GPIb/IX	—	—	—	—
—	—	Pe^a	GPIba	—	—	—	—
—	—	Oe^a	GPIIIa	—	—	—	—

Source: von dem Borne AEGKr, de Haas M, Simcek S, Porcelijn L, van der Schoot CE. Platelet and neutrophil alloantigens in clinical medicine. Vox Sang 1996;70(Suppl 3):34–40.

In addition to red cell and HLA system antigens, there are several antigen systems that are called platelet-specific (Table 9.11). More accurately, these antigens are present to a much greater extent on platelets than on other tissues, and so functionally they can be considered platelet-specific antigens. The antigens were discovered by studies of sera from mothers who delivered thrombocytopenic infants. The mother's sera reacted against platelets of the infant and the infant's father in a manner similar to red cell

Table 9.12 Clinical situations involving platelet-specific antigens and antibodies

---

Autoantibodies
    Autoimmune thrombocytopenia
    Drug-induced immune thrombocytopenia
Alloantibodies
    Neonatal alloimmune thrombocytopenia
    Posttransfusion purpura
    Refractoriness to platelet transfusion

---

hemolytic disease of the newborn. Since those initial clinical laboratory observations, much has been learned about the genetics and molecular basis of the antigens and their clinical significance.[55] The epitopes of these antigens are located on glycoproteins of the platelet membrane.[55] Not all of the platelet glycoproteins contain platelet-specific antigens. Much like red cell antigens, the initial names given to platelet-specific antigens often were related to the patients in whom the antibody was originally found. Thus, names such as PlA1 or Zw(a) were given, and in fact these terms refer to the same antigen. In 1990, a new nomenclature system was developed that used the prefix HPA for human platelet antigen and assigned a number to each locus followed by a letter to designate to each antigen. Thus, HPA 1a is the first antigen at the first locus. This antigen corresponds to the original antigen PlA1 (Table 9.11). At present there are five established antigen systems or loci, each with two antigens for a total of ten antigens. These antigens are located on four different glycoproteins (Table 9.11). In addition, four more antigen systems or loci, each involving one antigen, have been given provisional status (Table 9.11). Other individual antigens that appear to be platelet-specific have been reported but not yet classified (Table 9.11). As a result of increasing understanding of the molecular basis of platelet-specific antigens, it has been suggested that a new nomenclature system be developed that will better relate to the molecular basis of the antigens.[56] The HPA system is still in general use.

These platelet-specific antigens have clinical importance (see Chapter 12 and Table 9.12). They are targets for autoantibodies, alloantibodies, and drug-dependent antibodies.[55] These platelet-specific antibodies may cause autoimmune thrombocytopenia or several different clinical problems or diseases due to alloimmunization. Rather surprisingly, it appears that platelet-specific antigens and antibodies are not of major importance in alloimmunization to platelets and refractoriness to platelet transfusion (see Chapter 11). In addition to involvement in several clinical situations, some of the platelet-specific antigens are located on glycoprotein molecules that have other important functions. Platelet glycoproteins function as receptors in the hemostatic process and thus are involved in platelet aggregation and/or platelet adhesion to endothelial cells. It seems likely that future studies will demonstrate that abnormalities of these molecules cause alterations in platelet antigens or that altered platelet antigen strength or specificity may affect the structure or function of the cell.

GRANULOCYTES

Alloantigen systems of interest that might be found on granulocytes include red cell antigens, HLA antigens, and granulocyte-specific antigens. At one time, granulocytes were thought to contain ABH antigens on their surface. However, several studies have failed to demonstrate this.[57–60] Despite these in vitro data, it is also of interest to determine whether ABO incompatibility affects granulocytes in vivo. To study this, granulocytes labeled with [111]indium were transfused to patients who were receiving granulocyte transfusions. Transfused granulocytes demonstrated intravascular recoveries and survivals and migrated normally into skin chambers when injected into subjects who were ABO incompatible with the granulocyte donors.[61] Rh system antigens are also not present on granulocytes. Thus, the accumulated data indicate that ABO antigens are not present on granulocytes.

HLA-A, B, and C (class I) antigens are on the surface of granulocytes,[62,63] but the antigens are fewer in number than on lymphocytes.[64] It is possible that these HLA antigens are adsorbed onto the surface of granulocytes[65] rather than being an integral part of the membrane, but this is not established. It appears that HLA-D/DR antigens are not on granulocytes.[54]

Granulocytes also contain several alloantigen systems whose tissue distribution is limited to granulocytes (Table 9.13). This was first recognized by Lalezari in studies of sera obtained from patients with unexplained neutropenia.[66,67] From his early work, Lalezari proposed the nomenclature system used today. The letter N stands for neutrophil, a second letter stands for the gene locus (A, B, C, etc.), and a number stands for the antigen at that locus. Thus, the antigens are named NA1, NA2, NB1, etc. A total of seven antigens at five loci have been reported (Table 9.13). The clinical significance of these antigens is described in Chapters 12 and 14. This discussion will focus on the antigens and antibodies.

The N1 antigen was the first to be discovered.[66] The antibody defining this antigen was present in the serum of a woman who delivered an infant with transient neutropenia. Her serum reacted with the neutrophils of the infant and her husband in a situation similar to red cell HDN.[66,67] The NA2 and the NA null condition are now known also. During the past few years, very nice biochemistry and molecular genetics have provided a great deal of information about the NA antigens. NA-system antigens are present on the FcRIIIb portion of the Fc or gamma receptor of neutrophils.[68,69] The FcR molecule is a glycoprotein whose molecular weight varies with the NA phenotype because of the difference in the amount of carbohydrate side chains. The FcRIIIb is a phosphatidyl-inositol-glycan (PIG) anchored glycosylated protein. The FcRIIIb molecule has 233 amino acids and is expressed only on neutrophils but also can be found in plasma and body fluids in a soluble form.[70] The difference between NA1 and NA2 is four amino acids, apparently caused by one nucleotide difference in the gene. The gene is located on chromosome 1. Rare individuals lack both NA antigens and are thus NA null. These individuals lack the FcRIII molecule. Other antigens limited to granulocytes include NB, NC, ND, and NE (Table 9.13). In addition, there are several antigens that granulocytes share with other tissues. These include the 5(a) and (b), 9(a), and MART

Table 9.13 Neutrophil-specific and leukocyte antigens in "Caucasians"

System	Antigen	Glycoprotein	Phenotype frequency (%)	Gene frequency
Neutrophil-specific antigens				
NA	NA1	FcRIIIb	46	0.38
	NA2	FcRIIIb	88	0.63
NB	NB1	gp 56–64 kD	97	0.83
	NB2	gp 56–64 kD	32	0.17
Lan	Lan^a	FcRIIIb	>99	>0.91
Sar	Sar^a	FcRIIIb	>99	>0.91
Leukocyte antigens				
5	5a	70–95 kD	33	0.19
	5b	70–95 kD	96	0.82
9 = HMA	9^a = HMA1		69	0.44
	9^b = HMA2		81	0.56
Ond	Ond^a (E27)	CD11a (aL)	>99	>0.91
Mart	Mart^a	CD11b (aM)	99	0.91
SL	SL^a		66	

Source: von dem Borne AEGKr, de Haas M, Simcek S, Porcelijn L, van der Schoot CE. Platelet and neutrophil alloantigens in clinical medicine. Vox Sang 1996;70(Suppl 3):34–40.

antigens. They are of interest because they provide information about hematopoiesis and ontogeny and may be involved in clinical situations such as transfusion reactions or immune neutropenias.[62,63,71]

These granulocyte-specific antibody-antigen systems are involved in the pathophysiology of several clinical situations (Table 9.14). Both autoantibodies and alloantibodies have been identified, and each may cause severe clinical problems.[63,71] These situations include autoimmune neutropenia, alloimmune neonatal neutropenia (see Chapter 12), transfusion reactions (see Chapter 14), and granulocyte transfusions (see Chapter 11). One situation in which neutrophil-specific antibodies are not important is

Table 9.14 Clinical situations involving granulocyte-specific antigens and antibodies

Autoantibodies
    Autoimmune neutropenia
    Drug-induced immune neutropenia
Alloantibodies
    Alloimmune neonatal neutropenia
    Febrile transfusion reactions
    Transfusion-induced acute lung injury
    Poor response to granulocyte transfusion

bone marrow transplantation. We have demonstrated successful marrow engraftment of NA1-positive marrow in a patient with circulating anti-NA1.[72] This is consistent with evidence that these antigens are not present on promyelocytes, myeloblasts, and earlier uncommitted stem cells but become expressed during myeloid maturation.[73] Thus, the granulocyte-specific antigens can be thought of as differentiation antigens specific for this cell line and that become expressed during maturation of the cell.

REFERENCES

1. Daniels GL, Anstee DJ, Cartron JP, et al. Blood group terminology 1995: from the ISBT Working Party on Terminology for Red Cell Surface Antigens. Vox Sang 1995;69:265–279.
2. Mollison PL, Engelfriet CP, Contreras M. Blood transfusion. In: Clinical Medicine, 8th ed. Cambridge, MA: Blackwell Science Inc, 1987:613.
3. Daniels G. Human Blood Groups. Cambridge, MA: Blackwell Science Inc, 1995.
4. Widmann FK. Early observations about the ABO blood groups. Transfusion 1997;37:665–667.
5. Cook PJL, Roboon EB, Buckton KE, et al. Segregation of ABO, AK1 and ACONS in families with abnormalities of chromosome 9. Ann Hum Genet 1978;41:365.
6. Ferguson-Smith M, Aitken D, Turleau C, de Grouchy J. Localization of the human ABO:Np1:AK-1 linkage group by regional assignment of AK-1 to 9q34. Hum Genet 1976;34:35.
7. Yamamoto F, Clausen H, White T, Marken J, Hakomori S. Molecular genetic basis of the histo-blood group ABO system. Nature 1990;345:229.
8. Stroncek DF, Konz R, Clay ME, Houchins JP, McCullough J. Determination of ABO glycosyltransferase genotypes by use of the polymerase chain reaction and restriction enzymes. Transfusion 1995;35:231–240.
9. Levine P, Stetson R. An unusual case of intragroup agglutination. JAMA 1939;113:126.
10. Landsteiner K, Wiener AS. An agglutinable factor in human blood recognizable by immune sera for rhesus blood. Proc Soc Exp Biol Med 1940;43:223.
11. Wiener AS. Genetic theory of the Rh blood types. Proc Soc Exp Biol Med 1943;54:316.
12. Race RR. An "incomplete" antibody in human serum. Nature 1944;153:771.
13. Rosenfield RE, Allen FH Jr, Swisher SN, Kochwa S. A review of Rh serology and presentation of a new terminology. Transfusion 1962;2:287.
14. Moore S, Woodrow CF, McClelland DB. Isolation of membrane components associated with human red cell antigens Rho(D), (c), (E), and Fya. Nature 1982;295:529.
15. Gahmberg CG. Molecular identification of the human Rho(D) antigen. FEBS Lett 1982;140:93.
16. Cartron JP, Agre P. Rh blood group antigens: protein and gene structure. Semin Hematol 1993;30:193–208.
17. Saboori AM, Smith BL, Agre P. Polymorphism in the 32,000 Rh protein purified from Rh(D) positive and negative erythrocytes. Proc Natl Acad Sci USA 1988;85:4042.
18. Masouredis SP, Sudora EJ, Mahan L, Victoria EJ. Antigen site densities and ultrastructural distribution patterns of red cell Rh antigens. Transfusion 1976;16:94.
19. Nicolson GL, Masouredis SP, Singer SJ. Quantitative two-dimensional ultrastructural distribution of Rho(D) antigenic sites on human erythrocyte membranes. Proc Natl Acad Sci USA 1971;68:1416.
20. James NT, James V. Nearest neighbor analyses on the distribution of Rh antigens on erythrocyte membranes. Br J Haematol 1978;40:657.
21. Smith BL, Agre P. The erythrocyte membrane skeleton: site of the molecular defects of congenital anemias and the Rh antigens. In: Moore SB, ed. Progress in Immunohematology. Arlington, VA: American Association of Blood Banks, 1988:119.
22. Moore S, Green C. The identification of specific Rhesus polypeptide blood group ABH active glycoprotein complexes in the human red cell membrane. Biochem J 1987;244:735.
23. Bloy C, Blanchard D, Dahr W, et al. N-terminal sequence of blood group Rh(D) polypeptide and demonstration that the Rh(D), (c), and (E) antigens are carried by distinct polypeptide chains. Blood 1988;72:661–666.

24. Cherif-Zahar B, Mattei MG, Le Van Kim C, Bailly P, Cartron JP, Colin Y. Localization of the human Rh blood group gene structure to chromosome 1p34.3–1p36.1 region by in situ hybridization. Hum Genet 1991;86:98.

25. Le Van Kim C, Mouro I, Cherif-Zahar B, et al. Molecular cloning and primary structure of the human blood group RhD polypeptide. Proc Natl Acad Sci USA 1992;89:10925.

26. Colin Y, Cherif-Zahar B, Le Van Kim C, et al. Genetic basis of the Rh D-positive and Rh D-negative blood group polymorphism as determined by Southern analysis. Blood 1991;78:2747–2752.

27. Lee S, Zambas ED, Marsh WL, Redman CM. The human Kell blood group gene maps to chromosome 7q33 and its expression is restricted to erythroid cells. Blood 1993;81:2804.

28. Lee S, Zambas ED, Marsh WL, Redman CM. Molecular cloning and primary structure of Kell blood group protein. Proc Natl Acad Sci USA 1991;88:6353.

29. Redman CM, Marsh WL, Mueller KA, et al. Isolation of Kell-active protein from the red cell membrane. Transfusion 1984;294:176.

30. Redman CM, Avellino G, Pfeffer SR, et al. Kell blood group antigens are part of a 93,000 dalton red cell membrane protein. J Biol Chem 1986;261:9521.

31. Hadley TJ, David PH, McGinniss MH, Miller LH. Identification of an erythrocyte component carrying the Duffy blood group Fya antigen. Science 1984;223:597.

32. Masouredis SP, Sudora E, Mahan L, Victoria EJ. Quantitative immunoferritin microscopy of Fya, Fyb, Jka, U, and Dib antigen site numbers of human red cells. Blood 1980;56:969.

33. Miller LH, Mason SJ, Devorak JA, et al. Erythrocyte receptors for Plasmodium knowlesi malaria, Duffy blood group determinants. Science 1975;189:561.

34. Miller LH, Aikawa M, Johnson JG, Shiroishi T. Interaction between cytochalasin B-treated malarial parasites and erythrocytes: attachment and junction formation. J Exp Med 1979;149:172.

35. Geitvik GA, Hoyheim B, Gedde-Dahl T, et al. The Kidd (Jk) blood group locus assigned to chromosome 18 by close linkage to a DNA-RFLP. Hum Genet 1987;77:205–209.

36. Olives B, Neau P, Bailly P, et al. Cloning and functional expression of a urea transporter from human bone marrow cells. J Biol Chem 1994;269:31649–31652.

37. Eiberg H, Mohr J, Staub-Nielsen, Simonsen N. Genetics and linkage relationships of the C3 polymorphism: discovery of C3-Se linkage and assignment of LES-C3-DM-Se-PEPD-Lu synteny to chromosome 19. Clin Genet 1983;24:159–170.

38. Dahr W, Uhlenbruck G, Bird GW. Further characterization of some heterophile agglutinins reacting with alkali-labile carbohydrate chains of human erythrocyte glycoproteins. Vox Sang 1978;28:133.

39. Oriol R, Cartron J, Yvart J, et al. The Lewis system: new histocompatibility antigens in renal transplantation. Lancet 1978;1:574.

40. Chaplin H, Hunter VL, Malech AC, Kilzer P, Rosche ME. Clinically significant allo-anti- I in an I-negative patient with massive hemorrhage. Transfusion 1986;25:57.

41. Horuk R, Chitnis CE, Darbonne WC, et al. A receptor for the malarial parasite Plasmodium vivax: the erythrocyte cytokine receptor. Science 1993;261:1182–1184.

42. Smith BL, Preston GM, Spring FA, et al. Human red cell aquaporin CHIP. J Clin Invest 1994;94:1043–1049.

43. O'Neill GJ, Yang SY, Tegoli J, et al. Chido and Rodgers blood groups are distinct antigenic components of human complement C4. Nature 1978;273:688–690.

44. Tilley CA, Romans DG, Crookston MC. Localisation of Chido and Rodgers determinants to the C4d fragment of human C4. Nature 1978;276:713–715.

45. Telen MJ, Hall SE, Green AM, et al. Identification of human erythrocyte blood group antigens on decay accelerating factor (DAF) and an erythrocyte phenotype negative for DAF. J Exp Med 1988;167:1993–1998.

46. Rao N, Ferguson DJ, Lee SF, Telen MJ. Identification of human erythrocyte blood group antigens on the C3b/C4b receptor. J Immunol 1991;146:3502–3507.

47. Spring FA, Dalchau R, Daniels GL, et al. The In^a and In^b blood group antigens are located on a glycoprotein of 80,000 MW (the CDw44 glycoprotein) whose expression is influenced by the In (Lu) gene. Immunology 1988;64:37–43.

48. Chasis JA, Mohandas N. Red blood cell glycophorins. Blood 1992;80:1869–1879.

49. Spring FA, Gardner B, Anstee DJ. Evidence that the antigens of the YT blood group system are located on human erythrocyte acetylcholinesterase. Blood 1992;80:2136–2141.

50. Nowicki B, Labigne A, Moseley S, et al. The Dr hemagglutinin, afimbrial adhesins AFA- I and AFA-III, and F1845 fimbriae of uropathogeneic and diarrhea-associated Escherichia coli belong to a family of hemagglutinins with Dr receptor recognition. Infect Immunol 1990;58:279–281.

51. Johnson JR. Virulence factors in Escherichia coli urinary tract infection. Clin Microbiol Rev 1991;4:80–128.

52. Brown KE, Anderson SM, Young NS. Erythrocyte P antigen: cellular receptor for B19 parvovirus. Science 1993;262:114–117.

53. Dunstan RA, Simpson MB, Knowles RW, Rosse WF. The origin of ABO antigens on human platelets. Blood 1985;65:615.

54. Dunstan RA, Simpson MB, Sanfilippo FP. Absence of specific HLA-DR antigens on human platelets and neutrophils. Abstract. Blood 1984;64:85a.

55. Kunicki TJ, Newman PJ. The molecular immunology of human platelet proteins. Blood 1992;80:1386–1404.

56. Newman PJ. Nomenclature of human platelet alloantigens: a problem with the HPA system? Blood 1994;83:1447–1451.

57. Dunstan RA. Status of major red cell blood group antigens on neutrophils, lymphocytes and monocytes. Br J Haematol 1986;62:301–309.

58. Kelton JG, Bebenek G. Granulocytes do not have surface ABO antigens. Transfusion 1985;25:567–569.

59. Dunstan RA, Simpson MB, Borowitz M. Absence of ABH antigens on neutrophils. Br J Haematol 1984;60:651–657.

60. Gaidulis L, Branch DR, Lazar GS, Petz LD, Blume KG. The red cell antigens A, B, D, U, Ge, Jk3 and Yta are not detected on human granulocytes. Br J Haematol 1984;60:659–668.

61. McCullough J, Clay M, Loken M, Hurd D. Effect of ABO incompatibility on fate in vivo of [111]Indium granulocytes. Transfusion 1988;28:358.

62. Clay ME, Kline WE, McCullough J. Granulocyte antigens and antibodies: current concepts of detection and histocompatibility testing. In: Dutcher J, ed. Modern Transfusion Therapy. Boca Raton, FL: CRC Press 1990:182.

63. Clay ME, Stroncek DF. Granulocyte immunology. In: Anderson KC, Ness PM, eds. Scientific Basis of Transfusion Medicine: Implications for clinical practice. Philadelphia: W.B. Saunders Company, 1994;244–279.

64. Thompson JS. Antileukocyte capillary agglutinating antibody in pre- and post-transplantation sera. In: Rose NR, Friedman H, eds. Manual of Clinical Immunology. Washington, DC: American Society for Microbiology, 1976:868.

65. Minchinton RM, Waters AH, Malpas JS, et al. Platelet- and granulocyte-specific antibodies after allogeneic and autologous bone marrow grafts. Vox Sang 1984;46:125.

66. Lalezari P, Nussbaum M, Gelman S, Spaet TH. Neonatal neutropenia due to maternal isoimmunization. Blood 1960;15:236–243.

67. Boxer LA, Yokoyama M, Lalezari P. Isoimmune neonatal neutropenia. J Pediatr 1972;80:783.

68. Trounstine ML, Peitz GA, Yssel H, et al. Reactivity of cloned, expressed human FcRIII isoforms with monoclonal antibodies which distinguish cell type specific and allelic forms of Fc-gamma-RIII. Int Immunol 1990;2:303.

69. Ory PA, Clark MR, Kwoh EE, Clarkson SB, Goldstein IM. Sequences of complementary DNAs that encode the NA1 and NA2 forms of Fc receptor III on human neutrophils. J Clin Invest 1989;84:1688.

70. Huizinga TWS, Kleijer M, Tetteroo PAT, Roos D, von dem Born AEGKr. Bialletic neutrophil Na-antigen system is associated with a polymorphism on the phospho-inositol-linked Fc receptor III (CD16) Blood 1990; 75:213.

71. McCullough J, Clay ME, Press C, Kline W. Granulocyte Serology: a clinical and laboratory guide. Chicago: ASPC Press, 1988;83:112.

72. Warkentin PI, Clay ME, Kersey JH, et al. Successful engraftment of NA1 positive bone marrow in a patient with a neutrophil antibody, anti-NA1. Hum Immunol 1981;2:173.

73. Stroncek DF, Shapiro RS, Filipovich AH, Plachta LB, Clay ME. Prolonged neutropenia resulting from antibodies to neutrophil-specific antigen NB1 following marrow transplantation. Transfusion 1993;33:158.

LABORATORY DETECTION OF BLOOD GROUPS AND PROVISION OF RED CELLS

IMMUNOLOGIC MECHANISMS OF RED CELL DESTRUCTION

Almost all red cell antibodies are either IgM or IgG (see Chapter 9). Thus, these are the immunoglobulins of importance in considering red cell destruction. Immune destruction of red cells involves these two kinds of immunoglobulins, either with or without complement. Red cells containing bound IgG undergo accelerated clearance through the spleen, where Fc receptors of the phagocyte bind to the IgG molecules, leading to phagocytosis of the red cell. This process does not require complement. If the IgG-coated red cell also contains bound complement components, the binding and phago-cytosis are accelerated. In contrast, immune destruction of red cells coated with IgM depends on complement. IgM-coated red cells either are hemolyzed in the intravascular space or are cleared rapidly predominantly in the liver.

Complement can cause immune destruction of red cells in either of two ways: by accelerated clearance from the intravascular space by interacting with complement receptors in the fixed macrophage system primarily of the liver, or by direct intravascular lysis due to rupture of the cell membrane by complement components. Complement can be activated by either IgG or IgM. However, the exact mechanisms that determine the ability of different red cell antibodies to activate complement are not known. IgM is much more effective than IgG in activating complement, probably because the nature of the IgM molecule places several Fc receptor sites in close proximity. However, the situation is more complex than merely the number of Fc sites in close enough proximity to activate C1.[1] For instance, in general, anti-D (an IgG) is not effective in activating complement compared with anti-K or Jk^a (also IgG), which react

with antigens that actually have fewer antigen sites than D sites on the red cell.[1] Of IgG molecules, the subclasses of IgG1 and IgG3 are more effective in binding complement than IgG4.

The complement system involves several different proteins (complement components), the activation of which is influenced by a variety of inhibitors or proteases. Activation of C1 begins the complement cascade sequence leading to formation of the membrane attack complex (C5 to C9), which causes lysis of the red cell. Often the process does not proceed to completion of the membrane attack complex and cell lysis. However, red cells may be coated with certain complement components, which cause accelerated clearance of the red cells by interaction with complement receptors on cells of the fixed macrophage system. The first of these key steps is the activation of C3. After several activation and enzyme cleavage steps, the C3d fragment of C3 remains bound to the red cell membrane antigen-antibody complex. Red cells containing bound C3d undergo accelerated clearance in the liver by interaction with complement receptors in the fixed macrophage system. Intravascular hemolysis is the term applied to the destruction of red cells by the complement membrane attack complex. The red cell membrane is damaged, hemoglobin is released into the circulation, and the classic signs and symptoms of a hemolytic transfusion reaction occur (see Chapter 14). ABO incompatibility is the best example of red cell antibody-antigen reactions that cause this kind of hemolysis. Extravascular hemolysis is the term applied to red cell destruction caused by phagocytic cells of the fixed macrophage site. This occurs primarily in the spleen and is associated with an increase in bilirubin and its metabolites. In actuality, these are arbitrary distinctions, since complement may be involved in both intravascular and extravascular hemolysis and the degree or severity of hemolysis may be a factor in the symptoms and laboratory findings. For instance, red cells undergoing phagocytosis in the fixed macrophage system may be only partially engulfed and release some hemoglobin into the intravascular space, thus simulating intravascular hemolysis.

In practice, the red cell serologic tests for antibody identification and red cell compatibility are designed to enhance and speed the cell's reaction with IgM or IgG antibodies and to detect the reaction by looking for direct cell agglutination or using reagents or conditions to enhance red cell agglutination.

METHODS OF DETECTING RED CELL ANTIBODY-ANTIGEN REACTIONS

Factors That Affect Agglutination

Red cell agglutination occurs in two stages: first the antibody binds to the red cell surface; then the antibodies interact to bring the cells in approximation, and agglutination occurs. The first stage of agglutination is affected by temperature, pH of the medium, the affinity constant of the antibody, duration of incubation, ionic strength of the medium, and antigen-antibody ratio.[2] The second stage of agglutination is influenced by the distance between cells, the charge of molecules in the suspension, and membrane deformability, membrane surface molecules, and molecular structure. Many of the practical procedures used in the daily operation of a blood bank take advantage of these factors.

Techniques to Enhance Red Cell Antibody Detection

There are several techniques that can be used to enhance the antigen-antibody reaction. These techniques are based on the factors known to influence antibody-antigen reactions. The techniques are (a) use of high-protein medium, usually accomplished by adding albumin, (b) use of antihuman globulin (AHG) (see below), (c) enzyme treatment of the test red cells, (d) use of low-ionic strength solution (LISS), (e) use of polyethylene glycol, and (f) use of polybrene. Some of these techniques, such as use of AHG and LISS, can be combined.

Antihuman globulin serum   The cornerstone of red cell antibody detection is the use of antihuman globulin. Antihuman globulin is prepared from the serum of rabbits immunized with human IgG or human complement, usually the C3 component. These reagents have reactivity only against IgG or C3 and are called monospecific. Antihuman globulin can also be prepared as a blend of these sera. This antiglobulin serum is called polyspecific. Depending on the kind of antihuman globulin used, IgG and/or C3 can be detected on the surface of red cells. The original reports and use of antihuman globulin serum involved anti-IgG.[3] During the mid-1960s, several investigators began to describe the role of complement in red cell destruction.[4–6] It was established that some red cell antibodies caused red cell destruction by activating complement and that anti-complement activity in antiglobulin reagents could predict accelerated red cell destruction.[7–12] This led to several years of research and debate as to the value of anticomplement activity in antiglobulin reagents. The rationale was that the ability to detect not only IgG but also C3 on the red cell would enhance the likelihood of finding clinically significant antibodies. However, many clinically insignificant antibodies active at cold temperatures bind complement. Since these cold antibodies are present normally in many individuals, the addition of anti-C3 to antiglobulin serum led to many false-positive tests. Ultimately, a consensus developed that when anticomplement reagents are used for patient or donor antibody screening, there is a very high rate of detection of cold antibodies that are not clinically significant.[13] Thus, the practice has been abandoned.

Although detection of C3d bound to red cells is not helpful for compatibility testing, it is helpful in the evaluation of possible immune hemolytic anemia. For instance, some patients with warm antibody-type autoimmune hemolytic anemia, cold agglutinin syndrome, and drug-induced immune hemolytic anemias may have red cells that react only with reagents containing anti-C3d activity and not with anti-IgG reagents. These reagents are used in the direct antiglobulin test to determine whether anemia or accelerated red cell destruction may be due to complement activation and/or complement-binding antibodies.

Antihuman globulin serum can be used to demonstrate binding of IgG antibodies in several different techniques, including saline, high-protein, low-ionic strength solution, and polyethylene glycol (PEG). Antihuman globulin is not used in the polybrene test because of the nature of the agglutination reactions.

Low-ionic strength solution   At low-ionic strength, the ionized groups on red cell antigen and antibody molecules become more highly charged, and the attraction

between them increases. This is used as a method to enhance red cell antibody detection.[14,15] The solution used is phosphate-buffered saline with glycine added to reduce the ionic strength. Serum and red cells are incubated in the LISS at 37°C for only about 10 to 15 minutes, then the mixture is centrifuged and observed for agglutination. The LISS system is very effective in identifying red cell antibodies.[16-18] Advantages of the LISS system are increased sensitivity in detecting antibodies and the shortened incubation time, which reduces the overall time required for the compatibility test. The shortened time is an advantage when used in conjunction with the type and screen system, because on the rare occasions when blood is needed, it can be made available faster.

Polybrene   Hexadimethrine bromide or polybrene is thought to facilitate red cell agglutination by neutralizing the net negative charge between red cells and thus forming ionic bonds between the red cell and the polybrene. In the polybrene test, red cells and serum are incubated very briefly (about 1 minute) in a low-ionic strength solution to allow antibody binding, and then polybrene is added to promote aggregation. The red cells are resuspended and, if antibody binding has occurred, the cells fail to resuspend.[19] The polybrene method is sensitive and provides results more rapidly than other methods[20,21] but has not gained wide use. The system does not use antihuman globulin.

Polyethylene glycol   Polyethylene glycol is a polymer that is used to displace diluent molecules in solution, effectively increasing the antibody-antigen concentration and enhancing the reaction.[22,23] The PEG system uses a 20% solution of PEG in phosphate-buffered saline. Serum and red cells are incubated for about 15 minutes, and, after washing, antiglobulin serum is added. Originally PEG was proposed as a supplementary test to the identification of antibodies because there was a rather high false-positive rate with PEG.[22] Subsequent studies showed that PEG is more sensitive than LISS in detecting clinically significant antibodies but also had a higher false-positive rate (1.3% versus 0.1%).[23–26]

Enzymes   The antigens on test red cells can be modified by treating the cells with enzymes. The most popular enzymes are ficin, papain, and bromelin. The activity of some antigens is enhanced and others decreased (see Chapter 9). This can be especially helpful if multiple antibodies are suspected and one of the antigens is inactivated by enzymes.

Techniques for Detecting Red Cell Antigen-Antibody Reactions

Tube tests   Traditionally red cell testing has been carried out in tubes. Some large-scale screening studies or older laboratory methods involved testing on slides, but this has not been common in the United States for quite some time. Red cell agglutination in tube tests is observed macroscopically under strong light, usually by tipping the tube over a mirror. If agglutination is not observed using this macroscopic method, some technologists prefer to pour the cell suspension onto a slide and observe the mixture under a microscope to find very weak reactions. The largest study[27] of this issue

involved more than 200,000 antibody detection tests in patients. Antibodies that necessitated antigen-typed red cells were found in only seven patients (0.02%). Therefore, microscopic observation of antibody detection tests is not necessary.

Solid-phase tests   Solid-phase assays[28–30] are usually done in microtiter plates. The target antigen is fixed to the wells of the plate and the test serum or plasma is added. Often low-ionic strength solution is also used to enhance the antibody-antigen reaction. After incubation, the plates are washed. Reagent red cells coated with antihuman globulin are added, and if antibody was present in the test serum, the reagent red cells will adhere to the plate. The reaction can be read by a technologist or an automated plate reader. This system can be used for ABO and Rh typing and for antibody detection or identification, depending on the reagent red cells used to coat the plates.

Gel test   The gel test[31,32] is based on the principle of size exclusion. The gel is dextran acrylamide particles. The tubes come prefilled with gel and the test serum and/or reagent red cells are combined at the top of the tube. The reaction mixture is incubated and then centrifuged. The centrifugation drives the red cells into the gel. If antibody is present, large red cell agglutinates form and the red cells are trapped at the top of the gel column. The gel system can be used for ABO and Rh typing, red cell antibody detection, identification, and crossmatching.

Affinity column   Affinity columns[33] take advantage of the immunologic binding of IgG to staphylococcal protein G. The columns are composed of protein G bound to agarose. Test plasma or serum is combined with reagent red cells at the top of the tube but prevented from entering the agarose. The reaction mixture is incubated and then centrifuged. If antibody binding to the red cells has occurred, the IgG-coated red cells are trapped by the G protein at the top of the column. If agglutination has not occurred, the red cells not coated with IgG travel through the column and are found at the bottom.

RED CELL COMPATIBILITY TESTING

The term compatibility or pretransfusion testing refers to all procedures involved in providing for the patient blood products that "will have acceptable survival and will not cause clinically significant destruction of the recipient's own red cells."[34] The crossmatch is only one part of the compatibility or pretransfusion test (Table 10.1). All steps from the collection of the blood sample from the patient to the release of the blood component from the blood bank are important in providing a safe and effective transfusion.

For ABO typing, the methods involve incubation of red cells and antisera at room temperature for about 5 minutes, centrifugation, and observation of the cell suspension for agglutination. This can be done because the ABO antibodies react almost immediately at room temperature. For antibody detection more complex testing is necessary. Because antibodies in patients are more dangerous clinically, the antibody detection techniques used in testing patients' serum are usually different from those used for screening donor sera. For donor antibody detection, reagent red cells are usually

Table 10.1 Key steps in compatibility testing

ABO and Rh typing of donor red cells
Testing of donor serum for red cell antibodies
Identifying the patient, acquiring, and labeling patient blood sample
Reviewing patient and donor records
ABO and Rh testing of the recipient
Testing the recipient's serum for red cell antibodies
Identifying recipient red cell antibody if present
Selecting the proper blood component
Carrying out the major crossmatch
Labeling the blood component and completing all records

Adapted from Shulman IA, Petz LD. Red cell compatibility testing: clinical significance and laboratory methods. In: Petz L, Swisher S, Kleinman S, Spence R, Strauss R, eds. Clinical Practice of Transfusion Medicine. New York: Churchill Livingstone, 1996.

pooled, and no additives or enhancement reagents are used except for antihuman globulin (see Chapter 8). For patient testing, one of the enhancing methods is often used. For instance, testing might be done using enzyme-treated reagent red cells, or the media might be enhanced using albumin, LISS, or PEG. The increments improve the likelihood of detecting weak antibodies in the patient.

The results of the antibody detection test on the patient determines the crossmatching strategy to be used. If no antibody is detected, the crossmatch need involve only a method that will detect ABO incompatibility between the donor and recipient in an effort to avoid an ABO-incompatible transfusion. The results of the antibody detection test are considered valid for 3 months unless the patient has an experience, such as pregnancy or transfusion, that could stimulate red cell antibody formation. If an antibody is detected, the antibody should be identified (see below). Once the antibody is identified, the donor units can be typed for the corresponding antigen, and those units crossmatched to ensure compatibility between donor and recipient.

Positive identification of recipient and blood sample   The most common cause of a fatal hemolytic transfusion reaction is the administration of an ABO-incompatible unit of red cells. This often happens because of errors in collecting the original blood specimen from the patient or in administering the unit of blood to the wrong patient (see Chapters 13 and 14). Because of this, the acquisition of the blood sample for compatibility testing is extremely important. The procedures and techniques for obtaining the blood sample are described in Chapter 13. Labeling of the tubes to be used for the blood sample should occur at the patient's bedside, and great care should be taken to ensure that the blood sample is being obtained from the patient whose identity is being placed on the tube. This is done by asking patients to confirm their identity; for patients who are unable to communicate, each hospital should have a procedure to ensure the proper identity of the patient from whom the sample is being obtained.

Review of transfusion service records for results of previous testing of samples from the recipient   When the request for transfusion and blood sample is received in the blood bank laboratory, the first step is a review of blood bank records to determine

whether any blood samples have been received previously and any laboratory work carried out. If so, the patient's ABO and Rh blood types should be available in the records as well as the results of the antibody screening test. If the antibody screening test was positive, the identification of the antibody will also be available. These results do not substitute for proper laboratory testing of the new blood specimen but are used for comparison with the new results. If there are discrepancies in the ABO or Rh type, this must be resolved before blood can be released for transfusion. These discrepancies suggest a mix-up or misidentification of either the earlier or the present blood specimen. Antibodies present in previous blood samples may no longer be found because of natural changes in the strength of antibody activity. However, knowledge of antibodies previously present is important, because those antibodies could be expected to reappear quickly after transfusion of antigen-positive red cells. Thus, even though the antibody may no longer be present, the patient should receive red cells that lack the corresponding antigen to avoid a delayed hemolytic transfusion reaction (see Chapter 14).

ABO and Rh typing   Many clinical conditions and diseases may make interpretation of the results of ABO and Rh typing difficult. Careful attention to detail and the proper use and interpretation of controls is essential. The ABO and Rh type of the patient is confirmed on each blood sample used for pretransfusion testing to increase the safety of the transfusion by ensuring that the sample is from the correct patient. The ABO and Rh type of the donor blood will have been confirmed when the hospital received the blood from its regional blood supplier or by duplicate typing if the hospital collects its own blood supply.

Selection of blood components of appropriate ABO and Rh types   For routine transfusions, red cells are selected that are identical with those of the patient for the ABO and Rh(D) antigens. In some situations, such as massive bleeding or an emergent need for transfusion, red cells that are not ABO and Rh(D) identical may be used (see Chapter 12). When Rh-negative patients experience massive bleeding, it may be necessary to use Rh(D)-positive blood because of unavailability of Rh-negative red cells. This decision should be made by consultation between the blood bank physician and the attending physician. If necessary, Rh-negative red cells can be given to Rh-positive patients. Since Rh-negative red cells lack the D antigen, there will be no unusual adverse effect on the Rh-positive patient.

It may also be necessary to switch ABO types. When blood of a different ABO type is used, it is used as red cells, not whole blood, to avoid problems due to transfusion of antibodies contained in the plasma. Table 10.2 indicates the different ABO types of donor blood that can be used. Despite the small amount of plasma in the red cell unit, hemolysis due to passive transfusion of antibody in these units can occur. However, this is extremely rare, and the remote likelihood of such a problem should not interfere with making red cells available rapidly in urgent situations.

Antibody Detection Test (Indirect Antiglobulin or Coombs Test)

The antibody detection or screening process for testing donor blood is described in Chapter 8. Detection of antibodies in the recipient is even more important, because anti-

Table 10.2 ABO antigens, antibodies, and donors suitable for transfusion to patients of different ABO types

Gene	ABH antigen	ABO type	Antibody present	Preferable donor	Other acceptable donors*
A	A	A	B	A	O
B	B	B	A	B	O
H	H	O	A & B	O	None
A & B	A & B	AB	None	AB	A or B or O†

*If blood is used as red blood cells.
†Group A is preferable.

bodies in the patient are generally more dangerous than those in the donor. The antibody to cell or antigen ratio is higher when the antibody is in the patient because the donor antibody if present is diluted in the patient's entire blood volume.

In the antibody detection test the patient's serum is reacted with red cells from usually two normal individuals whose cells contain antigens reactive with all of the common clinically significant antibodies. The cells are usually purchased commercially and are subject to U.S. Food and Drug Administration (FDA) requirements for the antigens they contain and their strength of reactivity. The conditions of this test usually involve incubation of the patient's serum with test red cells suspended in saline or albumin followed by washing the red cells, adding antihuman globulin, centrifuging, and looking for agglutination. There is extensive literature describing the optimum technique for detecting different antibodies. The development of cardiac surgery involving hypothermia occurred during the years when new blood group antigens and antibodies were frequently being discovered. Some of these antibodies were optimally active at temperatures below normal body temperature (see Chapter 9). Thus, techniques were added to routine pretransfusion and compatibility testing to detect antibodies reactive in the cold. However, as more experience was gained, it became clear that it is not necessary to avoid cold-reacting antibodies for patients undergoing hypothermia during routine surgery.[35] In addition, almost all of the cold antibodies detected on routine testing were not clinically significant, and this test procedure was gradually eliminated.[36] Some of the other methods that may be used include treating the red cells with enzymes, extending the length of incubation, changing the serum to cell ratio, altering the incubation temperature, suspending the red cells in low-ionic strength solution, and using chemicals such as polybrene to enhance agglutination. Some of these techniques are used routinely by some blood banks; others are suitable for use only in reference laboratories for investigation of certain antibodies. The tests can be carried out in any of the tube, gel, solid-phase, or affinity systems described above. If the patient's serum contains an IgG antibody that reacts with an antigen on the red cells used in antibody screening tests, this will be detected using the antihuman

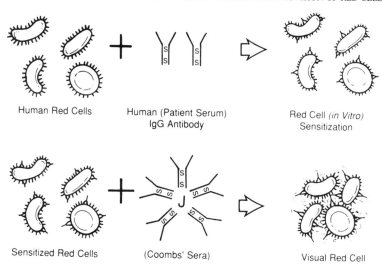

Human Red Cells   Human (Patient Serum)   Red Cell *(in Vitro)*
IgG Antibody   Sensitization

Sensitized Red Cells   (Coombs' Sera)   Visual Red Cell

Figure 10.1 Schematic illustration of crossmatch using antihuman globulin.
Source: After Harmening D. Modern blood banking and transfusion practices. Philadelphia, FA Davis, 1989.

IgG (Fig. 10.1). This is an extremely important test, since most clinically significant red cell antibodies are IgGs.

If an antibody is detected in the patient's serum, the antibody should be identified and red cells selected that lack the corresponding antigen if the antibody is clinically significant (see Chapter 9). This approach is preferable to selecting units of red cells that are compatible in a crossmatch without identifying the antibody. The antibody in the patient's serum may be too weak to react with red cells heterozygous for the antigen, and thus the crossmatch will appear to be compatible. However, transfusion of the red cells heterozygous for the antigen may result in accelerated destruction of the cells.

Crossmatch

Traditionally, the crossmatch involved testing the donor's red cells against the patient's serum in several different "phases" such as room temperature, after incubation at 37°C, and after the addition of antiglobulin serum. This group of methods was very effective in detecting all clinically significant antibodies. The reasons for failure of the system using saline and antiglobulin include weak antibodies, poorly reactive red cells, or the prozone phenomenon.[37] Experience then gradually established that the room temperature phase identified many antibodies (reactivity) that were not clinically significant.[36] Over a period of several years, the room temperature phase of testing was eliminated and the saline suspension test, along with an antiglobulin phase, was used to detect all clinically significant antibodies.

At about the same time as these methods were shifting and evolving, interest developed in using the antibody screening test more extensively instead of the crossmatch between patient's serum and donor cells.[38–41] Experience established that anti-

body screening could replace the antiglobulin phase of the crossmatch for patients in whom no antibody is detected in the antibody screening procedure.[42,43] Thus, for patients with no antibodies detected in the antibody screening test, the "crossmatch" is used to detect ABO incompatibility. This can be done with a simplified method involving a saline suspension medium and a short incubation of about 5 minutes.[42,43] It is important to allow this incubation period so that antibodies have time to react and to avoid false-negative tests due to the prozone phenomenon. Despite these shortcomings, the standard approach during the past few years has been to focus on the antibody screening procedure and, when it is negative, carry out a crossmatch designed to detect ABO incompatibility.[34]

In the major crossmatch, the recipient's serum is reacted with the intended donor's red cells, usually using a technique similar to that used in the antibody detection test. This involves incubation at 37°C and the use of antihuman globulin. Both antiglobulin reagents (polyspecific containing anti-IgG and anti-C3, or monospecific containing anti-IgG, only) are in routine use, but the detection of cell-bound C3d may lead to false-positive results, and some workers prefer to use the anti-IgG reagent. Various agents or procedural modifications may be used to attempt to enhance or speed antibody-antigen reactions. It appears that for patients in whom no antibodies are detected, a complete crossmatch is not necessary.[44] Thus, it is increasingly common to carry out a simplified crossmatch that confirms ABO compatibility if the patient has a negative antibody detection test and has not been pregnant or transfused within the preceding 3 months.[34,p. 28] However, this will not prevent the rare transfusion of an incompatible unit, since many blood group antigens of low frequency will not be present on the red cells used for antibody screening tests.

Labeling and issue of the appropriate blood products   Records of all laboratory tests should be made at the time the laboratory work is being done. At the completion of all laboratory testing, the records should be complete and the unit of red cells found to be compatible can be labeled and prepared for release for transfusion. Most blood banks today use bar code labeling systems, but whatever the nature of the label, a tag of some sort is attached to the unit. This "crossmatch tag" contains the patient's name, identification number, blood type, and the blood type and identification of the unit of red cells found to be compatible. Also, the tag contains the statement that this unit is compatible and suitable for transfusion to the specified recipient. Thus, the transfusionist can review the patient's identification, the identity of the unit of red cells, and the information on the crossmatch tag to ensure that the proper unit of red cells is being administered to the patient (see Chapter 13).

Minor Crossmatch

In the minor crossmatch, the donor's serum is reacted with the patient's red cells. This test was intended to detect antibodies in the donor that might cause hemolysis of the patient's red cells. Although a few such cases have been reported, this is very rare. The situation is now approached by carrying out an antibody detection test on the donor's serum at the time of donor blood processing. If donor antibodies are present, the unit is

either not used or the plasma is removed. Thus, the minor crossmatch is not necessary and is no longer used.

Computer Crossmatch

The next phase in the evolution of compatibility testing was the recognition that confirmation of ABO compatibility could be accomplished by methods other than laboratory tests. This led to the proposal for a "computer crossmatch."[45] In the "computer crossmatch" the laboratory test for ABO compatibility is replaced by a computer check of the records of the donor and patient. Safwenberg et al.[37] recently reported on 12 years of experience with computer crossmatches. The antibody screening methods evolved during the 12 years of data gathering. Initially the test used enzyme (bromelin)-treated reagent red cells, then an antiglobulin-phase tube test but no enzyme, and then an antiglobulin test carried out in a gel system. This represented a shift in emphasis of the screening procedure over the years from maximum sensitivity (with many false-positive reactions) to more specificity. Four different red cell suspensions were used as screening cells. The rate of alloantibody detection was about 1%. Combining all three of these antibody screening methods, the computer crossmatch system with antibody screening allowed 90% of the units to be released without a further laboratory crossmatch. There were no cases of hemolytic transfusion reactions due to failure of the system. The authors believe that the value of this approach is that it allows antibody screening to be carried out under more optimum conditions than in the crossmatch. The drawback is that the screening cells must be selected to contain the proper spectrum of antigens so that clinically significant antibodies will be detected. As the authors point out, this system will not detect a mislabeled unit, as happened once in their experience. Thus, the failure rate of the computer crossmatch in this study was 1/257,400 units.[37]

RED CELL ANTIBODY IDENTIFICATION

If the antibody screening test is positive, the antibody should be identified so that antigen-negative red cells can be selected for the crossmatch. Antibody identification is done using reagent red cells from several individuals (usually eight) selected to contain antigens corresponding to the clinically significant antibodies (Fig. 10.2). This group of reagent red cells is called a "panel." The technique used for identifying the antibody may be the same as that used for the antibody screening, or an alternative technique may be used. An alternative technique might be used because experience has established that method to be most effective locally, or because the screening test suggested a particular antibody specificity that is best demonstrated by a particular technique. It may be necessary to test the patient's serum against more than one panel or against sets of red cells especially selected to possess or lack certain antigens. In addition, since certain specific antibody-antigen reactions are known to be enhanced or inactivated by different conditions, these special tests may use techniques different from those used for antibody detection or the initial panel test. Examples of some of these special techniques are given below.

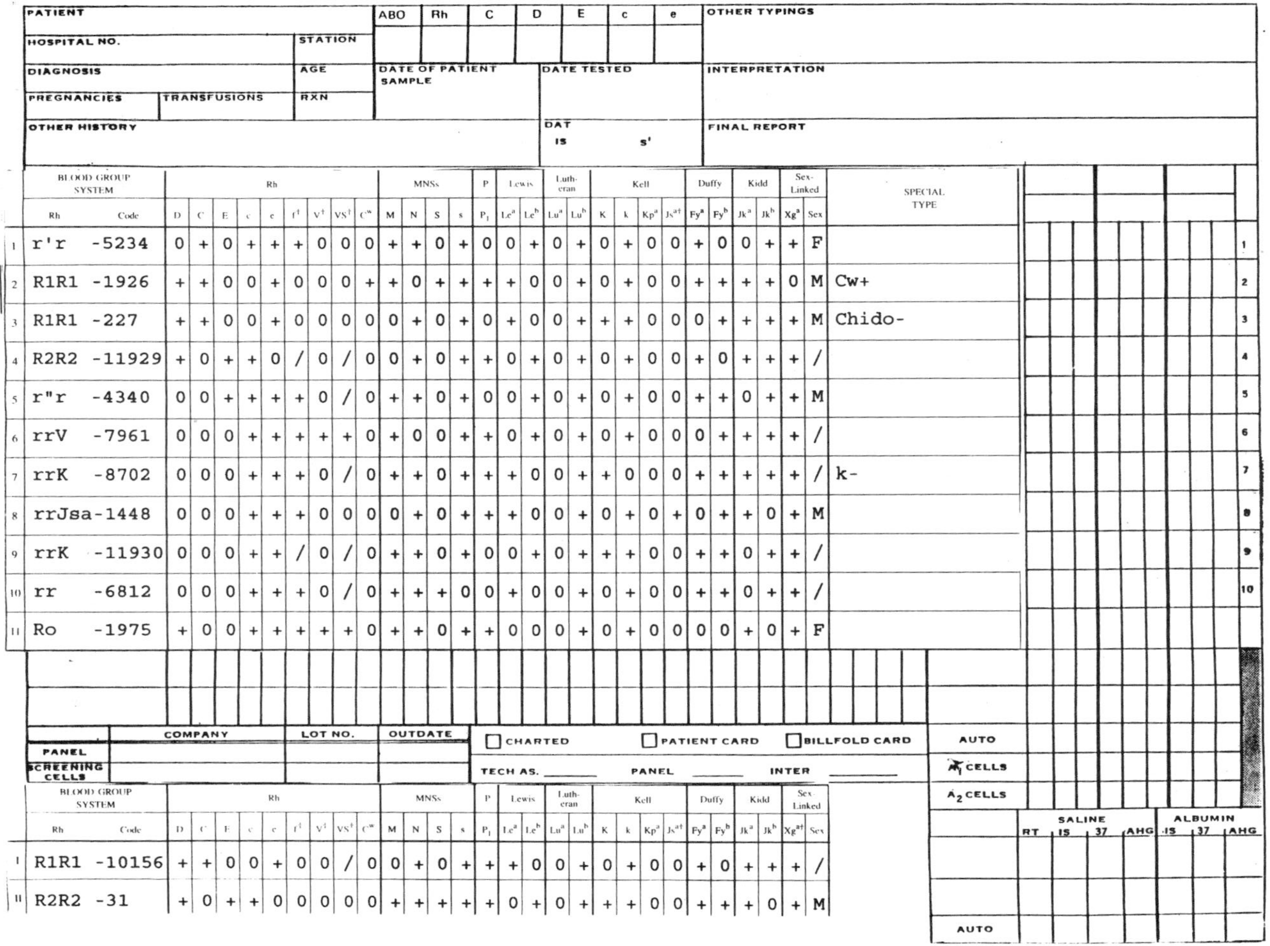

PATIENT		ABO	Rh						OTHER TYPINGS	
HOSPITAL NO.	STATION									
DIAGNOSIS	AGE		DATE OF PATIENT			DATE TESTED			INTERPRETATION	
PREGNANCIES	TRANSFUSIONS	RXN								
OTHER HISTORY						DAT			FINAL REPORT	

Panel — Blood Group System

	Rh Code	D	C	E	c	e	f(r')	r'	r"	V'	Vs'	Cʷ	M	N	S	s	P₁	Leᵃ	Leᵇ	Luᵃ	Luᵇ	K	k	Kpᵃ	Jsᵃ	Fyᵃ	Fyᵇ	Jkᵃ	Jkᵇ	Xgᵃ	Sex Linked Sex	Special Type
1	r'r -5234	0	+	0	+	+	+	+	0	0	0	0	+	+	0	+	0	0	+	0	+	0	+	0	0	0	0	0	0	+	F	
2	R1R1 -1926	+	+	0	0	+	0	0	0	0	0	+	+	0	+	+	+	+	0	0	+	0	+	0	0	+	0	+	+	0	M	Cw+
3	R1R1 -227	+	+	0	0	+	0	0	0	0	0	0	+	0	+	+	0	+	0	0	+	+	+	0	0	+	+	+	+	+	M	Chido-
4	R2R2 -11929	+	0	+	+	0	0	/	0	/	0	0	0	+	0	+	+	0	0	0	0	+	0	0	+	0	0	+	0	+	/	
5	r"r -4340	0	0	+	+	+	+	0	+	0	/	0	+	+	0	+	+	0	0	0	0	+	0	0	+	0	+	+	+	+	M	
6	rrV -7961	0	0	0	+	+	+	0	0	+	+	0	+	+	0	+	+	0	0	0	0	+	0	0	+	+	+	+	+	+	/	
7	rrK -8702	0	0	0	+	+	+	+	0	/	0	0	0	+	0	+	+	0	0	0	+	0	0	0	+	+	0	+	+	+	M	k-
8	rrJsa-1448	0	0	0	+	+	+	0	0	0	0	0	+	+	0	+	+	+	0	0	+	+	0	0	+	+	+	+	+	+	/	
9	rrK -11930	0	0	0	+	+	+	/	0	/	0	0	0	+	+	0	+	0	0	0	+	+	0	0	+	0	+	+	0	+	/	
10	rr -6812	0	0	0	+	+	+	0	0	0	0	+	+	+	+	0	0	0	0	0	+	+	0	0	+	+	0	0	0	+	/	
11	Ro -1975	+	0	0	+	+	+	+	+	+	0	0	+	+	0	+	+	0	0	0	+	0	0	+	0	0	+	+	0	+	F	

Screening Cells

	Rh Code	D	C	E	c	e	f(r')	r'	r"	V'	Vs'	Cʷ	M	N	S	s	P₁	Leᵃ	Leᵇ	Luᵃ	Luᵇ	K	k	Kpᵃ	Jsᵃ	Fyᵃ	Fyᵇ	Jkᵃ	Jkᵇ	Xgᵃ	Sex
I	R1R1 -10156	+	+	0	0	+	0	0	0	0	0	0	+	0	+	+	+	+	0	0	+	0	+	0	0	0	0	+	+	+	/
II	R2R2 -31	+	0	+	+	0	0	0	0	0	0	0	+	+	+	0	+	0	+	0	+	+	+	0	0	+	+	+	0	+	M

	SALINE		AHG	ALBUMIN		AHG
	RT	37	37	IS	37	IS

AUTO — A₁ CELLS — A₂ CELLS — AUTO

CHARTED — OUTDATE — LOT NO. — COMPANY — TECH AS. — PANEL — INTER — PATIENT CARD — BILLFOLD CARD

Figure 10.2 Example of a panel of reagent red cells used for antibody identification

Chemical Modification of Test Red Cells

Chloroquine can be used to elute IgG from red cells. This is of value in patients with a positive direct antiglobulin test. The IgG can be removed, making it possible to type the patient's red cells, which provides information about which antibodies the patient could produce. Test red cells can also be treated with dithiothreitol (DTT) to inactivate some antigens. DTT acts by disrupting sulfhydryl bonds, thus altering the tertiary structure of some antigens and rendering them less reactive. A third method of chemically treating red cells involves a reagent referred to as ZZAP. This combines the enzyme papain with DTT to inactivate Kell, MNSs, Duffy, Gerbich, and most LW, Cartwright, Dombrock and Knops antigens. This is probably a more effective way to inactivate red cell antigens than DTT alone. These strategies to inactivate certain known red cell antigens and then repeat the testing of the serum containing the unknown antibody can be a very helpful strategy for identifying red cell antibodies.

Enzymes and enhancement media   The use of enzymes to increase or decrease the reactivity of certain antigens and the use of enhancement media such as LISS, PEG, and polybrene have been described previously.

Neutralizing or inhibitor substances   Substances can be obtained commercially that inhibit certain antibody-antigen reactions. In trying to solve complex antibody problems, it may be easier to neutralize the antibody than to find a group of red cell suspensions that lack the suspected antigen. Examples of antigens for which this strategy can be used are P1, Lewis, and Chido/Rogers.

Sulfhydryl reagents for distinguishing IgG from IgM antibodies   Sulfhydryl reagents can be used to distinguish IgG from IgM antibodies.[46] DTT is most commonly used. The DTT cleaves the disulfide bonds between the subunit chains of IgM but does not affect the bonds between the monomers of IgG. This treatment of a serum containing a red cell antibody with DTT will inactivate an IgM but not an IgG antibody. This can be used conveniently in antibody identification.

Absorption   Absorption is of value primarily to remove cold-reactive antibodies that interfere with antibody identification. Absorption can be done using autologous red cells to remove cold-reactive antibody and the serum then tested at 37°C to detect warm-active alloantibodies. In patients suspected of having multiple alloantibodies, absorption can be done using allogeneic red cells selected to contain or lack specific combinations of antigens.

Elution   Elution is the process of removing bound antibody (usually IgG) from the red cell surface. This is done on red cells of patients who have a positive direct antiglobulin test. The recovered antibody in the eluate can then be identified using the same techniques that are used to test serum. Removing (eluting) bound antibody also makes it possible to type the patient's red cells to determine which antibodies the patient could form.

STRATEGIES FOR MAKING RED CELLS AVAILABLE FOR TRANSFUSION

Blood Availability

Red cell transfusions are used for replacement in chronic anemia and either controlled or uncontrolled blood loss. Transfusions for chronic anemia and controlled blood loss can be planned, and all of the steps described above can be carried out in an efficient, well-organized manner (Table 10.3). Most red cell transfusions are provided to patients who are relatively stable, and the process is uneventful and at a reasonable pace. The ABO and Rh typing, red cell antibody detection, and subsequent crossmatching, if the patient does not have any unexpected red cell antibodies, can be expected to take approximately 1 hour if other more urgent laboratory work does not interfere (Table 10.4). Thus, at best, red cells could be expected to be available within about an hour after receipt of the specimen and request forms in the blood bank. When patients experience acute blood loss, initial management is with intravenous fluids to maintain the blood volume (see Chapter 12), but there may be an urgent need for red cell replacement. For these situations, it is essential that the blood bank have policies, procedures, and systems in place to make red cells available quickly and safely. If a patient requires red cell transfusion sooner, there are several strategies that can be used to accomplish this. Each dif-

Table 10.3 Strategy for providing blood

Little Blood Loss, No Expected Transfusion
Type and screen
No antibody
No crossmatch
No blood set aside
Antibody present
Complete crossmatch
Blood set aside

Large Blood Loss, Transfusion Expected
Type and screen
No antibody
Crossmatch—ABO compatibility
Blood set aside
Antibody present
Crossmatch—complete
Blood set aside

Maximum (Standard) Surgical Blood Order
If excess blood, set aside
Increased waste
Increased costs
Anticipate number of units needed
Avoid over-ordering

Table 10.4 Time required to provide compatible RBCs in different situations

Emergency Method	Minutes
Complete compatibility test	60*
ABO, Rh type, and antibody screen	
Crossmatch	
Emergency crossmatch—previous sample	10
ABO crossmatch	
Emergency crossmatch—no previous sample	15
No crossmatch	10
ABO type specific	
No crossmatch	5
Universal donor	

*If antibody screen negative; if antibody screen is positive, time may be 120 minutes or much longer.

ferent strategy that shortens the time required to make red cells available involves eliminating some of the standard testing procedures. Because there is some possibility for increased risk of error or failure to detect red cell incompatibility, effective communication between the patient care team and the blood bank staff is essential. In this way, sound judgments can be made to balance the patient's clinical needs for urgent transfusion against the drawbacks of abbreviating the pretransfusion testing. The following sections describe the approaches to providing red cells under different conditions ranging from planned elective transfusion to the most urgent, life-threatening situations.

Standard or Maximum Surgical Blood Ordering

The amount of blood a hospital must maintain in its inventory is based on the amount ordered to be set aside (crossmatched), not the amount used. Thus, it is important to avoid ordering and sequestering excessive amounts of blood. To reduce this possibility, a structured approach to providing blood for elective surgery has developed over the last 20 years. Analysis of each hospital's blood usage for particular procedures is done to develop baseline data for that hospital. Alternatively, data is available from the literature describing the amount of expected blood use for different procedures. Based on these data, a standard or maximum amount of blood is defined for each type of surgical procedure.[47–50] This becomes the routine amount of blood that is crossmatched and set aside for a particular patient undergoing that procedure. This minimizes blood wastage by avoiding over-ordering blood and is referred to as the maximum or standard surgical blood order program.

Type and Screen

For surgical procedures in which blood is used rarely, if at all, blood is not crossmatched and sequestered for a particular patient, but instead the "type and screen" procedure is used.[41] In the type and screen, the patient's ABO and Rh blood types are deter-

mined and an antibody detection test is done. If no unexpected red cell antibodies are present and the patient is scheduled for a procedure in which blood is rarely used, no blood is set aside and no crossmatching is carried out. If the rare situation arises in which the patient requires a red cell transfusion, red cells can be provided either using the ABO crossmatch (which requires approximately 15 minutes) or, in an emergency, red cells ABO identical with the patient can be released without a crossmatch (Table 10.4). If an antibody is found in the antibody detection test, then the antibody is identified and the crossmatch technique to be used for that patient is defined. Often blood will be crossmatched and held for patients with complex antibodies in circumstances where the standard surgical blood request would not warrant this. Even though preparing blood for these patients involves additional work, it avoids the potential difficulties in making blood available quickly for patients who have red cell antibodies and for whom it may be difficult to locate red cells lacking the antigen in question and compatible in a crossmatch.

Emergency "Crossmatch"

When blood is needed urgently and a blood sample from the patient has been obtained earlier and is in the blood bank, the blood type and antibody screening result may already be known from testing of that sample. If no red cell antibody was found in the screening procedure, a unit of red cells that is ABO-identical with the patient can be selected and the ABO compatibility crossmatch can be performed in about 10 minutes.

If a blood specimen had not been obtained previously and the blood bank must determine the blood type on a new sample, this can be done within about 5 minutes and the proper ABO type unit selected and crossmatched as described above. This adds about 5 minutes to the time required, or a total of about 15 minutes for release of blood on an emergency basis. In this situation, however, an antibody screening test is not performed, and so it is possible that a red cell antibody other than ABO will be present and incompatible red cells could be transfused. When the ABO crossmatch is being set up in the laboratory, the antibody screening test will be set also. Often the antibody screening test result is known by the time the blood is released from the blood bank and transported to the patient's bedside. If an antibody is present, the blood bank technologist can telephone the patient care unit, and this information can be taken into consideration by the physician in deciding whether to continue the transfusion. Even when the antibody screening test is positive, it may be appropriate to continue the transfusion because of the patient's critical condition.

Uncrossmatched Red Cells

If red cells are needed urgently for a patient and it is not thought to be acceptable to wait approximately 10 to 15 minutes to obtain red cells that are ABO-identical with the patient and have undergone an ABO crossmatch, uncrossmatched red cells can be given. Whenever a crossmatch is not done, group O red cells are used. Usually Rh-negative red cells are selected, because the combination of O-negative red cells should avoid a hemolytic transfusion reaction to the most common clinically important red cell antibodies: anti-A or anti-B and anti-D. In the past, many hospitals attempted to main-

tain a small stock of O-negative red cells in the emergency department so that a transfusion could be started immediately. This practice is no longer used. The techniques for managing acute blood loss are much more effective today, and because the wastage of these red cells was very high, it is not practical to obtain an adequate supply of O-negative red cells for storage in emergency departments.

APPROACH TO THE PATIENT WITH AN INCOMPATIBLE CROSSMATCH

In compatibility testing when there is reactivity in the antibody detection test, serologic studies should be carried out to determine whether a red cell antibody is present. If a clinically significant antibody is identified, donor red cells typed and found to be negative for the corresponding antigen should be compatible when crossmatched. The blood bank staff will carry out these procedures and provide compatible blood, although additional time and blood samples may be necessary. For several reasons, this approach of identifying the antibody and selecting known antigen-negative red cells is preferable to merely crossmatching until compatible red cells are found. The panels used for red cell antibody identification do not represent random donors, and thus the antibody may react with a high proportion of donors, making it difficult to obtain compatible red cells. Some antibodies react in vitro only with red cells homozygous for the antigen but cause in vivo destruction of heterozygous red cells; and many sera that react in vitro do not signify potential in vivo red cell destruction. Thus, knowledge of the specificity of the red cell antibody and the character of anti-red cell reactivity improves the safety of the transfusion.

Some patients' serum reacts with many or even all of the donors tested. In this situation it is necessary to determine whether the patient has autoimmune hemolytic anemia. This is usually indicated by a positive direct antiglobulin test (DAT). The patient may or may not be anemic. The selection of blood for patients with autoimmune hemolytic anemia is discussed later. If the patient has a negative DAT and does not have autoimmune hemolytic anemia but the serum reacts with all donors' red cells tested, it must be determined whether an alloantibody is present against a high-frequency antigen or whether the reactivity is due to other non-red cell blood group factors. Examples of non-red cell blood group factors are abnormal proteins in the patient's plasma, high titers of normal cold agglutinins, and reactivity with test materials such as preservatives or antibiotics used in the test red cell suspension. If it is determined that the patient does have a high-frequency alloantibody, the clinical significance of the antibody determines whether it is preferable to obtain antigen-negative red cells. For instance, this is unnecessary for many antibodies that do not cause transfusion reactions, hemolysis, or accelerated clearance of red cells. If the alloantibody is expected to be clinically significant, most blood banks have local files of rare donors and, if necessary, national rare donor registries of the American Red Cross or American Association of Blood Banks can be contacted. In patients with a clinically significant high-frequency alloantibody, the decision as to whether to delay transfusion to obtain compatible antigen-negative red cells will depend on the patient's condition. If the patient's condition does not allow delay, an in vivo crossmatch can be done (see below). In situations where no specific antibody

has been identified, considerable emphasis has been placed on selecting the least incompatible donor units for transfusion. While it is unlikely that this is detrimental, there is no evidence that in these situations, red cells less reactive in vitro will have better survival in vivo.

IN VIVO RED CELL COMPATIBILITY TESTING

Occasionally, compatible donor red cells cannot be found either because the patient's serum contains an autoantibody that reacts with all donors' red cells or the serum contains an alloantibody against an extremely high-frequency antigen and cells lacking the antigen are not available. In these situations an "in vivo crossmatch" can be done. This involves labeling with ^{51}Cr a small volume (usually 5 mL or less) of the red cells to be transfused, injecting them, and determining the percent that survive 24 hours later.[51] In general, patients do not experience an acute hemolytic reaction if at least 85% of the donor red cells survive for 24 hours.[52] However, the 85% value should not be used as an arbitrary indication of a safe transfusion. Transfused red cells with lower 24-hour survivals in the in vivo crossmatch may have a better survival when the larger-volume transfusion is given, and occasional patients may experience severe hemolysis despite in vivo crossmatch results greater than 85%.[52] Thus, while an in vivo crossmatch may provide helpful information, it usually does not change the actual management of the patient.

LABORATORY INVESTIGATION OF POSSIBLE HEMOLYTIC DISEASE OF THE NEWBORN

Prior to approximately 1961, the red cell antibody titer and the history of the severity of affected infants in previous pregnancies were the only methods of predicting the severity of hemolytic disease of the newborn (HDN) in a present pregnancy. These measures were said to be only about 60% accurate in predicting the severity of HDN.[53] This situation was greatly improved by the development of a method for spectrophotometric analysis of amniotic fluid by Liley in 1961.[54] In this method, the amount of deviation in adsorbence of light at 450 nanometers from a line connecting the adsorbence at 350 to 700 nm is measured. This difference in adsorbence (ΔOD) measurement is then plotted on a chart based on the gestation stage of the pregnancy, and the position on the chart is used to predict the severity of HDN (Fig. 10.3). This proved to be an extremely accurate predictor of the severity of the disease.

In the late 1970s, ultrasound techniques became available for fetal assessment. This technique can make the diagnosis of fetal hydrops but not of impending hydrops. More recently, fetal umbilical blood sampling has been added to the ultrasound procedure.[55] This is the most accurate and effective means of determining the severity of HDN, because complete blood counts and other blood chemistry determinations can be made on these blood samples.

About 2 years after Liley introduced the technique for measuring amniotic fluid spectrophotometrically and predicting the severity of HDN, he reported a technique to

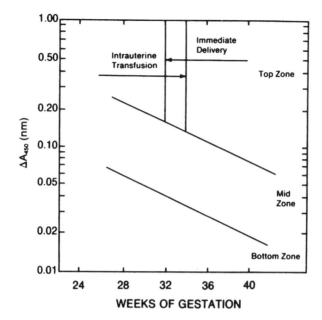

Reproduced with permission from reference 54.

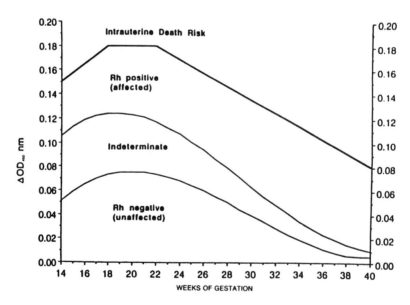

Figure 10.3 Liley graph. *(Source: Technical Manual, 12th ed. Bethesda, MD: American Association of Blood Banks, 1996:466–467.)*

Reproduced from Queenan JT, Tomai TP, ural SH, King JC. Deviation in amniotic fluid optical density at a wavelength of 45nm in Rh-immunized pregnancies from 14-40 weeks' gestation: a proposal for clinical management AM. J. Obstet Gynecol 1993,168:1370-1376.

Table 10.5 Steps in the evaluation of potential HDN

Type mother to be sure she is Rh negative
Type father to determine if he is Rh positive
Carry out antibody screening
    If the antibody screening test is positive, identify the antibody
    Titer the antibody
Repeat the titer at 16 to 18 weeks' gestation
If the titer rises or reaches a level beyond the acceptable limit, amniocentesis is indicated

transfuse severely affected infants.[56] The ultrasound visualization is used to guide a needle into the fetal peritoneal cavity, where the blood is transfused. This intraperitoneal transfusion procedure carried a general mortality of about 7% but greatly improved the prognosis for the most severely affected fetuses. More recently, with the introduction of fetal blood sampling techniques, it has become possible to provide direct intravascular transfusions to the fetus.[57]

The recommended approach to the diagnosis of HDN is briefly outlined in Table 10.5. After determining that the mother is Rh negative, it must be determined whether the father is Rh positive and whether the mother is already immunized. If an antibody is present, the titer is determined as a baseline for comparison of future samples. Another titer is obtained at about 16 to 18 weeks, because no treatment will be initiated before then. The subsequent titer is compared with the initial titer. Each laboratory establishes its own guidelines for significance of change in titers. Often an increase of two dilutions or a value of 1:16 are used, but these must be determined locally. If the titer changes more than that locally acceptable, then amniocentesis or fetal blood sampling are performed.

PLATELET COMPATIBILITY

Selection of ABO and Rh Type for Platelet Transfusion

ABO antigens are adsorbed onto the surface of the platelet and the recovery of A_1 platelets transfused into group O patients is decreased.[58] In patients with lymphocytotoxic antibodies against donor cells, the increment in peripheral blood platelet count has been reported to be the same[59] or reduced[60,61] following transfusion of HLA-matched ABO-incompatible platelets. Although the clinical importance of the ABO effect is not known, it is advisable to transfuse ABO-compatible platelets.[62] If ABO-compatible platelets are not available, ABO-incompatible platelets should be used rather than withholding platelet transfusion.

Incompatibility between the platelet donor plasma and recipient red cells usually is not clinically important because of the small volume of plasma (50 mL) from each individual platelet concentrate. If large numbers of platelet concentrates are being transfused to an adult or the patient is a small child, incompatible donor plasma may cause a positive direct antiglobulin test and red cell hemolysis (e.g., type O plasma contains anti-A and may react with a type A recipient's red cells). When ABO-compatible platelets are unavailable, consideration may be given to removing some plasma from

the platelet concentrate before transfusion or to selecting the platelet ABO type so that ABO-compatible plasma rather than compatible platelets is given. Red cell cross-matching is not necessary prior to platelet transfusion because the platelet concentrate usually contains about 0.5 mL of red cells.

Rh antigens are not found on platelets. However, patients may become immunized to Rh antigens from the red cells contaminating the platelet concentrate. The risk of forming anti-Rh(D) was first reported to be approximately 8% after 80 to 110 units of platelets.[63] However, a subsequent study showed no evidence of sensitization in 30 Rh-negative patients after extensive transfusion support with Rh-positive platelets.[64] In a more recent review of 73 Rh-negative oncology patients, nine (12%) became immunized to the D antigen after receiving a mean of 102 mL of Rh-positive red cells through platelet and granulocyte transfusions.[65] Because of the life-threatening nature of most cases of thrombocytopenia, platelets from Rh-positive donors can be administered to Rh-negative recipients. However, Rh-negative women of childbearing age with a non-malignant disease should not receive platelet concentrates from Rh-positive donors because of the effect of possible anti-Rh on future pregnancy. If Rh-positive platelets are given to such a patient, Rh immunization can be prevented by the administration of Rh immune globulin.

Rh-positive platelets have a normal survival in recipients with anti-Rh(D);[66] thus, the only concern is a possible transfusion reaction to Rh-positive red cells contained in the platelet concentrate. If the platelet concentrates are properly prepared, red blood cell contamination is 0.5 mL or less per unit, and thus a significant red cell hemolytic reaction would not be expected, even in a recipient with a preformed anti-Rh(D) antibody.

If an Rh-negative patient receives Rh-positive platelets, it may be desirable to attempt to prevent immunization. This can be done by giving the patient Rh immune globulin. Since one standard dose (1 mL) of Rh immune globulin will prevent immunization from up to 15 mL of Rh-positive red cells,[67] this should cover about 25 units of platelets (25 units × 0.5 mL = 12.5 mL red cells).

Red Cell Compatibility Testing for Platelet Transfusion

Compatibility testing is not usually done for platelet transfusions because of the small red cell content of the platelet concentrate. However, platelets also contain HLA antigens and platelet-specific antigens. Some patients may develop antibodies to these antigens following transfusion, pregnancy, or organ transplantation. When this occurs, transfused platelets have a decreased recovery and a shortened intravascular survival. These transfused platelets are therefore less effective in controlling hemorrhage. The management of these patients is discussed in Chapter 11.

GRANULOCYTE COMPATIBILITY

Compatibility Testing for Granulocyte Transfusion

Each granulocyte concentrate contains approximately 20 mL of red cells, and thus red cell compatibility testing must be done (see also Chapter 11). HLA and granulocyte antibodies can interfere with the ability of transfused granulocytes to circulate and

localize at sites of inflammation.[68] This problem could be overcome by carrying out leukocyte compatibility testing. However, technical problems make it impractical to do a leukocyte crossmatch of the patient's serum and donor's cells on the day of transfusion. Donors are usually selected by periodically screening the patient's serum against multiple granulocyte donors. Lack of an effective method of ensuring granulocyte compatibility is a major factor in the limited effectiveness of granulocyte transfusion.

REFERENCES

1. Petz LD, Swisher SN, eds. Clinical Practice of Transfusion Medicine, 2nd ed. New York: Churchill Livingstone, 1989.
2. Technical Manual, 12th ed. Bethesda, MD: American Association of Blood Banks, 1996.
3. Coombs RRA, Mourant AE, Race RR. A new test for the detection of weak and "incomplete" Rh agglutinins. Br J Exp Pathol 1945;26:225.
4. Stratton F. Complement in immunohematology. Transfusion 1965;5:211–215.
5. Mollison PL. Annotation—the role of complement in antibody-mediated red-cell destruction. Br J Haematol 1970;18:249–255.
6. Dacie JV, Crookston JH, Christenson WN. "Incomplete" cold antibodies: role of complement in sensitization to antiglobulin serum by potentially haemolytic antibodies. Br J Haematol 1957;3:77–87.
7. Sherwood GK, Haynes BF, Rosse WF. Hemolytic transfusion reactions caused by failure of commercial antiglobulin reagents to detect complement. Transfusion 1976;16:417.
8. Petz LD, Garratty G. Antiglobulin sera—past, present and future. Transfusion 1978;18:257.
9. Petz LD, Branch DR, Garratty G, et al. The significance of the anticomplement component of antiglobulin serum (AGS) in compatibility testing. Transfusion 1981;21:633.
10. Wright MS, Issitt PD. Anticomplement and the indirect antiglobulin test. Transfusion 1979;19:688–694.
11. Issitt PD, Issitt CH, Wilkinson SL. Evaluation of commercial antiglobulin sera over a two-year period. Part I. Anti-beta 1A, anti-alpha 2D, and anti-beta 1E levels. Transfusion 1974;14:93–108.
12. Garratty G, Petz LD. An evaluation of commercial antiglobulin sera with particular reference to their anticomplement properties. Transfusion 1971;11:79–88.
13. Milam JD. Laboratory medicine parameter—utilizing monospecific antihuman globulin to test blood-group compatibility. Am J Clin Pathol 1995;104:122–125.
14. Low B, Messeter L. Antiglobulin test in low-ionic strength salt solution for rapid antibody screening and crossmatching. Vox Sang 1974;26:53–61.
15. Elliot M, et al. Effect of ionic strength on the serologic behavior of red cell isoantibodies. Vox Sang 1964;9:396–414.
16. Moore HC, Mollison PL. Use of a low-ionic strength medium in manual tests for antibody detection. Transfusion 1976;16:291–296.
17. Wicker B, Wallas CH. A comparison of a low ionic strength saline medium with routine methods for antibody detection. Transfusion 1976;16:469–472.
18. Svoboda RK, Hafleigh EB, Grumet FC. LISS technique without room temperature phase: extensive transfusion service experience. Presented at the 31st Annual Meeting of the American Association of Blood Banks, New Orleans, LA, 1978.
19. Lalezari P, Jiang AF. The manual Polybrene test: a simple and rapid procedure for detection of red cell antibodies. Transfusion 1980;20:206–211.
20. Steane EA, Steane SM, Montgomery SR, Pearson JR. A proposal for compatibility testing incorporating the manual hexadimethrine bromide (Polybrene) test. Transfusion 1985; 25:540–44.
21. Fisher GA. Use of the manual Polybrene test in the routine hospital laboratory. Transfusion 1983;23:152–154.
22. Nance SJ, Garratty G. A new potentiator of red blood cell antigen-antibody reactions. Am J Clin Pathol 1987;87:63–65.
23. Wenz B, Apuzzo J. Polyethylene glycol improves the indirect antiglobulin test. Transfusion 1989;29:218–220.

24. DeMan AJ, Overbeeke MA. Evaluation of the polyethylene glycol antiglobulin test for detection of red blood cell antibodies. Vox Sang 1990;58:207–210.
25. Slater JL, Griswold DJ, Wojtyniak LS, Reisling MJ. Evaluation of the polyethylene glycol-indirect antiglobulin test for routine compatibility testing. Transfusion 1989;29:686–688.
26. Shirey RS, Boyd JS, Ness PM. Polyethylene glycol versus low-ionic-strength solution in pretransfusion testing: a blinded comparison study. Transfusion 1994;34:368–370.
27. Shulman IA. Controversies in red blood cell compatibility testing. In: Nance SJ, ed. Immune Destruction of Red Blood Cells. Arlington, VA: American Association of Blood Banks, 1989:171.
28. Plapp FV, Sinor LT, Rachel JM, Beck ML, Coenen WM, Bayer WL. A solid phase antibody screen. Am J Clin Pathol 1984;81:719–721.
29. Rachel JM, Sinor LT, Beck ML, Plapp FV. A solid-phase antiglobulin test. Transfusion 1985;25:224–226.
30. Sinor L. Advances in solid-phase red cell adherence methods and transfusion serology. Transfus Med Rev 1992;6:26–31.
31. Lapierre Y, Rigal D, Adam J, et al. The gel test: a new way to detect red cell antigen-antibody reactions. Transfusion 1990;30:109–113.
32. Malyska H, Weiland D. The gel test. Lab Med 1994;25:81–85.
33. Bjorck L, Kronvall GP. Purification and some properties of streptococcal protein G, a novel IgG-binding reagent. J Immunol 1984;133:969–974.
34. Standards for Blood Banks and Transfusion Services, 16th ed. Bethesda, MD: American Association of Blood Banks, 1994.
35. Schmidt PJ. Cold agglutinins and hypothermia. Arch Intern Med 1985;145:578. Letter.
36. Giblett ER. Blood group alloantibodies: an assessment of some laboratory practices. Transfusion 1977;17:299.
37. Safwenberg J, Hogman CF, Cassemar B. Computerized delivery control—a useful and safe complement to the type and screen compatibility testing. Vox Sang 1997;72:162–168.
38. Oberman HA, Barnes BA, Steiner EA. Role of the crossmatch in testing for serologic incompatibility. Transfusion 1982; 22:12–16.
39. Judd WJ. Are there better ways than the crossmatch to demonstrate ABO incompatibility? Transfusion 1991;31:192–194.
40. Napier JAF. Clinical annotation. The crossmatch. Br J Haematol 1991;78:1–4.
41. Boral LI, Henry JB. The type and screen: a safe alternative and supplement in selected surgical procedures. Transfusion 1977;17:163–168.
42. Heddle NM, O'Hoski P, Singer J, et al. A prospective study to determine the safety of omitting the antiglobulin crossmatch from pretransfusion testing. Br J Haematol 1992;81:579–584.
43. Pinkerton PH, Coovadia AS, Goldstein J. Frequency of delayed hemolytic transfusion reactions following antibody screening and immediate-spin crossmatch. Transfusion 1992;32:814–817.
44. Shulman IA, Nelson JM, Saxena S, et al. Experience with routine use of an abbreviated crossmatch. Am J Clin Pathol 1984;82:178.
45. Butch SH, Judd WJ, Steiner EA, Stoe M, Oberman HA. Electronic verification of donor-recipient compatibility: the computer crossmatch. Transfusion 1994;34:105–109.
46. Olson PR, Weiblen BJ, O'Leary JJ, Moscowitz AJ, McCullough J. A simple technique for the inactivation of IgM antibodies using dithiothreitol. Vox Sang 1976;30:149–159.
47. Friedman BA, Oberman HA, Chadwick AR, Kingdon KI. The maximum surgical blood order schedule and surgical blood use in the United States. Transfusion 1976;16:380–387.
48. Boyd PR, Sheedy KC, Henry JB. Use and effectiveness in elective surgery. Am J Clin Pathol 1980;73:694–699.
49. Mintz PD, Lauenstein K, Hume J, Henry JB. Expected hemotherapy in elective surgery. JAMA 1978;239:623–625.
50. Boral LI, Dannemiller FJ, Standard W, et al. A guideline for anticipated blood usage during elective surgical procedures. Am J Clin Pathol 1979;71:680–684.
51. International Committee for Standardization in Hematology. Recommended method for radioisotope red cell survival studies. Br J Haematol 1980;45:659.
52. Silvergleid AJ, Wells RP, Hafleigh EB, et al. Compatibility test using 51Cr-labeled red blood cells in crossmatched positive patients. Transfusion 1978;18:8.

53. Bowman JM, Pollock JM. Amniotic fluid spectrophotometry and early delivery in the management of erythroblastosis fetalis. Pediatrics 1965;35:815.

54. Liley AW. Liquor amnii analysis in the management of pregnancy complicated by rhesus immunization. Am J Obstet Gynecol 1961;82:1359–1370.

55. Daffos F, Capella-Pavlovsky M, Forestier F. Fetal blood sampling during pregnancy with use of a needle guided by ultrasound: a study of 606 consecutive cases. Am J Obstet Gynecol 1985;153:655.

56. Liley AW. Intrauterine transfusion of fetus in hemolytic disease. Br Med J 1963;2:1107.

57. Berkowitz RL, Chikara U, Goldberg JD, et al. Intrauterine intravascular transfusions for severe red blood cell isoimmunization: ultrasound guided percutaneous approach. Am J Obstet Gynecol 1986;155:574.

58. Aster R. Effect of anticoagulant and ABO incompatibility on recovery of transfused human platelets. Blood 1965;26:732.

59. Lohrman HP, Bull MI, Decter JA, et al. Platelet transfusions from HLA compatible unrelated donors to alloimmunized patients. Ann Intern Med 1974;80:9.

60. Duquesnoy RJ, Anderson AJ, Tomasulo PA, Aster RH. ABO compatibility and platelet transfusions of alloimmunized thrombocytopenic patients. Blood 1979;54:595–599.

61. Heal JM, Singal S, Sardisco E, Mayer T. Bacterial proliferation in platelet concentrates. Transfusion 1986;26:388–390.

62. Murphy S. ABO blood groups and platelet transfusion. Transfusion 1988;28:401.

63. Goldfinger D. McGinnis MH. Rh incompatible platelet transfusions—risks and consequences of sensitizing immunosuppressed patients. N Engl J Med 1971;284:942.

64. Lichtiger B, Surgeon J, Rhorer S. Rh-incompatible platelet transfusion therapy in cancer patients. Vox Sang 1983;45:139.

65. Baldwin ML, Ness PM, Scott D, et al. Alloimmunization to D antigen and HLA in D-negative immunosuppressed oncology patients. Transfusion 1988;28:330–333.

66. Pfisterer H, Thierfelder S, Kottusch H. Untersuchung menschlicher thrombocyten auf rhesus-antigen durch abbaustudien in vivo nach 51Cr-markierung. Klin Wochenschr 1967;45:519.

67. Pollack W, Ascari WQ, Kochesky RJ, et al. Studies on Rh prophylaxis. I. Relationship between doses of anti-Rh and size of antigenic stimulus. Transfusion 1971;11:333.

68. McCullough J, Clay M, Hurd D, Richards K, Ludvigsen C, Forstrom L. Effect of leukocyte antibodies and HLA matching on the intravascular recovery, survival and tissue localization of 111-indium granulocytes. Blood 1986;67:522.

CLINICAL USES OF BLOOD COMPONENTS

BLOOD COMPONENT THERAPY

The development of the closed plastic container system made it possible to separate blood into several of its components (see Chapters 1 and 5). As this plastic container technology was becoming available, it also became apparent that transfusion therapy was much more complicated than merely replacing the volume of shed blood with an equal volume of bank blood. A wide variety of patient situations emerged in which optimum transfusion medicine involved replacing only some components of the blood and, in some situations, replacing these components in ratios not ordinarily found in whole blood. This formed the basis of blood component therapy, in which specific parts or components of the blood are isolated, stored under conditions optimum for that component, and transfused to patients who need that specific component. This is accepted common transfusion medicine practice today, as illustrated in the discussions in the remainder of this chapter and also in Chapter 12.

TRANSFUSION OF COMPONENTS CONTAINING RED BLOOD CELLS

Physiology in Red Cell Transfusion Decisions

In the early 1900s, it was observed that surgical patients with hemoglobin levels less than 10 g/dL did poorly.[1] Mayo Clinic[2] surgeons who were studying anemia and oxygen transport recommended that a hemoglobin level of 8 to 10 g/dL be achieved prior to surgery. Although this original recommendation involved a range, the 10 g/dL became accepted in surgical practice and remained so for the next 40 years.[3] During the 1980s,

Table 11.1 Physiologic responses to anemia

Increased cardiac output
Decreased peripheral vascular resistance
Increased red blood cell release of oxygen
Increased heart rate, stroke volume, and contractility
Decreased blood viscosity

Source: Carson JL. Morbidity risk assessment in the surgically anemic patient. Am J Surg 1995;170:32S–36S.

with the development of invasive monitoring techniques, considerable advances were made in the understanding of oxygen delivery (D_{O_2}) and oxygen consumption (V_{O_2}). Also, as patient management techniques improved, it became increasingly clear that patients could survive with much lower hemoglobin concentrations than were previously believed to be possible. Thus, the indications for transfusion began to change. In considering these changes, it is helpful to briefly review the physiology of oxygenation of tissues and organs.

In response to anemia, several compensatory mechanisms increase oxygen delivery. These include a rightward shift of the oxyhemoglobin dissociation curve when the hemoglobin falls below 9.9 g/dL;[4] decreased peripheral vascular resistance due to the decrease in blood viscosity; and increased heart rate, cardiac stroke volume, and contractility, resulting in increased cardiac output when the hemoglobin falls below 8 to 10 g/dL[5–7] (Table 11.1). Coronary artery disease, congestive heart failure, pulmonary disease, peripheral vascular disease, and medications that affect the heart's ability to increase cardiac output (e.g., beta blockers) reduce the body's ability to compensate for anemia. Several measures have been proposed as indications for transfusion, including the hemoglobin level, the oxygen extraction ratio, the mixed venous partial pressure of oxygen ($P\bar{v}_{O_2}$), and mixed venous oxygen saturation ($S\bar{v}_{O_2}$). Others have suggested that the indications for transfusion should be based on both clinical and physiologic factors. These could include tachycardia, hypotension, oliguria, $S\bar{v}_{O_2}$ <60%, and $P\bar{v}_{O_2}$ <30 mm of mercury.[7] Thus, it is unlikely that a single hemoglobin value is adequate as an indicator for transfusion. Based on the work done during the 1980s and 1990s, an NIH consensus conference concluded than in addition to the hemoglobin, the patient's age, surgical procedure, diagnosis, presence of complicating factors such as those described above, anticipated volume of blood loss, and the cause of the anemia should be considered.[8] Most patients with hemoglobin concentrations of 10 g/dL or greater do not require transfusion, and most patients with a hemoglobin level less than 7 g/dL will benefit from transfusion.[8] Another set of suggested indications for red cell transfusion is shown in Table 11.2.[9] All of this experience indicates that red cells should not be transfused simply to increase the hemoglobin concentration unless there is a clinically defined need to improve oxygen availability. The management of acute blood loss is discussed in Chapter 12, but the most important principle is that blood volume should be restored first using volume expanders, not red cells. The indications of the need for red cell transfusion to provide increased oxygen availability are a combination of clinical and physiologic indicators as described above.

Table 11.2 Proposed clinical indicators for red cell transfusion

6 g/dL:	Patients with well-compensated chronic anemia; healthy (American Society of Anesthesiologists [ASA] Class I and some Class II) patients undergoing intentional hemodilution; and patients undergoing hypothermic cardiopulmonary bypass
8 g/dL:	Most postoperative coronary artery bypass graft patients, but not those with left ventricular hypertrophy, incomplete coronary revascularization, low cardiac output, poorly controlled tachycardia, or sustained fever
10 g/dL:	Patients whose cardiac output is unlikely to increase, with symptomatic cerebrovascular disease, or over age 65

Source: Robertie PG, Gravlee GP. Safe limits of isovolemic hemodilution and recommendations for erythrocyte transfusion. Int Anesthesiol Clin 1990;28:197–204.

Clinical Uses of Red Cells

The most common reason for transfusion is replacement of red cells for oxygen-carrying capacity. The need for increased oxygen delivery may arise due to acute blood loss or chronic anemia. Because of the heterogeneity of patients and clinical situations, there is no single standard indication for red cell transfusion. In deciding whether a patient requires red cell transfusion, the clinical condition of the patient is of primary importance; patients should not be transfused based only on their hemoglobin level.

Restoration of blood volume in acute blood loss   When there is sudden acute blood loss, the major threat to the patient is the loss of intravascular volume and resultant cardiovascular collapse. The amount of blood loss that can be tolerated without replacement depends on the condition of the patient (see Chapter 12). An otherwise healthy individual can tolerate the loss of up to half of the red cell mass without need for replacement.[10] The few studies that deal with the physiology of blood loss and the indications for red cell transfusion have been done in normal animals or essentially healthy humans. In most "normal" patients the loss of approximately 1,000 mL of blood can be replaced by colloid or crystalloid solutions alone.[11,12] However, the indications for transfusion in patients with cardiac disease, coronary atherosclerosis, or other vascular insufficiency are not known. Because many patients have some degree of cardiovascular compromise, they will require red cell replacement after smaller volumes of blood loss. The decision to transfuse red cells must take into consideration the patient's overall condition. If blood loss is judged sufficient to require transfusion, it is not necessary to wait until symptoms such as pallor, diaphoresis, tachycardia, or hypotension develop. Transfusion is with the standard red blood cell component from the stock supply of the blood bank.

Improvement of oxygen-carrying capacity   When anemia has developed over a long period of time, the patient adjusts to lower hemoglobin levels and may not require transfusion despite a very low hemoglobin level. There is no evidence that it is necessary to transfuse a patient to a "normal" hemoglobin prior to surgery,[8] nor is there any specific

hemoglobin value above which patients feel better or have better wound healing. In patients with chronic anemia, transfusion should be used only as a last resort, since it may suppress erythropoiesis.

Transfusion in preparation for surgery   It has become the custom of most anesthesiologists and surgeons to transfuse patients when the hemoglobin is 10 g/dL or less. There are no scientific or well-described clinical data to support this practice. It appears that many patients would not be at risk if transfusion was withheld until the hemoglobin was less than 7 g/dL.[8] In baboons subject to normovolemic anemia (exchange transfusion using dextran for replacement of red cells), death occurs at hematocrit levels of about 5%.[8,13,14] This decline in hemoglobin was accompanied by a linear decrease in mixed venous oxygen tension, an increase in extraction of oxygen from the red cells, and an increase in cardiac output, allowing oxygen consumption to remain unchanged until the hematocrit fell to 10% or less.[8] The authors concluded that the normal heart has a remarkable capacity to adjust to acute normovolemic anemia and suggested that most patients should not receive a transfusion unless the hemoglobin is 7 g/dL or less. Few patients, especially those with normal cardiac function, would require transfusions at hemoglobin levels of 10 g/dL. Transfusion to patients with hemoglobin between 7 and 10 g/dL should be based on clinical assessment of the particular patient.[13,14]

Uses of Specific Red Blood Cell Components

Red blood cells   Red cells are the component of choice for any patient with severe anemia. Most patients who require red cell replacement do not also need intravascular volume replacement. In patients who do need both intravascular volume and red cell replacement, crystalloid or colloid solutions, not human plasma, are the preferred solutions for intravascular volume replacement. These latter solutions have few, if any, adverse effects and their use allows the plasma from the original unit of whole blood to be used for the production of coagulation factor concentrate. Thus, almost all transfusions given for red cell replacement are red cells.

Whole blood   Whole blood is rarely used. Virtually all blood collected in the United States is separated into its components, and these are used for specific situations (see below and Acute Blood Loss in Chapter 12). Shed blood can be replaced with mixtures of separate components such as red cells and crystalloid or colloid solutions.

Leukocyte-depleted red cells   Multiparous women and patients who receive multiple transfusions may develop antibodies to leukocytes and platelets. These antibodies may be involved in many different clinical situations (Table 11.3) (see also Chapter 9). Because some of these situations are rather common, and others can be fatal, there is considerable interest in strategies for preventing alloimmunization to platelets and leukocytes and for avoiding the complications caused by immunization. The preparation of leukocyte-depleted components and the clinical situations in which these components are used are also described in other sections of this book (see Chapters 5, 12, and 14).

Table 11.3 Clinical situations involving leukocyte or platelet antibodies

Antibody	Clinical problem
Leukocytes	Acute graft rejection
	Inability to obtain compatible organ
	Rejection of transplanted marrow
	Febrile nonhemolytic transfusion reaction
	Poor response to granulocyte transfusion
Granulocytes	Refractoriness to platelet transfusion
	Alloimmune neonatal neutropenia
	Transfusion-related acute lung injury
	Febrile nonhemolytic transfusion reaction
	Poor response to granulocyte transfusion
Platelets	Refractoriness to platelet transfusion
	Alloimmune neonatal thrombocytopenia

When patients with leukocyte antibodies receive blood containing incompatible leukocytes, febrile transfusion reactions may occur[15] (see Chapter 14). These leukocyte reactions do not cause red blood cell hemolysis but can be extremely uncomfortable for the patient and are potentially fatal. Symptoms such as chills, fever, headache, malaise, nausea, vomiting, and chest or back pain may persist for up to 8 hours[16] and seem to be caused by immune damage to donor granulocytes. The frequency and severity of leukocyte transfusion reactions is directly related to the number of incompatible leukocytes transfused.[17] Therefore, leukocyte-depleted red cells are indicated for patients who have repeated febrile transfusions reactions.

Leukocyte-depleted red cells can be prepared by centrifuging an ordinary unit of red cells, by washing or freezing the red cells, or by filtering them (Table 11.4) (see Chapter 5). In the distant past, centrifugation, washing, and freezing were commonly used to prepare leukocyte-depleted red cells. Early versions of filters removed only granulocytes,[18] thus leaving about 25% to 35% of the leukocytes. About 15 years ago, filters were developed to remove microaggregates from citrated blood. When combined with centrifugation and cooling, this removed about 90% of the leukocytes from a unit of red cells while allowing routine collection and storage times and conditions.[19,20] This degree of leukocyte depletion is adequate to prevent most febrile transfusion reactions due to recipient antibodies reacting with donor leukocytes.[19,20] This remains a satisfactory approach today for the prevention of febrile nonhemolytic transfusion reactions.

Additional improvements have been made in blood filters during the past decade. The filters currently available remove more than 99% of the leukocytes, do not require priming, and allow high flow rates (see Chapter 5). These filters are effective in preventing alloimmunization and refractoriness to platelet transfusion (see Prevention of Alloimmunization and Platelet Refractoriness) and transmission of cytomegalovirus (see Cytomegalovirus-Safe Blood Components). Because of these advantages, the filters are becoming widely used and thus are readily available for use in patients who

Table 11.4 General comparison of methods of preparing leukocyte-depleted red cells for transfusion

Method	White cells removed (%)	Approximate no. WBCs remaining	Original red cells remaining (%)	Comment
Centrifugation	85	1×10^9	80	Product may contain dextran or hydroxyethyl starch; 24-h storage
Sedimentation (dextran)	95	0.9×10^9	90	24-h storage; product may contain dextran or hydroxyethyl starch
Freezing deglycerolizing	98	0.1×10^9	90	24-h storage
Washing	85	0.1×10^9	85	24-h storage
Spin cool filter	90	0.3×10^9	90	24-h storage
Nylon filter	65	1.5×10^9	88	Heparin required; 24-h storage
New-generation filters*	99	5×10^6	95	Bedside use

Source: McCullough J. Transfusion medicine. In: Handin RI, Lux SE, Stossel TP, eds. Blood—Principles & Practice of Hematology. Philadelphia: J.B. Lippincott, 1995:1947–2006.
*Refers to general results from several different manufacturers' filters that have become available during the late 1980s.

experience febrile transfusion reactions. Blood filtration is now the major and almost the only form of leukodepleted red cells in use. Because the filters remove about 99.9% of the leukocytes from the units of red cells or platelets, filtered red cells are effective in preventing febrile transfusion reactions[21-24] (see also Chapter 14). To summarize, the indications for leukodepleted red cells are as follows:

1. Prevention of alloimmunization to leukocytes and platelets
2. Prevention of transmission of cytomegalovirus
3. Treatment of patients with multiple febrile transfusion reactions
4. Prevention of immunomodulatory effects of transfusion

The kinds of patients who should receive leukodepleted red cells are those in whom the above factors are of potential concern. These include any patient with a disease potentially treated by marrow transplantation and those who will receive multiple transfusions during their life such as hemoglobinopathies. A specific suggested list of such patients is provided in Table 11.5.

Leukocyte-depleted red cells can be prepared by filtration in the blood bank laboratory soon after collection (prestorage filtration), in the blood bank immediately before

Table 11.5 Clinical situations in which leukodepleted red cells are recommended

---

Bone marrow or peripheral blood stem cell transplantation
Acute leukemia
Chronic leukemia
Congenital platelet function abnormalities
Congenital immune deficiency syndrome
Hematologic malignancies potentially treated with stem cell transplantation
Solid tumors potentially treated with stem cell transplantation
Intrauterine transfusions
Exchange transfusion for HDN
Hemoglobinopathy or thalassemia

---

transfusion (poststorage filtration), or at the bedside while the red cells are being transfused (bedside filtration). The advantages and disadvantages of each of these methods is discussed more fully in Chapter 5. While the proportion of leukodepleted units remains small, prestorage strategies require special orders to obtain the units from the supplier or the maintenance of a dual inventory in the hospital. Thus, bedside or blood bank filtration immediately before transfusion are the most common methods currently used. The bedside method is simple and is the most widely used today but may not provide the desired reproducibility.[25] The prestorage method may become more widely used as the number of leukocyte-depleted units increases.

Washed red cells   Washed red cells are composed of red cells suspended in an electrolyte solution (Table 11.4); most plasma, platelets, and leukocytes have been removed, although leukocyte removal is not as complete as with frozen deglycerolized red cells. After washing, the storage period is 24 hours because the washing has been carried out in an open system. Thus, washed cells are used only for specific indications and are not practical for the general inventory. Because the major advantage is the removal of the plasma by washing, washed red cells are indicated for patients who have reactions caused by plasma. For instance, patients with IgA deficiency can have severe, often fatal, anaphylactic reactions when exposed to plasma containing IgA (see Chapter 14). Although washed red cells have been used to prevent febrile reactions due to transfused leukocytes, the availability of high-efficiency filters for leukocyte removal eliminates this indication by providing another blood component with more extensive leukocyte depletion.

Frozen deglycerolized red blood cells   Frozen deglycerolized red cells are composed of essentially pure red cells suspended in an electrolyte solution (Table 11.4). Most of the plasma, platelets, and leukocytes have been removed by the washing step necessary to remove the glycerol cryoprotectant. Thus, the deglycerolized red cells have a 24-hour storage period, which is a major factor in the logistics of their use. The most important value of frozen red cells is that they can be stored for years, thus allowing development of a depot of red cells of rare types or for storage of autologous red cells. They have been used in the past as a leukocyte-poor red cell component instead of centrifuged,

filtered, or washed red cells. However, these uses are no longer recommended because of the availability of high-efficiency filters that provide a more leukodepleted component at lower cost and without a reduced storage period. There is no advantage of frozen red cells over washed red cells for patients who have reactions to plasma, because both components undergo a washing step that removes virtually all of the plasma.

Because of the extensive washing, there has been speculation that frozen deglycerolized red cells may have no risk of transmitting viruses such as hepatitis, HIV, or cytomegalovirus. One study[26] indicates that this may be true for cytomegalovirus. However, it would be preferable to see data confirming that frozen deglycerolized red cells have no risk of cytomegalovirus transmission before accepting this as established. Because more extensive and convincing data are available regarding the effectiveness of red cells leukodepleted by filtration in preventing CMV transmission, there is no reason to use frozen deglycerolized red cells for this purpose.

Effects of Red Blood Cell Transfusion

Circulation   When a unit of red cells or whole blood is transfused rapidly (within 30 to 60 minutes) to a patient with a normal blood volume, the blood volume is increased by the volume of the component. If the volume of blood transfused is very large or the patient has compromised cardiovascular function, the central venous pressure may increase. In most patients the intravascular volume remains about 10% above pretransfusion levels after 24 and even 48 hours.[27] Thus, patients who receive large volumes of blood or in whom cardiovascular function is compromised must be monitored for the effects of transfusion. If plasma alone is transfused, the blood volume may readjust more rapidly, returning to normal in 24 hours and often in only a few hours.[28] Some patients, such as those with chronic renal disease, may require prolonged periods to readjust their blood volume.[27]

Hemoglobin concentration   The effects of red blood cell transfusion on the recipient's hemoglobin concentration and hematocrit will be affected by the recipient's blood volume, pretransfusion hemoglobin level, clinical condition (stable, bleeding, etc.), and by the hemoglobin content of the donor unit. The rate of shift of water from the intravascular space and reequilibration of the intravascular volume will determine when after transfusion the hemoglobin value will reflect the new equilibrium. Because plasma may take up to 24 hours to exit the intravascular space, the new hemoglobin value may not be established until that time. The projected increase in hemoglobin concentration can be estimated. For instance, a hypothetical patient with a blood volume of 5,000 mL and hemoglobin concentration of 8 g/100 mL has a total of 400 g of hemoglobin. If a unit of red cells containing 60 g of hemoglobin (200 mL of red cells with hemoglobin of 30 g/dL and 100 mL of suspension medium) is transfused, the blood volume becomes 5,300, the total hemoglobin 460 g, and the hemoglobin concentration 8.7 g/dL. If the patient is able to readjust the blood volume to baseline levels within 24 hours, the result will be a 5,000 mL blood volume, 460 g of total hemoglobin, and a hemoglobin concentration of 9.2 g/dL.

Red cell production   It has been observed for many years that following transfusion to stable anemic patients, the hemoglobin returns to pretransfusion levels sooner than would be expected based on the life span of the transfused red cells.[27] In addition, there is a decrease in the reticulocyte count. Intentional transfusion programs for patients with thalassemia or sickle cell disease result in suppression of red cell production. Thus, transfusion of red cells results in a decrease in the recipient's red cell production rate, probably due to suppression of erythropoietin production as a result of the increased red cell mass.[27, p. 121] Thus, patients with a stable chronic anemia may receive less than the expected benefit from red cell transfusion, or the benefits may not be as long lasting as expected, since the patients' hemoglobin may fall to pretransfusion levels due to diminished production of their own red cells and the clearance of the transfused cells.

Survival of transfused red blood cells   The normal red cell has a life span of approximately 120 days. This is reflected after transfusion in the fact that approximately 1% of the donor cells are lost each day.[27] Each unit of blood contains red cells of all ages between 1 and 120 days. As the unit of blood is stored, the red cells continue to age, and the senescent red cells are removed from the circulation within 24 hours after transfusion. Thus, when stored blood is transfused, there is a slight decrease in the proportion of red cells surviving 24 hours after transfusion depending on the length of time the blood has been stored. For instance, approximately 80% of red cells stored in the anticoagulant AS-1 (Adsol) for 42 days survive following transfusion. These red cells then survive normally and are destroyed linearly with a mean half-life of 50 to 60 days.[27, p. 135] The survival of transfused red cells is also affected by the recipient's health and may be decreased in patients with active bleeding (and iatrogenic blood loss), hemolytic anemia due to defects extrinsic to the red cells (autoantibodies, hypersplenism), and chronic renal or liver failure.[27]

Immune System

It has been known since the 1970s that patients who received red cell transfusions experienced better renal graft survival than nontransfused patients.[29] This indicated that transfusion was associated with an immunomodulatory effect. Many studies during the past decade have suggested that this immunomodulatory effect may influence the rate of postoperative infection and the likelihood of cancer recurrence. A large number of studies have not resolved this issue.[30] At least one study has indicated that transfusion increases the likelihood of recurrence of malignancies of the colon,[31] while other studies have not found an effect of transfusion.[32,33] Similarly, there are studies showing that transfusion increases the likelihood of postoperative infection[34–37] and those finding no effect.[38] In animals and humans there is reason to believe that the immunomodulatory effect, if one exists, is due to the leukocytes contained in the transfusion components. Thus, interest has focused on the potential value of leukocyte-depleted components in preventing the immunomodulatory effect. The largest and most recent study of postoperative infection was a well-designed, controlled comparison of ordinary red cells compared to leukocyte-depleted red cells.[39] In that study, red cells depleted of leukocytes by

two different methods were both associated with higher rates of postoperative infection than no transfusions. Because of the clinical importance of this issue and the present confusing state of data, Blajchman called for a reanalysis of available data and a consensus conference to attempt to resolve this matter.[40] Although it seems likely that transfusion does cause an immune effect, the data are not yet adequate to recommend routine use of leukodepleted blood components for this purpose.

Leukocyte-Depleted Red Cells for Prevention of Graft versus Host Disease

Because there is no in vitro test to establish a patient's susceptibility for graft versus host disease (GVHD), nor is there a known threshold of leukocyte dose that will cause GVHD, leukocyte depletion is not an acceptable method for preventing transfusion-associated GVHD.

Bacterial Contamination of Units

Although some filters may remove some bacteria from units of whole blood,[41–48] there are many variables that can affect this situation. These include the type of filter, specific organism and their number, time of filtration, and conditions of filtration. Thus, filtration and leukodepletion should not be considered routine methods for removal of bacteria from contaminated units.

TRANSFUSION OF COMPONENTS AND DERIVATIVES CONTAINING COAGULATION FACTORS

Therapeutic agents containing coagulation factors can be prepared either from units of whole blood or from plasma by large-scale fractionation (see Chapter 5). The whole blood-derived components that can be used to replace coagulation factors are fresh frozen plasma, plasma, and cryoprecipitate. Plasma-derived products are factor VIII, factor IX, and antithrombin III (AT III) concentrates. Fibrin sealant or glue can be prepared either from units of whole blood or on a large scale from pools of plasma. In considering the use of coagulation components, it is convenient to separate situations requiring replacement of multiple factors from those requiring an isolated component.

Deficiency of Multiple Coagulation Factors

Prothrombin-complex deficiency The most common combination deficiency of coagulation factors involves those dependent on vitamin K for synthesis. This usually occurs as a result of liver disease or warfarin therapy. This type of coagulation disorder is best managed by treating the underlying condition with or without vitamin K administration. However, the coagulation factors can be replaced using plasma of any age, since these coagulation factors do not deteriorate during storage of whole blood

between 1°C and 6°C (see Chapter 5). Commercial concentrates containing factor IX (II, VII, IX, X) complex should not be used to replace an acquired deficiency of multiple factors because of the high hepatitis risk of these concentrates.[49]

Massive Transfusion

Bleeding due to multiple coagulation factor deficiency can occur in massive transfusion as a result of dilution of coagulation factors. Since virtually all red cell components today contain little plasma, deficiencies of multiple coagulation factors may develop in massive transfusion. Management of this situation is described more fully in Chapter 12, but if coagulation factor replacement is necessary in these patients fresh frozen plasma is usually used. Patients undergoing massive transfusion may also develop disseminated intravascular coagulation (DIC) due to the severity of the underlying problem. Thus, a bleeding diathesis may develop that is a combination of the dilutional coagulopathy of massive transfusion and the "consumption coagulopathy" of DIC.

Disseminated Intravascular Coagulation

Treatment of the underlying cause of the DIC is essential; without it, transfusion of blood components merely adds more substrate for the coagulation process. In mild forms of DIC, transfusion is usually not necessary. However, in the more extreme forms of disseminated intravascular coagulation, there is usually a deficiency of factors V and VIII, fibrinogen, and platelets. Replacement of coagulation factors in the management of DIC should be based on laboratory abnormalities and not on arbitrary formulas. When replacement is necessary, usually fresh frozen plasma is used to replace all factors.

Deficiency of Factor VIII

It is beyond the scope of this book to describe the management of patients with hemophilia A or congenital factor VIII deficiency. A brief description of the available products containing factor VIII and their use is presented. Factor VIII can be replaced with cryoprecipitate, fresh frozen plasma, or a number of factor VIII concentrates. With its discovery in the 1960s, cryoprecipitate became the mainstay of treatment for hemophilia A. Today, cryoprecipitate is used very little because of the availability of factor VIII concentrates.

The following approach can be used to determine the dose of different components. One unit of factor VIII equals the factor VIII activity of 1 mL of fresh normal pooled plasma. Factor VIII levels are usually reported as a percentage of normal. The intravascular recovery of factor VIII is close to 100%, so the amount of factor VIII required to achieve a specified factor VIII level can be estimated as follows:

Weight (kg) $\times$ 70 mL/kg = blood volume (mL) (adults)

Blood volume (mL) $\times$ (1 $-$ hematocrit) = plasma volume (mL)

Plasma volume (mL) $\times$ (desired factor VIII level % $-$ initial factor VIII %) = units factor VIII required

Example: To raise the factor VIII level to 50% in a 70-kg patient with a hematocrit of 40% and a factor VIII level of 0%:

$$70 \text{ kg} \times 70 \text{ mL/kg} = 4,900 \text{ mL}$$
$$4900 \text{ mL} \times (1 - .40) = 2,940 \text{ mL}$$
$$2,940 \text{ mL} \times .5 = 1,470 \text{ units}$$

If factor VIII concentrate is to be used, the number of units will be known from the manufacturer's quality control tests and vial labels. Thus the number of vials needed can be determined. If cryoprecipitate is to be used, each bag of cryoprecipitate contains about 100 units of factor VIII; thus in the above example 15 bags of cryoprecipitate will be required.

In cases where the initial factor VIII level is not known, it can be assumed to be 0% in a patient with severe classic hemophilia A. Since factor VIII is almost entirely intravascular, it can be assumed that virtually all of the injected factor VIII will be recovered. The half-life of factor VIII after transfusion is 8 to 12 hours, so it is usually necessary to repeat the factor VIII transfusion at 8- to 12-hour intervals to maintain hemostatic levels. Some hemophiliacs may have an inhibitor that causes a shortened half-life of factor VIII after transfusion. The calculations described above provide an estimate of the factor VIII level attained immediately after transfusion, and the dosage should be adjusted so that the minimum desired level is reached just prior to the next transfusion.

Example: If the desired minimum factor VIII level is 30% and the half-life of factor VIII is 12 hours, it is necessary to elevate the patient's initial factor VIII to 60% so that the level just before the next dose will be 30%. From the example above, the patient's plasma volume is 2,940 mL. The units required to elevate factor VIII to 60% are 2,940 mL $\times$ (60 − 0) or 1,764 units. Twelve hours later, half of the factor VIII remains, thus the factor VIII level is 30%. For the next dose of factor VIII, 2,940 $\times$ (.60 − .30) or only 882 units are required to elevate factor VIII to 60%. Once the dose of factor VIII is determined, the amount of cryoprecipitate or factor VIII concentrate necessary can be calculated easily. The duration of treatment with factor VIII depends on the type and location of the hemorrhage and the clinical response of the patient. Depending on the reason for administration of factor VIII, the dose may range from 25 to 50 units/kg, providing blood levels of factor VIII of 30% to 80%.[50]

Deficiency of Factor IX

Isolated inherited deficiency of factor IX (hemophilia B) is clinically similar to hemophilia A. Factor IX is stable in plasma when stored at 4°C or at −20°C. Thus, stored blood, liquid plasma, or fresh frozen plasma can be used to replace factor IX. However, it is difficult to replace large amounts of factor IX because of the volume of these components. Within the last few years, commercial preparations containing concentrated factor IX have become available and can be used when large amounts of factor IX must be administered. Factor IX is available in one of three forms: factor IX, factor IX complex (II, VII, IX, X), and activated factor IX complex. The approach to use of factor IX

is similar to that of factor VIII, except that since factor IX is distributed predominantly in the extravascular space, most of the injected dose will not be assayable in the blood. Recommended doses range from 15 to 40 units/kg depending on the clinical situation being managed.[50] The dose of factor IX must be repeated about every 12 hours as for factor VIII. In contrast to factor VIII concentrates, hepatitis is a major risk of transfusion of some factor IX concentrates.[49]

Hypofibrinogenemia

Hypofibrinogenemia may occur as an isolated inherited deficiency or may be associated with obstetric complications, disseminated intravascular coagulation, and some forms of cancer. In acquired hypofibrinogenemia, treatment should be directed toward the underlying cause of the disease rather than toward replacement of fibrinogen. Many physicians provide fibrinogen replacement during correction of the underlying disorder. Usually a fibrinogen level of 50 mg/dL will prevent spontaneous hemorrhage, and 100 mg/dL allows adequate hemostasis following trauma or surgery.[51] Cryoprecipitate is usually used as the source of fibrinogen for replacement therapy.[52] The dose of fibrinogen can be determined by either of the following methods: 100 mg fibrinogen per kilogram of body weight will raise the fibrinogen above 100 mg/dL;[51] or one bag of cryoprecipitate per 200 mL plasma volume will increase the fibrinogen to 100 mg/dL. Each bag of cryoprecipitate from a single donor contains approximately 200 mg of fibrinogen. The dose of fibrinogen for an adult is 6,000 to 8,000 mg, although this varies depending on the patient's fibrinogen level. Thus, usually about 30 bags of cryoprecipitate would be used. If cryoprecipitate is used as a source of fibrinogen, a quality-control program should be established by the blood bank so that its fibrinogen content will be known.

von Willebrand's Disease

Cryoprecipitate contains a substantial amount of the von Willebrand's factor from the original unit of blood. When replacement therapy is needed for these patients, multiple units of cryoprecipitate can be pooled. The usual dose of cryoprecipitate is one bag of cryoprecipitate per 10 kg body weight repeated every 8 hours.

Transfusion Techniques and Blood Group Compatibility of Components Used to Replace Coagulation Factors

In the transfusion of plasma components, procedures of patient and blood component identification, venipuncture, infusion solutions, and the use of filters are the same as those described for red blood cell transfusion (see Chapter 13). Since serious reactions may occur during the transfusion of plasma components, the attendant should obtain the patient's vital signs before initiating transfusion. The patient should be reevaluated approximately 15 minutes later to ensure that the transfusion is proceeding uneventfully and should be evaluated at the end of the transfusion to determine whether any adverse reaction has occurred. The rate of administration should be as rapid as possible but

depends on the patient's ability to tolerate the volume being transfused. Usually a unit of plasma with a volume of about 200 mL can be given in 30 minutes. Fresh frozen plasma need not be ABO identical but should be compatible with the recipient's red cells and can be given without regard to Rh type. Red cell compatibility testing is not necessary.

Cryoprecipitate should also be administered as ABO compatible. Although the volume of each unit is small, most therapy involves many units, and thus the total volume of plasma may be large. Cryoprecipitate can be administered without regard to Rh type. While compatibility testing is not necessary, ABO-incompatible cryoprecipitate and commercial concentrated preparations of factor VIII contain anti-A and anti-B, which may cause a positive direct antiglobulin test[53] and/or a hemolytic anemia if massive doses are administered. In addition, the recipient's fibrinogen may become elevated by the fibrinogen contained in cryoprecipitate if many units are given to patients who are not hypofibrinogenemic.

TRANSFUSION OF PLATELETS

The development of platelet therapy in transfusion medicine is described in Chapter 1, and the laboratory methods for the preparation of platelets and the production of platelets by apheresis are described in Chapters 5 and 7. Platelet transfusion therapy has made major contributions to the care of a variety of patients. Platelets may be transfused either to prevent bleeding (prophylactic) or to treat active bleeding. The decision whether to transfuse platelets depends on the clinical condition of the patient, the cause of the thrombocytopenia, the platelet count, and the functional ability of the patient's own platelets. The responses to platelet transfusion vary, and the strategies to deal with patients who fail to respond are complex. Most platelets are transfused to patients with transient thrombocytopenia due to chemotherapy for malignancy, including bone marrow transplantation.[54] Most platelet transfusions are used for the prevention of bleeding rather than the treatment of active bleeding (Table 11.6).

Prevention of Bleeding (Prophylaxis)

Hemorrhage has been the major cause of death in patients with bone marrow failure.[55] There is little risk of serious spontaneous hemorrhage when the platelet count is more than 20,000/μL, but the risk increases with lower platelet counts[56] Because of ethical concerns, very few controlled studies of prophylactic platelet transfusion were carried out when platelet therapy first became available. Several studies supported the use of prophylactic transfusions,[57–59] but other studies were not able to show a benefit of prophylactic platelet transfusion.[60,61] Despite the lack of substantial convincing clinical trial data, it became common practice for physicians to use platelet transfusions to prevent serious bleeding when the platelet count was less than 20,000/μL[54]

In an effort to better quantitate the risks of thrombocytopenia, occult blood loss in the stools was quantitated using chromium 51-labeled red cells in patients with different degrees of thrombocytopenia.[62] In stable thrombocytopenic patients, there was no increase in stool blood loss at platelet counts of 10,000/μL, and blood loss increased

Table 11.6 Situations in which platelet transfusion may be necessary

Decreased Production
Chemotherapy
Aplastic anemia
Irradiation
Increased Destruction
Disseminated intravascular coagulation
Thrombotic thrombocytopenia purpura
Cavernous hemangioma
Autoimmune thrombocytopenia
Drug-induced immune thrombocytopenia
Neonatal alloimmune thrombocytopenia
Dilution
Massive transfusion
Platelet Dysfunction
Exposure to certain drugs
Congenital platelet defects (name)
Damage due to extracorporeal devices
Extracorporeal membrane oxygenator
Cardiopulmonary bypass instruments
Metabolic effects
Uremia

Source: McCullough J. Transfusion medicine. In: Handin RI, Lux SE, Stossel TP, eds. Blood: Principles & practice of hematology. Philadelphia: J.B. Lippincott Company, 1995:1947–2006.

only when the platelet count reached 5,000/μL[62] During the late 1970s and 1980s considerable experience was gained in the management of thrombocytopenic patients, and this led to improvements in their outcome. Experience began to accumulate showing that patients could be maintained at platelet counts much lower than was previously believed to be possible. Serious bleeding usually occurred only when the platelet count was below 10,000/μL[63] and fatal bleeding is unlikely to occur at platelet counts above 5,000/μL[63–65] Gmur et al.[66] found that the threshold for prophylactic platelet transfusion could be 5,000/μL in uncomplicated patients, 10,000/μL in patients with fever or bleeding, and 20,000/μL in patients with coagulopathy or lesions. Based on analysis of 196 patients with acute leukemia, Aderka[65] proposed that prophylactic platelet transfusion was not necessary when the platelet count is greater than 10,000/μL. An NIH Consensus Conference recommended that the 20,000/μL value traditionally used for prophylactic platelet transfusion could be safely lowered for many patients.[67] A more recent summary of the data and recommendation by a prominent hematologist[68] began a major shift downward in the indications for prophylactic platelet transfusion. Now many physicians and hospital guidelines use platelet counts of 10,000 or 5,000/μL as the indication for transfusion to uncomplicated patients.

The usual dose of platelets in a prophylactic platelet transfusion is 1 unit per 10 kg patient weight per day. There is no evidence that use of large doses of platelets prophylactically to maintain the platelet count at higher levels is necessary. Some patients with stable but low platelet counts such as those with aplastic anemia or autoimmune thrombocytopenia have little evidence of bleeding and do not require prophylactic platelet transfusions at all.[62] The potential use of platelet growth factors to produce high-dose platelet concentrates may change platelet transfusion strategies (see Chapter 17).

Treatment of active bleeding   When considering platelet transfusion in a bleeding patient, data relating the bleeding time to the platelet count is helpful. With platelet counts below 100,000/μL, the bleeding time is increasingly prolonged, although it is only slightly prolonged when the platelet count is above 75,000/μL. Thus, platelet transfusions are not necessary for bleeding patients with a platelet count greater than 100,000/μL because they have a normal bleeding time.[69] The optimum platelet count to achieve in a bleeding patient is not known. In one study[70] of patients with platelet counts less than 100,000/μL and undergoing surgery, prophylactic platelet transfusions were given to those whose platelet count was less than 50,000/μL. Bleeding was similar in patients with counts less than 50,000/μL who received platelet transfusion and in those whose platelet count was greater than 50,000/μL but did not receive platelet transfusion. The bleeding did not relate to the platelet count but instead to the severity of the surgical procedure. Thus, platelet transfusion should be considered in actively bleeding patients with a platelet count less than approximately 50,000/μL. An attempt to achieve a level greater than 50,000/μL is recommended. If the patient's platelets are dysfunctional, such as due to drugs or uremia, the bleeding time may be much longer than would be expected based on the degree of thrombocytopenia. In such situations the decision to give a platelet transfusion is made on clinical grounds alone.

In patients with autoimmune thrombocytopenic purpura, the bleeding time also is prolonged when the platelet count is less than 100,000/μL[69] Spontaneous bleeding is not common in spite of the level of thrombocytopenia, possibly because the few platelets circulating are young and provide a shorter bleeding time than would be expected for that degree of thrombocytopenia.[69] These patients have platelet autoantibodies, and thus transfused platelets usually have a very short survival and limited effectiveness. Platelet transfusion may be effective in controlling serious active bleeding (e.g., during surgery), but is not recommended for prevention of bleeding. In patients with drug-induced immune thrombocytopenia, the offending drug should be discontinued and the patient closely observed. Because transfused platelets will have shortened survival, they are recommended in these cases only for treatment of severe thrombocytopenia with active hemorrhage.

Outcome of Platelet Transfusion

There is a dose-response effect from platelet transfusion.[71,72] Within 1 hour after transfusion, the platelet count increases by approximately 10,000/μL when 1×10^{11} platelets are transfused into a 70-kg patient.[72,73] Since a platelet concentrate usually

contains approximately 0.7×10^{11} platelets, this should cause a platelet count increase of 5,000 to 10,000/μL in an average-sized adult. Thus, in an adult with 1.8m^2 body surface area, if it is desired to elevate the platelet count from 5,000 to 40,000/μL, seven units of platelet concentrate would be required ([40,000 − 5,000] ÷ 5,000 = 7). Another, simpler way to determine the dose of platelets is to give one platelet concentrate per 10 kg of body weight. This should increase the platelet count by approximately 40,000/μL. The 1-hour posttransfusion platelet count is an excellent predictor of an effective platelet transfusion.[73] If a very accurate determination of the response to platelet transfusion is needed, the 1-hour corrected count increment or the percent recovery can be determined. Today, the corrected count increment (CCI) is most commonly used. The CCI is calculated as follows:

$$CCI = \frac{(\text{Posttransfusion} - \text{Pretransfusion Platelet Count}) \times (\text{Body Surface Area})}{\text{No. of Platelets Transfused}}$$

The expected CCI is about 15,000/mL $\times$ 10^{11} platelets transfused per square meter of body surface area. If the CCI is less than 5,000 to 7,500, the patient is considered to be refractory. If platelet recovery is used as an indicator, the expected result is about 65%, because some of the platelets normally are sequestered in the spleen.

ABO and Rh in Platelet Transfusion

It appears that ABO antigens are on platelets. These antigens consist of type II chains intrinsic to the platelet and type I chains representing the soluble ABH antigens normally found in plasma and adsorbed onto the surface of the platelet.[74] More than 30 years ago, it was shown that when ^{51}Cr-labeled group A platelets were transfused to normal group O volunteers, the recovery was reduced to one-third of that occurring following ABO-compatible transfusions.[75] The higher the ABO isoagglutinin titers, the greater the reduction in recovery of transfused platelets. This ABO effect was later substantiated clinically in several studies. Duquesnoy[76] reported a 23% reduction in recovery when platelets from HLA-matched donors were transfused to alloimmunized patients who were ABO incompatible with the donor platelets. Skogen et al.[77] reported two group O patients who were refractory to platelets transfused from group A donors but not from platelets transfused from group O donors. Heal et al.[78] reported a 41% decrease in the recovery of A- or B-incompatible platelets compared to ABO-compatible platelets transfused to HLA-matched refractory patients. Similar observations were also reported by Brand et al.[79] Ogasawara et al.[80] also reported a patient in whom there was a poor response to some but not all ABO-incompatible platelets. The transfusions providing a poor response were from donors with high expression of A or B antigens. All of these studies substantiate the concept that if platelets containing ABH antigens are transfused into patients with circulating antibody directed against those antigens, the intravascular recovery of the transfused platelets is substantially decreased. However, another aspect of platelet ABO incompatibility makes this situation even more interesting. Heal et al.[78] also observed an 18% decreased recovery of transfused platelets when the incompatibility involved transfusion of ABO antibody directed against the recipi-

ent's ABO antigens (e.g., group O platelets transfused to a group A patient). Recent studies have suggested a possible mechanism for the pathophysiology of ABO incompatibility as it affects response to platelet transfusion. It is postulated that the ABO effect is due to the formation of circulating immune complexes by soluble ABO substance and ABO antibodies.[81] This can occur with the antigen-antibody complexes from either donor or recipient antibody and donor or recipient ABO substance. Thus, the reduced platelet recovery due to circulating immune complexes can occur when the ABO incompatibility is either the "major" or "minor" type.[81]

The results of the Duquesnoy study[76] have been interpreted by some to mean that ABO incompatibility need not be considered in platelet transfusion. However, the specific conclusions of those authors dealt with whether ABO incompatibility should preclude the use of ABO-incompatible HLA-matched platelets for refractory patients. They concluded that, although there was a definite effect of ABO incompatibility in reducing posttransfusion survival, this was not of a magnitude that would contraindicate transfusion of ABO-mismatched but HLA-matched platelets. The emphasis, however, was on the overriding value of HLA matching but that ABO incompatibility definitely reduced the effect of the transfusion. Thus, although there has been some skepticism, it now seems clear that ABO incompatibility is associated with reduced posttransfusion platelet recovery.[75–85]

A separate consideration involving the ABO system and platelet transfusion is the potential administration of large volumes of ABO-incompatible plasma if transfusions involve "minor" incompatibility (e.g., group O platelets transfused to a group A patient). As described above, it appears that this may reduce the survival of the transfused platelets, but another concern is the potential for hemolysis when large amounts of ABO-incompatible antibody are transfused. This has been reported,[86,87] and it is now common to limit the volume of ABO-incompatible plasma a patient can receive. This can be in terms of a percentage of the patient's estimated blood volume or an absolute volume limit. For instance, we limit adults to no more than 1 liter of ABO-incompatible plasma per week. It is recognized that a rare unit may have a very high titer, but this approach seems to be satisfactory.

Rh antigens are not present on the platelet surface. However, the few red cells contained in the platelet concentrate can lead to immunization, and thus Rh must be considered in platelet transfusion. In Rh-negative oncology patients, reported rates of immunization to the D antigen range from 0% to 18%.[88–91] Because oncology and bone marrow transplant patients receive a large number of platelet transfusions, it is usually not possible to provide all Rh-negative platelets for Rh-negative patients. Thus, it is common to provide platelets to these patients without regard to Rh type. $Rh_o(D)$ immune globulin (RhIG) is not administered to prevent alloimmunization. Even when patients develop circulating anti-D, this antibody does not interfere with the circulation of Rh(D)-positive platelets.[92] Rh-negative platelets are recommended for patients who can be expected to receive only a few platelet transfusions and who may have long-term survival with the potential to become pregnant in the future. Examples of such patients are women of childbearing age undergoing cardiovascular or orthopedic surgery or experiencing acute trauma or complications of pregnancy. If Rh-negative platelets are not available, transfusion should not be delayed. Instead, RhIG can be administered to

prevent alloimmunization. The dose of RhIG can be determined from the number of units of platelets that patient receives. For instance, since most therapeutic doses of platelets (e.g., one single donor unit, or six pooled random donor units) contain less than 1 mL of red cells (see Chapter 5), one standard dose of 300 μg of RhIG is sufficient.

Lack of Response to Platelet Transfusion (Refractoriness)

Many patients do not attain the expected posttransfusion increment in platelet count; these patients are said to be "refractory" to platelet transfusion. This is one of the major problems in platelet transfusion. Refractoriness to platelet transfusion can be caused by many factors, some related to the patient and some related to the platelet concentrate. Another way of categorizing the reasons for refractoriness is immune versus nonimmune factors. It is often difficult to separate these, but in one study nonimmune factors were present alone in 67% of patients and coexisted with immune factors in an additional 21% of patients.[93]

Factors related to the patient   In patients who have platelet antibodies, such as those with autoimmune thrombocytopenic purpura or patients who are immunized to antigens of the HLA system, survival of circulating platelets is extremely brief, sometimes only a matter of minutes.[61] Splenomegaly also causes sequestration of platelets and a reduced posttransfusion increment.[94] In a careful study of 941 platelet transfusions to 133 patients, Bishop et al.[95] found the following factors were associated with a poor response to platelet transfusion: disseminated intravascular coagulopathy, amphotericin administration, palpable spleen, presence of HLA antibody, presence of platelet antibody, status after marrow transplantation, and fever (Table 11.7). Active bleeding was previously thought to be associated with a reduced response to platelet transfusion; however, this was not found to be true in Bishop's study. Thus, patients can be refractory because of alloimmunization (HLA and/or platelet antibodies) or nonimmune factors. The exact proportions of refractory patients resulting from alloimmunization and nonimmune factors is not known. In some studies, refractoriness is clearly associated

Table 11.7 Clinical factors associated with a reduced response to platelet transfusion

Disseminated intravascular coagulation
Fever
Amphotericin receipt
Palpable spleen
HLA antibodies
Platelet-specific antibodies
Marrow transplant

Source: Bishop JF, McGrath K, Wolf MM, et al. Clinical factors influencing the efficacy of pooled platelet transfusions. Blood 1988;71:383.

with the presence of HLA antibodies,[73,96] although there is not a generally accepted laboratory test that defines with high precision refractoriness due to alloimmunization. However, many of these patients also have one or more clinical factors present that could account at least partly for the refractoriness. Thus, in practice it is very difficult to determine whether a patient is refractory due to immune or nonimmune factors, and this affects the strategy used to manage these patients.

In the past the incidence of refractoriness was rather high. In one study, about 38% of patients who received multiple platelet transfusions (such as those with acute leukemia or undergoing bone marrow transplantation) become refractory to platelets.[97] This occurred after approximately nine transfusions involving 61 units of platelets. It appears that patients who become refractory do so after relatively few transfusions, and some patients do not become refractory regardless of the number of transfusions.[97] However, the incidence of platelet refractoriness seems to be changing. In a more recent study of newly diagnosed acute myelogenous leukemia patients, only about 15% became refractory after the first 8 weeks of therapy.[98] This may be a result of changing transfusion practices (described under Prevention of Alloimmunization and Platelet Refractoriness, below).

Factors related to the platelet concentrate: ABO antigens   ABO incompatibility may reduce the intravascular recovery and survival of transfused platelets. This is discussed in detail above. Therefore, patients who are refractory to platelet transfusion should receive a trial of at least two ABO-identical platelet transfusions.

Factors related to the platelets: age of the platelets   Another cause of reduced recovery of transfused platelets is the transfusion of platelets near the end of their storage period. Lazarus et al.[99] demonstrated that platelets stored for longer than 24 hours provided a substantially reduced posttransfusion increment. Although there are not extensive data on this topic, it is generally accepted that platelets near the end of their 5-day storage period may provide less of an increment than fresh platelets; therefore, in determining whether a patient is refractory, at least one transfusion of platelets about 24 hours old should be provided.

Strategies for Managing Patients Refractory to Platelet Transfusion

HLA matching for platelet transfusion   If the use of ABO-matched platelets of approximately 24 hours' storage fails to produce a satisfactory increment, efforts should be made to use platelets that are matched to the recipient. During the 1960s it was observed that in refractory patients, platelets from HLA-identical siblings provided a good response.[100] Later it was shown that HLA-identical platelets from unrelated donors were also beneficial.[101] This still provided matched platelets for only a limited number of patients because of the small chance of finding an HLA-identical donor in the random population. The use of HLA-matched platelets became practical when it was shown that good responses could be obtained when the donor platelets were only partially matched.[102–104] Many blood banks have large files of HLA-typed volunteer

donors so that HLA-matched platelets can be located for most patients. However, most HLA-matched platelets obtained from unrelated donors have some antigens mismatched with the patient. Although the average response to these partially matched transfusions is similar to that from fully matched, HLA-identical transfusions, 20% to 50% of HLA-matched transfusions do not provide a satisfactory response.[102–106] Also, since these patients require frequent platelet transfusions, many donors who are matched to the patient must be available to sustain the patient for days or a few weeks.[107]

Platelet Crossmatching for Platelet Transfusion

In HLA-matched transfusions there is a 20% to 50% failure rate.[102–106] Thus, there is a great potential for any method that might improve on these results. One approach that should be effective is crossmatching the patient's serum and the potential donor's cells. The development of this approach was slow for many years because the platelet antibody detection techniques were complex and did not lend themselves to rapid response on a large scale with relatively low cost. While it appears that in most patients HLA antibodies are responsible for refractoriness, platelet-specific antibodies may sometimes be involved. Because the relative roles of platelet-specific and HLA antibodies have not been clear, this further complicates the choice of the optimum method for crossmatching.[106]

There has been great variability in the experience with platelet crossmatching.[105] The positive predictive value of platelet crossmatching ranged from 73% to 100% and the negative predictive value, from 52% to 92% in 10 studies summarized by Heal et al.[78] Many of these studies were retrospective, and some of the prospective studies did not use fresh platelets.[105] In comparing four platelet crossmatch techniques, McFarland and Aster found the best results using a monoclonal anti-IgG assay.[108] Moroff et al.[105] compared HLA matching and platelet crossmatching in 73 patients. Although platelet refractoriness is often associated with the presence of lymphocytotoxicity antibodies in the patient's serum, Moroff et al.[105] were unable to demonstrate lymphocytotoxic antibodies in 55% of the patients in their study who were refractory to platelet transfusion and had no obvious clinical causes for the refractoriness. Both HLA matching and platelet crossmatching provided similar degrees of successful 1-hour corrected count increments (40% to 60%). If transfusions only with the HLA matching of grade A or Bu were considered, HLA matching was superior to platelet crossmatching. However, Moroff et al.[105] concluded that a similar number of successful transfusions could be obtained by either HLA matching or platelet crossmatching. Tasato[109] found that a platelet migration inhibition assay predicted platelet transfusion responses but that granulocytotoxicity, microleukoagglutination, and capillary leukoagglutination were not helpful. Filip et al.[110] found that serotonin release, platelet factor 3 release, and platelet aggregometry were unsatisfactory methods for platelet crossmatching, but Freedman[111] reported that a platelet immunofluorescence technique predicted a successful outcome of platelet transfusion in 90% of cases; Kickler,[112] using a modified microtiter method, also found outstanding predictability of a successful 1-hour CCI with a compatible platelet crossmatch. Heal et al.[78] also found that a microtiter

platelet crossmatch procedure was the most important of many factors studied in determining an effective platelet transfusion in refractory patients. However, none of these methods was suitable for general use and none gained wide practical application.

During the last several years, a solid-phase red cell adherence assay was developed specifically for platelet crossmatching.[113] This method has overcome the previous barriers of test complexity and speed of results. In clinical use, the method predicted a successful transfusion outcome in 97% of patients with no clinical factors to cause nonimmune platelet destruction.[114] Successful prediction of transfusion response using the solid-phase red cell adherence assay was confirmed by O'Connell et al.[115] and also by Friedberg,[116] who, in a separate study of 962 single-donor platelet transfusions to 71 refractory patients, showed that the solid-phase red cell adherence assay was superior to HLA matching. This method is coming into more widespread use because of its effectiveness and practicality.

Other Approaches to the Refractory Patient

Other strategies that have been attempted include plasma exchange,[117] treatment of the patient's plasma with a staphylococcal protein A column,[118] and administration of cyclosporine. These methods are not usually successful and are not recommended. Case reports have shown a beneficial effect of intravenous immunoglobulin in improving the response to platelet transfusion in alloimmunized refractory patients,[119,120] but another larger, more definitive study found no benefit[121] and recommended against its use.

A Practical Approach to the Patient Refractory to Platelet Transfusion

The lack of a response to platelet transfusion is often associated with bleeding. These patients are usually quite ill with problems such as fever, sepsis, disseminated intravascular coagulopathy, or viral infections. Whether patients with similar clinical problems but who are responsive to platelets have fewer bleeding problems has not been established. However, because refractoriness is often associated with bleeding and a poor outcome, it is important to define the steps that can be taken to improve the response to transfusion in these patients.

Clinical factors such as infection that might cause refractoriness should be sought and, if present, appropriate treatment should be initiated to correct them. Additional simple steps that should be attempted include the transfusion of ABO-identical platelets and platelets less than 24 hours old. The techniques for platelet transfusion should be reviewed to be sure the platelets are not being damaged or lost because of improper handling after leaving the blood bank, use of incorrect filters, or improper storage conditions after leaving the blood bank. An additional step is to be certain that the platelet concentrates contain an adequate number of platelets. This can be done by checking the routine quality control testing that the blood bank carries out. If questions continue, the platelet count and content of the specific concentrates being used for the patient can be determined. If these measures fail, platelets that are matched to the recipient should be used. This can be accomplished by HLA matching donor and recipient or by using platelets that are compatible in a crossmatch. Most HLA-matched platelets obtained

from unrelated donors will not be matched for all four of the HLA-A and HLA-B locus antigens, and thus there will be some degree of antigen mismatch between the patient and donor. Although the average response to these partially matched transfusions is similar to that from fully matched HLA-identical transfusions, about 30% of HLA-matched transfusions do not provide a satisfactory response.[102–106] Also, since these patients require frequent platelet transfusions, many donors who are matched to the patient must be available to sustain the patient for days or a few weeks.[107] For many patients this may not be practical. An additional or alternative approach is to crossmatch the patient's serum and the potential donor's cells. As described above, the success rate is similar to HLA-matched transfusions. Thus, it seems as if either HLA matching or platelet crossmatching can be used to obtain about the same effect. One practical difference is that usually crossmatched platelets can be obtained more rapidly than HLA-matched platelets because crossmatching is done on platelets already collected and available in inventory, whereas HLA-matched donors must be located and scheduled for donation.[105] A practical suggested strategy for dealing with patients who are refractory to platelet transfusion is as follows:

1. Treat any correctable clinical factors present that may cause platelet refractoriness. Until these factors are eliminated, recognize that any of the steps listed below may not be effective.
2. Ensure that the patient is receiving the correct dose of platelets.
3. Give at least one test transfusion of platelets that are not more than 48 hours old and preferably less than 24 hours old.
4. Ensure that platelets being transfused are ABO identical.
5. If these steps have failed and transfusion is urgently needed, give transfusions of either crossmatch-compatible or HLA-matched platelets, whichever is available soonest. Give at least one and preferably two or three such transfusions.
6. Continue to use either crossmatched or HLA-matched platelets until the desired increment is obtained.
7. Determine whether the patient has HLA or platelet-specific antibodies or both. This may be of value in making future decisions about platelet transfusion if the patient does not respond to HLA-matched or crossmatched platelets.

Some patients do not respond to either HLA-matched or crossmatched platelets. Often these are patients in whom marrow grafting has failed or who have graft versus host disease, are septic, or are experiencing other severe complications of cytopenia. The transfusion strategies for these patients should be based on a discussion between the patient's attending physician and the transfusion medicine physician. One approach is increasing the dose of platelets to two or even three single-donor or 20 to 30 random-donor units per day. While this may enable the physicians to feel that they are doing something helpful, usually the patients fail to achieve a substantial increase in platelet count. It is not known whether the transfusions are helpful despite the lack of increase in circulating platelets. Other strategies for the management of refractoriness that have not generally been effective are mentioned above.

Reducing the Volume of the Platelet Concentrate

The dose of platelets necessary in some situations may result in a volume of plasma in the platelet concentrate that is too large for the patient to safely tolerate. Examples of these situations are transfusion to small children or the need for large doses of platelets to average-sized adults. In such situations, the platelet concentrate can be centrifuged and excess plasma removed safely anytime during the 5-day storage period.[122] It is important that the centrifugation technique be gentle and that the laboratory gain some experience with the technique to ensure that there is not excessive damage to platelets before attempting this for patient therapy.

Prevention of Alloimmunization and Platelet Refractoriness

Because of the difficulty in managing patients who are refractory to platelet transfusion, there is considerable interest in preventing alloimmunization. Immunization may occur due to pregnancy but is also thought to be caused by the leukocytes contained in the platelet and red cell transfusions patients receive.[123,124] Although the exact mechanism of alloimmunization has not been defined, it appears that intact viable leukocytes present HLA class I and II antigens for processing.[125] Thus, strategies to modify the transfusion products have been attempted. In general, these strategies have involved limiting the number of donor exposures, removing the leukocytes, or treating the components to render the leukocytes nonimmunogenic. Gmur et al.[126] demonstrated that use of non-HLA-matched single-donor platelet concentrates reduced the incidence of alloimmunization (HLA), prolonged the time to immunization, reduced the incidence of refractoriness, and prolonged the time to refractoriness. However, because of the role of leukocytes, the expense of single-donor platelet concentrates in some centers, and the remarkable improvements in blood filtration systems, leukodepletion has become the major approach to preventing alloimmunization. Now there is a very substantial body of data that establishes that leukodepletion reduces the incidence of alloimmunization and delays and/or reduces the onset of refractoriness.[126–132] Clinical trials are difficult to accomplish perfectly, and many of these studies have one or another shortcoming; however, there is little disagreement that leukodepletion is effective. This has recently been confirmed in the largest prospectively randomized trial reported. In this study[98] of more than 500 newly diagnosed acute leukemia patients, the use of leukodepleted red cells and platelet concentrates reduced the incidence of alloimmunization. There was no difference between pooled random-donor and single-donor platelet concentrates, suggesting that the important factor is the reduction of the leukocyte exposure rather than the number of different donors.

With the availability of new blood filtration systems, the issue has arisen whether to filter the components at the time they are produced in the laboratory "prestorage" or later at the bedside. Although prestorage filtration may be more effective in preventing transfusion reactions (see Chapter 14), and one report suggests that prestorage filtration may be more effective for prevention of alloimmunization,[133] another report showed no benefit from bedside filtration in prevention of alloimmunization and refractoriness.[134] However, at present the data are not sufficiently extensive to allow a conclusion as to whether prestorage filtration is superior to bedside filtration for the prevention of alloimmunization and platelet refractoriness.[135]

Another strategy proposed for the prevention of alloimmunization is the treatment of the platelet concentrates with ultraviolet light. Considerable work during the past few years has established that ultraviolet radiation inhibits the ability of lymphocytes to either proliferate or stimulate in a mixed lymphocyte culture.[136] Subsequent studies have established that UV-B light does not interfere with platelet function in vitro[136,137] or in vivo[138] at doses that will abrogate lymphocyte function. In mice, UV-B treatment of platelets reduced the alloantigenicity of transfused leukodepleted platelets,[139] and non-leukoreduced transfused platelets.[140] Practical systems were developed for UV irradiation of platelet concentrates,[141] and UV-irradiated platelet concentrates were included in the TRAP study.[98] In that study, UV-irradiated platelets reduced the incidence of alloimmunization but no more so than filtered leukodepleted platelets.[98] Thus, although this approach appears to be effective in preventing alloimmunization, it is not currently used and no systems are licensed by the FDA for routine blood bank use.

GRANULOCYTE TRANSFUSION

There is an inverse relationship between the granulocyte count and the presence of infection. As the granulocyte count falls below 1,000/mL, there is an increased risk of infection,[142] which is further increased by the duration of granulocytopenia.[143] The increasingly common and aggressive treatment of patients with hematologic malignancies and aplastic anemia has made granulocytopenia common. During the early 1970s, almost 80% of deaths in patients with bone marrow failure were due to infection.[55,142] Because of the success of platelet transfusion in the management of hemorrhage due to thrombocytopenia, there was considerable interest in transfusion of granulocytes for the management of infection in granulocytopenic patients. Because of the small number of granulocytes in the peripheral blood of normal humans, collection of cells for transfusion was not practical. Initial studies of granulocyte transfusion involved cells obtained from patients with chronic myelogenous leukemia. During the late 1960s and early 1970s, several blood cell separators were devised to allow collection of approximately 4×10^{10} granulocytes from patients with chronic myelogenous leukemia and 1×10^{10} granulocytes from normal donors by leukapheresis.[144] These cells function normally in vitro and have normal in vivo survival and migration to sites of infection.[144,145] Granulocytes for transfusion have also been prepared by isolating the buffy coat from units of fresh whole blood. This has usually been done for transfusion of neonates (see Chapter 12), because they do not require the larger dose of cells produced by leukapheresis. Recently, it has been suggested that a sufficient dose of granulocytes for adults can be obtained by pooling the buffy coats from 15 to 18 units of blood less than 12 hours after collection and such transfusions can be effective.[146] However, there is little experience with this technique, and no large clinical studies of its use have been reported.

A variety of patients have been involved in clinical studies of granulocyte transfusions, including those with acute leukemia, chronic leukemias, aplastic anemia, Hodgkin's disease, lymphoma, and solid tumors.[147] Patients with fever of unknown origin do not experience improvement as a result of granulocyte transfusion.[148] Most clinical trials of granulocyte transfusion involve patients with Gram-negative bacteremia,[147] and there is little information regarding other organisms. There is also little

information that collates the site of infection other than bacteremia with response to granulocyte transfusion.[147] A series of studies in the 1970s established that granulocyte transfusion provided improved survival in patients with documented Gram-negative sepsis who remained granulocytopenic for at least 10 days.[149,150] Some additional data indicated that granulocytes may be helpful in patients with other kinds of documented infections (either Gram positive or Gram negative) and granulocytopenia of more than 10 days' duration.[150]

However, today most patients can be expected to respond to antibiotics, and granulocyte transfusion is rarely used for bacterial infections. Granulocyte transfusion should not be initiated for at least 96 hours after the onset of clinical signs or symptoms of an infection. This allows transfusions to be given only to patients who do not respond to antibiotics. Many of the patients who do not respond have severe (less than $100/\mu L$) and prolonged neutropenia. The fever may be due to documented or assumed fungal infection,[151,152] which requires amphotericin therapy. When signs and symptoms of infection persist in these patients, granulocyte transfusions are often used. No clinical trials have documented the effectiveness of granulocyte transfusion for fungal infections, although animal[153] and clinical[154] studies support their use, and granulocytes do kill fungi in vitro.

The minimum dose of granulocytes required for clinical efficacy has not been established. There have been encouraging results from the use of approximately 5×10^9 granulocytes per square meter per day;[149] however, this represents less than 5% of the total daily granulocyte production by normal humans. Thus, most investigators believe it is necessary to transfuse at least 1×10^{10} granulocytes per day. The minimum number of transfusions necessary for improvement differs depending on the patient's clinical status. Granulocyte transfusion should be used as a course of treatment similar to antibiotics. Monitoring clinical symptoms and signs, such as temperature elevation, as a means of deciding daily whether to use granulocyte transfusions can be misleading and will create logistical problems with procurement of granulocytes. Just as antibiotics would not be discontinued on the basis of brief clinical improvement, granulocyte transfusions once initiated should be continued daily until the patient's general condition has stabilized and improved. In general, it is advisable to consider a course of granulocyte transfusion therapy as lasting at least 7 days.

Most experience with granulocyte transfusion involves treatment of existing infection. At one time, there has been considerable interest in the use of granulocytes to prevent infection in granulocytopenia patients. However, prophylactic granulocyte transfusions are not helpful in this regard for newly diagnosed patients with acute myelogenous leukemia.[155]

Hematopoietic growth factors such as granulocyte colony-stimulating factor (G-CSF) have been used to stimulate granulocyte production in neutropenic patients. Stimulation of normal blood donors increases the level of circulating granulocytes and increases the yield of granulocytes.[156,157] This can provide a dose of up to 10^4 granulocytes, or four times the doses used in the studies of the 1970s. By combining the use of corticosteroids and G-CSF, the level of circulating granulocytes can be increased further to about $40,000/\mu L$, compared with about $30,000/\mu L$ with G-CSF alone.[158] This should further increase the yield of granulocytes for transfusion. Whether the availabil-

ity of these strategies to obtain substantially greater granulocyte doses for transfusion will initiate a new phase of clinical trials of granulocyte transfusions remains to be determined. This will probably depend on whether there is a large enough group of patients that are unresponsive to present antibiotic regimens and with a reasonable expectation of survival to make such clinical trials practical.

Granulocyte transfusion of septic neonatal patients is described in Chapter 12.

CYTOMEGALOVIRUS-SAFE BLOOD COMPONENTS

Cytomegalovirus (CMV) can be transmitted by blood transfusion with a severe, even fatal result. Transfusion-transmitted CMV disease can be prevented by using blood components that do not transmit CMV. This can be accomplished using CMV antibody-negative blood components or components leukodepleted by filtration. This section describes the indications for CMV-free blood components in different situations.

Most individuals previously infected with CMV are no longer infectious but they have antibodies to CMV. Unfortunately, there is no simple, effective test that can be used to distinguish CMV antibody-positive blood donors who are infectious. Providing blood components that do not contain anti-CMV is a well-established method of preventing transfusion-transmitted CMV disease (see below). Because a substantial portion of blood donors are CMV antibody positive, providing CMV antibody-negative blood components is sometimes difficult, especially as the indications for CMV-free blood components have increased. Attempts to improve the testing methods to identify only the infectious units have not been successful. Alternatively, because it is presumed that leukocytes are the reservoir of CMV in asymptomatic blood donors, prevention of transfusion-transmitted CMV has been attempted using leukodepleted components. Several small studies[159,160] and one large controlled trial[161] have established that leukodepleted components are as effective as antibody-negative components in preventing transfusion-transmitted CMV. Leukodepleted and antibody-negative components can be considered equivalent and used interchangeably depending on logistical considerations of each transfusion service.

Neonates

Landmark studies by Yaeger and colleagues[162] established that neonates weighing less than 1,200 g born to CMV-negative mothers were at substantial risk of developing CMV disease if they received blood from CMV antibody-positive donors. Serious disease or death occurred in 50% of the infected neonates. These observations have been supported by some other studies but not by others. This is not surprising because of the large variation in the prevalence of CMV in blood donors in different parts of the United States. It has been suggested that at least some of the differences between the studies mentioned above could be a changing incidence of transfusion-transmitted CMV infection due to differences in techniques of CMV testing of donated blood, less use of fresh blood components, more use of plasma containing CMV antibodies, and a changing donor population because of HIV and non-A, non-B hepatitis screening

practices. Because the magnitude of this problem varies considerably, the incidence of CMV disease in neonates should be established locally to determine whether CMV-free blood components should be provided.

Pregnant Women

CMV infection of the fetus is a severe clinical problem that can cause growth and mental retardation, hepatitis, deafness, intracranial calcifications, and bleeding diathesis. Congenital CMV infection due to primary infection in the mother is usually more serious than infections due to recurrent maternal CMV infection.[163] Thus, it is prudent to avoid primary CMV infection in pregnant women. Although there have been no specific clinical studies of this situation, it is advisable to provide CMV-free blood to pregnant women or for intrauterine transfusion of the fetus.[164]

Kidney Transplantation

CMV disease is common in renal transplant recipients, occurring in 60% to 90% of patients. Because it can be very serious, causing graft rejection or even death, its prevention is important. The cause of CMV disease in these patients may be (a) reactivation of latent previous CMV infection; (b) acquisition of CMV from the donor organ; or (c) acquisition of CMV from blood transfusion. The prevalence of CMV ranges from 30% to 70% in the blood donor population,[165] and most renal transplant patients will have received previous transfusions, further increasing the proportion of them who have previous CMV infection. Thus, reactivation of a previous infection is by far the most common cause of CMV disease in these patients.[166,167]

Approximately 77% of CMV antibody-negative patients who receive a kidney from a CMV antibody-positive donor develop CMV infection, compared with 8% to 20% in similar patients who receive a kidney from a CMV antibody-negative donor but receive CMV antibody-positive blood transfusions.[166,167] If a CMV antibody-negative patient receives a kidney from a CMV antibody-negative donor and then receives CMV antibody-negative blood components, the likelihood of developing CMV infection is almost zero.[167] Thus, it is advisable to provide CMV-free blood components for these latter patients.

Renal transplant patients with anti-CMV may develop CMV disease due to acquisition of a second strain of the virus from the donor organ.[168] Acquisition of a second strain of CMV from blood transfusion has not been reported. Thus, providing CMV-free blood components for patients with anti-CMV to avoid transmitting a new CMV strain is not recommended unless this is shown to be a larger clinical problem than it now appears.

Bone Marrow Transplantation

CMV disease is a major complication of marrow transplantation. CMV disease is a more frequent and severe problem in marrow transplantation patients because they are more severely immunosuppressed than solid organ recipients. CMV disease occurs in 40% to 50% of patients undergoing allogeneic marrow transplantation, and it is an important source of posttransplant mortality.[169] As with renal transplantation, the

majority of CMV disease in marrow transplantation patients occurs in patients with CMV antibody and is probably due to reactivation of virus from a previous infection, not to acquisition of a new strain.[170] However, in CMV antibody-negative patients who receive marrow from a CMV antibody-negative donor, the risk of developing CMV infection is approximately 40%.[170] The likelihood of these patients acquiring CMV infection is almost eliminated by the use of CMV antibody-negative blood components.[161,170,171] Thus, it is customary to provide CMV-free blood components to CMV antibody-negative marrow transplantation patients whose marrow donor is CMV antibody negative. Providing CMV antibody-negative blood components for marrow transplantation patients may be difficult in areas with a large marrow transplantation program and a high CMV prevalence in the donor population. Other approaches currently under study for the prevention of CMV infection include the use of CMV intravenous immunoglobulin,[172,173] ordinary intravenous immunoglobulin,[174] or leukocyte-poor blood components.[159–161,175,176] The intravenous immunoglobulin is extremely expensive and the availability of CMV intravenous immunoglobulin is limited.

Since most CMV disease occurs in marrow transplant patients who are CMV antibody positive, extension of the use of CMV antibody-negative blood components to potential marrow transplant patients who are CMV antibody-negative has been suggested. Thus, they would not become infected with CMV as a result of transfusions received earlier in their disease and before entering a marrow transplantation program. This practice has not been shown to be necessary or cost-effective in clinical studies; however, it is gaining in popularity.

Heart, Heart-Lung, Liver, and Pancreas Transplantation

Very few data are available describing CMV infections in recipients of heart, heart-lung, liver, or pancreas transplantations. One small study of heart transplant patients demonstrated that CMV infection was transmitted by either the donor heart or blood components.[177] When both the donor organ and all blood components were CMV antibody-negative, CMV infection was prevented in heart[177] as well as in liver[178] transplant recipients. A more recent study of heart transplantations found a very low (1.5%) incidence of CMV infection.[179] Although the data are not extensive and are somewhat conflicting for these transplant situations, the patients are immunosuppressed, and CMV infection is a clinical problem that can be prevented by the use of CMV antibody-negative blood components. This practice is advisable in CMV antibody-negative patients who receive an organ from a CMV antibody-negative donor. CMV infections in CMV antibody-positive heart transplant patients are the result of reactivation of latent virus,[180] and therefore the use of CMV-free blood components is not indicated for these patients.

Acquired Immune Deficiency Syndrome

Acquired immune deficiency syndrome (AIDS) patients have severely impaired immune function, and CMV infections are an important clinical problem for them. Thus, use of CMV antibody-negative blood components is indicated for CMV antibody-negative AIDS patients, although no clinical trials have been done to form the basis for this

practice. The same potential extension of the use of CMV antibody-negative blood components mentioned for potential marrow transplant patients also applies to individuals infected with HIV-1. That is, use of CMV antibody-negative blood components for CMV antibody-negative patients infected with the HIV virus but currently asymptomatic. This would prevent the development of latent CMV infection in these patients, which could reactivate later when AIDS develops. The cost-effectiveness and practicality of this approach have not been established, and at present the use of CMV-free components for these patients is not recommended.

Severe Combined Immune Deficiency (Congenital)

There are no specific studies or data regarding prevention of CMV infection in patients with congenital severe combined immune deficiency by the use of CMV antibody-negative components. However, because these patients are severely immunocompromised, provision of CMV-free blood components is the usual transfusion practice.

Patients Receiving Extensive Chemotherapy

As more varied chemotherapy regimens are used, patients are experiencing greater drug-induced immunosuppression. However, in general, CMV infection has not been an important clinical problem in these patients. Since there is no good way of determining the level of immune function at which patients become increasingly susceptible to CMV infection, the use of CMV-free blood components is not recommended in these patients.

IRRADIATED BLOOD COMPONENTS

Graft-Versus-Host Disease

Graft versus host disease (GVHD) is a serious, often fatal disease that occurs when there are histocompatibility differences between the donor and recipient, the recipient receives immunocompetent donor cells, and the recipient is unable to reject the donor cells. GVHD was originally identified in immunodeficient children,[181-184] but the more common situation in which GVHD occurs is in bone marrow transplantation,[185] and it is now clear that GVHD can occur in a wide variety of immunocompromised patients. In marrow transplantation, GVHD is caused by the immunocompetent marrow donor cells,[185] whereas in blood transfusion, viable lymphocytes contained in blood components can cause fatal GVHD in susceptible patients. The hallmark features of GVHD are involvement of skin, liver, gastrointestinal tract, bone marrow, and lymphoid system.[186] There are some clinical differences between GVHD associated with marrow transplantation and transfusion-associated GVHD; these are illustrated in Table 11.8.

The majority of cases of GVHD occur in immunocompromised patients such as those with congenital immunodeficiency, those undergoing marrow transplantation, or those who have received extensive myeloablative therapy.[187-191] However, recently cases of transfusion-associated GVHD have been reported in apparently immunocom-

Table 11.8 Clinical and pathologic comparison of graft versus host disease associated with bone marrow transplantation (BMTA-GVHD) and transfusions (PT-GVHD)

Manifestation	BMTA-GVHD	PT-GVHD
Time sequence	35–70 days	2–30 days
Skin rash	+	+
Constitutional symptoms	Profound	Mild to moderate
Liver enzyme elevation	+	+
Pancytopenia	Rare to minimal	Almost always
Bone marrow hypoplasia or aplasia	Negative	Positive
Occurrence of GVHD	70%	0.1–1.0%
Response to therapy	80–90%	None
Mortality	10–15%	90–100%

Source: Brubaker DB. Transfusion-associated graft-versus-host disease. Hum Pathol 1986;17:1085–1088.

petent patients.[192–197] It appears that this occurs when the donor is HLA homozygous and haploidentical with the recipient. In this situation, although the recipient may be immunocompetent, the donor cells would not be recognized as foreign and thus would not be rejected. If the donor cells are immunocompetent, they proliferate, causing transfusion-associated GVHD. Possibly some of these patients were somewhat immunocompromised, but there is a very high incidence (approximately 1:600) of transfusion-associated GVHD in patients undergoing heart surgery in Japan.[197,198] This has been attributed to the high incidence of HLA homozygosity in the Japanese population.[195–198] Transfusion-associated GVHD has also been reported when patients receive transfusions of fresh components such as platelets from first-degree relatives.[192,196] Since there is a higher likelihood that these relatives will share an HLA haplotype with the patients, this same mechanism of an HLA-homozygous donor who is haploidentical with the patient has been proposed to account for these cases of transfusion-associated GVHD in immunocompetent patients.

Irradiation of Blood Components

To prevent transfusion-associated GVHD, blood components are subjected to radiation, which interferes with the ability of lymphocytes to proliferate. Blood components can be successfully irradiated using either gamma radiation or x-rays. Both of these methods damage the lymphocytes by forming electrically charged particles or ions that alter the DNA, making the lymphocyte unable to proliferate.[199] Ultraviolet irradiation is not an effective method of damaging lymphocytes to prevent GVHD because, although the rays will damage lymphocytes, they cannot penetrate the plastic containers used to store blood products. Hospitals that provide very few irradiated units may do this using x-ray instruments, but blood banks that provide large numbers of irradiated products usually do this with a dedicated instrument. These instruments usually use ^{137}Cs or ^{60}Co as the source of the radioactivity. These blood irradiators may contain different amounts of isotope, and this affects the length of time required to irradiate the blood components.

Also, different irradiation devices contain radiation chambers of different sizes, and thus there are differences in the number of units of blood components that can be irradiated.

The optimum minimal dose of radiation necessary has evolved over the years. Following early experiences with transfusion-associated GVHD, a minimum dose of 3,000 rads was recommended.[182] The occurrence of transfusion-associated GVHD in several individuals who received blood components supposedly irradiated with at least 1,500 rads[187,200,201] has focused attention during the past few years on the configuration of the blood containers in the irradiated field, the distribution of radiation within the field, and quality control methods to ensure that the desired dose was actually being administered.[199]

A survey of irradiation practices revealed that doses range from 1,500 to 5,000 rads, with 97% of institutions using between 1,500 and 3,000 rads.[202] Considerations in selecting a dose include the ability of that dose to interfere with lymphocyte proliferation, the effect on the cells being given for therapeutic purposes, and the clinical experience with blood components subjected to the doses selected. A very low dose of radiation interferes with lymphocyte response to allogeneic cells. Gamma irradiation at a dose of only 500 rads will abolish lymphocyte proliferation in mixed lymphocyte culture.[203,204] Irradiation with 1,500 to 5,000 rads reduces the incorporation of ^{14}C-thymidine into mitogen-stimulated lymphocytes by 85% to 98.5%.[205] Doses of up to 5,000 rads do not have an adverse effect on red cells, platelets, or granulocytes.[205,206] Red cell survival in vivo and in certain in vitro assays are normal after irradiation with up to 10,000 rads.[206] Granulocyte chemotaxis may be slightly reduced by even 500 rads, but this does not become significant until irradiation with greater than 10,000 rads.[204] Very high doses such as 40,000 rads are required to interfere with phagocytosis and microbial killing.[204,206,207] In vitro platelet function studies have generally been normal following irradiation with up to 5,000 rads.[205] However, at this dose there is a 33% reduction in in vivo recovery and diminished correction of the bleeding time by irradiated platelets.[206] However, since Button et al.[206] did not observe a difference in the platelet increment following transfusion of irradiated compared with nonirradiated platelets, they concluded that 5,000 rads was a clinically acceptable dose. Studies involving lower doses of irradiation such as 2,500 or 3,000 rads showed normal in vivo survival[208,209] and posttransfusion increments.[210] Thus, it appears that at the doses of radiation generally in use there is no interference with platelet function or survival.

One difficulty in selecting a radiation dose is the lack of a definitive in vitro assay to establish a clinically effective dose. The dose of radiation to prevent transfusion-associated GVHD was originally selected using the mixed lymphocyte culture (MLC) assay. During the past few years, the limiting dilution assay (LDA) has been proposed as a better indicator of the effects of irradiation on lymphocytes because the LDA detects a reduction in viable T cells of 5 $\log_{10}$, compared to a reduction of 1 to 2 $\log_{10}$ detectable by the MLC assay.[199,211] Studies using the limiting dilution assay showed that a radiation dose of 2,500 rads completely eliminated T-lymphocyte growth,[212] and, based on this experience, the U.S. Food and Drug Administration (FDA) has recommended a minimum dose of 2,500 rads.[213]

Storage of Irradiated Components

In almost all of the studies on irradiation of blood components the cells were studied shortly after irradiation. As the use of irradiated blood components has increased, interest has developed in irradiating the components after collection and storing them for use days or weeks later. Red cells have reduced but acceptable in vivo survival when stored for 42 days following irradiation,[214] and others have also found reduced but acceptable survival rates following storage periods of 21 or 28 days. An additional consideration is that doses of 2,000 or 3,000 rads to units of red cells result in potassium levels two and three times normal after storage for 4 to 5 days.[215,216] This suggests that leakage of potassium from the red cells occurred during postirradiation storage, perhaps resulting from irradiation damage to the red cell membrane or the sodium-potassium pump. This has led some blood banks to wash red cells that have been stored for several days after irradiation. However, in a thorough review of the situation Strauss concluded that washing is not necessary for most clinical situations.[217] Based on these studies, red cells can be stored for only 28 days after irradiation.

Quality Control of Irradiation

Quality control of blood irradiators is extremely important to ensure that the components receive the expected dose. Moroff et al.[199] have proposed the following as appropriate quality control measures for blood irradiation:

1. Use of qualitative indicators to confirm that irradiation was performed as intended.
2. Periodic measurement over the delivered dose using appropriate dosimetric techniques.
3. Periodic surveys to detect isotope leakage.
4. Daily confirmation of timer accuracy.

Because there is no reduction in platelet recovery and survival when previously irradiated platelets are stored,[218] platelets can be irradiated and stored for the normal 5 days. Red cells that have been irradiated can be frozen, stored, and thawed with no reduction in in vivo red cell recovery.[219] The effect of irradiating frozen red cells is not known, and although some authors[199] believe it is acceptable to irradiate frozen components, it seems more advisable to irradiate these components either before freezing or after deglycerolization.

Leukocyte Depletion to Prevent GVHD

Because blood filters are very effective in removing leukocytes, the question has arisen as to whether blood filtration might be an alternative to irradiation for prevention of GVHD. Present blood filters remove up to 99.9% of the leukocytes from red cells and plasma, resulting in fewer than 5×10^6 leukocytes per unit.[220,221] However, differences in patient size and in the degree of immunocompetence make it impossible based on available information to predict a minimum GVHD-producing dose of leukocytes for each patient. Because irradiation is almost completely effective in preventing transfusion-associated GVHD, there is no motivation to develop alternative GVHD

prevention methods and almost no willingness by physicians to undertake clinical trials. This is particularly true since, although on average filters produce components that contain fewer than 5×10^6 leukocytes, a small percentage of units contain considerably more leukocytes.[25] Thus, filtration is not an acceptable approach to prevention of transfusion-associated GVHD.

Because it is difficult to quantitate cellular immunity, there are no in vitro assays that define the degree of immunodeficiency that makes a patient susceptible to transfusion-associated GVHD. Even if better assays were available, these probably would not be helpful because the degree of HLA matching between the patient and blood donor may be a factor in the likelihood of transfusion-associated GVHD. In the situations described below, patients are so severely immunocompromised that transfusion-associated GVHD is very likely unless blood components are irradiated.

Indications for Irradiated Components

Fetus Fatal GVHD can occur from viable lymphocytes in blood used for intrauterine or exchange transfusion.[222, 223] All blood components used for these indications should be irradiated. Components transfused to these patients after delivery should also be irradiated.

Neonates Although neonates do not have adult levels of immune competence, there are very few reports of transfusion-associated GVHD in neonates (see Chapter 12). There is no evidence that newborns who do not have a congenital immunodeficiency are at increased risk of developing transfusion-associated GVHD. Routine irradiation of blood components for all neonates is not recommended.[224] However, it has been proposed that infants whose birth weight is less than 1,250 g should receive irradiated components because of their underdeveloped immune system.[225]

Congenital immune deficiency Patients with severe combined immunodeficiency syndrome or Wiskott-Aldrich syndrome have severe defects in immunity. These patients have a very high likelihood of developing transfusion-associated GVHD, even from one unit of fresh plasma,[183] and should receive irradiated blood components. Patients suspected of having congenital immune deficiency should receive irradiated components until the diagnosis is refuted.

Allogeneic bone marrow transplantation These patients are severely immunocompromised by the irradiation with or without chemotherapy given to prepare them for the transplant and in many situations to eradicate residual disease. The GVHD that commonly follows allogeneic bone marrow transplantation is caused by viable lymphocytes in the donor marrow.[185] Irradiation of all blood components has become routine; however, as a result there are no data describing the risk of development of transfusion-associated GVHD in allogeneic bone marrow transplant recipients. It can be presumed that the risk would be extremely high, and so irradiated blood components are used routinely.[185] Unless the patient has a disease that would necessitate the use of irradiated blood products, these are not necessary for bone marrow transplant patients until the transplant preparative regimen is begun. Prior to that time, the blood components should be selected based on the patient's underlying disease.

Autologous bone marrow transplantation Although there may be some differences in the irradiation and chemotherapy preparation for autologous compared with allogeneic bone marrow transplantation, patients undergoing autologous bone marrow transplantation are severely immunocompromised. Because the use of irradiated blood components was an established practice in allogeneic bone marrow transplantation, it has been adopted for autologous bone marrow transplantation without clinical or laboratory study.

There are several other clinical situations in which isolated cases of transfusion-associated GVHD have been reported and for which some medical centers use irradiated blood components, but there is no consensus on recommended practice.

If transfusions are provided before or during the stage of peripheral blood stem cell collection, irradiation avoids the potential that transfused viable donor lymphocytes could be ultimately transfused to the patient with the stem cell transplant. Although no such cases have been reported, irradiation avoids this theoretical situation.[226]

Hematologic malignancies Some patients with acute leukemia, lymphoma, or Hodgkin's disease and receiving chemotherapy, often along with radiation, have developed transfusion-associated GVHD.[188-190,227-230] Often these patients have received granulocyte transfusions. The risk of transfusion-associated GVHD in these patients has been estimated to be between 0.1 and 1.0%,[231] but this risk is difficult to determine because of the lack of comprehensive follow-up studies. The data currently available are insufficient to establish whether blood components for these patients should be routinely irradiated.

Aplastic anemia These patients usually do not have defective cellular immunity. There have not been documented cases of transfusion-associated GVHD due to transfusion of normal cells. Thus, the use of irradiated blood components is not necessary.

Solid tumors One patient with neuroblastoma and one with glioblastoma have developed transfusion-associated GVHD.[191,227] Some treatment protocols for these patients result in rather severe immune system compromise; however, the data are not adequate to recommend irradiation of blood products for these patients except in therapy involving severe immune deficiency.

Acquired immune deficiency syndrome Despite the fact that these patients have severely impaired immune function, no cases of transfusion-associated GVHD have been reported. This may be because these patients receive irradiated blood components in some centers. However, the risk for AIDS patients of developing transfusion-associated GVHD is not known.

Granulocyte transfusions During the 1970s, there was concern that granulocyte transfusion posed a greater risk of transfusion-associated GVHD than other cellular blood components.[229] However, this was probably due to the increased risk of transfusion-associated GVHD from transfused chronic myelogenous leukemia cells,[230] not normal donor cells. Thus, there is no need to routinely irradiate granulocyte concentrates obtained from normal donors. The decision to irradiate granulocytes should be based on

the patient's underlying condition. Chronic myelogenous leukemia cells are rarely used for transfusions, but if they are used, they should be irradiated.

Noncellular blood components Transfusion-associated GVHD has occurred in patients with congenital immune deficiency following transfusion of fresh liquid plasma[181–183] but has not been reported to be caused by previously frozen components, fresh frozen plasma, or cryoprecipitate. These components contain fragments of leukocytes but few, if any, viable lymphocytes. They would not be expected to cause transfusion-associated GVHD. Although irradiation of fresh frozen plasma and cryoprecipitate is probably not necessary, many blood banks do irradiate these components to avoid clerical errors in which a cellular blood component might not be irradiated when necessary.

Components from partially HLA-matched, related, or unrelated donors Several years ago, some cases of transfusion-associated GVHD occurred after transfusion from relatives who were partially HLA-matched with the patient[182,183,227] or from unrelated but partially HLA-matched donors.[188] This raised the theoretical concern that transfusion-associated GVHD might develop in patients not severely immunocompromised if there was partial HLA matching between the patient and the blood donor. However, since most of the patients involved in these reports were severely immunocompromised, this remained a theoretical concern until 1989. Then several reports appeared suggesting this situation might be more common than previously believed. Thaler et al.[192] reported transfusion-associated GVHD apparently caused by fresh blood donated by children in two immunocompetent patients who underwent cardiac surgery. In each case one of the blood donors was homozygous for an HLA class I antigen haplotype shared with the recipient. Thus, the recipient would not have recognized the HLA class I antigens as foreign. There have now been additional reports of transfusion-associated GVHD in Japan in patients who received fresh blood after cardiac surgery, in a woman who was transfused following delivery,[193] in a cardiac surgery patient in New York,[194] and in a Japanese woman transfused after cholecystectomy.[195] The apparent high incidence of this situation in Japan may be due to the rather high frequency of certain HLA antigens in the Japanese, with the resulting likelihood that a random unrelated donor may be partially HLA-matched with the recipient. The incidence of transfusion-associated GVHD in immunocompetent patients in the United States is not known. There is no evidence that this is a problem when unrelated donors are used; however, the increasing use of directed donors who are related to the patient may increase the likelihood of transfusion-associated GVHD. The problem can be prevented by irradiating the blood components donated by first-degree relatives of the patient.

FIBRIN SEALANT (GLUE)

Since the early part of this century, various crude forms of fibrinogen have been used to attempt to control localized bleeding.[232] Fibrin sealant or glue refers to the use of fibrinogen in some form along with thrombin as a topical adhesive to control bleeding.[233]

Table 11.9 Composition of fibrin sealant

Source	Human fibrinogen (mg/mL)	Human factor XII (U/mL)	Human thrombo-poietin (U/mL)	Bovine aprotinin (KIU/mL)	Virus-inactivated fibrinogen	Virus-inactivated thrombin
IMMUNO AG (Austria)	70–115	10–50 (Europe) <1 (USA)	4 and 500 (Europe) 500 (USA)	3000	Two-step vapor heat at 60/80°C	Two-step vapor heat at 60/80°C
Centeon Pharma GmbH (Germany)	65–115	40–80	400–600	900–1100	Wet heat, 10 hours at 60°C	Wet heat, 10 hours at 60°C
LFB-Lille (France)	115	10–30	500	3000	SD*	SD
SNBTS (Scotland)	40	10	200	None	Dry heat 72 hours at 80°C	SD
Haemacure Biotech (Canada)	50–70	20–40	150–250	None	SD, nanofilter dry heat,1 hour at100°C	SD, nanofilter dry heat, 1 hour at100°C
Baxter/American Red Cross (USA)	100	24	300	None	SD	SD, nanofilter
Melville Biologics (USA)	50–95	3–5	200	None**	SD,UVC†	SD, UVBC

Source: Levitsky S. Further information on the fibrin sealant conference. Transfusion 1996;36:845. Letter to the editor.
*Solvent-detergent treatment.
**0.1 M epsilon amino caproic acid as excipient.
†Ultraviolet C light.

There is no one specifically defined fibrin glue product. For several years, many blood banks have dispensed cryoprecipitate in syringes along with thrombin for use by surgeons.[234] More pure forms of fibrinogen are now being produced with chemical additives.[233] The composition and characteristics of five of these products are listed in Table 11.9. All contain fibrinogen, factor XIII, and human thrombin. They are reconstituted with saline at 37°C within about 10 minutes.[232] Currently all of these products are experimental drugs in the United States, although it appears that one or more may be licensed by the FDA soon.

Fibrin sealant may be used for either its hemostatic or its adhesive properties. To achieve hemostasis, surgeons use fibrin sealant (*a*) to deal with microvascular bleeding in cardiovascular surgery to reduce mediastinal drainage, (*b*) to seal synthetic vascular grafts, (*c*) to seal bleeding surfaces of the liver or spleen, (*d*) in maxillofacial surgery, (*e*) for sealing dura, and (*f*) for peripheral nerve repair.

Controlled trials have demonstrated that fibrin sealant significantly reduces the time required to achieve hemostasis in vascular surgery,[235] improves hemostasis after operation following cardiac operations,[236] and reduces blood loss from vascular cannulation in neonates.[232] The adhesive properties of fibrin sealant are used to promote the union of middle ear bones in otolaryngologic surgery, to enhance skin grafting, to seal bronchopulmonary fistulas, and as a matrix for repair of bone defects.[232]

Since fibrin glue is made from human plasma, transmission of diseases might occur. The likelihood of this is not known[233] but seems to be quite low.[232] All of the commercially prepared products involve at least one viral inactivation step, and it is hoped that this will render these products free of viral disease transmission. When fibrin sealants are prepared locally from cryoprecipitate, the product should be considered to have the same risk of disease transmission as other blood components. Fibrin sealant has been associated with the development of antibodies to the bovine thrombin it contains as well to factor V.[234,237]

REFERENCES

1. DaCosta JC, Kalteyer FJ. The blood changes induced by the administration of ether as an anesthetic. Ann Surg 1901;34:329–360.
2. Adams RC, Lundy JS. Anesthesia in cases of poor surgical risk: some suggestions for decreasing the risk. Surg Gynecol Obstet 1942;74:1011–1019.
3. Clark JH, Nelson W, Lyons C, et al. Chronic shock: the problem of reduced blood volume in the chronically ill patient. Ann Surg 1947;125:618.
4. Rodman T, Close HP, Purcell MK. The oxyhemoglobin dissociation curve in anemia. Ann Intern Med 1960;52:295–309.
5. Whitaker W. Some effects of severe chronic anemia on the circulatory system. Q J Med 1956;25:175–309.
6. Roy SB, Bhatia ML, Mathur VS, Viramani S. Hemodynamic effects of chronic severe anemia. Circulation 1963;28:346–356.
7. Varat MA, Adolph RJ, Fowler NO. Cardiovascular effects of anemia. Am Heart J 1972;83:415–426.
8. National Institutes of Health Consensus Conference. Perioperative red blood cell transfusion. JAMA 1988;260:2700–2703.

9. Robertie PG, Gravlee GP. Safe limits of isovolemic hemodilution and recommendations for erythrocyte transfusion. Int Anesthesiol Clin 1990;28:197–204.
10. Hillman RS. Acute blood loss anemia. In: Beutler E, Lichtman MA, Coller BS, et al., eds. Williams Hematology. 5th ed. New York: McGraw Hill Inc., 1995:704–708.
11. Gollub S, Svigals R, Bailey CP, et al. Electrolyte solutions in surgical patients refusing transfusion. JAMA 1971;215:2077.
12. Rigor B, Bosomworth P, Ruth BF Jr. Replacement of operative blood loss of more than 1 liter with Hartmann's solution. JAMA 1968;203:111.
13. Welch HG, Meehan KR, Goodnough LT. Prudent strategies for elective red blood cell transfusion. Ann Intern Med 1992;116:393.
14. American College of Physicians. Practice strategies for elective red blood cell transfusion. Ann Intern Med 1992;115:403.
15. McCullough J, Clay ME, Press C, Kline W. Granulocyte Serology: A clinical and laboratory guide. Chicago: ASPC Press, 1988:83–112.
16. Brittingham TE, Chaplin H. Febrile transfusion reactions caused by sensitivity to donor leukocytes and platelets. JAMA 1957;165:819.
17. Perkins HA, Payne R, Ferguson J, et al. Nonhemolytic febrile transfusion reactions: quantitative effects of blood components with emphasis on isoantigenic incompatibility of leukocytes. Vox Sang 1966;11:578.
18. Greenwalt TJ, Gajewski M, McKenna JL. A new method for preparing buffy coat-poor blood. Transfusion 1962;2:221–229.
19. Snyder EL, Bookbinder M. Role of microaggregate blood filtration in clinical medicine. Transfusion 1983;23:460–470.
20. Wenz B. Microaggregate blood filtration and the febrile transfusion reaction: a comparative study. Transfusion 1983;23:95–98.
21. Snyder EL. Clinical use of white cell-poor blood components. Transfusion 1989;29:568.
22. Class FHJ, Smeenk RJT, Schmidt R, et al. Alloimmunization against the MHC antigens after platelet transfusions is due to contaminating leukocytes in the platelet suspension. Exp Hematol 1981;9:84.
23. Eernisse JG, Brand A. Prevention of platelet refractoriness due to HLA antibodies by administration of leukocyte-poor blood components. Exp Hematol 1981;9:77.
24. Schiffer CA, Dutcher JP, Aisner J, et al. A randomized trial of leukocyte depleted platelet transfusion to modify alloimmunization in patients with leukemia. Blood 1980;56:182a. Abstract.
25. Kao KH, Mickel M, Braine HG, et al. White cell reduction in platelet concentrates and packed red cells by filtration: a multicenter trial. Transfusion 1995;35:13–19.
26. Brady MT, Milam JD, Anderson DC, et al. Use of deglycerolized red blood cells to prevent posttransfusion infection with cytomegalovirus in neonates. J Infect Dis 1984;150:334.
27. Mollison PL, Engelfriet CP, Contreras M. Blood transfusion. In: Clinical Medicine, 8th ed. Cambridge, MA: Blackwell Science, 1987:613.
28. Sharpey-Schafer EP, Wallace J. Retention of injected serum in the circulation. Lancet 1942;1:699.
29. Opelz G, Sengar DPS, Mickey MR, et al. Effect of blood transfusions on subsequent kidney transplants. Transplant Proc 1973;5:253.
30. Vamvakas EC. Transfusion-associated cancer recurrence and postoperative infection: meta-analysis of randomized, controlled clinical trials. Transfusion 1996;36:175–186.
31. Heiss MM, Mempel W, Delanoff CC, et al. Blood transfusion-modulated tumor recurrence: first results of a randomized study of autologous versus allogeneic blood transfusion in colorectal cancer surgery. J Clin Oncol 1994;12:1859–1867.
32. Busch OR, Hop WC, Hoynck van Papendrecht MA, et al. Blood transfusions and prognosis in colorectal cancer. N Engl J Med 1993;328:1372–1376.
33. Houbiers JG, Brand A, van de Watering LM, et al. Randomised controlled trial comparing transfusion of leukocyte-depleted or buffy-coat-depleted blood in surgery for colorectal cancer. Lancet 1994;344:573–578.
34. Mezrow CK, Bergstein I, Tartter PI. Postoperative infections following autologous and homologous blood transfusions. Transfusion 1992;32:27–30.

35. Murphy P, Heal JM, Blumberg N. Infection or suspected infection after hip replacement surgery with autologous or homologous blood transfusions. Transfusion 1991;31:212–217.

36. Heiss MM, Mempel W, Jauch KW, et al. Beneficial effect of autologous blood transfusion on infectious complications after colorectal cancer surgery. Lancet 1993;342:1328–1333.

37. Jensen LS, Anderson AJ, Christiansen PM, et al. Postoperative infection and natural killer cell function following blood transfusion in patients undergoing elective colorectal surgery. Br J Surg 1992;79:513–516.

38. Ness PM, Walsh PC, Zahurak M, et al. Prostate cancer recurrence in radical surgery patients receiving autologous or homologous blood. Transfusion 1993;32:31–36.

39. Houbiers JG, van de Velde CJ, van de Watering LM, et al. Transfusion of red cells is associated with increased incidence of bacterial infection after colorectal surgery: a prospective study. Transfusion 1997;37:1226–1234.

40. Blajchman MA. Allogeneic blood transfusions, immunomodulation, and postoperative bacterial infection: do we have the answers yet? Transfusion 1997;37:121–125.

41. Buchholz DH, AuBuchon JP, Snyder EL, et al. Removal of Yersinia enterocolitica from AS-1 red cells. Transfusion 1992;332:667–672.

42. Wenz B, Burns ER, Freundlich LF. Prevention of growth of Yersinia enterocolitica in blood by polyester fiber filtration. Transfusion 1992;32:663–666.

43. Hogman CF, Gong J, Hambraeus A, et al. The role of white cells in the transmission of Yersinia enterocolitica in blood components. Transfusion 1992;32:654–657.

44. Kim DM, Brecher ME, Bland LA, et al. Prestorage removal of Yersinia enterocolitica from red cells with white-cell-reduction filters. Transfusion 1993;33:520–523.

45. Wenz B, Ciavarella D, Freundlich LF. Effect of prestorage white cell reduction of bacterial growth in platelet concentrates. Transfusion 1993;33:520–523.

46. Nusbacher J. Yersinia enterocolitica and white cell filtration. Transfusion 1992;32:597–600.

47. Rawal BD, Vyas GN. Complement mediated bactericidal action and the removal of Yersinia enterocolitica by white cell filters. Transfusion 1993;33:536. Letter.

48. Gong J, Hogman CF, Hambraeus A, et al. Transfusion associated Serratia marcescens infection: studies of the mechanism of action. Transfusion 1993;33:802–808.

49. Factor IX complex and hepatitis. Food Drug Admin Drug Bull 1976;6:22.

50. Petz LD, Swisher SN, eds. Clinical Practice of Transfusion Medicine, 2nd ed. New York: Churchill Livingstone, 1989.

51. Corrigan JJ. Hemorrhagic and Thrombotic Disease in Childhood and Adolescence. New York: Churchill Livingstone, 1985.

52. Ness PM, Perkins HA. Cryoprecipitate as a reliable source of fibrinogen replacement. JAMA 1979;241:1690.

53. Rosati LA, Barnes B, Oberman H, Penner J. Hemolytic anemia due to anti-A in concentrated hemophilic factor preparations. Transfusion 1970;10:139.

54. McCullough J, Steeper TA, Connelly DP, Jackson B, Huntington S, Scott EP. Platelet utilization in a university hospital. JAMA 1988;259:2414.

55. Hersch EM, Bodey GP, Nies BA, Freireich EJ. Causes of death in acute leukemia: a ten year study of 414 patients from 1954–1963. JAMA 1965;193:105.

56. Gaydos LA, Freireich EJ, Mantel N. The quantitative relation between platelet count and hemorrhage in patients with acute leukemia. N Engl J Med 1962;266:905.

57. Roy AJ, Jaffe N, Djerassi I. Prophylactic platelet transfusions in children with acute leukemia: a dose-response study. Transfusion 1973;13:283.

58. Higby DJ, Cohen E, Holland JF, Sinks L. The prophylactic treatment of thrombocytopenic leukemia patients with platelets: a double blind study. Transfusion 1974;14:440.

59. Soloman J, Bokefkamp T, Fahey JL, et al. Platelet prophylaxis in acute non-lymphocytic leukemia. Lancet 1978;1:267.

60. Murphy S, Litwin S, Herring LM, et al. Indications for platelet transfusion in children with acute leukemia. Am J Hematol 1982;12:347.

61. Slichter SJ. Controversies in platelet transfusion therapy. Annu Rev Med 1980;31:509.

62. Slichter S, Harker LA. Thrombocytopenia: mechanisms and management of defects in platelet production. Clin Haematol 1978;7:523.
63. Patten E. Controversies in transfusion medicine. Prophylactic platelet transfusion revisited after 25 years: con. Transfusion 1992;32:381.
64. Belt RJ, Leite C, Haas CD, Stephens RL. Incidence of hemorrhagic complications in patients with cancer. JAMA 1978;239:2571–2574.
65. Aderka D, Praff G, Santo M. Bleeding due to thrombocytopenia in acute leukemias and reevaluation of the prophylactic platelet transfusion policy. Am J Med Sci 1986;291:147–151.
66. Gmur J, Burger J, Schanz U, Fehr J, Schaffner A. Safety of stringent prophylactic platelet transfusion policy for patients with acute leukaemia. Lancet 1991;338:1223–1226.
67. Consensus Development Conference. Platelet transfusion therapy. JAMA 1987;257:1777–1780.
68. Beutler E. Platelet transfusions: The 20,000/μL trigger. Blood 1993;81:1411–1413.
69. Harker LA, Slichter SJ. The bleeding time as a screening test for evaluation of platelet function. N Engl J Med 1972;287:155.
70. Bishop JF, Schiffer CA, Aisner J, Matthews JP, Wiernik PH. Surgery in acute leukemia: a review of 167 operations in thrombocytopenic patients. Am J Hematol 1987;26:147.
71. Gaydos LA, Freireich EJ, Mantel N. The quantitative relation between platelet count and hemorrhage in patients with acute leukemia. N Engl J Med 1962:266:905.
72. Freireich EJ, Kliman A, Gaydos LA, et al. Response to repeated platelet transfusion from the same donor. Ann Intern Med 1963;50:277.
73. Daly PA, Schiffer CA, Aisner J, Wiernik PH. Platelet transfusion therapy: one-hour posttransfusion increments are valuable in predicting the need for HLA-matched preparations. JAMA 1980;243:435.
74. Dunstan RA, Simpson MB, Knowles RW, Rosse WF. The origin of ABO antigens on human platelets. Blood 1985;65:615–619.
75. Aster RH. Effect of anticoagulant and ABO incompatibility on recovery of transfused human platelets. Blood 1965;26:732–743.
76. Duquesnoy RJ, Anderson AJ, Tomasulo PA, Aster RH. ABO compatibility and platelet transfusions of alloimmunized thrombocytopenic patients. Blood 1979;54:595–599.
77. Skogen B, Rossebo Hansen B, Husebekk A, Havnes T, Hannestad K. Minimal expression of blood group A antigen on thrombocytes from A2 individuals. Transfusion 1988;28:456–459.
78. Heal JM, Blumberg N, Masel D. An evaluation of crossmatching, HLA, and ABO matching for platelet transfusions to refractory patients. Blood 1987;70:23–30.
79. Brand A, Sintnicolaas K, Claas FHJ, Eernisse JG. ABO antibodies causing platelet transfusion refractoriness. Transfusion 1986;26:463–466.
80. Ogasawara K, Ueki J, Takenaka M, Furihata K. Study on the expression of ABH antigens on platelets. Blood 1993;82:993–999.
81. Heal JM, Masel D, Rowe JM, Blumberg N. Circulating immune complexes involving the ABO system after platelet transfusion. Br J Haematol 1993;85:566–572.
82. Carr R, Hutton JL, Jenkins JA, Lucas GF, Amphlett NW. Transfusion of ABO- mismatched platelets leads to early platelet refractoriness. Br J Haematol 1990;75:408.
83. Murphy S. ABO blood groups and platelet transfusion. Transfusion 1988;28:401–402.
84. Lee EJ, Schiffer CA. ABO compatibility can influence the results of platelet transfusion: results of a randomized trial. Transfusion 1989;29:384.
85. Heal JM, Masel D, Blumberg N. Interaction of platelet Fc and complement receptors with circulating immune complexes involving the ABO system. Vox Sang 1996;71:205–211.
86. Pierce RN, Reich LM, Mayer K. Hemolysis following platelet transfusions from ABO- incompatible donors. Transfusion 1985;25:60–62.
87. Lasky L, Warkentin P, Ramsay N, Kersey J, McGlave P, McCullough J. Hemotherapy in patients undergoing blood group incompatible bone marrow transfusion. Transfusion 1983;23:277–285.
88. Goldfinger D, McGinnis MH. Rh incompatible platelet transfusions—risks and consequences of sensitizing immunosuppressed patients. N Engl J Med 1971;284:942.
89. Baldwin ML, Ness PM, Scott D, Braine H, Kickler TS. Alloimmunization to D antigen and HLA in D-negative immunosuppressed oncology patients. Transfusion 1988;28:330–333.

90. McLeod BC, Piehl MR, Sassetti RJ. Alloimmunization to RhD by platelet transfusions in autologous bone marrow transplant recipients. Vox Sang 1990;49:185–189.

91. Lichtiger B, Surgeon J, Rhorer S. Rh-incompatible platelet transfusion therapy in cancer patients. Vox Sang 1983;45:139.

92. Pfisterer H, Thierfelder S, Kottusch H, Stich W. Untersuchung menschlicher thrombocyten auf Rhesus-antigene durch abbaustudien in vivo nach 51Cr-markierung. Klin Wochenschr 1967;45:5519–5522.

93. Doughty HA, Murphy MF, Metcalfe P, et al. Relative importance of immune and non-immune causes of platelet refractoriness. Vox Sang 1994;66:200–205.

94. Aster RH, Jandl JH. Platelet sequestration in man. II. Immunological and clinical studies. J Clin Invest 1964;43:856.

95. Bishop JF, McGrath K, Wolf MM, et al. Clinical factors influencing the efficacy of pooled platelet transfusions. Blood 1988;71:383.

96. Dutcher JP, Schiffer CA, Aisner J, Wiernik PH. Long-term follow-up of patients with leukemia receiving platelet transfusions: identification of a large group of patients who do not become alloimmunized. Blood 1981;58:1007.

97. Dutcher JP, Schiffer CA, Aisner J, Wiernik PH. Alloimmunization following platelet transfusion: the absence of a dose-response relationship. Blood 1981;57:395.

98. TRAP Trial Study Group. A randomized trial evaluating leukocyte-reduction and UV-B irradiation of platelets to prevent alloimmune platelet refractoriness. N Engl J Med. In press.

99. Lazarus HM, Herzig RH, Warm SE, Fishman DJ. Transfusion experience with platelet concentrates stored for 24 to 72 hours at 22°C. Transfusion 1982;22:39.

100. Yankee RA, Grumet FC, Rogentine GN. Platelet transfusion therapy: the selection of compatible platelet donors for refractory patients by lymphocyte HLA typing. N Engl J Med 1969;281:1208.

101. Grumet FC, Yankee RA. Long-term platelet support of patients with aplastic anemia—effect of splenectomy and steroid therapy. Ann Intern Med 1970;73:1–7.

102. Lohrman HP, Bull MI, Decter JA, et al. Platelet transfusions from HLA compatible unrelated donors to alloimmunized patients. Ann Intern Med 1974;80:9.

103. Duquesnoy RJ, Filip DJ, Rodey GE, et al. Successful transfusion of platelets "mismatched" for HLA antigens to alloimmunized thrombocytopenic patients. Am J Hematol 1977;2:219.

104. Duquesnoy RJ, Vieira J, Aster RH. Donor availability for platelet transfusion support of alloimmunized thrombocytopenic patients. Transplant Proc 1977;9:519.

105. Moroff G, Garratty G, Heal JM, et al. Selection of platelets for refractory patients by HLA matching and prospective crossmatching. Transfusion 1992;32:633.

106. McFarland JG, Anderson AJ, Slichter SJ. Factors influencing the transfusion response to HLA-selected apheresis donor platelets in patients refractory to random platelet concentrates. Br J Haematol 1989;73:380–386.

107. Bolgiano DC, Larson EB, Slichter SJ. A model to determine required pool size for HLA-typed community donor apheresis programs. Transfusion 1989;29:306.

108. McFarland JG, Aster RH. Evaluation of four methods for platelet compatibility testing. Blood 1987;69:1425–1429.

109. Tasato G, Appelbaum FR, Trapani RJ, Dowling R, Deisseroth AB. Use of in vitro assays in selection of compatible platelet donors. Transfusion 1980;20:47–53.

110. Filip DJ, Duquesnoy RJ, Aster RH. Predictive value of cross-matching for transfusion of platelet concentrates to alloimmunized recipients. Am J Hematol 1976;1:471–479.

111. Freedman J, Hooi C, Garvey MB. Prospective platelet crossmatching for selection of compatible random donors. Br J Haematol 1984;56:9–18.

112. Kickler TS, Ness PM, Braine HG. Platelet crossmatching: a direct approach to the selection of platelet transfusions for the alloimmunized thrombocytopenic patient. Am J Clin Pathol 1988;90:69–72.

113. Rachel JM, Sinor LT, Tawfik OW, et al. A solid-phase red cell adherence test for platelet cross-matching. Med Lab Sci 1985;42:194–195.

114. Rachel JM, Summers TC, Sinor LT, Plapp FV. Use of a solid phase red blood cell adherence method for pretransfusion platelet compatibility testing. Am J Clin Pathol 1988;90:63–68.

115. O'Connell BA, Lee EJ, Rothko K, Hussein MA, Schiffer CA. Selection of histocompatibility apheresis platelet donors by cross-matching random donor platelet concentrates. Blood 1992;79:527–531.

116. Friedberg RC, Donnelly SF, Boyd JC, Gray LS, Mintz PD. Clinical and blood bank factors in the management of platelet refractoriness and alloimmunization. Blood 1993;81:3428–3434.

117. Bensinger WI, Buckner C, Clift RA, Slichter SJ, Thomas ED. Plasma exchange for platelet alloimmunization. Transplantation 1986;41:602–605.

118. Christie DJ, Howe RB, Lennon SS, Sauro SC. Treatment of refractoriness to platelet transfusion by protein A column therapy. Transfusion 1993;33:234–242.

119. Kekomaki R, Elfenbein G, Gardner R. Improved response of patients refractory to random-donor platelet transfusions by intravenous gamma globulin. Am J Med 1984;73:199–203.

120. Junghans RP, Ahn YS. High-dose intravenous gamma globulin to suppress alloimmune destruction of donor platelets. Am J Med 1994;73:204–208.

121. Schiffer CA, Hogge DE, Aisner J, et al. High-dose intravenous gammaglobulin in alloimmunized platelet transfusion recipients. Blood 1984;64:937–940.

122. Moroff G, Friedman A, Robkin-Kline L, Gautier G, Luban NLC. Reduction of the volume of stored platelet concentrates for use in neonatal patients. Transfusion 1984;24:144–146.

123. Claas FHJ, Smeenk RJT, Schmidt R, van Steenbrugge GJ, Eernisse JG. Alloimmunization against the MHC antigens after platelet transfusions is due to contaminating leukocytes in the platelet suspension. Exp Hematol 1981;9:84–89.

124. Meryman HT. Transfusion-induced alloimmunization and immunosuppression and the effects of leukocyte depletion. Trans Med Rev 1989;3:180.

125. Schiffer CA. Prevention of alloimmunization against platelets. Blood 1991;77:1–4.

126. Gmur J, von Felten A, Osterwalder B, et al. Delayed alloimmunization using random single donor platelet transfusions: a prospective study in thrombocytopenic patients with acute leukemia. Blood 1983;62:473–479.

127. van Marwijk Kooy M, van Prooijen HC, Moes M, et al. Use of leukocyte-depleted platelet concentrates for the prevention of refractoriness and primary HLA alloimmunization: a prospective, randomized trial. Blood 1991;77:201–205.

128. Saarinen UM, Kekomaki R, Siimes MA, Myllyla G. Effective prophylaxis against platelet refractoriness in multitransfused patients by use of leukocyte-free blood components. Blood 1990;75:512–517.

129. Andreu G, Dewailly J, Leberre C, et al. Prevention of HLA immunization with leukocyte-poor packed red cells and platelet concentrates obtained by filtration. Blood 1988;72:964–969.

130. Novotny VMJ, van Doorn R, Witvliet MD, et al. Occurrence of allogeneic HLA and non-HLA antibodies after transfusion of prestorage filtered platelets and red blood cells: a prospective study. Blood 1995;85:1736–1741.

131. Sniecinski I, O'Donnell MR, Nowicki B, Hill LR. Prevention of refractoriness and HLA- alloimmunization using filtered blood products. Blood 1988;71:1402–1407.

132. Sintnicolaas K, van Marwijk Kooij M, van Prooijen HC, et al. Leukocyte depletion of random single-donor platelet transfusions does not prevent secondary human leukocyte antigen-alloimmunization and refractoriness: a randomized prospective study. Blood 1995;85:824–828.

133. Blajchman MA, Bardossy L, Carmen RA, et al. An animal model of allogeneic donor platelet refractoriness: the effect of the time of leukodepletion. Blood 1992;79:11371–11375.

134. Williamson LM, Wimperis JZ, Williamson P, et al. Bedside filtration of blood products in the prevention of HLA alloimmunization. A prospective randomized study. Blood 1994;83:3028–3035.

135. Heddle NM, Blajchman MA. The leukodepletion of cellular blood products in the prevention of HLA-alloimmunization and refractoriness to allogeneic platelet transfusions. Blood 1995;85:603–606.

136. Deeg HJ. Transfusions with a tan: prevention of allosensitization by ultraviolet irradiation. Transfusion 1989;29:450–455.

137. Kahn RA, Duffy BF, Rodey GG. Ultraviolet irradiation of platelet concentrate abrogates lymphocyte activation with affecting platelet function in vitro. Transfusion 1985;25:547–550.

138. Deeg HJ, Aprile J, Graham TC, Appelbaum FR, Storb R. Ultraviolet irradiation of blood prevents transfusion-induced sensitization and marrow graft rejection in dogs. Blood 1986;87:537–539.

139. Grana NH, Kao KJ. Use of 8-methoxypsoralen and ultraviolet-A pretreated platelet concentrates to prevent alloimmunization against class I major histocompatibility antigens. Blood 1991;77:2530–2537.

140. Kao KJ. Effects of leukocyte depletion and UVB irradiation on alloantigenicity of major histocompatibility complex antigens in platelet concentrates: a comparative study. Blood 1992;80:2931–2937.

141. Capon SM, Sacher RA, Deeg JH. Effective ultraviolet irradiation of platelet concentrates in teflon bags. Transfusion 1990;30:678–681.
142. Bodey GP, Buckley M, Sath YS, Freireich EJ. Quantitative relationships between circulating leukocytes and infection in patients with acute leukemia. Ann Intern Med 1966;64:328.
143. Gurwith MJ, Brunton JL, Lank BA, et al. Granulocytopenia in hospitalized patients. I. Prognostic factors and etiology of fever. Am J Med 1978;61:121.
144. McCullough J. Leukapheresis and granulocyte transfusion. CRC Crit Rev Clin Lab Sci 1979;10:275.
145. Freireich EJ, Levin RH, Wang J. The function and gate of transfused leukocytes from donors with chronic myelocytic leukemia in leukopenic recipients. Ann NY Acad Sci 1965;113:1081.
146. Belardinelli A, Belletti D, Nucci S, Tazzari PL, Conte R. Granulocyte transfusion: is there a role for buffy coats in the current management of infected neutropenic adult patients? Vox Sang 1996;70:45–46.
147. Strauss RG. Therapeutic neutrophil transfusions: are controlled studies no longer appropriate? Am J Med 1978;65:1001.
148. Alavi JB, Roat RK, Djerassi I, et al. A randomized clinical trial of granulocyte transfusions for infection of acute leukemia. N Engl J Med 1977;296:706.
149. Graw RH Jr, Herzig G, Perry S, Henderson ES. Normal granulocyte transfusion therapy. Treatment of septicemia due to gram-negative bacteria. N Engl J Med 1972;287:367.
150. Herzig GP, Graw RG Jr. Granulocyte transfusions for bacterial infections. In: Brown EB, ed. Progress in Hematology, vol 9. New York: Grune & Stratton, 1975:207.
151. Degregorio MW, Lee WMF, Linker CA, et al. Fungal infections in patients with acute leukemia. Am J Med 1982;73:543.
152. Young LS. Nosocomial infections in the immunocompromised adult. Am J Med 1981;70:398.
153. Ruthe RC, Ansersen BR, Cunningham BL, Epstein RB. Efficacy of granulocyte transfusions in the control of systemic candidiasis in leukopenic host. Blood 1978;52:493.
154. Raubitschek AA, Levin AS, Stites DP, et al. Normal granulocyte infusion therapy for aspergillosis in chronic granulomatous disease. Pediatrics 1973;51:230.
155. Strauss RG, Connett JE, Gale RP, et al. A controlled trial of prophylactic granulocyte transfusion during initial induction. N Engl J Med 1981;305:597.
156. Bensinger WI, Price TH, Dale DC, et al. The effects of daily recombinant human granulocyte-colony-stimulating factor administration on normal granulocyte donors undergoing leukapheresis. Blood 1993;81:1883–1888.
157. Caspar CB, Seger RA, Burger J, Gmur J. Effective stimulation of donors for granulocyte colony-stimulating factor. Blood 1993;81:2877–2871.
158. Liles WC, Juang JE, Llewellyn C, et al. A comparative trial of granulocyte-colony-stimulating factor and dexamethasone, separately and in combination, for the mobilization of neutrophils in the peripheral blood of normal volunteers. Transfusion 1997;37:182–187.
159. Gilbert GL, Hudson IL, Hayes JJ. Prevention of transfusion-acquired cytomegalovirus infection in infants by blood filtration to remove leukocytes. Lancet 1989;1:1228.
160. Murphy MF, Grint PCA, Hardiman AE, Lister TA, Waters AH. Use of leukocyte-poor blood components to prevent primary cytomegalovirus (CMV) infection in patients with acute leukemia. Br J Haematol 1988;70:253.
161. Bowden RA, Slichter SJ, Sayers M, et al. A comparison of filtered leukocyte-reduced and cytomegalovirus (CMV) seronegative blood products for the prevention of transfusion-associated CMV infection after marrow transplant. Blood 1995;86:3598–3603.
162. Yaeger AS, Grumet FC, Hafleigh EB, et al. Prevention of transfusion-acquired cytomegalovirus infections in newborn infants. J Pediatr 1981;98:281.
163. Stagno S, Pass RF, Dworsky ME, et al. Congenital cytomegalovirus infection: the relative importance of primary and recurrent maternal infection. N Engl J Med 1982;306:945.
164. Adler SP. Neonatal cytomegalovirus infections due to blood. CRC Crit Rev Clin Lab Sci 1985;23:1.
165. Tegtmeier GE. Cytomegalovirus and blood transfusion. In: Dodd RY, Barker LF, eds. Infection, Immunity, and Blood Transfusion, vol 182. New York: Alan R Liss, 1985:175.
166. Glenn J. Cytomegalovirus infection following renal transplantation. Rev Infect Dis 1981;3:1151.
167. Rubin RH, Tolkoff-Rubin NE, Oliver D, et al. Multicenter seroepidemiologic study of the impact of cytomegalovirus infection on renal transplantation. Transplantation 1985;40:243.

168. Chou S. Acquisition of donor strains of cytomegalovirus by renal-transplant recipients. N Engl J Med 1986;314:1418.

169. Miller W, Flynn P, McCullough J, et al. Cytomegalovirus infection after bone marrow transplantation: an association with acute graft-vs-host disease. Blood 1986;67:1162.

170. Bowden RA, Sayers M, Flournoy N, et al. Cytomegalovirus immune globulin and seronegative blood products prevent primary cytomegalovirus infection after marrow transplantation. N Engl J Med 1986;314:1006.

171. Miller WJ, McCullough J, Balfour HH, et al. Prevention of cytomegalovirus infection following bone marrow transplantation: a randomized trial of blood product screening. Bone Marrow Transplant 1991;7:227–234.

172. Condie RM, O'Reilly RJ. Prevention of cytomegalovirus infection by prophylaxis with an intravenous, hyperimmune, native, unmodified cytomegalovirus globulin. Am J Med 1984;76:134.

173. Meyers JD, Leszczynski J, Zaia JA, et al. Prevention of cytomegalovirus infection by cytomegalovirus immune globulin after marrow transplantation. Ann Intern Med 1983;98:442.

174. Winston DJ, Ho WG, Lin C, et al. Intravenous immunoglobulin for modification of cytomegalovirus infections associated with bone marrow transplantation. Am J Med 1984;76:128.

175. Gilbert GL, Hudson IL, Hayes JJ. Prevention of transfusion-acquired cytomegalovirus infection in infants by blood filtration to remove leucocytes. Lancet 1989;1:1228.

176. Murphy MF, Grint PCA, Hardiman AE, Lister TA, Waters AH. Use of leukocyte-poor blood components to prevent primary cytomegalovirus (CMV) infection in patients with acute leukemia. Br J Haematol 1988;70:253.

177. Preiksaitis JK, Rosno S, Grumet C, Merigan TC. Infections due to herpes viruses in cardiac transplant recipients: role of the donor heart and immunosuppressive therapy. J Infect Dis 1983;147:1974.

178. Rakela J, Wiesner RH, Taswell HF, et al. Incidence of cytomegalovirus infection and its relationship to donor-recipient serologic status in liver transplantation. Transplant Proc 1987;19:2399.

179. Preiksaitis JK, Grumet FC, Smith WK, Merigan TC. Transfusion-acquired cytomegalovirus infections in cardiac surgery patients. J Med Virol 1985;15:283.

180. Adler SP, Baggett J, McVoy M. Transfusion-associated cytomegalovirus infections in seropositive cardiac surgery patients. Lancet 1985;743.

181. Hathaway WE, Githens JH, Blackburn WR, et al. Aplastic anemia, histiocytosis and erythrodermia in immunologically deficient children: probable human runt disease. N Engl J Med 1965;271:953–955.

182. Park BH, Good RA, Gate J, et al. Fatal graft-versus-host reaction following transfusion of allogeneic blood and plasma in infants with combined immunodeficiency disease. Transplant Proc 1974;6:385.

183. Douglas SD, Fudenberg HH. Graft versus host reaction in Wiskott-Aldrich syndrome: antemortem diagnosis of human GVH in an immunologic deficiency disease. Vox Sang 1969;16:172.

184. Hathaway WE, Githen JA, Blackburn JR, et al. Aplastic anemia, histiocytosis and erythroderma in immunologically deficient children. N Engl J Med 1965;273:953–955.

185. Thomas ED, Storb R, Clift RA, et al. Bone-marrow transplantation. N Engl J Med 1975;292:832.

186. Wagner JE, Vogelsang GB, Beschorner WE. Pathogenesis and pathology of graft-versus host disease. Am J Pediatr Hematol Oncol 1989;11:196–212.

187. Dobrynski W, Thibodeau S, Truitt RL, et al. Third-party-mediated graft rejection and graft-versus-host disease after T-cell-depleted bone marrow transplantation as demonstrated by hypervariable DNA probes and HLA-Dr polymorphism. Blood 1989;74:2285–2294.

188. Weiden PL, Zuckerman N, Hansen JA, et al. Fatal graft-versus-host disease in a patient with lymphoblastic leukemia following normal granulocyte transfusions. Blood 1981;57:328.

189. Siimes MA, Koskimies S. Chronic graft-versus-host disease after blood transfusions confirmed by incompatible HLA antigens in bone marrow. Lancet 1982;1:42.

190. Lowenthal RM, Menon C, Challis DR. Graft-versus-host disease in consecutive patients with acute myeloid leukemia treated with blood cells from normal donors. Aust NZ J Med 1981;11:179.

191. Woods WG, Lubin BH. Fatal graft versus host disease following a blood transfusion in a child with neuroblastoma. Pediatrics 1981;67:217.

192. Thaler M, Shamiss A, Orgad S, et al. The role of blood from HLA-homozygous donors in fatal transfusion-associated graft-versus-host disease after open-heart surgery. N Engl J Med 1989;321:25.

193. Sheehan T, McLaren KM, Brettle R, Parker AC. Transfusion-induced graft-versus-host disease in preg-

nancy. Clin Lab Haematol 1987;9:205.

194. Arsura EL, Bertelle A, Minkowitz S, Cunningham JN, Crob D. Transfusion-associated graft-versus-host disease in a presumed immunocompetent patient. Arch Intern Med 1988;148:1941.

195. Otsuka S, Kunieda K, Hirose M, et al. Fatal erythroderma (suspected graft-versus-host disease) after cholecystectomy. Transfusion 1989;29:544.

196. Sakakibara T, Ida T, Mannouji E, et al. Post-transfusion graft-versus-host disease following open-heart surgery. J Cardiovasc Surg 1989;30:687–691.

197. Juji T, Takahashi K, Shibata Y. HLA-homozygous donors and transfusion-associated graft-versus-host disease. N Engl J Med 1990;332:107. Letter.

198. Juji T. Post transfusion GVHD. Vox Sang 1996;70:24–25.

199. Moroff G, Leitman SF, Luban NLC. Principles of blood irradiation, dose validation and quality control: a practical approach. Transfusion. In press.

200. Lowenthal RM, Challis DR, Griffiths AE, et al. Transfusion-associated graft-versus-host disease: report of a case following administration of blood. Transfusion 1993;33:524–529.

201. Sproul AM, Chalmers EA, Mills KI, et al. Third party mediated graft rejection despite irradiation of blood products. Br J Haematol 1992;80:251–252.

202. Anderson KC, Goodnough LT, Sayers M, et al. Variation in blood component irradiation practice: implications for prevention of transfusion-associated graft-versus-host disease. Blood 1991;77:2096–2102.

203. Leitman SF, Holland PV. Irradiation of blood products: indications and guidelines. Transfusion 1985;25:293.

204. Sprent J, Anderson RE, Miller JFAP. Radiosensitivity of T and B lymphocytes. II. Effect of irradiation on response of T cells to alloantigens. Eur J Immunol 1974;4:204.

205. Valerius NH, Johansen KS, Nielsen OS, et al. Effect of in vitro x-irradiation on lymphocyte and granulocyte function. Scand J Hematol 1981;27:9.

206. Button LN, DeWolf WC, Newburger PE, Jacobson MS, Kevy SV. The effects of irradiation on blood components. Transfusion 1981;21:419.

207. Holley TR, Van Epps DE, Harvey RL, et al. Effect of high doses of radiation on human neutrophil chemotaxis, phagocytosis, and morphology. Am J Pathol 1974;75:61.

208. Greenberg ML, Chanana AD, Cronkite, et al. Extracorporeal irradiation of blood in man: radiation resistance of circulating platelets. Radiat Res 1968;35:147.

209. Read EJ, Kodis C, Carter CS, Leitman SF. Viability of platelets following storage in the irradiated state. A pair-controlled study. Transfusion 1988;23:446–450.

210. Duguid JKM, Carr R, Jenkins JA, et al. Clinical evaluation of the effects of storage time and irradiation on transfused platelets. Vox Sang 1991;60:151–154.

211. Moroff G, Luban NLC. Prevention of transfusion-associated graft-versus-host disease. Transfusion 1992;32:101–103. Editorial.

212. Pelszynski M, Moroff G, Luban N, et al. Dose dependent lymphocyte inactivation in red blood cell (RBC) units with gamma irradiation. Transfusion 1991;31(Suppl):17S. Abstract.

213. Center for Biologics Evaluation and Research. License amendments and procedures for gamma irradiation of blood products. Bethesda, MD: U.S. Food and Drug Administration, July 22, 1993.

214. Davey RJ, McCoy NC, Yu M, et al. The effect of prestorage irradiation on posttransfusion red cell survival. Transfusion 1992;32:525–528.

215. Ramirez AM, Woodfield DG, Scott R, McLachlan J. High potassium levels in stored irradiated blood. Transfusion 1987;27:444. Letter.

216. Rivet C, Baxter A, Rock G. Potassium levels in irradiated blood. Transfusion 1989;29:185. Letter.

217. Strauss RG. Routine washing of irradiated red cells before transfusion seems unwarranted. Transfusion 1990;30:675–677.

218. Read EJ, Kodis C, Carter CS, Leitman SF. Viability of platelets following storage in the irradiated state. Transfusion 1988;28:446–450.

219. Suda BA, Leitman SF, Davey RJ. Characteristics of red cells irradiated and subsequently frozen for long-term storage. Transfusion 1993;33:389–392.

220. Freedman JJ, Blajchman MA, McCombie N. Canadian Red Cross Society symposium on leukodepletion: report of proceedings. Transfus Med Rev 1994; 8:1–14.

221. Chambers LA, Garcia LW. White blood cell content of transfusion components. Lab Med 1991;22:857–860.
222. Parkman R, Mosier D, Umansky I, et al. Graft-versus-host disease after intrauterine and exchange transfusions for hemolytic disease of the newborn. N Engl J Med 1974;290:359.
223. Bohm N, Kleine W, Enzel U. Graft-versus-host disease in two newborns after repeated blood transfusions because of Rhesus incompatibility. Beitr Pathol 1977;160:381.
224. Strauss RG. Practical issues in neonatal transfusion practice. Am J Clin Pathol 1997;107 (Suppl 1):S57–S63.
225. Mintz PD, Luban NLC. Irradiated blood components. Am J Clin Pathol 1997;107:252. Letter to the Editor.
226. Benson K. Irradiated blood components. Am J Clin Pathol 1997;107:251. Letter to the Editor.
227. Schmidmeier W, Feil W, Gebhart W, et al. Fatal graft-versus host reaction following granulocyte transfusions. Blut 1982;45:115.
228. Cohen D, Weinstein H, Mihm M, Yankee R. Nonfatal graft-versus-host disease occurring after transfusion with leukocytes and platelets obtained from normal donors. Blood 1979;53:1053.
229. Ford JM, Lucey JJ, Cullen MH, et al. Fatal graft-versus-host disease following transfusion of granulocytes from normal donors. Lancet 1976;2:1167.
230. Schwarzenberg L, Mathe G, Amiel JL, et al. Study of factors determining the usefulness and complications of leukocyte transfusions. Am J Med 1967;43:206.
231. von Fliedner V, Higby DJ, Kim U. Graft-versus-host reaction following blood transfusion. Am J Med 1982;72:951.
232. Alving BM, Weinstein MJ, Finlayson JS, Menitove JE, Fratantoni JC. Fibrin sealant: summary of a conference on characteristics and clinical uses. Transfusion 1995;35:783–790.
233. Gibble JW, Ness PM. Fibrin glue, the perfect operative sealant? Transfusion 1990; 30:741–747.
234. Cmolik BL, Spero JA, Magovern GJ, Clark RE. Redo cardiac surgery: late bleeding complications from topical thrombin-induced factor V deficiency. J Thorac Cardiovasc Surg 1993;105:222–228.
235. Milne AA, Murphy WG, Reading SJ, Ruckley CV. A randomized trial of fibrin sealant in peripheral vascular surgery. Vox Sang 1996;70:210–212.
236. Rousou J, Levitsky S, Gonzales-Lavin L, et al. Randomized clinical trial of fibrin sealant in patients undergoing resternotomy or reoperation after cardiac operations; a multicenter study. J Thorac Cardiovasc Surg 1989;97:194–203.
237. Berruyer M, Amiral J, Ffrench P, et al. Immunization by bovine thrombin used with fibrin glue during cardiovascular operations. J Thorac Cardiovasc Surg 1993;105:892–897.

TRANSFUSION THERAPY IN SPECIFIC CLINICAL SITUATIONS

ACUTE BLOOD LOSS

Physiology and Therapy

The signs, symptoms, and physiologic changes that occur in association with different degrees of blood loss are rather well known. Loss of approximately 10% of the blood volume causes few symptoms (Table 12.1) and is what happens thousands of times each day when people donate blood for transfusion. Loss of up to 20% may still not cause unusual signs or symptoms when the patient is at rest, although there is usually tachycardia with exercise. When up to 30% of the blood volume has been lost without replacement, hypotension and tachycardia often develop, but at rest there may still be few signs or symptoms (Table 12.1). With blood loss exceeding 30%, there are serious signs and symptoms of cardiovascular compromise. These include tachycardia with a weak pulse, hyperpnea, hypotension, decrease in central venous pressure and cardiac output, and cold clammy skin.

When patients experience acute blood loss, the primary need is for volume replacement. This need is more urgent the greater the extent of the blood loss. Initially blood loss depletes the intravascular space, and only later is there a shift of fluid from the extravascular into the intravascular space. Thus, early in the blood loss situation, attention can be focused on replacing intravascular space losses, and this can be accomplished easily using crystalloid solutions such as isotonic saline or Ringer's lactate.[1] As blood loss continues, fluid shifts from the extravascular space to compensate for the decreased intravascular volume. Because crystalloid solutions are distributed into the

Table 12.1 Reaction to acute blood loss of increasing severity

Volume lost up to		Clinical signs
% TBV*	mL**	
10	500	None. Rarely see vasovagal syncope in blood donors.
20	1,000	With the patient at rest it is still impossible to detect volume loss. Tachycardia is usual with exercise, and a slight postural drop in blood pressure may be evident.
30	1,500	Neck veins are flat when supine. Postural hypotension and exercise tachycardia are generally present, but the resting, supine blood pressure and pulse still can be normal.
40	2,000	Central venous pressure, cardiac output, and arterial blood pressure are below normal even when the patient is supine and at rest. The patient usually demonstrates air hunger; a rapid, thready pulse; and cold, clammy skin.
50	2,500	Severe shock, death.

Source: Hillman RS. Acute blood loss anemia. In: Beutler E, Lichtman MA, Coller BS, et al., eds. Williams Hematology, 5th ed. New York: McGraw Hill, Inc. 1995:704–708.
*TBV, total blood volume; **mL of blood lost.

extravascular space as well, it is necessary to administer two to three times the amount of crystalloid as the volume lost. If large volumes of crystalloids are given, there is a risk of fluid overload, especially in the elderly. There has been a debate on whether the use of colloid solutions is preferable, since these solutions would maintain the intravascular oncotic pressure without providing the large amount of extra fluid[2]. The solutions are compared in Table 12.2. The results of clinical studies have not resolved this issue.[3] Crystalloid solutions are recommended as the initial treatment of acute blood loss. If blood loss continues and represents a substantial portion of the blood volume, colloid solutions can be added. The colloid solutions used are 5% human serum albumin, hydroxyethyl starch (HES), or 5% plasma protein fraction (see Chapters 2 and 5). These products provide replacement of the volume lost on an equal basis, and HES may actually provide a slightly larger volume replacement than the volume administered.

Table 12.2 Comparison of crystalloid and colloid solutions

	Crystalloid	Colloid
Intravascular retention	Poor	Good
Peripheral edema	Common	Possible
Pulmonary edema	Possible	Possible
Easily excreted	Yes	No
Allergic reactions	Absent	Rare
Cost	Inexpensive	Expensive

Source: Stehling L. Fluid replacement in massive transfusion. In: Jefferies LC, Brecher ME, eds. Massive Transfusion. Bethesda, MD: American Association of Blood Banks, 1994:1–16.

The symptoms that occur with blood loss are the result of blood volume depletion, not depletion of red cell mass. Several compensatory mechanisms act to maintain blood flow to and oxygenation of the brain and heart. These mechanisms include adrenergic nervous system stimulation, release of vasoactive substance, hyperventilation, shift of fluid from intracellular to extracellular space, shift of fluid from the interstitial to the intravascular space, and renal conversion of water and electrolytes. Two major points deserve emphasis: (*a*) because the manifestations of acute blood loss are due to hypovolemia, early and aggressive replacement of intravascular volume is essential; and (*b*) unless the patient has a very low initial hemoglobin concentration or has severely impaired cardiovascular function, red cell replacement is not necessary during initial therapy of acute blood loss. Also, resuscitation with blood is not practical because of logistic difficulties. With the shift to blood component therapy, whole blood is rarely available, and it is impractical to maintain an adequate stock of "universal donor" group O negative red cells for every situation. Thus, the initial management of acute blood loss is as described here. If blood loss continues, the situation becomes one of massive transfusion and then there are additional therapeutic considerations.

Blood Bank Procedures

In the management of acute blood loss, effective communication between the physicians or key personnel on the patient care team and the blood bank is essential. Blood bank personnel are well aware that there may be situations in which there is an urgent need for blood, and each blood bank should have a procedure for the rapid release of red cells.[4] Busy emergency departments usually have well-defined plans for these situations; however, when acute blood loss occurs in other situations, clinical care personnel may be less familiar with the policies and procedures necessary for rapid, safe provision of blood components. In these situations, clear, concise, and informative communication from the physician to the blood bank and the blood bank to the physician is essential. To avoid frivolous release of incompletely crossmatched or noncrossmatched red cells, the blood bank personnel will usually ask questions about the patient situation. It is essential that a physician take responsibility for the situation and clearly indicate the urgent nature of the patient's situation to the blood bank personnel. After the emergency has passed, the physician will be expected to sign a form taking responsibility for the emergency release of the blood. The most important feature of the communication is for the clinical care team to provide the blood bank with a clear, concise assessment of the situation and the anticipated blood needs. Initially it may be difficult to predict the needs, and so continuing communication is important. The blood bank has a variety of ways to respond depending on the patient's needs.

First, a blood specimen should be obtained and sent to the blood bank for emergency type and crossmatch. An ABO and Rh type can be performed quickly and blood of the same type as the patient can be selected. This blood can be released under an emergency crossmatch procedure, which requires approximately 15 minutes. Thus, partially crossmatched blood of the patient's type can be available quickly. Blood released using this emergency crossmatch procedure involves shortening the incubation of the patient's serum and the donor's red cells. Usually this is done in a way to detect only ABO incompatibility, since that is usually the most disastrous kind of transfusion reac-

tion. In the past, blood was often released without any crossmatch. Today, most blood banks have simplified procedures to carry out a rapid crossmatch that will detect ABO incompatibility in a very few minutes to avoid compromising patient care. If it is considered necessary to release blood without a crossmatch and if the blood bank has a sample of the patient's blood, the ABO type can be determined quickly and ABO type-specific blood released without a crossmatch. Usually Rh-positive blood would be chosen, since 85% of patients will be Rh-positive and the inventory of Rh-negative blood is limited. In some situations, Rh-negative blood may be used depending on the hospital's inventory and the age and sex of the patient. When the patient's ABO type is not known, group O red cells are used. This has led to the designation of group O Rh-negative individuals as a universal donor, since these red cells would not be hemolyzed by either anti-A, anti-B, or any Rh(D) antibody present in the patient and would not immunize patients to the D antigen. Group O Rh-negative (universal donor) red cells do not avoid the potential risk that the recipient may have another red cell antibody or a red cell autoantibody, and so hemolysis or transfusion reactions can occur following transfusion of group O Rh-negative "universal donor" red cells. Stocking O Rh-negative red cells routinely in emergency departments is neither necessary, practical, or appropriate. The red cells may not be stored properly, and there may not be a system of checks for release of the units—practices that can lead to serious problems. In addition, there is not an adequate national supply of O negative red cells to provide these for every emergency department. Techniques of fluid management and resuscitation are so highly developed today that patients can be maintained for the very few minutes required to obtain red cells from the blood bank.

Changing Blood Types

During acute blood loss or massive transfusion, the supply of the patient's specific blood type in the hospital may not be sufficient to meet the need. Thus, it may be necessary to change blood types. The factors that should be considered include (a) the patient's immediate clinical condition, (b) the patient's overall diagnosis, (c) the patient's blood type, (d) the hospital's blood inventory, (e) responsiveness of the blood supplier, and (f) the supplier's blood inventory.

Patients with less common types of AB or B can be switched to the more common type A (from AB) or O (from B). This switch means that patients will be receiving plasma containing ABO-incompatible antibodies. Although most of the plasma is removed in the production of red blood cells, transfusion of large amounts of ABO-incompatible blood can provide sufficient antibody to cause a positive direct antiglobulin test and/or hemolysis. Appropriate monitoring of these patients involves testing for ABO antibody, performing a direct antiglobulin test, and observing the patient for a decrease in hemoglobin not attributable to other causes.

For Rh-negative patients, it may be necessary to convert to Rh-positive blood. If these patients also have the less common ABO types (AB or B), converting only the Rh type but continuing to use the patient's own ABO type may not provide much additional blood. Thus, if the clinical situation indicates a continuing need for a large amount of blood, it is usually advisable to switch AB or B negative patients to A or O positive red

cells. For A or O negative patients, the only option is to switch to A or O positive red cells. If the supply of Rh-negative red cells is inadequate to meet the patient's needs, there should be no hesitancy in switching to Rh-positive red cells. It is most important to deal with the patient's immediate transfusion needs and address the possibility of Rh immunization later. In women of childbearing age, Rh immune globulin can be used to prevent immunization (see Chapter 10).

Once the patient is stabilized, bleeding is controlled, and blood inventory is adequate, consideration can be given to switching the patient back to his or her original type. The major criterion for this switch is the absence of circulating ABO antibody incompatible with the patient's original type. In this situation, the crossmatch should be incompatible. The patient's serum should be tested in the antiglobulin phase or by an equally sensitive method to ensure the absence of free ABO-incompatible antibody. There is a theoretical concern that in the absence of free ABO antibody, antibody bound to the patient's red cells could re-equilibrate and coat the newly transfused cells, thereby reducing their survival. It is not known that this occurs, and the presence or absence of free antibody is a suitable indicator of safety.

MASSIVE TRANSFUSION

Massive transfusion may occur in several circumstances, such as (*a*) replacement of the patient's blood volume during a 24-hour interval, (*b*) transfusion of more than 20 units of red cells in 24 hours, (*c*) replacement of more than 50% of the patient's blood volume in 3 hours, or (*d*) blood loss more than 150 mL/minute in an adult. The potential complications of massive transfusion are the results of the biochemical and functional characteristics of stored blood (Table 12.3) (see Chapter 5). Most red cells are suspended in an additive solution to optimize the quality of cells and length of storage. This means that virtually all of the plasma and platelets have been removed, and thus in massive transfusion of red cells these other blood components are not replaced. These changes in stored red cells, as well as the citrate content and cold temperature, create potential for substantial complications (Table 12.4) when large volumes are transfused rapidly.

Table 12.3 Changes in red blood cell units during storage

Decreased pH
Increased affinity of hemoglobin for oxygen
Decreased red cell deformability
Hemolysis
Increased potassium concentration
Increased ammonia concentration
Increased phosphate concentration
Development of microaggregates
Deterioration of platelets
Decrease in factors V and VIII
Release of vasoactive substances
Denaturation of proteins

Table 12.4 Potential complications of massive transfusion

Thrombocytopenia
Coagulopathy
Hypothermia
Acidosis
Poor oxygen dissociation
Hypocalcemia
Hyperkalemia
Adult respiratory distress syndrome due to microaggregates
Hyperammonemia
Plasticizer toxicity

Coagulopathy

Well-defined coagulation disorders can be identified in one-half to two-thirds of patients receiving a massive transfusion.[5–7] Several clinical studies substantiate that thrombocytopenia is the most common coagulation abnormality in patients receiving a massive transfusion.[6,7] The platelet count is usually inversely related to the number of units of blood transfused.[6] Transfusion of large amounts of blood depleted of platelets and coagulation factors may create deficiencies in the recipient because of dilution of the recipient's blood with this depleted stored blood. In addition, the hemostatic process that occurs in the bleeding patient consumes the patient's own platelets and coagulation factors and compounds the depletion state. Usually factor VIII is rapidly replaced by the patient, and factor V levels do not fall below that needed for hemostasis. Measurement of fibrinogen, which is not depleted in stored blood, is also often helpful as an aid in diagnosing disseminated intravascular coagulopathy (DIC),[6,7] but in general the prothrombin time (PT), partial thromboplastin time (PTT), and bleeding time are not helpful in elucidating the cause of abnormal bleeding,[6,8] because there is little relation between the level of coagulation factors and bleeding.[6,9] Predetermined standard schemes for transfusion of platelets[10] or fresh frozen plasma[9] or both[7] are not effective clinically. Patients undergoing massive transfusions should be followed closely with PT, PTT, fibrinogen, and platelet count. If coagulation abnormalities or thrombocytopenia develops, these deficiencies should be replaced with the appropriate blood components based on the degree of abnormality observed. In a busy general acute care hospital, these patients may account for a substantial portion of blood use.[11]

Hemoglobin Function

Pioneering studies during the late 1960s established that the level of 2,3-diphosphoglycerate (DPG) controls the release of oxygen from hemoglobin.[12,13] During blood bank storage, red cell DPG levels decline[14] (see Chapter 5). This is associated with a shift in the oxygen dissociation curve of hemoglobin to increase oxygen binding and decrease the ability to release oxygen to the tissues.[15] Although DPG levels are regen-

erated and oxygen dissociation returns to nearly normal about 24 hours after transfusion,[16] there has been concern that massive transfusion of DPG-depleted red cells might result in poor oxygen delivery. The clinical importance of this has been more difficult to determine than expected.[17] Studies have shown that animals can compensate very well for DPG-depleted red cells if the hematocrit and blood volume are maintained.[18,19] In humans, cardiac output and oxygen extraction are far more important than the small contribution to oxygenation made by increased levels of DPG. Thus, it appears that in most humans moderate depletion of DPG is tolerated. In patients with anemia or compromised cardiopulmonary function low DPG levels may be detrimental, but there is little evidence supporting this.

Hypocalcemia

The likelihood of development of hypocalcemia due to the infusion of large amounts of citrate during massive transfusion has been overemphasized.[20] Routine administration of calcium during massive transfusion is probably not necessary. Up to one unit of red cells can be administered every 5 minutes to adults with normal body temperature and not in shock.[21] Of primary concern regarding hypocalcemia are its cardiovascular effects, which occur before hypocalcemia is severe enough to cause coagulopathy. The effects of rapid citrate infusion are described in more detail in Chapter 7.

Hypothermia

If large amounts of cold blood are transfused rapidly, hypothermia may result. Then cardiac arrhythmia may occur and oxygen and energy requirements are increased, metabolism of citrate and lactate are impaired, potassium is released from the intracellular space, and the affinity of hemoglobin for oxygen is increased.[22] Thus, in massive transfusion, warming of blood to approximately 37°C is necessary (see Chapter 13).

Acid-Base Balance

Stored blood contains an acid load, primarily due to citric acid and lactic acid. This may be an exaggerated problem because patients undergoing massive transfusion may have a metabolic acidosis. However, worsening acidosis is often related to the inability to control hemorrhage and shock. Routine administration of alkalinizing agents in these patients gives an additional sodium load and might shift the oxygen dissociation curve to impair the release of oxygen from red cells. Thus, use of alkalinizing agents should be based on specific results of monitoring the patient rather than predetermined arbitrary schedules.

Microaggregates

The standard blood filters have a pore size between 170 and 230μm. During the 1970s, it was recognized that microaggregates of 20 to 120μm composed of platelets, leukocytes, and fibrin strands develop in stored blood.[23] It was believed that these were impor-

tant causative factors in the development of adult respiratory distress syndrome (ARDS), and thus microaggregate filters were developed. As the pathophysiology of ARDS was better understood, it became clear that this is a complex situation and that microaggregates are not the primary cause. These filters are available and are used in some centers, but they do not achieve substantial leukocyte reduction; the increasing use of leukodepleted components is eliminating the need for microaggregate filters.

Plasticizers

Plasticizers from the bags accumulate in red cell components during storage[24] and can be found in tissues of multitransfused patients.[25,26] However, there is no evidence that transfusion of this material causes clinical problems.[27]

Electrolytes

Potassium, ammonia, and phosphate levels are elevated in stored blood, but this does not cause clinical problems,[28] with the possible exception of the transfusion to neonates of stored blood with high potassium levels (see Pediatric Patients, below).

Blood Types

Occasionally it may be necessary to change to a different blood group in massive transfusion. The patient's history and clinical situation should be considered as well as the potential blood supply. It is sometimes more desirable to switch Rh types (for instance, from Rh negative to positive) than to switch ABO group. This is discussed under Acute Blood Loss above.

CARDIOVASCULAR SURGERY

Patients undergoing cardiopulmonary bypass often develop thrombocytopenia, platelet function abnormalities, and abnormal blood coagulation due to depletion of factors V, VII, VIII, and IX.[29–33] The coagulation and platelet abnormalities are thought to be caused by hemodilution, activation of platelets by the cardiopulmonary bypass instruments, fibrinolysis, inadequate neutralization of heparin, and alteration of von Willebrand factor.[30] However, most patients do not experience unusual bleeding, and the extent of bleeding is not associated with these hemostatic abnormalities.[29–33] Thus, the routine transfusion of plasma components or platelets following cardiopulmonary bypass is not indicated.[33] Although there is considerable variability in transfusion practices in these patients,[34] patients who develop excessive bleeding should be managed like any other surgical patients; that is, transfusion is indicated if the platelet count is less than $50,000/\mu L$ or if a severe platelet function defect is present.[35] The problem is that it can be presumed that all patients will have some degree of platelet dysfunction following cardiopulmonary bypass, so it is essential to determine whether excessive

bleeding is caused by platelet dysfunction or anatomic problems. The routine use of fresh frozen plasma or cryoprecipitate is not necessary, although the use of desmopressin acetate may reduce blood loss in patients undergoing complex cardiovascular procedures.[36]

The volume of blood lost by patients undergoing cardiopulmonary bypass is now relatively small, usually one to six units.[34] This blood can be replaced using routine red cell components according to usual blood bank practices. Because the red cells may undergo some trauma in the bypass instrument, it is advisable that not all units of red cells be near the end of their storage period. However, the use of units that have been stored for different periods of time is usual blood bank practice.

BONE MARROW TRANSPLANTATION

The overall important role of the blood bank in a marrow transplantation program has been summarized in several reports during the past few years.[37–39] Blood transfusion is an essential part of marrow transplantation. These patients use considerable amounts of blood components and place a substantial demand on the blood bank[37] (Table 12.5). Patients who are candidates for or are undergoing marrow transplantation have unique transfusion requirements. This is because of the need to minimize the likelihood of alloimmunization, the severe immunosuppression these patients undergo, their temporary inability to produce blood cells, and the fact that their blood type may change and they may become a temporary or permanent chimera. Since transfusion therapy may differ before and after transplant, these situations will be considered separately.

Pretransplant

Before transplant, bone marrow transplant patients are not immunosuppressed and thus may become alloimmunized to leukocytes or platelets following transfusion. This alloimmunization may cause transfusion reactions but, more importantly, may interfere with engraftment or with platelet transfusions needed during the transplant period. The presence of HLA antibodies is associated with marrow graft rejection,[40] and pretransplant transfusions are associated with decreased patient[41] or graft survival.[42] Thus, patients with aplastic anemia should be evaluated quickly and marrow transplantation, if indicated, done as quickly as possible to minimize the number of pretransplant transfusions. The problems of platelet refractoriness is discussed in Chapter 11, and febrile nonhemolytic transfusion reactions in Chapter 14. A considerable amount of data has accumulated over the past few years indicating that leukocyte depletion is effective in reducing the likelihood of alloimmunization following transfusion (see Chapters 11 and 14).

The indications for transfusion of the various blood components are the same as indications for other relatively stable anemic, thrombocytopenic, or leukopenic patients. Because of the potentially serious adverse effect of transfusion on marrow engraftment and survival in these patients, transfusion should be given only after careful consideration of the patient's condition. In fact, Storb and Weiden[43] have recom-

Table 12.5 Blood component utilization by patients undergoing bone marrow transplantation at the University of Minnesota

	Related				Unrelated				Autologous			
	% Transfused	Total used	# Units range	# Units median	% Transfused	Total used	# Units range	# Units median	% Transfused	Total used	# Units range	# Units median
Red blood cells	98	1077	0–75	18	100	856	6–93	15	100	1124	4–95	14
Peds red blood cells	1	1	0–1	0	13	3	0–1	0	8	7	0–3	0
Fresh frozen plasma	30	311	0–47	0	51	415	0–115	2	15	628	0–167	0
Peds fresh frozen plasma	9	4	0–1	0	16	5	0–1	0	5	4	0–2	0
Cryoprecipitate	9	115	0–36	0	16	104	0–24	0	9	256	0–184	0
Random platelet	89	2800	0–235	36	76	2311	0–977	17	74	1757	0–188	14
Apheresis platelet	98	2017	0–115	24	100	1460	4–172	32	100	1740	3–77	21

	Related				Unrelated				Autologous			
	% Transfused	Total used	# Units range	# Units median	% Transfused	Total used	# Units range	# Units median	% Transfused	Total used	# Units range	# Units median
Apheresis platelet (split)	54	70	0–8	1	27	27	0–7	0	17	12	0–2	0
HLA platelet	26	118	0–37	0	35	213	0–41	0	22	136	0–30	0
Granulocytes	7	34	0–8	0	16	147	0–52	0	6	46	0–10	0
Granulocyte platelets	5	42	0–27	0	16	54	0–31	0	1	16	0–16	0
CMV-negative product	37	2248	0–277	0	19	1969	0–1258	0	38	1342	0–219	0
Leukocyte removal	40	1673	0–342	0	30	1703	0–1168	0	31	1462	0–351	0

Source: McCullough J. Collection and use of stem cells; role of transfusion centers in bone marrow transplantation. Vox Sang 1994;67(Suppl 3):35–42.

mended that prophylactic platelets be given only when the platelet count is less than 5,000/μL. For patients who require red cell or platelet transfusions before transplantation, the following is recommended:

1. Red cells should be depleted of leukocytes. This is usually done by filtration. In the past, either washing or freezing and deglycerolizing was sometimes used to prepare leukocyte-depleted red cells, but present filters are more effective and convenient (see Chapters 5 and 11).
2. Platelet concentrates should be depleted of leukocytes. This can be done by filtration or by certain apheresis collection procedures (see Chapter 7).
3. The use of single-donor instead of pooled random-donor platelet concentrates should be considered. It has been thought that use of single-donor platelets might delay alloimmunization by limiting the number of donor exposures. However, the largest, most recently completed study did not show a difference in the rate of alloimmunization between single-donor and pooled random-donor platelet concentrates.[44]
4. Family members should not be used as blood or component donors (before transplant) because of the risk of alloimmunization and an unsuccessful marrow graft.[43]

Patients with inborn errors of metabolism or other nonmalignant diseases rarely require transfusion before marrow transplantation. If transfusion is necessary, these patients should be managed similarly to patients with aplastic anemia. Patients with malignancies who will undergo bone marrow transplantation usually have received multiple transfusions during the initial chemotherapy of their underlying disease. However, the effects of this on subsequent marrow engraftment are not as severe as for aplastic anemia patients because the chemotherapy is extremely immunosuppressive. Thus, transfusion therapy for these patients can be that necessitated by their chemotherapy. No modifications are necessary because they may become bone marrow transplant candidates in the future. However, transfusions from family members should be avoided.[43] These patients usually have no transfusion requirements in the immediate pretransplant period, because they are in hematologic remission.

Posttransplantation

Because of the severe immunosuppression caused by the pretransplant preparative regimen, fatal graft versus host disease can occur due to transfusion of viable lymphocytes in blood components.[45] Transfusion-related graft versus host disease can be prevented by irradiating all blood components with at least 2,500 rads (see Chapter 11).

About 20 days elapse between transplantation and marrow engraftment, although this period is becoming more variable as different sources of stem cells are used for transplantation. The return of production of different blood cell lines varies, so although the duration of transfusion therapy may range from 2 to 6 weeks, the need for different components varies with different types of transplants (Table 12.5). Almost all patients require platelet and red cell transfusions, but since marrow transplantation does not usu-

ally interfere with the production of coagulation factors, transfusions of fresh frozen plasma and cryoprecipitate are necessary only if complications such as disseminated intravascular coagulopathy develop. Although marrow transplant patients are severely neutropenic, granulocyte transfusions are not usually necessary.

The indications for the transfusion of blood components are the same as those for other kinds of patients. Because of their complex situation these patients may place a major demand on the blood bank for blood components, especially platelets (Table 12.5). Even though these patients are recovering from severe immunosuppression as part of the preparative regimen for the transplant, they can become alloimmunized after transplantation.[37,46] Thus, transfusion practices must take this possibility into account. The red cells used can be routine red cell components, although it is becoming common practice to use leukodepleted red cells to minimize the likelihood of inducing alloimmunization. Another unique consideration in the transfusion management of marrow transplant patients is the source of platelets. Either random-donor or single-donor (apheresis) platelets can be used. Some authors have advocated the use of single-donor platelets to delay alloimmunization and platelet refractoriness;[47,48] however, it is not established whether this practice has any overall benefit to the patient. The largest and most recently completed study was carried out in newly diagnosed patients with acute myelogenous leukemia and showed no difference in the rate of alloimmunization between pooled random-donor and single-donor platelets.[44] Since alloimmunization is caused by leukocytes contained in the blood components, leukodepletion has been used as another strategy to reduce alloimmunization. Results of studies of leukodepleted platelet concentrates have suggested this strategy is effective.[49–54] The large-scale TRAP study of newly diagnosed acute leukemia patients showed that leukodepletion of red cells and platelets is associated with significant reduction in alloimmunization.[44] Thus, leukodepletion of all blood components has become the standard practice for marrow transplant patients.

If patients become refractory to platelet transfusion, HLA-matched platelets from an unrelated or family donor can be used. Many marrow transplant programs use family members as donors following the transplant, because they may be partially HLA matched and they are readily available and motivated to donate often. This and other approaches to the management of patients refractory to platelet transfusion are described in more detail in Chapter 11. Another unique feature of bone marrow transplant patients is that the marrow donor is available as a potential platelet donor. Platelets are occasionally obtained from the marrow donor if the patient is refractory and experiencing serious bleeding problems, but this decision requires considerable thought because of ethical considerations regarding the donor.

ABO- and Rh-Incompatible Transplants

ABO incompatibility between donor and recipient does not preclude marrow transplantation,[55–58] because it appears that hematopoietic stem cells lack ABH antigens.[57] ABO-incompatible transplants may be done when there is patient antibody directed against donor cells (major incompatibility; i.e., patient O, donor A) or donor antibody directed against the patient's red cells (minor incompatibility; i.e., patient A, donor O).

Table 12.6 Theoretical immunohematologic consequences of ABO-incompatible bone marrow transplants

Minor ABO Incompatibility

Anticipated problems
Graft versus host disease
Immune hemolysis at the time of infusion of the donor marrow caused by anti-A and anti-B in the plasma of the marrow product
Unanticipated problem
Immune hemolysis of delayed onset caused by red cell antibodies produced by the donor marrow

Major ABO Incompatibility

Anticipated problems
Failure of stem cell engraftment
Delay in onset of hematopoiesis, especially erythropoiesis
Acute hemolysis at the time of infusion of the donor marrow
Delayed onset of hemolysis associated with persistence of anti-A and/or anti-B after transplantation
Hemolysis of infused red cells of donor type
Hemolysis of red cells produced by the engrafted marrow
Unanticipated problem
Mixed hematopoietic chimerism

Source: Petz LD. Immunohematologic problems associated with bone marrow transplantation. Transfus Med Rev 1987;1:86.

Each of these situations has unique potential complications that present challenges to the transfusion service[58] (Table 12.6). In general, blood components given near the time of bone marrow transplantation should be compatible with both the donor and the recipient to minimize the chance of red cell hemolysis. Therefore, it may be necessary to use components of different ABO types at different times during the patient's course (Fig. 12.1). These situations are described more completely below.

When ABO-incompatible marrow is to be transfused into a patient with circulating antibodies against the donor's ABO type (e.g., A marrow into O patient), hemolysis of the red cells in the marrow can be expected. Some years ago, plasma exchange was used to reduce the level of circulating antibody in the recipient, but this was of only temporary value and high titers of antibody returned quickly, leading to hemolysis.[59] This problem is now avoided by processing the marrow to remove the red cells (see Chapter 18). Following transplant and after engraftment, the patient will become type A but cannot begin to receive type A red cells until the circulating anti-A has disappeared (Fig. 12.1). Anti-A persists longer than anti-B.[60] Thus, even after the transfusion of type A marrow, the patient continues to receive type O red cells containing additional anti-A that can slow the appearance of type A red cells. Usually, this does not lead to active hemolysis. If red cell engraftment is unexpectedly delayed, this is more likely the result of persistence of the patient's original antibodies than the transfusion of additional antibodies. Currently used red cell storage solutions contain very

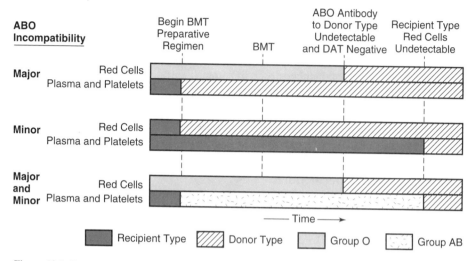

Figure 12.1. Recommended ABO type of blood components for use in ABO-incompatible bone marrow transplants. *(Modified from McCullough J, Lasky LC, Warkentin PI. Role of the blood bank in bone marrow transplantation. In: Advances in Immunobiology: Blood Cell Antigens and Bone Marrow Transplantation. New York: Alan R. Liss, Inc., 1984:379–412.)*

little of the original donor's plasma, and so this is not usually a major source of antibody; washing red cells to remove this antibody is not necessary. If delayed red cell engraftment is occurring, the titer of anti-A should be determined and a direct antiglobulin test done to determine if high levels of circulating anti-A are hemolyzing newly forming A red cells. Although it is rare, these original patient ABO antibodies may remain for many months.[61] In making the decision when to convert to the new donor ABO type for red cell transfusion, we follow the procedure described earlier for massive transfusion by using the crossmatch to determine when all circulating antibody has disappeared. If the crossmatch technique is one that is sensitive to ABO antibodies, that is a satisfactory indicator of the safety to begin transfusing the new donor ABO type red cells.

Conversely, in a "minor" incompatible marrow transplant (e.g., O donor and A recipient), there are two dangers. First, the transfusion of large volumes of incompatible plasma with the marrow at the time of transplant may cause hemolysis. This can be avoided by removing the plasma from the marrow, much the same as converting whole blood into packed red cells (see Chapter 18). The second potential problem is the continued production of antibody by the new donor lymphocytes while there are original patient cells continuing to circulate.[62] Thus, the group O donor cells may begin to produce anti-A while original patient A red cells remain, leading to hemolysis. This can be alleviated by red cell exchange transfusion if necessary. Hemolysis of original patient type O red cells by "passenger lymphocytes" in the marrow seems to be a greater problem in unrelated marrow transplants, even leading to hemolysis of group O red cells as well as the incompatible A or B red cells.[63]

Rh-mismatched transplants are also successful, even when Rh-positive marrow is transplanted to patients with anti-D.[64] When an Rh-positive patient receives Rh-negative marrow, some original patient Rh-positive red cells circulate for weeks after transplant. Some of these patients have developed anti-D.[58] It is not known whether avoidance of Rh-positive blood components in the posttransplant period would prevent this. However, we suggest converting to the use of Rh-negative red cells at the time of transplant. When an Rh-negative patient receives Rh-positive marrow, no cases of Rh immunization have been reported. These patients can receive Rh-positive blood products after transplant.

Posttransplant Chimeric States

After transplantation, the development of a chimeric state (a combination of donor and original patient cells) has been reported to occur following 17%[65] and 58%[66] of cases. Thus, this is not an uncommon occurrence, and the chimeric state may be long lasting.[62] In Petz's[65] series of 172 patients, 41% of those who originally had a chimerism maintained the chimerism for 2 or more years. All other patients ultimately assumed the new donor's type.

Immune Cytopenias following Marrow Transplantation

Because of asynchrony in the reappearance of different cell (especially lymphocyte) populations, apparent "autoimmune" cytopenias have been reported. These include autoimmune hemolytic anemia,[67] thrombocytopenia, and granulocytopenia.[68] These conditions have been reported after both allogeneic and autologous transplants. Only in autologous transplants would cytopenia truly be autoimmune. In allogeneic transplants, Anderson[37] proposes that the cytopenias are probably due to "transient immune system imbalance common to both allografts and autografts." In addition, either donor or recipient red cell, platelet, or HLA antibodies may reactivate soon after transplantation,[69] occasionally leading to transient cytopenias of various kinds.

Intravenous Immune Globulin

Since patients are severely immunodeficient after bone marrow transplantation, infections with opportunistic organisms are a major problem. The recent availability of intravenous immune globulin (IVIG) provides a new approach to the prevention or treatment of some of these infections. Varicella-zoster immune globulin has been shown to prevent varicella-zoster virus infections in other immunosuppressed patients[70] and can be used if marrow transplant patients are exposed to varicella. Cytomegalovirus intravenous immune globulin[71,72] or ordinary intravenous immune globulin[73] may prevent cytomegalovirus (CMV) infections in bone marrow transplant patients, but this is not used because of the effectiveness of CMV-safe blood components (see Chapter 11). The largest use of IVIG in marrow transplant patients is for its potential value in reducing general infections and possible role in modifying graft versus host disease. Studies are under way to establish the role of immune globulins in bone marrow transplant patients, but at present this group of patients represents a very large use of IVIG.

SOLID ORGAN TRANSPLANTATION

Blood component use in patients receiving solid organ transplants is modest, with the exception of liver transplant patients (Table 12.7). This was particularly true during the early days of liver transplantation, when transfusion episodes involving 50 to 75 units of red cells and larger numbers of other components were not uncommon. For instance, between 1981 and 1985 at the University of Pittsburgh, where liver transplants were pioneered, these patients accounted for 0.01% of admissions but 20% of red cell, 25% of platelet, and 37% of fresh frozen plasma usage.[74] Patients may require transfusion before, during, or after transplantation, although the situations are not as different as in marrow transplantation and usually there are not differences in the type of blood components used at these different times.

Traditionally, kidney recipients required a considerable number of transfusions prior to transplantation because of the anemia associated with end-stage renal disease. With the availability of erythropoietin this has decreased dramatically (see Chapter 17). During the 1960s and early 1970s, transfusions were minimized to reduce the likelihood of alloimmunization to HLA antigens and the resulting difficulty obtaining a kidney transplant. This resulted in patients being maintained at very low hemoglobin levels, which contributed to their general state of poor health. In 1973, a landmark study showed that kidney graft survival was better in patients who received transfusions than in nontransfused patients.[75] Separate studies showed that in patients receiving a kidney from a living related donor, pretransplant transfusions from the intended kidney donor were associated with improved graft survival.[75,76] Both of these observations led to the change in practice to intentionally transfuse patients prior to transplantation.[77] Despite a large number of studies, the biologic mechanism that accounts for the transfusion effect has not been defined. This was the first clinical indication in humans that blood transfusion has an immunologic effect, and a debate is active today as to whether

Table 12.7 Mean blood components transfused during transplant surgery (ranges of reported means in parentheses)

n*	Organ	Red cells	Platelet concentrates**	FFP	Cryoprecipitate
13	Kidney	<1 (0–2)	0 (0–0.1)	0	0
13	Heart	3.0 (1–6)	2.7 (0–10.5)	3.0 (0–8)	1.4 (0–5)
12	Liver (adult)	17.3 (6–37.1)	21.8 (3–58)	23.1 (11–42.5)	15.3 (0–40)
11	Liver (pediatric)	7.1 (1–13.7)	7.1 (1.1–23)	6.8 (0–17.2)	5.6 (0.27)
6	Lung	3.4 (1–7)	1.9 (0–6.4)	1.2 (0–2.7)	1.8 (0–5)

Source: Danielson CF. Transfusion support and complicating coagulopathies in solid organ transplantation. In: Hacke E, AuBuchon J, eds. Advances in Transplantation. Bethesda, MD: American Association of Blood Banks, 1993:45.

*n = The number of institutions providing data. In some cases, the values supplied by the institution were estimates or a range was given. In these cases, the estimate or mean of the range has been used.

**Includes platelets, pheresis; each platelet, pheresis was considered equivalent to six platelet concentrates.

transfusion is associated with increased postoperative infection and increased likelihood of recurrence of malignancy (see Chapter 14).

Transfusion practice for kidney transplant patients changed again during the mid-1980s. The use of cyclosporine for immunosuppression and other improvements in patient care increased patient and graft survival rates to a level where a beneficial effect of blood transfusion was no longer apparent.[78] In addition, the growing concern about transfusion-transmitted diseases caused elimination of intentional pretransplant transfusions, and in most centers a reversion to a more conservative use of transfusions. When end-stage renal disease patients awaiting transplant require transfusion, this involves only red cells to maintain hemoglobin levels. If red cell transfusion is necessary during end-stage renal disease and before transplantation, leukocyte-poor red cells are used to reduce the likelihood of HLA alloimmunization and resulting difficulty obtaining a compatible kidney for transplant. During the perioperative and postoperative periods red cell transfusions may be necessary to replace operative blood loss or maintain the hemoglobin level. If complications develop involving bleeding, sepsis, etc., transfusion of other blood components can be given based on the specific needs of the patient.

Patients undergoing liver transplantation have more extensive requirements for replacement not only of red cells but also of coagulation factors and platelets. Most transplant programs use intraoperative salvage to reduce the use of allogeneic red cells. The liver disease itself usually results in coagulopathy before transplantation due to decreased synthesis of factors and slower clearance of inhibitors. In some patients, plasma exchange may be used to improve the coagulation status before surgery. The manipulations of the liver, the anhepatic phase, and the insertion of the new liver interfere with coagulation factor synthesis and cause activation of the coagulation system. There is considerable information in the literature about the changes in the coagulation system, but the impact on transfusion medicine is that there is need for coagulation factor and platelet replacement. Fresh frozen plasma is used as the source of coagulation factors, and cryoprecipitate is used as a source of fibrinogen. Some programs have planned algorithms for the use of specific combinations of blood components.

The impact of cardiopulmonary surgery on the coagulation system and the needs for component transfusion are well known. Factors that influence hemostasis include the type of bypass instrument, the prime solution, duration of bypass, use of hypothermia, and heparinization. Usually the coagulation alterations are not sufficient to account for excessive bleeding. Cardiopulmonary bypass also alters platelet function and number.[31,79–82] The platelet defects are probably more related to excessive bleeding in these patients than to coagulopathy. Nevertheless, routine platelet transfusion is not necessary, because most patients undergoing cardiac transplant do not experience excessive bleeding and do not require substantial numbers of red cells (Table 12.7).

The use of CMV-negative blood for solid organ transplant patients is discussed in Chapter 11. CMV-negative patients undergoing solid organ transplants who receive an organ from a CMV antibody-negative donor should receive CMV-negative components.

Although viable lymphocytes are administered in the transplanted organs and the patients are immunosuppressed, graft versus host disease is rare following solid organ transplantation. Thus, irradiation of blood components is not routine, although its use

may be increasing.[83] Another version of graft versus host disease is the development of red cell antibodies by donor "passenger lymphocytes" directed against the patient's red cells. This is discussed more fully below.

Blood Group Antibodies Following Solid Organ Transplantation

Lymphocytes in transplanted organs (passenger lymphocytes) may produce antibodies in the recipient. This phenomenon usually occurs in situations in which the donor was producing the antibodies prior to transplantation.[84] ABO is the blood group system most commonly involved. When a group O donor organ is transplanted into a group A or B recipient, the corresponding anti-A or anti-B appears in the recipient's circulation about 70% of the time; following heart-lung transplants, 40%; following liver transplants, 15%; and 15% following kidney transplants.[85] These ABO antibodies are usually IgG, appear 1 or 2 weeks following transplantation, and disappear after a few weeks. The antibodies may cause a positive direct antiglobulin test and varying degrees of hemolysis—in some situations quite severe.[86,87] If hemolysis is severe, the patient can be treated with plasma exchange or preferably red cell exchange providing new red cells of the donor type.

Other blood group antibodies that have been produced by passenger lymphocytes include Rh, Kell, Kidd, and platelet antibodies.[84] Usually this occurs when the donor has been previously immunized and is making the antibody at the time of transplantation.

NEONATES

During the first weeks of life, the red cell mass decreases in most infants; because of the common nature of this change, it is referred to as "physiologic" anemia of infancy. Usually the minimum hemoglobin value of approximately 9 g/dL occurs at 10 to 12 weeks of age. In premature infants, however, there is a larger and earlier decline in red cell mass, with the hemoglobin decreasing to 7 g/dL or less. It appears that the more severe fall in hemoglobin in premature infants is caused by diminished erythropoietin (EPO) production in these patients.[88] It appears that the reduced production of EPO in response to anemia is because in premature infants much of the EPO is produced in the liver, which is less responsive than the kidney to hypoxia.

Because the anemia of prematurity is due to erythropoietic deficiency, it would seem that administration of erythropoietin would be beneficial. Strauss[89] summarized 14 studies of the use of EPO to treat the anemia of prematurity; he recommends that EPO be administered to infants with a birth weight between 0.8 and 1.3 kg who are in stable condition and able to take oral iron. He concluded that the data are inadequate to support the use of EPO in other premature infants at this time and that if EPO is to be administered, it should be done as a part of a research protocol.

Transfusion of very small patients presents some unique considerations.[90] The anemia of prematurity is often exacerbated by blood removal for laboratory studies. The smaller the neonate, the more likely he or she will receive a transfusion. Neonates may require any of the blood components that are available for adults.

Red Blood Cell Transfusions

Neonates may require red blood cell transfusions or exchange transfusion for hyperbilirubinemia, correction of symptomatic neonatal anemia, or acute or chronic blood loss. The decision to transfuse a newborn should be based on symptoms such as the infant's weight gain or fatigue during feeding, signs such as tachycardia or tachypnea, and laboratory values such as hemoglobin, reticulocyte count, and presence of nucleated red cells on the blood smear.[91] Although there are no exact requirements, premature infants with symptomatic anemia are usually given red cell transfusions for hematocrits of 23% to 25%; those with a moderate degree of cardiopulmonary disease or undergoing major surgery are transfused when the hematocrit is 30%; and those with severe cardiopulmonary disease are transfused when the hematocrit falls to 40%.[89] Each transfusion is usually 15 mL/kg. Blood drawn for laboratory tests is a common cause for red blood cell transfusion. Replacement transfusions for each blood sample collected are not recommended routinely but instead should be based on the neonate's hemoglobin value and clinical condition. Sacher et al.[92] recommend replacement transfusion when (a) more than 5% of the neonate's blood volume has been removed in less than 10 days or (b) when there has been a 10% reduction in the infant's blood volume and the infant's initial hematocrit was 50% or greater. Red blood cell transfusions for neonates can be given as packed red cells. Usually red cells less than 7 days of age are used to avoid transfusing supernatant containing high levels of potassium and lactic acid. Red cells, as currently produced by most blood banks, are suspended in a medium containing glucose, sodium, adenine, mannitol, citrate, and phosphate. Although there have been no reports of complications caused by transfusing these materials to neonates, there is very little information on this subject. There is no specific indication for routine use of frozen, thawed, or washed red cells.

Pretransfusion Testing

Because the neonate's immune system is not fully functional, any blood group antibodies in the neonate are those of the mother. Thus, a blood sample is usually obtained from both the mother and the newborn. The ABO and Rh types of both are determined and the mother's serum is tested for the presence of unexpected (non-ABO) red blood cell antibodies. If a clinically significant antibody is present, the mother's serum is usually used for subsequent compatibility testing for the neonate because her serum should have higher levels of antibody. If no unexpected red blood cell antibodies are present, no additional compatibility testing is required[4] during that hospital stay because of the remote possibility that the neonate would form a new red blood cell antibody.[93] This approach applies if the neonate has received only group O Rh-negative red cells or red cells of group O and of the neonate's original Rh type.

Red Cell Products Used for Neonatal Transfusion

Blood banks have devised several ways to provide small volumes of blood components while not wasting the remainder of the original donor unit. These techniques may

involve multiple-bag systems, dispensing components in syringes, or using specially collected small units. One common approach is to collect one O negative unit into a quadruple bag, separate the unit into four parts, and use each of these for one patient for several days. Once each of these small units is entered it will have only a 24-hour dating period unless a sterile docking device is used. Another approach is to use one unit of O negative red cells for all patients being transfused on that day. This makes available very fresh blood but increases the number of donor exposures for the infant. These different "minimal donor exposure" programs are described more fully in Chapter 6. Regardless of which method of storing the red cells is used, many blood banks provide the red cells to the patient care unit in syringes rather than the plastic bag used for storage. The blood is removed from the bag through a sample site coupler. The syringe must be properly labeled and the red cells transfused soon because the syringe is not a blood storage container and the conditions and suitable storage period for these syringes have not been extensively studied. Walking donor programs are not recommended because they are associated with serious problems.[94]

Techniques of Administering Blood to Neonates

Most neonates require only a small volume of the component being transfused (usually less than 20 mL). The administration devices usually available were designed to handle large volumes of blood. Thus, the devices may lead to wastage of a large proportion of the components. Several additional factors unique to transfusion of small volumes of blood to neonates may cause hemolysis. These include flow monitoring devices, viscosity of the red cell units, filters, flow rates, tubing size, needle size, and pressure systems. The problem of wastage has been minimized by use of small tubing sets and infusion pumps to control the transfusion of small volumes, and most neonatal units have developed very effective methods of administering blood components. Red cells should be administered through a 23 or 25 gauge needle. It is not necessary to warm the blood routinely, but the rate of transfusion must be controlled to avoid rapid transfusion of large volumes of cold blood. Rapid transfusion of viscous red cells through some filters under pressure can cause hemolysis. Thus, careful attention to these details is important, and it is important that the blood bank have close interaction with the neonatal patient care unit to review the techniques of blood administration to ensure proper handling of the components. Techniques for the transfusion of blood components are described in more detail in Chapter 13.

CMV-Negative Blood Components

Neonates of less than 1,500 g birth weight are at increased risk of CMV infection from blood transfusions.[95] Thus, it is common to provide CMV-negative cellular blood components for such patients. However, American Association of Blood Banks Standards[4] recommend this for infants under 1,200 g when the mother or infant is CMV negative and only if local data indicate that transfusion-transmitted CMV disease is a problem. For a more detailed discussion, see Chapter 11.

Irradiated Blood Components

Because neonates do not have a fully developed immune response, there has been concern that transfused blood components could cause graft versus host disease in neonates. Some physicians have recommended the routine use of irradiated blood components to prevent graft versus host disease in neonates. Many thousands of neonates have received transfusions of unirradiated blood components without developing graft versus host disease, although a few cases in neonates have been reported.[96,97] Almost all of these patients had an underlying clinical problem that would today be an indication for irradiated blood components.[98] Because there is little evidence that this is a clinical problem, irradiation of blood components for all routine transfusions to neonates is not done in most neonatal care centers. Recently, however, irradiation of blood for neonates has been recommended for infants whose birth weight is 1,250 g because of their underdeveloped immune system.[99]

Platelet Transfusions

Neonates may require platelet transfusions for most of the same reasons as adults and additional ones such as neonatal alloimmune thrombocytopenia, infection-related thrombocytopenia, thrombocytopenia due to maternal problems (idiopathic thrombocytopenic purpura, systemic lupus erythematosus, etc.), respiratory distress syndrome, phototherapy, polycythemia, necrotizing enterocolitis, and certain congenital diseases such as Wiskott-Aldrich syndrome. The indications for platelet transfusions in neonates may be somewhat different than for adults. Some neonatologists prefer to administer prophylactic platelet transfusions to severely ill premature infants when the count falls below $50,000/\mu L$[100] Neonates can receive platelet transfusions in a volume and dose based on the size and platelet count of the patient. There are several ways to determine the recommended dose: (*a*) one unit of platelets per 10 kg body weight, (*b*) four units of platelets per square meter body surface area, or (*c*) 10 mL of platelet concentrate per kilogram body weight. Thus, neonates will usually require less than one unit of a platelet concentrate prepared from a unit of whole blood. If a higher than usual post-transfusion count is desired, the platelet unit can be centrifuged and concentrated to provide a larger dose of platelets in the volume desired for transfusion. This "volume reduction" does not adversely affect platelet recovery or function.[101,102]

Platelets should be ABO and Rh identical with the patient.

Granulocyte Transfusions

Neonatal sepsis is a rather frequent occurrence that has a mortality ranging from 3% in term infants to 90% in infants weighing less that 1 kg.[103] The abnormal function and number of neutrophils in newborns may contribute to the incidence and severity of newborn sepsis.

Granulocyte transfusions have been reported to be helpful in patients who are neutropenic (less than $3,000/\mu L$) and have an inadequate marrow response.[104] Since it is often impractical to do a bone marrow examination to determine marrow reserve, some have suggested that marrow reserves are depleted if more than 70% of circulating

neutrophils are immature forms[104] and that this be used as an indication for granulocyte transfusion in these patients. Strauss[103] reviewed 11 reports of granulocyte transfusions in neonates and concluded that "the role of granulocyte transfusion in neonatal sepsis is unclear." It appears that granulocyte transfusions may be beneficial for neutropenic patients with sepsis when the cells were obtained by automated apheresis instruments.[103] Strauss recommends that each institution evaluate its results and, if they are unsatisfactory, consider a program to provide granulocyte transfusions. A major practical problem is that granulocyte transfusions to neonates are usually needed urgently, but lack of good preservation techniques makes them difficult to obtain because a stock inventory is not maintained. Either granulocytes obtained by leukapheresis or those separated from whole blood have been used, but the logistical problems have never been satisfactorily solved, and granulocyte transfusions are not widely used for neonates.

EXCHANGE TRANSFUSION OF THE NEONATE

There are many indications for exchange transfusion in the neonate, including hyperbilirubinemia, sepsis, disseminated intravascular coagulopathy (DIC), polycythemia, respiratory distress syndrome, hyperammonemia, anemia, toxin removal, thrombocytopenia, and sickle cell disease.[105] In the past, hemolytic disease of the newborn (HDN) due to the Rh(D) antigen was the most common reason for exchange transfusion, and so this general discussion will focus on that situation. Most of the considerations and potential complications also apply to exchange transfusion in neonates with other conditions. The objectives of exchange transfusion in HDN are (*a*) correction of anemia, (*b*) reduction of bilirubin concentration, and (*c*) replacement of Rh-positive red cells with Rh-negative cells. The use of Rh immune globulin has greatly reduced the incidence of HDN. Because there are substantial risks of exchange transfusion, considerable attention has been devoted to defining the indications for exchange. Those that apply to exchange because of blood group incompatibility are the most well described.[91] The cord hemoglobin could be one indicator, but this is not helpful because severely affected infants will have received an intrauterine transfusion affecting the cord hemoglobin value. A cord indirect bilirubin value greater than 4 mg/dL or an indirect bilirubin of 20 mg/dL within the first 72 hours of life is often used. For infants with cord indirect bilirubin values less than 4 mg/dL, the rate of change of the indirect bilirubin is another indication. Changes of 0.15 to 0.2 mg/dL/hour or total bilirubin of 0.6 mg/dL/hour during the first 12 hours have been used.

The exchange transfusion is usually done via the umbilical vein. If the procedure is being carried out on a child of a few days of age, a peripheral vein can also be used. When the umbilical vessels are available, both the artery and the vein can be cannulated; then the vein can be used for transfusion and the artery for withdrawal, thus making an isovolemic exchange possible. Alternatively, the umbilical vein is used for both withdrawal and transfusion using a three-way stopcock and "push-pull" discontinuous technique. The maximum volume of blood withdrawn at one time depends on the blood volume and the condition of the infant. In a discontinuous exchange of a stable infant,

aliquots of 10 to 20 mL may be done, but the aliquot should not exceed 5% to 10% of the patient's blood volume.[106] A one blood volume exchange should remove about 65% of the original intravascular constituent and a two blood volume exchange about 85%. The exchange transfusion should require about 1 to 1½ hours.

Most blood banks do not have whole blood available, and thus exchange transfusion is usually done with red cells that are only a few days old. Using relatively fresh red cells is important to provide red cells containing maximum levels of DPG. Red cells as they are currently prepared are usually suspended in additive solutions containing glucose and adenine (see Chapter 5). Red cells suspended in the anticoagulant preservative CPDA-1 have been used satisfactorily for exchange transfusion.[105,107] The initial hemoglobin, the desired final hemoglobin, and the volume intended for exchange will determine the hematocrit of the blood to be used for the exchange. The hematocrit of the blood used for exchange can be adjusted to elevate the hemoglobin in anemic patients. Formulas are available for this calculation.[107] The red cells can be reconstituted by adding 5% normal serum albumin if it is desired to lower the hematocrit. An additional benefit of the albumin is that it binds bilirubin and thus may improve the effectiveness of the exchange transfusion, although it also increases the osmotic pressure and thus must be used cautiously. If necessary, because of coagulopathy, fresh frozen plasma can be used to reconstitute the red cells to provide coagulation factors during the exchange transfusion.

Another consideration due to the composition of the blood component being used for exchange is the possibility of hyperglycemia from the high glucose content of the red cell units. This may cause insulin release and a rebound hypoglycemia. Thus, blood glucose must be monitored. The citrate used as the anticoagulant in the red cell units may lead to hypocalcemia, so physicians often give supplemental calcium.[105] These infants may also metabolize citrate slowly due to poor liver function and experience acidosis, but additional buffers are not used because this may cause a later alkalosis.[105]

There are a number of potential complications of exchange transfusion (Table 12.8). Because of the underdeveloped immune system in neonates, blood used for exchange transfusion in these patients should be irradiated (see Chapter 11). Also, because these patients may be poorly oxygenated, red cells used for exchange should not contain hemoglobin S. Thus, it is necessary to screen these units of red cells for hemoglobin S to avoid using blood that might have been collected from a donor with sickle trait. These potential complications can be avoided or minimized by careful technique, selection of the optimum blood component, and good general patient care. Since many of these patients are quite ill and unstable, exchange transfusion can be a risky procedure.

PEDIATRIC PATIENTS

Pediatric patients may require transfusion for reasons similar to those described for adults but with some additional unique situations, primarily in the newborn period. The other conditions leading to transfusions in pediatric patients are inherited disorders of hemoglobin, which are discussed below. Any of the blood components described for

Table 12.8 Potential complications of exchange transfusion

Infection
    Bacterial
    Viral
Metabolic
    Hyperglycemia
    Rebound hypoglycemia
    Hypocalcemia (due to citrate anticoagulant in the exchange blood)
    Hyperkalemia (if older red cells are used)
    Late-onset alkalosis
    Hypernatremia
Cardiac
    Volume overload
    Cardiac arrest
Hematologic
    Hemolysis
    Thrombocytopenia
    Neutropenia
    Coagulopathy
General
    Graft versus host disease
    Hypothermia

transfusion to adults may be used in children. Transfusion of red cell products may be necessary for red cell mass replacement to maintain oxygen delivery to the tissues. The usual dose of red cells is 2.5 to 5 mL per kilogram, which should elevate the hemoglobin about 1 g/dL in a stable patient. Coagulopathy may be present due to hemorrhagic disease of the newborn, DIC, massive transfusion, liver disease, major surgery, or many other conditions. If coagulation factor replacement is necessary, the usual dose of fresh frozen plasma is 10 to 15 mL/kg body weight.[108] This dose should be adequate to control bleeding in most situations unless severe DIC is present. Cryoprecipitate can be used to replace fibrinogen or factor VIII. The usual dose is one donor unit (bag) per 3 to 5 kg body weight. Another approach is one bag of cryoprecipitate per 100 mL plasma volume.[108] This should raise the fibrinogen level to 200 mg/dL, which provides adequate hemostasis for trauma or surgery.

The risks of bleeding in thrombocytopenic pediatric patients are thought to be similar to those in adults, but pediatric patients may need platelet transfusions because of maternal idiopathic thrombocytopenic purpura (ITP), neonatal alloimmune thrombocytopenia, infections, maternal drug ingestion, treatment of malignancy, or congenital syndromes involving megakaryocytic hypoplasia. A random donor platelet concentrate should increase the platelet count by 8,000 to 10,000/μL in a 70-kg adult with about 1.7 m^2 body surface area.[109] Thus, the expected response to platelet transfusion can be calculated using the formula previously described (see Chapter 11). Another approach to determining the dose of platelets is that one unit of random donor platelet concentrate per 10 kg recipient body weight should elevate the platelet count approximately 40,000/μL. A third alternative method of determining the dose of platelets is 1 unit per 2,500 g body weight.

Because of the size of pediatric patients, the techniques of transfusion and the doses of components are often different from those for adults. This means that the volumes of blood components being transfused to neonates and pediatric patients may be considerably smaller than those for adults, and the equipment for transfusion may be different. One issue is the size of the needle used for transfusion. For adults it is recommended that needles for transfusion be no smaller than 21 gauge. Hemolysis can occur from high or very low flow rates and with smaller needles, especially when older stored blood is used.[107] However, citrated blood stored about 24 hours has been administered through 27 gauge needles with no hemolysis.[110] Thus, the use of butterfly or angiocatheter needles of 22 to 27 gauge is acceptable. In patients who will receive many transfusions during a course of therapy (i.e., bone marrow transplantation or chemotherapy), indwelling catheters such as Broviac or Hickman may be used for transfusion.[106] All blood products should be filtered, and filters with small internal volumes are now available.[107] For small patients receiving small volumes of blood, it is customary to control the rate of transfusion by using a constant-infusion or syringe pump. In general, these devices work well for this purpose,[107] but the particular brand of device should be tested to ensure accuracy and lack of hemolysis. Because of the immature thermoregulatory systems in newborns and the importance of temperature control in many pediatric patients, it is often desirable to warm the blood during transfusion. A drawback of many blood warming devices is the large volume of blood required to prime the system and the resultant loss of blood remaining in the system. If these systems are used, the volume of blood obtained from the blood bank must take into account this extra need to fill the warming device. One approach for syringe transfusion is to place the syringe in the incubator with the infant for 15 to 30 minutes, at which time the blood will be suitably warmed. It is important to ensure that the incubator temperature is not greater than about 37°C to avoid hemolysis. Guidelines regarding solutions for use in transfusing blood components are similar to those for transfusion of adults. An excellent summary of the policies along with specific procedures for the techniques for transfusion of neonates and pediatric patients can be found in reference 107.

TRANSFUSION THERAPY IN HEMOGLOBINOPATHIES

Sickle Cell Disease

Clinical indications for transfusion   Most patients with sickle cell disease (SCD) are asymptomatic even with hemoglobin concentrations as low as 6 g/dL. Thus, transfusion is not used to manage chronic steady-state anemia. Uncomplicated painful crises, minor surgery not involving general anesthesia, and minor infections are also usually not considered indications for transfusion. However, there are several situations in which red cell transfusion is indicated in these patients (Table 12.9). In these situations, the goal of transfusion is to reduce intravascular sickling by diluting or replacing the patient's sickled cells with nonsickling red cells from a normal donor. The major complications of SCD are aplastic crisis, stroke, acute pain syndrome, infection (especially with pneumococci), acute splenic sequestration, priapism, and chronic leg ulcers. Since acute sickle cell crises rarely occur when the hemoglobin S is maintained below 45% to 50% total hemoglobin, some patients are kept on an ongoing transfusion program to main-

Table 12.9 General indications for transfusion in sickle cell anemia

To improve oxygen-carrying capacity and transport in patients with:
  Physiologic derangement
  Fatigue and dyspnea (usually Hb < 50 g/L)
  Acute or chronic hypoxia (PO_2 < 65 mm Hg)
To decrease the concentration of HbS, thereby improving microvascular perfusion in acute situations such as:
  Life-threatening events including infection
  Acute, impending, or suspected cerebrovascular accidents
  Acute splenic or hepatic sequestration crises
  Acute priapism
  Acute progressive lung disease
  Fat embolization following fractures
  Preparation for surgery
  Intractable acute events, including painful crises
  Prior to injection of contrast material
To maintain HbS level below 0.3 total Hb for chronic conditions such as:
  After cerebrovascular accidents
  For leg ulcers
  During pregnancy
  For decreased performance status and disability due to recurrent acute complications
  In chronic organ failure

Source: Brettler DB. Inhibitors of factor VIII: detection and treatment. In: Hackel E, Westphal RG, Wilson SM, eds. Transfusion Management of Some Common Heritable Blood Disorders. Bethesda, MD: American Association of Blood Banks, 1992:56.

tain hemoglobin A levels between 50% and 70% total hemoglobin. This can usually be accomplished by transfusing 10 to 15 mL/kg (for children) or 1 to 2 units (for adults) every 2 to 4 weeks.

In transfusing patients with SCD, the blood viscosity must be considered as well as the proportion of hemoglobin S. When the proportion of hemoglobin is stable, the blood viscosity increases as the hematocrit increases, causing a decline in effective oxygen delivery in the hematocrit range of 20% to 40%.[111] Thus, in some situations exchange transfusion may be preferred over simple transfusion.

Red cell exchange transfusion is used for acute situations in which it is desired to decrease the level of hemoglobin S and increase the level of hemoglobin A rapidly.[112–114] It is usually desirable to reduce the hemoglobin S to less than 30% of the total hemoglobin, although it is also important not to elevate the hematocrit excessively, since blood viscosity begins to increase above hemoglobin levels of 14 to 15 g/dL. Formulas are available for determining the volume of blood necessary to reduce hemoglobin S below 30% from various starting hematocrits.[115] Exchange transfusions can be carried out by using a three-way stopcock, syringes, and a "push-pull" technique or by using semiautomated blood cell separators and a technique similar to plasma exchange.[112–114]

Pregnancy increases the likelihood of complications and sickle cell crises. Prophylactic transfusion to maintain hemoglobin S levels below 80% of total hemoglobin are now often part of the management of these patients,[116–118] although some[119,120]

believe that improvements in the general care of pregnant SCD patients make prophylactic transfusions indicated only for selected patients.

Surgery—especially procedures involving general anesthesia—increases the likelihood of complications of sickle cell disease, and thus preoperative prophylactic transfusion might be effective. Preoperative transfusion can be used to reduce the hemoglobin S level to 60% or less and to elevate the total hemoglobin to about 11 g/dL.[121–123] However, the clinical benefits of these transfusions are not as clearly established as for pregnancy. If the surgical procedure is expected to be complicated or general anesthesia prolonged, transfusion is more likely to be used.

Red cell antibodies   Many SCD patients form red cell antibodies as a result of transfusion. Often multiple antibodies are present, making it very difficult to find compatible red cells.[124–127] It is difficult to determine whether SCD patients are more likely than others to form red cell antibodies, because SCD patients receive many units of blood over a long period of time, and appropriate control groups are not available. Immunization may also be increased because most of the red cells the patients receive are from donors of a different ethnic or racial group with some differences in antigen frequency, thus leading to the patients' being exposed to antigens that they lack.[124] Garraty[125] concludes that red cell antibody formation is more common among SCD patients, but regardless of this point, there is considerable debate about the selection of donors for SCD patients. Since most SCD patients do not form red cell antibodies, standard blood bank operations—in which no special donor-recipient matching is done—can be followed, and when red cell antibodies occur, appropriate antigen-negative red cells are used.[126,127] However, locating antigen-negative red cells may be quite difficult for some patients with multiple antibodies, and this can delay transfusion. An alternative strategy is to avoid antibody formation by using red cells matched for the antigens most likely to cause immunization.[124,128–130] These would include antigens in the Rh, Kell, Duffy, and Kidd systems. Although the optimum strategy has been debated for two or three decades, there is no general agreement, and the approach is usually determined locally.

Transfusion reactions   Transfusion reactions may be confusing in SCD patients, because some symptoms of a transfusion reaction such as fever, sickle cell crisis pain, or arthralgias may be caused by the sickle cell disease. Since some patients have multiple antibodies, making it difficult to find compatible red cells, there may be additional concern as to whether acute or delayed hemolysis is occurring. A particular issue in SCD patients is the occasional occurrence of hemolysis in the absence of demonstrable red cell antibodies.[125,131,132] Thus, there is considerable benefit to avoiding febrile nonhemolytic transfusion reactions. This can be done by using leukodepleted blood components (see also Chapters 11 and 14).

Components   Standard red cell components are satisfactory for transfusion to SCD patients. For acute crises, it may be desirable to use red cells less than 1 week old to provide maximal oxygen-carrying capacity immediately after transfusion. It is preferable to avoid transfusing sickle-trait red cells, especially during a crisis. The hypoxia and acidosis in the patient may be adequate to cause sickling of the sickle-trait red cells,

thus adding to rather than alleviating the problem. In addition, the combination of homozygous and heterozygous sickle hemoglobin and hemoglobin A may complicate monitoring the results of transfusion. Thus, red cells to be used for SCD patients should be free of sickle-trait hemoglobin.

Thalassemia

Patients with thalassemia were transfused as little as possible until the early 1960s, when studies revealed that children whose hemoglobin was maintained at 8 g/dL or greater had better growth, less hepatosplenomegaly, fewer bone abnormalities, and less cardiac enlargement. This led to the use of "hypertransfusion," in which the hemoglobin is maintained at 9 g/dL or greater,[133,134] or "supertransfusion" programs, which maintain the hemoglobin at 11.5 g/dL or greater.[90] The supertransfusion program is thought to almost completely suppress the patient's own hematopoiesis without increasing the transfusion requirements after the initial transfusion.[90]

Transfusion requirements for thalassemia patients usually are 80 to 150 mL/kg per year.[135] There is some debate on the benefit of the supertransfusion program, and it is not clear whether maintaining the hemoglobin at the higher level (11.5 g/dL) provides an overall benefit.

Ordinary red cells can be used for the transfusions. There has been some question of whether the reduced 2,3-DPG in stored red cells would result in tissue hypoxia and increased production of red cells. There is little evidence that this actually occurs. A more common problem is the development of febrile or allergic transfusion reactions in these multitransfused patients. The febrile reactions can be avoided by using leukocyte-depleted red cells. Allergic reactions are usually caused by plasma proteins and, if not controlled by antihistamines, may necessitate the use of washed red cells.

Red cell alloantibodies   These multitransfused patients may, as expected, develop red cell alloantibodies.[126] The considerations about whether to provide red cells matched for some antigens or to await the development of antibodies is similar to those for SCD patients.

Neocytes

Many patients, especially those with hemoglobinopathies, require ongoing transfusion therapy and may become iron overloaded. Iron chelation and removal and supertransfusion strategies have been used in these patients. Another approach is the transfusion of red cell units enriched with younger cells (neocytes) so that the transfusion requirements would be reduced. These neocyte units have increased the interval between transfusion by about 13 days (from 30 to 43 days)[90] and have provided a 41% increase in intravascular survival.[136] Neocyte units are usually prepared by cytapheresis using blood cell separators and thus are expensive. It is not clear whether the advantages of neocytes will be sufficient to warrant their broad use in the therapy of patients requiring repeated transfusions.

One method of preparing neocytes uses an elongated, funnel-shaped bag that allows better isolation of neocytes from the top of the red cell portion.[137] In a trial of neocytes produced using this system, Spanos et al.[138] found a 69% greater use of red cell units but a 20% mean reduction in the volume of red cells transfused.

HEMOPHILIA AND VON WILLEBRAND'S DISEASE

Hemophilia A (Factor VIII Deficiency)

The blood components and derivatives containing coagulation factors VIII and IX are described in Chapter 2, and the use of these products to replace coagulation factors is also discussed in Chapter 11. For patients with mild hemophilia, minor procedures or dental work may be managed using desmopressin acetate to stimulate endogenous release of factor VIII.[139] In more severe cases or for major bleeding episodes or major procedures, factor VIII concentrates are used. For early treatment of minor bleeding episodes, patients can keep factor VIII concentrates at home and are taught self-injection techniques. This early treatment of bleeding episodes minimizes the complications and greatly increases convenience for the patient.

About 15% of patients with severe hemophilia develop inhibitors that are alloantibodies that inhibit the procoagulant activity of the factor VIII molecule. These antibodies react with different epitopes on the factor VIII molecule.[139] The treatment of bleeding episodes in hemophilia patients with inhibitors depends on the severity of the bleeding episode, the severity of the hemophilia, and the response of the patient to factor VIII. The different alternatives for treatment are use of (a) large doses of factor VIII, (b) activated or nonactivated prothrombin complex concentrates, (c) plasma exchange, (d) porcine factor VIII, (e) recombinant factor VIIa, (f) and/or immunosuppression with cytotoxic agents or IVIG.[139]

Hemophilia B (Factor IX Deficiency)

For the treatment of factor IX deficiency or hemophilia B, coagulation factor concentrates containing factor IX are available, and this has simplified treatment of these patients. One of the major complications of treatment of factor VIII or factor IX deficiency with concentrates is the development of inhibitors. This occurs more frequently in factor VIII-deficient than in factor IX-deficient patients.

von Willebrand's Disease

von Willebrand's factor is present in the plasma in a wide range of multimers. The high-molecular weight multimers are the most hemostatic. Patients with von Willebrand's disease can be managed either by stimulation of endogenous production of von Willebrand's factor in those mildly affected or by replacement of the deficient coagulation factor in those severely affected. The former is accomplished by the administration

of desmopressin acetate. The blood component used to replace von Willebrand's factor is cryoprecipitate. Each bag of cryoprecipitate contains a substantial amount of von Willebrand's factor, and so the usual dose is 1 unit per 10 kg body weight every 12 hours. Cryoprecipitate is preferred over fresh frozen plasma because of the higher content of high-molecular weight multimers in cryoprecipitate.

AUTOIMMUNE HEMOLYTIC ANEMIA

The types of autoimmune hemolytic anemia are shown in Table 12.10. These patients often require transfusion. It is time consuming to find compatible red cells, and after considerable effort all red cell units may be incompatible. Therefore, the laboratory work to locate red cell units suitable for transfusion should be initiated early in the patient's course, even if at the time transfusion does not seem to be indicated. The decision to transfuse a patient with autoimmune hemolytic anemia should be based on the severity of the anemia, whether the anemia is rapidly progressive, and the associated clinical findings.[140] In newly diagnosed patients with autoimmune hemolytic anemia, the hemoglobin should be measured frequently to determine whether the anemia is stable or progressing. Transfusion is not recommended unless the hemoglobin is in the range of 5 to 8 g/dL. Many of these patients will compensate for their anemia, especially on bed rest in the hospital, and transfusion is not necessary. When the anemia becomes severe, cardiovascular or neurologic symptoms are those usually seen. This may involve angina, cardiac failure, mental confusion, weakness, or obtundation. Transfusion is indicated for such patients.

Although autoimmune hemolytic anemia patients are experiencing hemolysis, they usually do not experience signs or symptoms of an acute hemolytic transfusion reaction.[140] However, transfusion in patients with autoimmune hemolytic anemia involves risks in addition to those usually associated with transfusion. The unique potential complications of transfusion in autoimmune hemolytic anemia patients are increased hemolysis and congestive heart failure. The increased hemolysis can occur because, since red cell destruction is a mass-action phenomenon, the number of red cells (red cell mass) destroyed increases as the total-body red cell mass is increased by transfusion. Transfusion may also cause congestive heart failure due to circulatory overload if the patient has poor cardiac reserve.

If transfusion is indicated, the two goals of compatibility testing are to select red cells that will survive at least as long as the patient's own cells and to avoid transfusing red cells that are incompatible with any clinically significant alloantibodies the patient may have.

In the serologic investigation of autoimmune hemolytic anemia patients, ABO and Rh typing can usually be done without difficulty, although proper controls must be used, especially with the Rh typing, to ensure that the results are not obscured by spontaneous agglutination caused by the autoantibody (see Chapter 10). There are particular problems in the serologic investigation of patients with cold antibody-type autoimmune hemolytic

Table 12.10 Autoimmune hemolytic anemia

IgG Antibody Type

Infections
    Postviral autoimmune hemolytic anemia of childhood
    Infectious mononucleosis
    HIV-1 infection
Immune deficiency states
    Hypogammaglobulinemia
    Wiskott-Aldrich syndrome
    Dysgammaglobulinemia
Neoplasms of the immune system
    Lymphocytic disorders
        Chronic lymphocytic leukemia
        Non-Hodgkin's lymphoma
    Hodgkin's disease
    Plasma cell disorders
        Waldenström's macroglobulinemia
        Multiple myeloma
Diseases of immune dysfunction
    Systemic lupus erythematosus
    Scleroderma
    Rheumatoid arthritis
    Sjögren's syndrome
    Immune thrombocytopenia (Evans' syndrome)
Miscellaneous diseases
    Pernicious anemia
    Thyroiditis
    Ulcerative colitis
    Ovarian tumors and cysts
    Other tumors
Idiopathic

IgM Warm Antibody Type

Idiopathic
Lymphocytic malignancies

IgM Cold Antibody Type

Infectious
    EBV-infectious mononucleosis
    Mycoplasma pneumoniae
    Listeria monocytogenes
Idiopathic
Malignancies
    Lymphocytic malignancies
Adenocarcinomas
Benign monoclonal B-cell gammopathy

Source: Adapted from Rosse W. In: Handin RI, Lux SE, Stossel TP, eds. Blood: Principles and practice of hematology. Philadelphia: J.B. Lippincott Company, 1995:1831.

anemia (see Chapter 10). The cold-reacting autoantibody may cause red cell agglutination even at warmer temperatures, thus making the routine test methods inaccurate. If the patient has not been transfused recently, it is advisable to type his or her red cells for other clinically significant antigens as an aid in identifying any alloantibodies potentially present. Knowledge of the antigens the patient lacks will also aid in the identification of antibodies that may form in the future.

Selecting the red cell units that will have optimum survival may be difficult. The patient's serum will react with red cells from all donors because the autoantibodies have a broad spectrum of reactivity. The autoantibody may obscure alloantibodies present in the patient's serum. It is usually not possible to obtain red cells for transfusion that are compatible (negative crossmatch). The risk is that the broad, nonspecific reactivity will obscure an alloantibody, so laboratory testing is designed to detect this problem and select units that lack the antigen corresponding to any alloantibody present. In the absence of an alloantibody, the nonspecific reactivity from the patient's autoantibody makes the crossmatch incompatible but usually does not cause red cell destruction in excess of that already occurring because of the patient's disease. The patient's serum is also studied to determine whether the autoantibody has any blood group specificity. If the autoantibody has blood group specificity, selection of donor red cells lacking the corresponding antigen may provide cells that survive better than the patient's,[140] although the data to support this practice are not convincing. Even when the autoantibody has blood group specificity, it is not always possible to provide red cells that lack the corresponding antigen. For instance, it is not advisable to give Rh-positive red cells to an Rh-negative patient only to avoid an apparent autoantibody specificity. Another example is that if the autoantibody has anti-e specificity and the patient is Rh negative, it will be difficult to locate Rh-negative red cells that lack the e antigen (e.g., type as cdE/cdE), because this is an unusual Rh phenotype. Instead the common Rh-negative phenotype cde/cde would be used.

Several serologic techniques are also available to detect alloantibodies that might be present from previous transfusions or pregnancy. These techniques use two approaches: removing the autoantibody from the patient's red cells to determine which antigens the patient lacks and thus might be immunized against; and absorbing the patient's serum using autologous red cells or those known to possess certain combinations of antigens to try to identify an underlying alloantibody. These techniques are discussed in Chapter 10. If any clinically significant alloantibodies are present, red cells selected for transfusion should lack the corresponding antigen.

Because of the autoantibodies, red cells from all donors will have a shortened survival. Despite this hemolysis, patients with autoimmune hemolytic anemia do not require unusual or special red cell components. The usual packed red cells are satisfactory. It is advisable to choose units that are not toward the end of their storage life so as to obtain the maximum benefit from the transfusion by avoiding loss of senescent red cells. It may also be advisable to use leukocyte-depleted red cells to avoid a possible febrile transfusion reaction, which might be confused with a hemolytic reaction and might (at least temporarily) interrupt the transfusion. There is no reason to use frozen deglycerolized red cells for autoimmune hemolytic anemia patients.

The serologic evaluation is different (see Chapter 10) in patients with cold-type autoimmune hemolytic anemia compared to those with warm-type anemia; however, the considerations in transfusing these patients are similar. One unique issue for patients with cold-type anemia is the need to be sure that the blood is warmed before transfusion to avoid hemolysis due to the cold active antibody. Blood warming is discussed in Chapter 13.

PREGNANT WOMEN

Anemia is common during pregnancy; however, these patients rarely require transfusion. When transfusion is necessary it is usually because of some other complicating factor or disease. The choice of blood components then is based on the specific reason for the transfusion (i.e., acute blood loss, sickle cell disease, etc.). It is recommended that pregnant patients who are CMV negative or whose CMV status is unknown receive CMV-free blood components because of the severe effects that acute CMV infection of the mother can have on the fetus (see Chapter 11).

ACQUIRED IMMUNE DEFICIENCY SYNDROME

The hematologic complications of acquired immune deficiency syndrome (AIDS) are anemia, thrombocytopenia, leukopenia, lupus-like coagulation inhibitors, and DIC caused by either the disease itself or the antiviral agents used for therapy.

Anemia

The anemia in AIDS patients is similar to the anemia of chronic disease; it is characterized by a low reticulocyte count and adequate iron stores. Anemia is probably due to ineffective erythropoiesis, possibly because of the effect of HIV infection on erythroid maturation or the release of cytokines that inhibit erythroid maturation.[141,142] The decision to transfuse these patients is similar to the decision for other patients with chronic anemias and is based on symptoms and hemoglobin level. When red cell transfusion is used, standard red blood cells are satisfactory. The use of irradiated blood components for AIDS patients is discussed in Chapter 11.

Thrombocytopenia

The thrombocytopenia in AIDS patients may be due to increased platelet-associated immunoglobulin,[143] circulating immune complexes bound to the platelet surface,[143] antibodies that cross-react with platelet surface glycoproteins,[144] or an effect of the viral infection of megakaryocytes.[145] Because in general the thrombocytopenia is thought to be on an immunologic basis, platelet transfusions are generally not indicated. Instead corticosteroids, immunoglobulins, or splenectomy are preferred treatment in patients whose thrombocytopenia poses a major problem. Platelet transfusions may be used in emergencies, as would be the case for autoimmune thrombocytopenic purpura.

Leukopenia

The lymphocyte, neutrophil, and monocyte-macrophage cell lines may all be affected in AIDS patients. However, transfusion therapy for these leukopenic situations is not generally used.

Lupus Anticoagulant

AIDS patients with lupus anticoagulant should be managed as any other patient with a lupus anticoagulant. Prophylactic treatment is not necessary.

Disseminated Intravascular Coagulopathy

AIDS patients with DIC should also be managed like others with DIC. If the process is severe, plasma exchange is indicated. These patients may pose a potential problem during plasma exchange because of the known infectious plasma. This is discussed more fully in Chapter 19.

AUTOIMMUNE THROMBOCYTOPENIA

Autoimmune thrombocytopenia patients have platelet IgG autoantibodies that bind to platelets and cause accelerated platelet destruction by interacting with Fc receptors on macrophages. This also results in a severely shortened intravascular survival of transfused platelets. Despite very low platelet counts, most patients with autoimmune thrombocytopenia do not require platelet transfusion.[146] It has been suggested that these patients have a population of young platelets, which provide better hemostasis than would be expected based on their platelet count.[146] For instance, when autoimmune thrombocytopenic patients undergo splenectomy, platelet transfusions are rarely required.[147] There are many therapies available for these patients, including corticosteroids, splenectomy, the androgen danazol, vinca alkaloids, immunosuppressives such as cyclophosphamide or azathioprine, and IVIG. The intravenous form of Rh immune globulin (Rh-IVIG) may also be effective in Rh-positive patients.[148]Although a more recent study indicates that this therapy is effective only in nonsplenectomized patients.[151] Although the survival of transfused platelets is reduced in these patients, platelet transfusion should be administered if serious life-threatening hemorrhage occurs, even though the transfused platelets may survive for only a few minutes or hours.[149] Some of these transfusions will cause a short but measurable increase in the platelet count.[150]

NEONATAL ALLOIMMUNE THROMBOCYTOPENIA

Neonatal alloimmune thrombocytopenia is estimated to occur 1 in 5,000 live births. It is the platelet analog of hemolytic disease of the newborn. In neonatal alloimmune thrombocytopenia, the mother becomes immunized to an antigen that she lacks but the

fetus has inherited from the father. Alloimmunization is usually due to the platelet antigen HPA1 (PlA1), but many other platelet-specific antigens have been involved (see Chapter 9). Maternal IgG antiplatelet antibodies then cross the placenta and cause thrombocytopenia in the fetus.[152] Mortality rates of approximately 15% have been reported,[153] primarily due to intracranial hemorrhage either before birth or during vaginal delivery. Testing of sera of pregnant women at risk of delivering a baby with neonatal alloimmune thrombocytopenia is helpful if an antibody is detected, but failure to find platelet antibody does not ensure that the baby's platelet count will be normal.[154]

If neonatal alloimmune thrombocytopenia is diagnosed during pregnancy, fetal platelet counts can be obtained. If the fetus is severely thrombocytopenic the mother can be treated with IVIG.[155] If necessary, intrauterine platelet transfusions can be given,[155] although this is not usually necessary because the fetus is usually not at risk until labor begins. If thrombocytopenia is present at the time of delivery, a cesarean section can be done to minimize the trauma to the infant. If the infant is severely thrombocytopenic at birth with a platelet count below 50,000/µL or serious hemorrhage, treatment should be initiated. Treatment can involve transfusion of platelets lacking the offending antigen or exchange transfusion to remove the offending antibody. Platelets lacking the antigen can be obtained from the mother, although the plasma containing the antibody should be removed before transfusion and the platelets resuspended in saline or AB plasma. Because of the small size of the infant, an adequate number of platelets can be obtained from one unit of whole blood; apheresis is not necessary. However, it may be difficult for the mother to donate a unit of blood because of postpartum anemia or logistic reasons if the infant has been transferred to another hospital. The antibody most commonly responsible for neonatal alloimmune thrombocytopenia is anti-PlA1. Most large blood banks have a few PlA1-negative donors available to provide compatible platelets if laboratory facilities are available to quickly determine the serologic specificity of the antibody or if this is known in advance. The half-life of IgG is approximately 21 days, and so more than one platelet transfusion may be necessary in severely affected infants. Alternatively, exchange transfusion can be done using techniques similar to those recommended for HDN. However, since it is impossible to remove all of the antibody, and there can be serious complications from exchange transfusion, management using platelet transfusions is usually preferable to exchange transfusion.

ALLOIMMUNE NEONATAL NEUTROPENIA

This is the neutrophil analog of HDN and neonatal alloimmune thrombocytopenia. It is extremely rare; only a few cases have been reported in the literature and there are no estimates of its incidence. Patients usually are discovered because they develop infection of a circumcision site or the perineal area. Cases due to several different neutrophil-specific antibodies have been reported.[156] Although these infants can be given granulocytes obtained from a whole blood donation by the mother, the very short half-life of granulocytes limits the effectiveness of this approach. Thus, exchange transfusion is the recommended approach for these patients. Alloimmune neonatal neutropenia is discussed more fully in Chapter 10.

RARE BLOOD TYPES

There is no universal definition of a rare blood type. For clinical transfusion purposes this usually refers to an individual who lacks a blood group antigen that is present in very high frequency in the normal population. This means that the individual will almost certainly be exposed to the antigen if he or she receives a transfusion or becomes pregnant. Almost all of these patients will have circulating antibody against the antigen, which is what brings them to the attention of the blood bank. Thus, the first question is whether the antibody is clinically significant and likely to cause accelerated destruction of red cells. In general, antibodies that react in vitro at body temperature (37°C) may be clinically significant, although many such antibodies are not. Reference texts should be consulted in making the decision. Use of an in vivo crossmatch may be helpful (see Chapter 10). If the antibody is clinically significant, efforts should be made to obtain red cells that lack the antigen. If such compatible donors are not available through the local blood supplier, donors can be sought from the American Association of Blood Banks and the American Red Cross, who maintain national registries of rare blood donors. Considerable planning may be necessary to obtain the red cells, especially if the donors live in other cities. If the transfusion is to replace blood loss during elective surgery, it may be necessary to plan the surgery around the availability of blood. Red cells from some rare donors may be available only in the frozen state, which may create additional problems if the transfusion is for anticipated but uncertain blood loss. To avoid wasting rare red cells and also avoid transfusing the patient unnecessarily, close communication between the blood bank and the clinician is essential.

If the need for transfusion is urgent, it is helpful to consider in greater detail the likely clinical effect of the antibody. If the antibody can be expected to cause a somewhat shortened red cell survival but little or no acute hemolysis or symptoms, the decision might be made to use incompatible red cells, at least to maintain the patient until antigen-negative compatible red cells can be located.

Patients with rare blood types who do not have an antibody occasionally become known to the blood bank. For those patients red cells negative for the rare antigen of concern are not necessarily provided. The decision to use antigen-negative red cells for nonimmunized patients should be based on the clinical significance of the antibody the patient might produce, the antigenicity of the antigen, the patient's current medical condition, and the likelihood that the patient will require transfusion or may become pregnant in the future.

REFERENCES

1. Maier RV, Carrico CJ. Developments in the resuscitation of critically ill surgical patients. Adv Surg 1986;19:271.
2. Shine KI, Kuhn M, Young LS, Tillisch JH. Aspects of the management of shock. Ann Intern Med 1980;93:723.
3. Stehling L. Fluid replacement in massive transfusion. In: Jefferies LC, Brecher ME, eds. Massive Transfusion. Bethesda, MD: American Association of Blood Banks, 1994:1–16.

4. Standards for Blood Banks and Transfusion Services, 16th ed. Arlington, VA: American Association of Blood Banks, 1994.

5. Faringer PD, Mullins RJ, Johnson RL, Trunkey DD. Blood component supplementation during massive transfusion of AS-1 red cells in trauma patients. J Trauma 1993;34:481–488.

6. Counts RB, Haisch C, Simon TL, Maxwell NG, Heimbach DM, Carrico CJ. Hemostasis in massively transfused trauma patients. Ann Surg 1979;190:91.

7. Mannucci PM, Federici AB, Sirchia G. Hemostasis testing during massive blood replacement: a study of 172 cases. Vox Sang 1982;42:113.

8. Wilson RF, Dulchavsky SA, Soullier G, Beckman B. Problems with 20 or more blood transfusions in 24 hours. Am Surg 1987;53:410.

9. Martin DJ, Lucas CE, Ledgerwood AM, et al. Fresh frozen plasma supplement to massive red blood cell transfusion. Ann Surg 1985;202:505.

10. Reed RL, Ciavarella D, Heimbach, DM, et al. Prophylactic platelet administration during massive transfusion. Ann Surg 1986;203:40.

11. Sawyer PR, Harrison CR. Massive transfusion in adults. Vox Sang 1990;58:199–203.

12. Benesch R, Benesch RE. Intracellular organic phosphates as regulators of oxygen release by haemoglobin. Nature 1969;221:618–622.

13. Chanutin A, Curnish RR. Effect of organic and inorganic phosphates on the oxygen equilibrium of human erythrocytes. Arch Biochem 1967;121:96–102.

14. Miller LD, Oski FA, Diaco JF, et al. The affinity of hemoglobin for oxygen: its control and in vivo significance. Surgery 1970;68:187–195.

15. Valtis DJ, Kennedy AC. Defective gas-transport function of stored red blood-cells. Lancet 1954;1:119–125.

16. Beutler E, Wood L. The in vivo regeneration of red cell 2,3 diphosphoglyceric acid (DPG) after transfusion of stored blood. J Lab Clin Med 1969;74:300.

17. International Forum. What is the clinical importance of alterations of the hemoglobin oxygen affinity in preserved blood—especially as produced by variations of red cell 2,3 DPG content? Vox Sang 1978;34:111–127.

18. Collins JA. Abnormal hemoglobin-oxygen affinity and surgical hemotherapy. In: Collins JA, Lundsgaard-Hansen P, eds. Surgical Hemotherapy. New York: S. Karger, 1980:46.

19. Spector JI, Zaroulis CG, Pivacek LE, Emerson CP, Valeri CR. Physiologic effects of normal- or low-oxygen-affinity red cells in hypoxic baboons. Am J Physiol 1977;232:H79–H84.

20. Perkins HA, Snyder M, Thagher C, Rolfs MR. Calcium ion activity during rapid exchange transfusion with citrated blood. Transfusion 1971;11:204.

21. Fakhry SM, Sheldon GF. Massive transfusion in the surgical patient. In: Jefferies LC, Brecher ME, eds. Massive Transfusion. Bethesda, MD: American Association of Blood Banks, 1994:17–42.

22. Collins JA. Problems associated with the massive transfusion of stored blood. Surgery 1974;75:274.

23. Snyder EL, Bookbinder M. Role of microaggregate blood filtration in clinical medicine. Transfusion 1983;23:460–470.

24. Jaeger RJ, Rubin RJ. Migration of a phthalate ester plasticizer from polyvinyl chloride blood bags into stored human blood and its localization in human tissues. N Engl J Med 1972;287:1114–1118.

25. Hillman LS, Goodwin SL, Sherman WR. Identification and measurement of plasticizer in neonatal tissues after umbilical catheters and blood products. N Engl J Med 1975;292:381–386.

26. Plonait SL, Nau H, Maier RF, Wittfoht W, Obladen M. Exposure of newborn infants to di-(2-ethylhexyl)-phthalate and 2-ethylhexanoic acid following exchange transfusion with polyvinylchloride catheters. Transfusion 1993;33:598–605.

27. Rubin RJ, Ness PM. What price progress? An update on vinyl plastic blood banks. Transfusion 1989;29:3358–3361.

28. Wilson RF, Binkley LE, Sabo FM, et al. Electrolyte and acid-base changes with massive blood transfusions. Am Surg 1992;58:535–545.

29. Bick RL. Hemostasis defects associated with cardiac surgery, prosthetic devices, and other extracorporeal circuits. Semin Thromb Hemost 1980;11:249.

30. Gelb AB, Roth RI, Levin J. Changes in blood coagulation during and following cardiopulmonary bypass. Am J Clin Pathol 1996;106:187–199.

31. Harker LA, Malpass TW, Branson HE, et al. Mechanism of abnormal bleeding in patients undergoing cardiopulmonary bypass: acquired transient platelet dysfunction associated with selective alpha-granule release. Blood 1980;56:824–834.

32. Milam JD, Austin SF, Martin RF, et al. Alteration of coagulation and selected clinical chemistry parameters in patients undergoing open heart surgery without transfusions. Am J Clin Pathol 1981;76:155–162.

33. Simon TL, Akl BF, Murphy W. Controlled trial of routine administration of platelet concentrates in cardiopulmonary bypass surgery. Ann Thorac Surg 1984;37:359–364.

34. Goodnough LT, Johnston MF, Toy PT. The variability of transfusion practice in coronary artery bypass surgery. Transfusion Medicine Academic Award Group. JAMA 1991;265:86–90.

35. Goodnough LT, Johnston MF, Ramsey G, et al. Guidelines for transfusion support in patients undergoing coronary artery bypass grafting. Transfusion Practices Committee of the American Association of Blood Banks. Ann Thorac Surg 1990;50:675–683.

36. Salzman EW, Weinstein MJ, Weintraub RM, et al. Treatment with desmopressin acetate to reduce blood loss after cardiac surgery. N Engl J Med 1986;314:1402.

37. Anderson KC. The role of the blood bank in hematopoietic stem cell transplantation. Transfusion 1992;32:272–285.

38. McCullough J. The role of the blood bank in transplantation. Arch Pathol Lab Med 1991;115:1195–1200.

39. McCullough J, Lasky LC, Warkentin PI. Role of the blood bank in bone marrow transplantation. In: Advances in Immunobiology: Blood cell antigens and bone marrow transplantation. New York: Alan R. Liss, Inc., 1984:379–412.

40. Storb R, Prentice RL, Thomas ED. Marrow transplantation for treatment of aplastic anemia: an analysis of factors associated with graft rejection. N Engl J Med 1977;296:61.

41. Storb R, Thomas ED, Buckner CD, et al. Marrow transplantation in 30 "untransfused" patients with severe aplastic anemia. Ann Intern Med 1980;92:30.

42. Champlin RE, Horowitz MM, van Bekkum DW, et al. Graft failure following bone marrow transplantation for severe aplastic anemia: risk factors and treatment results. Blood 1989;73:606.

43. Storb R, Wieden PL. Transfusion problems associated with transplantation. Semin Hematol 1981;18:163.

44. TRAP Trial Study Group. A randomized trial evaluating leukocyte-reduction and UV-B irradiation of platelets to prevent alloimmune platelet refractoriness. N Engl J Med 1997. In press.

45. Thomas ED, Storb R, Clift RA, et al. Bone-marrow transplantation. N Engl J Med 1975;292:832.

46. Klingemann HG, Self S, Banaji M, et al. Refractoriness to random donor platelet transfusions in patients with aplastic anaemia: a multivariate analysis of data from 264 cases. Br J Haematol 1987;66:115–121.

47. Gmur J, von Felten A, Osterwalder B, et al. Delayed alloimmunization using random single donor platelet transfusions: a prospective study in thrombocytopenic patients with acute leukemia. Blood 1983;62:473–479.

48. Sintnicolaas K, Vriesendorp HM, Sizoo W, et al. Delayed alloimmunization by random single donor platelet transfusions. A randomized study to compare single donor and multiple donor platelet transfusions in cancer patients with severe thrombocytopenia. Lancet 1981;1:750–754.

49. Fisher M, Chapman JR, Ting A, Morris PJ. Alloimmunization to HLA antigens following transfusion with leukocyte-poor and purified platelet suspensions. Vox Sang 1985;49:331–335.

50. Murphy MF, Metcalfe P, Thomas H, et al. Use of leukocyte-poor blood components and HLA-matched-platelet donors to prevent HLA alloimmunization. Br J Haematol 1986;62:529–534.

51. Brand A, Claas FHJ, Voogt PJ, Wasser MN, Eernisse JG. Alloimmunization after leukocyte-depleted multiple random donor platelet transfusions. Vox Sang 1988;54:160–166.

52. Andreu G, Dewailly J, Leberre C, et al. Prevention of HLA immunization with leukocyte-poor packed red cells and platelet concentrates obtained by filtration. Blood 1988;72:964–969.

53. Sniecinski I, O'Donnell MR, Nowicki B, Hill LR. Prevention of refractoriness and HLA alloimmunization using filtered blood products. Blood 1988;71:1402–1407.

54. Saarinen UM, Kekomaki R, Siimes MA, Myllyla G. Effective prophylaxis against platelet refractoriness in multitransfused patients by use of leukocyte-free blood components. Blood 1990;75:512–517.

55. Gale RP, Feig S, Ho W, et al. ABO blood group system and bone marrow transplantation. Blood 1977;50:184.

56. Buckner CP, Clift RA, Sanders JE, Thomas ED. The role of a protective environment and prophylactic granulocyte transfusion in marrow transplantation. Transplant Proc 1978;10:255.

57. Hershko C, Gale RP, Ho W, Fitchen J. ABH antigens and bone marrow transplantation. Br J Haematol 1980;44:65.
58. Lasky L, Warkentin P, Ramsay N, Kersey J, McGlave P, McCullough J. Hemotherapy in patients undergoing blood group incompatible bone marrow transfusion. Transfusion 1983;23:277–285.
59. Warkentin PI, Yomtovian R, Hurd D, Brunning R, Swanson J, Kersey JH, McCullough J. Severe delayed hemolytic transfusion reaction complicating an ABO-incompatible bone marrow transplantation. Vox Sang 1983;45:40–47.
60. Wernet D, Mayer G. Isoagglutinins following ABO-incompatible bone marrow transplantation. Vox Sang 1992;62:176–179.
61. Barge AJ, Johnson G, Witherspoon R, Torok-Storb B. Antibody-mediated marrow failure after allogeneic bone marrow transplantation. Blood 1989;74:1477–1780.
62. Hows J, Beddow K, Gordon-Smith E, et al. Donor-derived red blood cell antibodies and immune hemolysis after allogeneic bone marrow transplantation. Blood 1986;67:177–181.
63. Gajewski JL, Petz LD, Calhoun L. Hemolysis of transfused group O red blood cells in minor ABO-incompatible unrelated-donor bone marrow transplants in patients receiving cyclosporine without post-transplant methotrexate. Blood 1992;79:3076–3085.
64. Berkman EM, Caplan SN. Engraftment of Rh positive marrow in a recipient with Rh antibody. Transplant Proc 1977;9:215.
65. Petz LD. Immunohematologic problems associated with bone marrow transplantation. Transfus Med Rev 1987;1:86–92.
66. Hill RS, Peterson FB, Storb R, et al. Mixed hematologic chimerism after allogeneic marrow transplantation for severe aplastic anemia is associated with a higher risk of graft rejection and a lessened incidence of acute graft-versus-host disease. Blood 1986;67:811–816.
67. Klumpp T, Caliguri MA, Rabinowe SA, Soiffer RJ, Murray C, Ritz J. Autoimmune pancytopenia following allogeneic bone marrow transplantation. Bone Marrow Transplant 1990;6:445–447.
68. Minchinton RM, Waters AH, Malpas JS, Starke I, Kendra JR, Barrett JA. Platelet- and granulocyte-specific antibodies after allogeneic and autologous bone marrow grafts. Vox Sang 1984;46:125–135.
69. Wernet D, Schnaidt M, Northoff H. Reactivation of recipient antibody to blood cell antigens soon after allogeneic bone marrow transplantation. Vox Sang 1996;71:212–215.
70. Gershon AA, Steinberg S, Brunell PA. Zoster immune globulin: a further assessment. N Engl J Med 1974;290:243.
71. Condie RM, O'Reilly RJ. Prevention of cytomegalovirus infection by prophylaxis with an intravenous, hyperimmune, native, unmodified cytomegalovirus globulin. Am J Med 1984;76:134.
72. Meyers JD, Leszczynski J, Zaia JA, et al. Prevention of cytomegalovirus infection by cytomegalovirus immune globulin after marrow transplantation. Ann Intern Med 1983;98:442.
73. Winston DJ, Ho WG, Lin C, et al. Intravenous immunoglobulin for modification of cytomegalovirus infections associated with bone marrow transplantation. Am J Med 1984;76:128.
74. Nusbacher J. Blood transfusion support in liver transplantation. Transfus Med Rev 1991;5:207–213.
75. Opelz G, Sengar DPS, Mickey MR, et al. Effect of blood transfusions on subsequent kidney transplants. Transplant Proc 1973;5:253.
76. Opelz G, Terasaki PI. Improvement of kidney-graft survival with increased numbers of blood transfusions. N Engl J Med 1978;299:799.
77. Salvatierra O Jr, Vincenti F, Amend W, et al. Deliberate donor-specific blood transfusions prior to living related renal transplantation. A new approach. Ann Surg 1980;192:543–552.
78. Opelz G. Improved kidney graft survival in non-transfused recipients. Transplant Proc 1987;19:149–152.
79. Bick RL. Alterations of hemostasis associated with cardiopulmonary bypass: pathophysiology, prevention, diagnosis, and management. Semin Thromb Hemost 1976;3:59–82.
80. Mammen EF, Koets MH, Washington BC, et al. Hemostasis changes during cardiopulmonary bypass surgery. Semin Thromb Hemost 1985;11:281–292.
81. McKenna R, Bachmann F, Whittaker B, et al. The hemostatic mechanism after open-heart surgery. J Thorac Cardiovasc Surg 1975;70:298–308.
82. de Leval MR, Hill JD, Mielke CH, et al. Blood platelets and extracorporeal circulation. J Thorac Cardiovasc Surg 1975;69:144–151.
83. Anderson KC, Goodnough LT, Sayers M, et al. Variation of blood component irradiation practice: implications for prevention of transfusion-associated graft-versus-host disease. Blood 1991;77:2096–2102.

84. Ramsey G. B-cell-mediated graft-versus-host disease in transplantation. Vox Sang 1996;70(Suppl 3): 74–77.
85. Ramsey G. Red cell antibodies arising from solid organ transplants. Transfusion 1991;31:76–86.
86. Hunt BJ, Yacoub M, Amin S, Devenish A, Contreras M. Induction of red blood cell destruction by graft-derived antibodies after minor ABO-mismatched heart and lung transplantation. Transplantation 1988;46:246–249.
87. Minakuchi BJ, Toma H, Takahashi K, Ota K. Autoanti-A and -B antibody induced by ABO unmatched blood group kidney allograft. Transplant Proc 1985;17:2297–3000.
88. Brown MS, Garcia JF, Phibbs RH, et al. Decreased response of plasma immunoreactive erythropoietin to "available oxygen" in anemia of prematurity. J Pediatr 1984;105:793.
89. Strauss R. Current issues in neonatal transfusions. Vox Sang 1986;51:1–9.
90. Propper RD, Button LN, Nathan DG. New approaches to the transfusion management of thalassemia. Blood 1980;55:55.
91. Wolfe LC. Neonatal anemia. In: Handin RI, Stossel TP, Lux SE, eds. Blood: Principles and practice of hematology. Philadelphia: J.B. Lippincott Company, 1995:2105–2130.
92. Sacher RA, Luban NLC, Strauss RG. Current practice and guidelines for the transfusion of cellular blood components in the newborn. Transfus Med Rev 1989;3:39.
93. Ludvigsen CW, Swanson JL, Thompson TR, McCullough JJ. The failure of neonates to form red blood cell alloantibodies in response to multiple transfusions. Am J Clin Pathol 1987;2:250.
94. Oberman HA. Transfusion of the neonatal patient. Transfusion 1974;14:183.
95. Yaeger AS, Grumet FC, Hafleigh EB, et al. Prevention of transfusion-acquired cytomegalovirus infections in newborn infants. J Pediatr 1981;98:281.
96. Parkman R, Mosier D, Umansky I, et al. Graft-versus-host disease after intrauterine and exchange transfusions for hemolytic disease of the newborn. N Engl J Med 1974;290:359.
97. Bohm N, Kleine W, Enzel U. Graft-versus-host disease in two newborns after repeated blood transfusions because of Rhesus incompatibility. Beitr Pathol 1977;160:381.
98. Strauss RG. Practical issues in neonatal transfusion practice. Am J Clin Pathol 1997;107(Suppl 1): S57–S63.
99. Mintz PD, Luban NLC. Irradiated blood components. Am J Clin Pathol 1997;107:252. Letter to the Editor.
100. Strauss RG. Transfusion therapy in neonates. Am J Dis Child 1991;145:904–991.
101. Simon TL, Sierra ER. Concentration of platelet units into small volumes (rapid communications). Transfusion 1984;24:173–175.
102. Moroff G, Friedman A, et al. Reduction of the volume of stored platelet concentrates for neonatal use. Transfusion 1982;22:427.
103. Strauss RG. Management of the septic or neutropenic neonate. In: Capon SM, Chamber LA, eds. New Directions in Pediatric Hematology. Bethesda, MD: American Association of Blood Banks, 1996:121–139.
104. Christensen RD, Rothstein G, Anstall HB, et al. Granulocyte transfusions in neonates with bacterial infection, neutropenia, and depletion of mature marrow neutrophils. Pediatrics 1982;70:1.
105. Seibel M, Gross S. Exchange transfusion in the neonate. In: Kasprisin DO, Luban NLC, eds. Pediatric Transfusion Medicine, vol. 1. Boca Raton, FL: CRC Press, 1987:43–52.
106. Warkentin PI. Transfusion therapy for the pediatric oncology patient. In: Kasprisin DO, Luban NLC, eds. Pediatric Transfusion Medicine, vol 2. Boca Raton, FL: CRC Press, 1987:19–49.
107. Butch SH, Coltre MA. Techniques of transfusion. In: Kasprisin DO, Luban NLC, eds. Pediatric Transfusion Medicine, vol 1. Boca Raton, FL: CRC Press, 1987:91–135.
108. Corrigan JJ. Hemorrhagic and Thrombotic Disease in Childhood and Adolescence. New York: Churchill Livingstone, 1985.
109. Freireich EJ, Kliman A, Gaydos LA, et al. Response to repeated platelet transfusion from the same donor. Ann Intern Med 1963;50:277.
110. Herrera AJ, Corless J. Blood transfusions: effects of speed of infusion and of needle gauge on hemolysis. J Pediatr 1981;99:757.
111. Sharon BI, Honig GR. Management of congenital hemolytic anemias. In: Rossi EC, Simon TL, Moss GS, eds. Principles of Transfusion Medicine. Baltimore: Williams & Wilkins, 1991:131–149.

112. Key TC, Horger EO III, Walker EM Jr, Mitchum EN. Automated erythrocytopheresis for sickle cell anemia during pregnancy. Am J Obstet Gynecol 1980;138:731–737.

113. Klein HG, Garner RJ, Miller DM, et al. Automated partial exchange transfusion in sickle cell anemia. Transfusion 1980;20:578–84.

114. Kleinman S, Thompson-Breton R, Breen D, et al. Exchange red blood cell pheresis in pediatric patient with severe complications of sickle cell anemia. Transfusion 1981;21:443–446.

115. Cohen AR. Transfusion therapy for disorders of hemoglobin. In: Kasprisin DO, Luban NLC, eds. Pediatric Transfusion Medicine. Boca Raton, FL: CRC Press, Inc., 1997;2:51–83.

116. Morrison JC, Schneider JM, Whybrew WD, et al. Prophylactic transfusions in pregnant patients with sickle hemoglobinopathies: benefit versus risk. Obstet Gynecol 1980;274–280.

117. Cunningham FG, Pritchard JA, Mason R. Pregnancy and sickle cell hemoglobinopathies: results with and without prophylactic transfusion. Obstet Gynecol 1983;62:419–424.

118. Miller JM Jr, Horger EO III, Key TC, Walker EM Jr. Management of sickle hemoglobinopathies in pregnant patients. Am J Obstet Gynecol 1981;141:237–241.

119. Charache S, Scott J, Niebyl J, Bonds D. Management of sickle cell disease in pregnant patients. Obstet Gynecol 1980;55:407–410.

120. Koshy M, Burd L, Wallace D, et al. Prophylactic red cell transfusions in pregnant patients with sickle cell disease. N Engl J Med 1988;319:1447–1452.

121. Janik J, Seeler RA. Perioperative management of children with sickle hemoglobinopathy. J Pediatr Surg 1980;12:117–120.

122. Morrison JC, Whybrew WD, Bucovaz ET. The use of partial exchange transfusion preoperatively in patients with sickle cell hemoglobinopathies. Am J Obstet Gynecol 1978;132:59–63.

123. Fullerton MW, Philippart AI, Sarnaik S, Lusher JM. Preoperative exchange transfusion in sickle cell anemia. J Pediatr Surg 1981;16:297–300.

124. Vichinsky EP, Earles A, Johnson RA, et al. Alloimmunization in sickle cell anemia and transfusions of racially unmatched blood. N Engl J Med 1990;322:1617–1621.

125. Garratty G. Severe reactions associated with transfusion of patients with sickle cell disease. Transfusion 1997;37:357–359. Editorial.

126. Coles SM, Klein HG, Holland PV. Alloimmunization in two multi-transfused patient populations. Transfusion 1981;21:462–466.

127. Sarnaik S, Schornack JL, Lusher JM. The incidence of development of irregular red cell antibodies in patients with sickle cell anemia. Transfusion 1986;26:249–252.

128. Ambruso DR, Githens JH, Alcorn R, et al. Experience with donors matched for minor blood group antigens in patients with sickle cell anemia who are receiving chronic transfusion therapy. Transfusion 1987;27:94–99.

129. Blumberg N, Ross K, Avila E, Peck K. Should chronic transfusions be matched for antigens other than ABO and Rho(d)? Vox Sang 1984;47:205–208.

130. Sandler SG, Mallory D, Wolfe JS, Byrne P, Lucas DM. Screening with monoclonal anti-Fy3 to provide blood for phenotype-matched transfusions for patients with sickle cell disease. Transfusion 1997;37:393–397.

131. King KE, Shirey RS, Lankiewicz MW, Young-Ramsaran J, Ness PM. Delayed hemolytic transfusion reactions in sickle cell disease: simultaneous destruction of recipients' red cells. Transfusion 1997;37:376–381.

132. Petz LD, Calhoun L, Shulman IA, Johnson C, Herron RM. The sickle cell hemolytic transfusion reaction syndrome. Transfusion 1997;37:382–392.

133. Wolman IJ. Transfusion therapy in Cooley's anemia: growth and health as related to long-range hemoglobin levels: a progress report. Ann NY Acad Sci 1974;119:736.

134. Necheles TF, Chung S, Sabbah R, Whitten D. Intensive transfusion therapy in thalassemia major: an eight-year follow-up. Ann NY Acad Sci 1974;232:179.

135. Platt OS. The sickle syndromes. In: Handin RI, Lux S, Stossel TP, eds. Blood: Principles and practice of hematology. Philadelphia: J.B. Lippincott Company, 1995:1645–1700.

136. Bracey AW, Klein HG, Chambers S, Corash L. Ex vivo selective isolation of young red blood cells using the IBM-2991 cell washer. Blood 1983;61:1068.

137. Simon TL, Sohmer P, Nelson EJ. Extended survival of neocytes produced by a new system. Transfusion 1989;29:221–225.

138. Spanos T, Ladis V, Palamidou F, et al. The impact of neocyte transfusion in the management of thalassaemia. Vox Sang 1996;70:217–223.

139. White GC. Coagulation factors V and VIII: normal function and clinical disorders. In: Handin RI, Stossel TP, Lux SE, eds. Blood: Principles and practice of hematology. Philadelphia: J.B. Lippincott Company, 1995:1151–1179.

140. Petz LD, Swisher SN, eds. Clinical Practice of Transfusion Medicine, 2nd ed. New York: Churchill Livingstone, 1989.

141. Spivak J, Barnes DC, Fuchs E, et al. Serum immunoreactive erythropoietin in HIV-infected patients. JAMA 1989;261:3104–3107.

142. Zhang Y, Harada A, Bluethmann H, et al. Tumor necrosis factor (TNF) is a physiologic regulatory of hematopoietic cells: increase of early hematopoietic progenitor cells in TNF receptor p55-deficient mice in vivo and potent inhibition of progenitor cell proliferation by TNF in vitro. Blood 1995;86:2930–2937.

143. Karpatkin S. Immunologic thrombocytopenic purpura in HIV-seropositive homosexuals, narcotic addicts, and hemophiliacs. Semin Hematol 1988;25:219–229.

144. Battaieb A, Fromont P, Louache F, et al. Presence of cross-reactive antibody between HIV and platelet glycoproteins in HIV-related immune thrombocytopenic purpura. Blood 1992;80:162–169.

145. Louache F, Bettaieb A, Henri A, et al. Infection of megakaryocytes by HIV in seropositive patients with immune thrombocytopenic purpura. Blood 1991;78:1697–1705.

146. Harker LA, Slichter SJ. The bleeding time as a screening test for evaluation of platelet function. N Engl J Med 1972;287:155.

147. Schwartz SI, Bernard RP, Adams JT, Bauman AW. Splenectomy for hematologic disorders. Arch Surg 1970;101:338.

148. Bussel JB, Graziano JN, Kimberly RP. Intravenous anti-D treatment of immune thrombocytopenic purpura: analysis of efficacy, toxicity, and mechanism of effect. Blood 1991;77:1884–1893.

149. Aster RH, Jandl JH. Platelet sequestration in man. II. Immunological and clinical studies. J Clin Invest 1964;43:856.

150. Baumann MA, Menitove JE, Aster RH, Anderson T. Urgent treatment of idiopathic thrombocytopenic purpura with single-dose gammaglobulin infusion followed by platelet transfusion. Ann Intern Med 1986;104:808–809.

151. Scaradavou A, Woo B, Woloski BMR, et al. Intravenous anti-D treatment of immune thrombocytopenic purpura: experience in 272 patients. Blood 1997;89:2689–2700.

152. McIntosh S, O'Brien RT, Schwartz AD, Pearson HA. Neonatal isoimmune purpura: response to platelet infusions. J Pediatr 1973;82:1020–1027.

153. Pearson HA, Shulman NR, Marder VJ, Cone TE. Isoimmune neonatal thrombocytopenia purpura: clinical and therapeutic considerations. Blood 1964;23:154.

154. McFarland JG, Frenzke M, Aster RH. Testing of maternal sera in pregnancies at risk for neonatal alloimmune thrombocytopenia. Transfusion 1989;29:128.

155. Bussel JB, McFarland JG, Berkowitz RL. Antenatal management of fetal alloimmune and autoimmune thrombocytopenia. Transfus Med Rev 1990;14:149–162.

156. Lalezari P. Alloimmune neonatal neutropenia. In: Engelfriet CP, von Loghem JJ, von dem Borne AEGKr, eds. Immunohematology. Amsterdam: Elsevier Science Publishers, 1984:178.

THIRTEEN

TECHNIQUES OF BLOOD TRANSFUSION

Transfusion-related fatalities other than those due to disease transmission are estimated to occur once in 100,000 patients who receive a transfusion or once in 600,000 transfusions.[1] It is estimated that one in 12,000 units of blood is administered to the wrong patient.[2] The most common cause of transfusion-related fatality reported to regulatory agencies is hemolytic transfusion reaction.[1,2] The most common cause of an acute hemolytic transfusion reaction is ABO incompatibility, and this is usually the result of "management" error.[1,2] The incidence of ABO-incompatible transfusions is one in 10,000 to 40,000.[1-4] It appears that despite improvements in blood safety and the increasingly sophisticated technology used in the operation of blood centers and clinical laboratories, this error rate has remained relatively unchanged for years. Most of these management errors occur outside of the blood bank in the process of obtaining blood samples or administering the transfusion (Table 13.1).[1] "Blood given to the wrong person" was the most common of all the errors.[1] This is not a problem resulting from the urgent need to transfuse patients during surgery, since about two-thirds of these errors occurred outside of the operating suite. Nurses were most often involved, but nurses along with physicians or physicians alone were also responsible for the errors.

Because many of these steps at which fatal errors occur are part of the process of administering the transfusions, it is essential that blood transfusions be administered according to clearly defined procedures that are well understood and carried out by qualified personnel. Each hospital should have its own specific blood administration procedures and should designate the individuals authorized to administer blood components. Blood components are prescription drugs and thus can be administered only on the written order of a physician. The physician's order should include the blood component to be administered, any special requirements, the rate of administration, and any other instructions for care of the patient during the transfusion.

Table 13.1 Types of errors leading to transfusion-related fatalities

Failure to properly identify the recipient when the blood sample is collected for compatibility testing
Incorrect labeling of the properly collected sample
Improper labeling of tubes when testing is carried out in the laboratory
Use of an incorrect sample in the laboratory
Recording results in the incorrect record within the laboratory
Placing the compatibility tag on the incorrect unit
Releasing the unit to the incorrect patient
Administering correctly labeled and tested unit to the incorrect patient

Source: From information in Sazama K. 355 reports of transfusion-associated deaths. Transfusion 1990;30:583; and Linden JV, Paul B, Dressler KP. A report of 104 transfusion errors in New York State. Transfusion 1992;32:601–606.

OBTAINING CONSENT FOR TRANSFUSION

Once it has been determined that a blood transfusion is necessary, the procedure should be explained to the patient to minimize his or her apprehension and to obtain the patient's consent. In the past, a discrete consent for transfusion was usually not obtained. Increased awareness of the risks of transfusion on the part of physicians and patients has drawn attention to this and altered the extent to which consent for transfusion is obtained.[5,6] Acquiring consent for transfusion is now a requirement of the Joint Commission on Accreditation of Healthcare Organizations. As a result, most hospitals are now updating and improving the process for obtaining this consent. The elements of the consent are rather standard and include the nature, severity, and probability of risks and the general time frame in which they can be expected.[5] An additional step that can occur along with the consent process is the documentation of the reason for transfusion. This is increasingly important, as lawsuits contend that a transfusion that caused a complication may not have been necessary. This also provides an opportunity to describe the alternatives to transfusion or the ramifications to refusing a transfusion.[5] At present there is great variation in how consent is obtained. This ranges from the physician discussing transfusion with the patient, to use of printed material, to nurses discussing transfusion with the patient, to incorporation of information in general consent materials or inclusion of information in care protocols. The process may be documented by a note in the medical record, a discrete consent form, or as part of another consent form such as that used for consent for a surgical procedure. Although a single approach cannot be defined, it seems clear that physicians will be expected to ensure that patients understand the risks of transfusion and any alternatives to homologous donor blood that might be available.

OBTAINING THE BLOOD SAMPLE FOR COMPATIBILITY TESTING

One of the most common errors that leads to the administration of incompatible red cells is mislabeling the blood sample to be used for compatibility testing.[1,2] Wenz[7] describes three basic identification systems that can be used for specimen collection and control.

These are wristbands, dedicated transfusion systems, and mechanical barriers. In the wristband system, the hospital wristband and unique hospital number are the basis for identifying the patient and relating laboratory work and the transfusion of blood components. Unfortunately, errors in the availability or accuracy of wristbands are common, occurring on average in 5% of wristbands and varying from 1% to 60% in different hospitals.[7] These errors include absence of the wristband or errors in the information it contains. In the dedicated transfusion system, a separate wristband, request form, and labels are associated with unique preprinted numbers linking all of these items. In the mechanical barrier system, a unique number is assigned to the patient, and this number must be entered into a device that opens a mechanical barrier to the use of the unit.[4] This system has been reported to reduce potential transfusion accidents.[4,7] The system is not widely used at present, possibly because it still requires that staff members write the unique number on tubes being obtained for compatibility testing.

Each hospital should have a specific written procedure for this, and individuals collecting blood samples for compatibility testing should be familiar with and follow that procedure. Typically this involves the person collecting the sample to check the identifying information on the patient's wristband against the blood request form. Charts or tags on the bed are not suitable for identifying the patient. One of the most crucial steps is that the label should be applied to the blood specimen at the patient's bedside and the label should indicate the patient's full name and hospital number. The label on the specimen should also identify the phlebotomist. The blood sample should also be checked when it arrives in the blood bank to be sure that all required information is completed. It is not acceptable to change or "correct" information on a specimen label. If there is any doubt about the specimen or the information on the label, a new specimen should be obtained. The blood sample should not be obtained from an arm being used for the infusion of intravenous fluids, because these may alter the blood specimen and invalidate the crossmatch. If the blood sample is being obtained from an indwelling catheter, the catheter must be properly irrigated to clear it of any solutions being infused before the blood sample for compatibility testing is collected. One recommended procedure is to flush the line with 5 mL of saline and then withdraw a volume of blood twice the amount that is in the line before obtaining the sample for testing.

BLOOD ADMINISTRATION SETS AND FILTERS

Red cells, platelets, granulocytes, fresh frozen plasma, and cryoprecipitate are administered through a filter because fibrin clots and other particulate debris may be present. Traditional blood administration sets have contained filters with a pore size of approximately 170 to 250 μm. During the 1970s, it was recognized that microaggregates of 20 to 120 μm composed of platelets, leukocytes, and fibrin strands develop in stored blood.[8] It was believed that an important factor in the development of adult respiratory distress syndrome (ARDS) that often accompanied massive transfusion was the lodging of blood microemboli in the pulmonary microcirculation (see Chapter 14). As a result, several commercial microaggregate filters were developed and their use was advocated routinely in patients receiving a massive transfusion. As the pathophysiology of ARDS was better understood, it became clear that this is a complex situation and that microaggregates are

not the primary cause. Factors such as shock and complement activation were thought to be important. Clinical laboratory studies have never established the effectiveness of these microaggregate filters in preventing ARDS.[9] These filters are more expensive than standard blood filters, and at least some microaggregate filters had lower maximum flow rates than standard blood filters. There has been considerable debate as to the role of microaggregates in ARDS and the optimum uses for these microaggregate filters. Because these filters are costly, their indiscriminate use is not recommended. These filters are available and are used in some centers or for some patients in whom microaggregates are thought to be a problem (e.g., cardiovascular surgery), but the microaggregate filters do not achieve substantial leukocyte reduction. The increasing use of leukocyte-reduced components is eliminating the need for microaggregate filters.

Febrile transfusion reactions can be prevented by less expensive filters. Leukocyte reduction may delay or prevent alloimmunization and platelet refractoriness in some patients;[10–13] however, the optimal cost-effective strategy and patient population are not known.[9] Leukocyte reduction also prevents transmission of some cell-associated viruses such as cytomegalovirus,[14–16] These are new indications for blood filtration, that are causing the increasing use of leukodepletion filters (see Chapters 5, 11 and 12).

Hospitals have policies for the length of time that different types of vascular access devices can be left in place. Some indwelling catheters remain in place for long periods. Intravenous infusion sets using needles for the short-term administration of drugs or blood are usually not left in place for long periods. This is especially true for infusion sets used to transfuse blood components, because there are several features that increase the potential for problems. A small percentage of units of blood components contain some bacteria (see Chapter 14); the administration set is at room temperature, which can facilitate bacterial growth; and fibrin strands and blood cellular debris accumulate, providing an excellent milieu for bacterial growth. Therefore, the blood filter, intravenous tubing, and other special drip chambers, if used, should be discarded immediately after the blood component has been transfused. When giving consecutive units of blood or components, the filter and intravenous tubing should be discarded periodically. Although there is not a definitive number of units or amount of time that a filter can be used, a new filter and tubing are usually used after the transfusion of about two units of red cells or components. Another arbitrary limitation sometimes used is to change the filter sets after about 4 hours.

VENOUS ACCESS AND THE VENIPUNCTURE

Blood components are administered intravenously. Usually this involves a peripheral vein, but for patients in intensive care units or those receiving many intravenous fluids and blood components over a long period (e.g., marrow transplantation), central venous catheters may be used. When using peripheral veins, a vein should be selected that will be large enough to accommodate the needle but is comfortable for the patient. Veins in the antecubital fossa are most accessible and widely used. However, transfusion in these veins limits the patient's ability to flex the elbow during the transfusion. If only one or two units of components are to be given and the expected duration of transfusion is a

few hours, the antecubital fossa site is preferred. Veins in the forearm or hand are equally suitable, although venipuncture in these areas may be more difficult or painful for the patient. The veins tend to "roll" and the skin is tougher, sometimes making venipuncture more difficult. For venipuncture using peripheral veins, either steel needles or plastic catheters are used.

The venipuncture should be started before or at the time the blood component is being obtained from the blood bank so that the component can be transfused immediately after it arrives at the patient care unit, thus minimizing the chance of improper storage after leaving the blood bank.

The administration set should be cleared of air before the venipuncture. The venipuncture can be performed with a needle attached to a syringe or attached directly to the blood administration set. Red cells should be administered using a needle of 19 gauge or larger. Other blood components such as platelets, cryoprecipitate, fresh frozen plasma, and blood derivatives can be administered through smaller needles. Needles as small as 23 gauge thin wall can be used to administer red cells to small patients or adults with small veins. The disadvantage of these small needles for adult patients is the prolonged time required to complete the transfusion. Transfusion of red cells under pressure through these small-lumen needles can cause hemolysis,[17] and thus this cannot be used as a method of speeding the transfusion. The flow rate through small-lumen needles can be increased somewhat by diluting the red cells with saline. The transfusion of blood components through a central line that is being used to measure central venous pressure is not recommended. If blood or components are administered through this line, the manometer should be disconnected and the intravenous tubing cleared of the blood components prior to obtaining the central venous pressure reading.

INFUSION SOLUTIONS

The common use of additive solutions for red cell storage (see Chapter 5) has resulted in lower hematocrit and viscosity of red cell components, and there is less concern about slow flow than during the 1970s and 1980s. Thus, there is less need to add solutions to units of red cells to improve the flow characteristics. This need does sometimes still arise for exchange transfusion or other special transfusion situations. Sodium chloride injection (normal saline) is the solution most commonly used in the transfusion of blood components containing red cells, platelets, or leukocytes. Other solutions that are satisfactory are 5% normal serum albumin, plasma protein fraction, or ABO-compatible plasma. Certain calcium-free electrolyte solutions can be used; however, these do not have the advantages of plasma or albumin, but they cost more than saline and so their use is uncommon. Other solutions can cause hemolysis or red cell clumping and interfere with the success of the transfusion. In vivo hemolysis of red cells exposed to various intravenous solutions seems to be primarily dependent on the amount of red cell swelling that occurs in vitro.[18] Five percent dextrose in water is not satisfactory for filling or flushing blood administration sets, because red cell clumping and swelling with subsequent hemolysis may occur.[19] Lactated Ringer's solutions may cause clot formation because they contain calcium, which will recalcify the anticoagulated blood. Other

hypotonic sodium chloride solutions also cause red cell swelling and are not recommended. Great care must be taken to ensure that drugs that are toxic to blood components are not infused through the same administration set as the blood component.

Medications are never added directly to the blood component or infused simultaneously through the same intravenous line. The blood component must be clamped off and the intravenous line cleared with saline prior to administering intravenous medications.

IDENTIFICATION OF THE PATIENT AND BLOOD COMPONENT

Ensuring that the correct unit of blood component arrives at the patient care unit in good condition and is administered to the patient begins when the component is released from the blood bank. Blood components may be transported from the blood bank to the patient care unit either by a mechanical transport system or by personnel who hand carry the components. If a mechanical transport system is used, the technologist releasing the blood from the blood bank must ensure that the correct unit is being sent. This involves checking the request to determine that the component being released is what was ordered, reviewing the name, identification number, ABO and Rh type of the recipient and donor unit, the results of the compatibility test, and the appearance of the unit. If the component is to be transported by personnel, the same procedure is followed, but in addition the individual usually reviews the identity of the unit and the patient with the blood bank staff member who releases the unit. The blood bank staff member also records the name of the person to whom the component is being released. Each institution has specific policies defining the personnel authorized to receive blood components and transport them to the patient care unit. These should define their responsibilities for identifying the unit and describe proper handling techniques to ensure that the unit is not damaged during transport.

Before beginning the transfusion, it is extremely important to correctly identify the patient and the blood component, because this is the last opportunity to detect any clerical errors. This is one of the most common steps at which errors are made that result in fatal transfusion reactions.[1-3] It is ideal for two persons to carry out the steps involved in cross-checking the information. This is done by one person reading aloud the patient's name and identification number from either the patient identification bracelet or the compatibility tag on the component. The second person reads the information on the opposite tag or bracelet to determine that all information matches. This is also the stage at which the medical record is checked to confirm that the component about to be administered was actually ordered by the patient's physician.

STARTING THE TRANSFUSION

All supplies and equipment should be accumulated before initiating the transfusion. The patient should be asked whether there are any questions and the nurse should attempt to establish an atmosphere of rapport and assurance. The medical record should be checked to determine that the transfusion was ordered and that the correct component is being administered. Baseline vital signs (temperature, pulse, and blood pressure)

are obtained and recorded. If premedications were ordered, it should be determined that they have been administered and that ample time has elapsed for them to be effective.

Blood components, except platelets and thawed cryoprecipitate, should be stored in a regulated blood bank refrigerator until immediately before transfusion. Because there is an interval between the removal of the red cells from the refrigerator and the initiation of the transfusion, it is important to have policies and procedures to cover this period. Since it is impossible to monitor the temperature of the blood while it is outside the blood bank, it is customary for the blood bank to establish a time limit within which the blood may be out of the control of the blood bank and still be suitable for use. After 45 minutes' exposure to room temperature, the surface temperature of a unit of red cells reaches about 10°C, and after 60 minutes the core temperature is 10°C.[20] The length of time that red cells can be out of the blood bank refrigerator is established by each hospital but is usually between 30 and 60 minutes. Thus, if the transfusion cannot be started within 30 minutes after the blood arrives at the patient care unit, the blood should be returned to the blood bank for further storage. Blood components should not be placed in a refrigerator in the patient care area or near a window, since freezing and thawing or overheating from sunshine may cause red cell hemolysis.

Platelets are stored at room temperature, but this does not mean that they can be handled carelessly. During storage in the blood bank, the platelet concentrate undergoes continuous gentle agitation. If the platelets are left undisturbed for prolonged periods, the pH may rise and damage may occur. Also, the platelets must not be exposed to hot or cold temperatures, as might occur if they are left in the sunlight or near a cold window. Thus, the platelet transfusion should be started promptly. Similarly, fresh frozen plasma or cryoprecipitate should not be exposed to extreme cold or warm temperatures during the interval between leaving the blood bank and administration to the patient, as exposure to these temperatures may reduce their effectiveness.

RATE OF TRANSFUSION

The rate of transfusion depends on the clinical condition of the patient and the component being transfused. Most patients who are not in congestive heart failure or in danger of fluid overload tolerate the transfusion of one unit of red cells in 1 to 2 hours. To minimize the severity of a transfusion reaction or the amount of blood hemolyzed if this is going to occur, the first 25 to 50 mL of the component should be transfused slowly and the patient monitored. If no adverse reaction occurs, the rate can be increased. The transfusion should be completed in less than 4 hours because of the dangers of bacterial proliferation,[21,22] which may occur as the blood warms to room temperature.

WARMING OF BLOOD

It is not necessary to warm blood before transfusion for most patients. Very rapid transfusion of large amounts of cold blood does increase the incidence of cardiac arrest.[23] Therefore, it is recommended that blood be warmed in the following circumstances: (*a*) for massive transfusions or when the administration rate is greater than 50 mL/minute

for 30 minutes or more; (*b*) for exchange transfusion of a newborn; and (*c*) for patients with potent cold agglutinins. If blood must be warmed prior to transfusion, this should be done using a blood-warming device designed specifically for blood transfusion.[24] Blood can be warmed in a thermostatically controlled water bath, in a dry heat device with a warming plate, or in a heat exchanger with a hot water jacket. These devices usually maintain the temperature at approximately 35°C to 38°C, but always less than 42°C. They have a thermometer to monitor the temperature and sound an audible alarm if the temperature is reaching 42°C. Hemolysis may occur when blood is subjected to temperatures greater than 42°C. Blood should never be warmed by placing it near a radiator, heater, or stove. Microwave instruments have not been satisfactory for warming red cells because they cause focal overheating and red cell hemolysis.[25,26]

INFUSION PUMPS

Electromechanical pumps that precisely control the flow rate are valuable for the transfusion of neonates or of small children or adults. There are two basic types of infusion pumps. One uses a screw mechanism to advance the plunger on a syringe. This is suitable for transfusion of small volumes of blood to neonates or very small patients. The second type uses a peristaltic or roller pump to control blood flow through the tubing in the administration set. Some pumps of this latter type require a special tubing set. One consideration when using these pump devices is that if the lumen of the needle or catheter is small, the pressure caused by the pump can cause hemolysis.[17,27] Thus, the rate of flow being controlled by the pump must take into account the lumen size of the needle. Before using a particular device, it is important to determine that the manufacturer has established that the device can be used safely for control of blood transfusion. Nursing staff should be trained in the proper use of infusion pumps.

A separate method of providing pressure to speed the rate of transfusion is to place the blood container inside a pressure bag or pressure duff specifically designed for this purpose. The pressure bag is inflated, causing pressure against the blood container and increasing the flow out of the blood container. This is simple and effective but has the drawback of poor control of the exact amount of pressure being applied. Excessive pressure can cause rupture of the blood container or hemolysis if the lumen of the needle is inadequate for the amount of pressure being applied. If these devices are to be used, the blood should be transfused through a needle or catheter with a lumen of at least 18 gauge.

NURSING CARE OF PATIENTS RECEIVING A TRANSFUSION

Effective nursing care is important for patients receiving transfusions of all blood components, including platelets, plasma products, cryoprecipitate, and albumin, as well as red cells. The nurse can reduce the patient's anxiety by answering any remaining questions and establishing rapport with the patient. If premedication is to be given, this should be done and adequate time allowed for the medication to take effect. All sup-

plies and equipment should be accumulated so that starting the transfusion can begin efficiently, thus also adding reassurance to the patient. During the first 15 minutes, the rate of transfusion should be slow: approximately 2 mL/minute. This will minimize the volume transfused if the patient experiences an immediate reaction. The nurse should observe the patient during at least the first 5 minutes of the transfusion, then return after 15 minutes to ensure that the transfusion is proceeding uneventfully. If so, the rate of flow can be increased to that ordered by the physician. Baseline values for temperature, pulse, respirations, and blood pressures should be obtained before beginning the transfusion and should be determined every hour until 1 hour posttransfusion. At the completion of the transfusion, the nurse should record whether any adverse reaction occurred.

TRANSFUSION TECHNIQUES FOR CHILDREN AND NEONATES

The selection of components for and special transfusion needs of children and neonates are described in Chapter 12. Issues related to obtaining informed consent, obtaining the pretransfusion blood sample, identifying the patient and the component, delivering infusion solutions, starting the transfusion, and administering nursing care during the transfusion are similar to those described above for adults. However, because of their size, neonatal patients and small children require special attention to the methods of administering the transfusion. The volume of component being administered is usually small, and for neonates the red cells may be contained in a syringe rather than the usual plastic bag.

Transfusion in small patients is usually accomplished using scalp vein needles or catheters ranging in size from 22 to 27 gauge. Hemolysis can occur when red cells with a high hematocrit are forced by pressure through small-bore needles. The age of the stored red cells may also be a factor, as some studies show that red cells stored longer are more likely to hemolyze than fresher red cells. The difficulty is to determine the relationship among these factors. There is no exact limit that can be specified for each possible combination of needle size, flow rate, hematocrit, and blood storage time. Thus, it is advisable to use the largest size needle practical, to dilute the red cells to a hematocrit of about 60% if possible, and to administer the red cells slowly, usually less than 10 mL/hour. The older the red cells, the more important each of these factors becomes. The use of infusion pumps is described above.

A relatively large amount of blood in relation to the volume transfused may be used to fill the "dead space" of the tubing sets. Shorter tube sets are available to reduce this wastage. Also, a few smaller filters are available to reduce the amount of blood required to fill this space. One concern has been that microaggregates that form in stored blood might be a particular problem for neonates because they could pass into the systemic circulation via a patent foramen ovale or intrapulmonary shunting. This is not considered to be a problem, because neonates are usually transfused with blood that has not been stored for long periods and thus does not contain many microaggregates.

When a small volume of blood component is being transfused, this can be measured using a buret in the tubing set. Some sets are available that are designed specifi-

cally for neonates and contain a buret, a small-volume filter, and short tubing to minimize the volume of component necessary for the dead space.

Because the volume of blood being transfused to small patients is also small, it may seem as if warming the blood is unnecessary. However, the relationship of the volume being transfused to the patient's total blood volume and the rate of transfusion must be considered. Usually for replacement transfusion, the flow rates are not rapid and the blood need not be warmed because it approaches room temperature during the transfusion. However, even for small volumes of blood, warming may be necessary. Many of the standard blood warming devices have adapters or small inserts that reduce the volume necessary to fill the device.

TRANSFUSION IN THE NONHOSPITAL SETTING

Program Rationale

The increasing emphasis on health care cost reduction is shifting more health care into the nonhospital setting. As a part of this shift, more transfusions are provided in the outpatient setting.[28,29] Additional impetus for transfusion in the nonhospital setting is the growing population of elderly patients and those with chronic debilitating diseases. In many situations, the nonhospital setting is a major clinic that functions almost as part of the hospital. However, there are many other situations in which the possibility of providing out-of-hospital transfusions is considered. These include individual physicians' offices or clinics not part of a hospital, the patient's home, or a nursing or long-term care facility. This section deals with the provision of transfusions in a non-health care facility such as the patient's home where other experienced health care personnel, equipment, and care systems are not available. The blood for these out-of-hospital transfusion programs can be provided from either a hospital blood bank or a community blood center.

Administrative Issues

The development and implementation of an out-of-hospital transfusion program (OHTP) should be led by transfusion medicine and blood bank personnel and developed through the structure of the hospital medical staff and hospital administration. There are a number of technical, medical, legal, and administrative issues that must be addressed (Table 13.2). As all of these issues are reviewed by transfusion medicine and blood bank professionals, interaction should occur with appropriate hospital medical staff committees and administrative groups. A recommendation can then be made to these groups for formal approval of the OHTP and the provision of blood to the OHTP by the hospital blood bank or community blood center. As part of this decision-making and approval process, the legal risks and compliance with applicable state and local laws should be evaluated by the hospital or blood center's risk management personnel. At present there are no specific federal regulations of OHTPs, but all procedures are

Table 13.2 Issues for consideration in establishing an out-of-hospital transfusion program

Nature of the organization providing the program
Standard operating procedures to be used
Qualifications of staff
Staff training program
Patient and specimen identification systems
Mechanism for obtaining emergency assistance
Management of adverse reactions
Requirement (if any) for other people to be in attendance with the patient
Transportation systems and containers for components
Limits (if any) on the number and volume of components to be transfused
Use of transfusion equipment and devices such as filters, blood warmers, and infusion pumps
Follow-up information to be obtained
Nature of record systems

expected to conform with applicable sections of the Code of Federal Regulations. Some states such as New York have developed regulations for OHTPs.

A suggested minimum list of standard operating procedures (SOPs) is shown in Table 13.3. Once an OHTP is in place and operating, a system should be in place and individuals designated as responsible to monitor the OHTP to ensure that the program is operating as expected.

Table 13.3 Standard operating procedures for out-of-hospital transfusion programs

Selection of suitable patients
Patient identification
Indication for the transfusion of various components
Proper blood administration
Monitoring of the nursing staff
Blood administration techniques
Storage conditions
Use of infusion pumps or blood warmers
Posttransfusion follow-up
Disposal of blood components
Patient premedication
Emergency measures
Medications available
Basic nursing instructions
Ambulance availability
Physician availability
Management of transfusion reactions

Source: Snyder EL. Medical aspects of home blood transfusion: a view from the hospital. In: Friday JL, Kasprisin CA, Issitt LA, eds. Out of Hospital Transfusion Therapy. Bethesda, MD: American Association of Blood Banks, 1994.

Patients

Patients with hemophilia A have been receiving home therapy with coagulation factor concentrates for years. This has proven to be safe and extremely effective. Transfusion of other blood components such as red cells, platelets, or plasma carries additional risks, and therefore the OHTP is more complex. OHTP can be extremely helpful for chronically ill debilitated patients, especially those who are not ambulatory and would require automobile or ambulance transportation to the hospital to receive the transfusion. Patients should be evaluated by a physician and the decision for transfusion made as part of the physician's care of the patient. A written order for the transfusion must be provided according to the policies of the OHTP. OHTP may provide a convenient service for patients with end-stage malignancy; acquired immune deficiency syndrome; inflammatory, collagen vascular, neuromuscular, or other debilitating diseases; hemoglobinopathies; end-stage renal disease; myelodysplasia; chronic low-grade bleeding; or chronic hemolysis. Patients should be stable, not acutely ill, and with satisfactory cardiovascular and respiratory function and fluid balance. Many OHTPs require that patients have been transfused previously with a similar component in the hospital and have been free of adverse reaction following that transfusion.

Informed Consent

All transfusions involve risk, but out-of-hospital transfusions involve some additional risks because they do not occur in a health care facility. The patient must be informed that receiving a transfusion in a non-health care facility carries additional risks. The informed consent document should specify these risks and include all of the issues ordinarily covered in consent for blood transfusion that is obtained in the hospital setting (see Obtaining Consent for Transfusion, above).

Pretransfusion Compatibility Samples and Testing

Because such a large portion of transfusion fatalities are due to clerical errors or errors in patient or sample identification, these steps are extremely important parts of the pretransfusion testing process. The OHTP procedures must describe exactly how the patient will be identified and the personnel who will be authorized to collect blood samples for pretransfusion compatibility testing. The process of identifying the patient at the time of transfusion is discussed below. Some OHTPs use a unique patient identification system such as an arm band or other commercial system to identify the patient and connect the sample identification to that patient. In the hospital setting, it is often possible to require that two different individuals participate in different steps of the patient identification, but with OHTPs this is not practical. Thus, extra careful attention to these procedures is important. The blood samples must be labeled at the bedside at the time of collection. The samples also must be properly stored until they are returned to the laboratory for pretransfusion testing. This may involve having a cooler or some other container available if a long interval is projected before the samples are taken to the laboratory.

The pretransfusion compatibility testing methods themselves need not be any different for OHTP than for transfusion provided in the hospital. Because the transfusion is provided in a nonhospital setting where the management of adverse reactions is more difficult, some OHTPs prefer that the serologic testing be more extensive than usual. For instance, there may a request for a more sensitive antibody screening method or the use of a larger number of screening cells to minimize the likelihood of missing a clinically significant antibody to a low-frequency antigen. If the patient is new to the OHTP, two different blood samples may be required. One can be obtained when the patient is evaluated for transfusion and a decision is made to provide the transfusion, and the second obtained just before the unit to be transfused is obtained from the blood bank or blood center. This does involve two separate trips by OHTP staff to the patient's location, and this adds to the cost. Some OHTPs may be unwilling to transfuse patients who have red cell alloantibodies. However, if this is a well-documented alloantibody, the serologic studies are clear and the red cell compatibility test employs proper methods, there is no reason to refuse to provide OHTP for these patients.

Thus, in general, the serologic methods used in OHTP are no different from those used for hospital-based transfusions. Because of the special surroundings for out-of-hospital transfusions, extra attention is directed to patient and sample identification.

Transporting Components

The OHTP agency must have policies and procedures for the handling, preservation, and transportation of blood components from a hospital blood bank or community blood center to the site of the transfusion. Red cell components must be maintained between 1°C and 6°C and platelet concentrates between 20°C and 24°C. For transport of red cell components properly packed with ice, shipping containers are available that are suitable for maintenance of these temperature ranges. However, the OHTP must have data documenting that the containers meet these requirements and establishing the maximum length of time that the type of shipping container will maintain a satisfactory temperature range. Usually thawed fresh frozen plasma or cryoprecipitate is not transfused in the nonhospital setting, and so the issue that they are required to be stored between 1°C and 6°C does not arise. Often a portable insulated cooler such as those used to carry beverages to picnics can be packed with wet ice and can serve very well for transporting red cell components. Red cells should never be stored in the home refrigerator or freezer. These refrigerators are not designed to provide the proper temperature control and also may pose a risk of spreading transfusion-transmitted disease to members of the family.

Some transfusion episodes may involve administration of two units of red cells to the patient, and these can be released from the blood bank together and transported in the same container as long as the documentation of the container establishes its ability to maintain the proper temperature range for more than one unit. If the OHTP agency is obtaining blood for more than one patient at the same time, it might be desirable to place each patient's red cells in a separate small shipping container. If red cells for more than one patient are transported in the same shipping container, the OHTP agency's SOPs must clearly describe the methods used to ensure that the correct units of red cells

are removed from the shipping container for each patient. When the shipping container is packed and ready for release, this should be documented by blood bank or blood center personnel.

Transfusion Techniques

Generally, the maximum numbers of components that are transfused to a patient in one day are as follows: red cells, 2 units; pooled platelet concentrates, 10 units; single-donor apheresis platelet concentrates, 1 or 2 units; fresh frozen plasma, 3 units.[28] The total volume for each of these components would be 500 to 600 mL, thus minimizing the possibility of fluid overload. Patients who require larger volumes of transfusions are generally sufficiently ill that transfusion in the hospital is preferable.

The patient's physician should indicate as part of the order for the transfusion the rate at which the component should be administered. Ordinarily, for a unit of red cells this is approximately 2 hours. In the hospital, transfusions must be completed within 4 hours of the unit being removed from the controlled-temperature storage condition. This requirement also applies to out-of-hospital transfusions. If it is necessary to transfuse the unit extremely rapidly, this suggests that the patient is sufficiently ill that the procedure should be carried out in a hospital. Usually a standard blood administration set and filter are used. If units of red cells have not been leukocyte reduced at the time of preparation, a leukocyte reduction filter may be used to reduce the likelihood of a transfusion reaction. It should not usually be necessary to warm the blood, because this is done only when the rate of transfusion is very rapid. If such rapid transfusion is necessary, the transfusion should be carried out in the hospital setting. Blood should never be warmed in the home or nonhospital setting under warm tap water or in a microwave oven. It also should not be necessary to use a mechanical infusion pump, although this certainly can be done to control the rate if necessary. If an infusion pump is to be used, its safety and appropriateness for this purpose must be previously documented. The infusion solutions used before transfusion in the nonhospital setting should be the same as those used when transfusions are carried out in the hospital.

Nursing Care

The facility in which the transfusion will be given should be evaluated when the nurse arrives. This includes the availability of another responsible adult, telephones, access for emergency personnel, and even such things as road access to the home in case it is necessary to request an emergency vehicle.

The nursing care of patients receiving a transfusion outside the hospital is similar to that provided to patients in the hospital. Vital signs (temperature, pulse, and blood pressure) are obtained before starting the transfusion, after 15 minutes of transfusion, every hour until the transfusion is completed, and then once more about one hour after completion of the transfusion. Because the nurse is in constant attendance during the transfusion, patients receiving out-of-hospital transfusions are probably monitored more closely than many patients who receive transfusions in the hospital. Any unexplained clinically important deviations of the vital signs or the appearance of signs or symptoms

of a transfusion reaction should be managed as described in Chapter 14. The most important first steps are to stop the transfusion and maintain an open intravenous line while the patient is being evaluated. The SOPs of the OHTP must include specific instructions for the management of reactions in this setting. Because other hospital facilities are not available, usually the transfusion is discontinued and not restarted. In general, the management of these situations is much more cautious and conservative than would be the case in the hospital setting.

In an effort to avoid febrile nonhemolytic transfusion reactions that might prevent completion of the transfusion, leukocyte-reduced red cells are often used in the nonhospital setting when they might not be indicated in the hospital setting. Although this involves an increased cost for each unit, the overall reduction in costs by minimizing the likelihood of an unsuccessful transfusion may outweigh these extra costs for the leukocyte-reduced red cells.

Another approach to minimizing the possibility of febrile nonhemolytic transfusion reactions is the routine prophylactic premedication with diphenhydramine hydrochloride, and acetaminophen.

Posttransfusion Follow-up

There is sometimes disagreement among transfusion medicine physicians and patient care physicians regarding the amount of posttransfusion follow-up. In general, a hematocrit, platelet count, or coagulation test (depending on the component transfused) is done at some reasonable interval after a transfusion in the hospital setting. This is part of the overall quality assurance program to determine that the therapy has been effective and that the components have accomplished their intended objective. However, to obtain these laboratory studies in patients in a nonhospital setting requires an additional nursing visit with the attendant expense. Many patient care physicians prefer to monitor the patient clinically and obtain the follow-up laboratory work much later than would be the case in a hospital and when other procedures or blood samples are being obtained from the patient as part of the patient's general care. This issue should be debated when the OHTP is established and the policies determined at that time. One approach is to establish some maximum interval at which a follow-up blood sample will be obtained. This establishes that follow-up will be done but may provide more latitude to incorporate this follow-up into other patient care procedures and thus minimize the inconvenience to the patient and the cost of extra nursing visits.

Another unique issue in OHTP is the importance of educating those who will be with the patient about possible transfusion reactions that may occur after the nurse leaves.

Disposal of "Used" Components

An important issue is the safe disposal of used transfusion materials such as blood containers, IV tubing, needles, and blood-soaked gauze or bandages. Ideally, the nurse administering the transfusion collects all of these materials in suitable containers and returns them to the hospital for appropriate disposal. Alternatively, the OHTP agency

may have its own disposal system. If the program involves returning the used materials to the hospital blood bank, a system should be in place to document the return of this material and its proper disposal.

Quality Assurance

An effective quality assurance program is even more important for OHTP than for in-hospital transfusion, because the transfusion occurs outside of the hospital and problems may not be recognized due to the unavailability of medical personnel. The effective quality program begins with the usual important activities such as standard operating procedures, use of qualified staff, effective staff training, accurate and complete documentation and record keeping, a system to monitor the program, and a plan for handling unexpected adverse events.[29] It has been suggested that, at a minimum, the hospital or blood center should involve itself in the following: patient and sample identification, patient selection, indications for transfusion, handling of biohazardous waste, and transfusion reactions.[29]

REFERENCES

1. Sazama K. 355 reports of transfusion-associated deaths. Transfusion 1990;30:583.
2. Linden JV, Paul B, Dressler KP. A report of 104 transfusion errors in New York State. Transfusion 1992;32:601–606.
3. Baele PL, DeBruyere M, Deneys V, et al. Bedside transfusion errors. Vox Sang 1994;66:1117–1121.
4. Mercuriali F, Inghilleri G, Colotti MT, et al. Bedside transfusion errors: analysis of 2 years' use of a system to monitor and prevent transfusion errors. Vox Sang 1996;70:16–20.
5. Widmann FK. Informed consent for blood transfusion: brief historical survey and summary of a conference. Transfusion 1990;30:460
6. Sazama K. Practical issues in informed consent for transfusion. Am J Clin Pathol 1997;107:S72–S74.
7. Wenz B, Mercuriali M, AuBuchon JP. Practical methods to improve transfusion safety by using novel blood unit and patient identification systems. Am J Clin Pathol 1997;107:S12–S16.
8. Snyder EL, Bookbinder M. Role of microaggregate blood filtration in clinical medicine. Transfusion 1983;23:460–470.
9. Snyder EL. Clinical use of white cell-poor blood components. Transfusion 1989;29:568.
10. Class FHJ, Smeenk RJT, Schmidt R, et al. Alloimmunization against the MHC antigens after platelet transfusions is due to contaminating leukocytes in the platelet suspension. Exp Hematol 1981;9:84.
11. Eernisse JG, Brand A. Prevention of platelet refractoriness due to HLA antibodies by administration of leukocyte-poor blood components. Exp Hematol 1981;9:77.
12. Schiffer CA, Dutcher JP, Aisner J, et al. A randomized trial of leukocyte depleted platelet transfusion to modify alloimmunization in patients with leukemia. Blood 1980;56:182a. Abstract.
13. Sniecinski I, O'Donnell MR, Nowicki B, Hill LR. Prevention of refractoriness and HLA- alloimmunization using filtered blood products. Blood 1988;71:1402.
14. Gilbert GL, Hudson IL, Hayes JJ. Prevention of transfusion-acquired cytomegalovirus infection in infants by blood filtration to remove leukocytes. Lancet 1989;1:1228.
15. Murphy MF, Grint PCA, Hardiman AE, Lister TA, Waters AH. Use of leukocyte-poor blood components to prevent primary cytomegalovirus (CMV) infection in patients with acute leukemia. Br J Haematol 1988;70:253.
16. Bowden RA, Slichter SJ, Sayers M, et al. A comparison of filtered leukocyte-reduced and cytomegalovirus (CMV) seronegative blood products for the prevention of transfusion-associated CMV infection after marrow transplant. Blood 1995;86:3598–3603.

17. Wilcox GJ, Barnes A, Modanlou H. Does transfusion using a syringe infusion pump and small gauge needle cause hemolysis? Transfusion 1981;21:750–751.
18. DeCesare WR, Bove JR, Ebaugh FG Jr. The mechanism of the effect of iso- and hyperosmolar dextrose-saline solutions on in vivo survival of human erythrocytes. Transfusion 1964;4:237.
19. Ryden SE, Oberman HA. Compatibility of common intravenous solutions with CPD blood. Transfusion 1975;15:250.
20. Pick P, Fabijanic J. Temperature changes in donor blood under different storage conditions. Transfusion 1971;11:213–215.
21. Braude AI, Carey FJ, Siemienski J. Studies of bacterial transfusion reactions from refrigerated blood: the properties of cold growing bacteria. J Clin Invest 1955;34:311.
22. Braude AI. Transfusion reactions from contaminated blood: their recognition and treatment. N Engl J Med 1958;258:1289.
23. Boyan CP, Howland WS. Cardiac arrest and temperatures of bank blood. JAMA 1963;183:58–60.
24. Iserson KV, Huestis DW. Blood warming: current applications and techniques. Transfusion 1991;31:558–571.
25. McCullough J, Polesky HF, Nelson C, Hoff T. Iatrogenic hemolysis: a complication of blood warmed by a microwave device. Anesth Analg 1972;1:102–106.
26. Staples PJ, Griner PF. Extracorporeal hemolysis of blood in a microwave blood warmer. N Engl J Med 1971;285:317–319.
27. Burch KJ, Phelps SJ, Constance TD. Effect of an infusion device on the integrity of whole blood and packed red cells. Am J Hosp Pharm 1991;48:92–97.
28. Snyder EL. Medical aspects of home blood transfusion: a view from the hospital. In: Friday JL, Kasprisin CA, Issitt LA, eds. Out of Hospital Transfusion Therapy. Bethesda, MD: American Association of Blood Banks, 1994.
29. Evans CS. Out-of-hospital transfusion. Transfusion 1997;37:756–767.

FOURTEEN

COMPLICATIONS OF TRANSFUSION

Despite its lifesaving role, there are risks associated with blood transfusion. The complications of transfusion can be categorized as immunologic and nonimmunologic (Table 14.1). The immunologic complications involve various forms of what are usually thought of as transfusion reactions, but more recently there is an increased interest in the immunomodulation effects of transfusion. Nonimmunologic complications are usually caused by the physical effects of the blood component or the transmission of disease. Many of the complications of transfusion are caused by the leukocytes contained in the blood components (Table 14.2). This chapter considers all of these complications except transmission of disease, which is discussed in Chapter 15.

It is difficult to determine a single value for the overall risk from a transfusion. Adverse effects during or shortly after completion of the transfusion occur after about 1% to 3% of transfusions. The incidence of long-term or later adverse effects of transfusion are more variable because many of these are the result of disease transmission, the likelihood of which depends on the prevalence of the diseases in the donor population, the natural history of the patient's basic disease, and the extent of follow-up care the patient receives. It has been estimated that almost 20% of transfusions result in some kind of adverse effect, with about 0.5% of these considered serious.[1] Walker[1] estimated that the most common adverse event that accounted for about 10% of those described was alloimmunization to leukocytes or platelets, followed by cytomegalovirus seroconversion (7%) and alloimmunization to red cells (1%)[1] (Table 14.3). De Christopher and Anderson[2] also estimated that the most common adverse event is

Table 14.1 Complications of transfusion

Transfusion Reactions	
Red cell hemolysis	Antibodies in patient or donor
Febrile	White blood cells in component
Transfusion-related acute lung injury	White blood cells or cytokines in components
Allergic	Plasma proteins in components
Anaphylactic	Plasma proteins (IgA) in component
Disease Transmission	
Viral	Caused by contaminated component
Bacterial	Caused by contaminated component
Parasitic	Caused by contaminated component
Graft versus Host Disease	
	Caused by viable lymphocytes
Immunization or Immune Modulation	
White cells	Febrile reaction; platelet refractoriness
Platelets	Febrile reaction; platelet refractoriness
Red cells	Hemolytic reaction
Graft acceptance	Caused by white cells
Cancer recurrence	Caused by white cells
Postoperative infection	Caused by white cells
Other Adverse Effects	
Circulatory overload	Caused by whole blood
Citrate toxicity	Caused by citrate anticoagulant
Bleeding tendency	Massive transfusion
Electrolyte imbalance	May cause arrhythmia
Hemosiderosis	Caused by chronic transfusions
Embolism	Air or particles
Cord blood	May cause arrhythmia

alloimmunization to leukocyte or platelet antigens but that this occurs after about 1% of units (Table 14.3). These two sets of data are estimates not based on careful follow-up of a defined group of patients, but they are relatively consistent in most of their estimates. The short-term fatality rate following transfusion is about 1 to 1.2 per 100,000 patients who receive a transfusion.[3] This amounts to approximately 35 transfusion-related deaths per year in the United States not including deaths that occur years after the transfusion due to disease transmission. There are several scientific developments during the past few years that are opening exciting new ways of thinking about certain complications of transfusions. These are the role of biological response modifiers in hemolytic transfusion reactions, the role of cytokines in febrile nonhemolytic transfusion reactions, and the immunomodulatory effect of transfusion.

Table 14.2 Adverse effects of leukocytes in blood components

Immunologic Effects
Alloimmunization
Febrile nonhemolytic transfusion reactions
Refractoriness to platelet transfusion
Rejection of transplanted organs
Graft versus host disease
Transfusion-related acute lung injury
Immunomodulation
Increased bacterial infections
Increased recurrence of malignancy

Infectious Disease
Cytomegalovirus
HTLV-I
Epstein-Barr virus

IMMUNOLOGIC COMPLICATIONS OF TRANSFUSION RESULTING IN TRANSFUSION REACTIONS

Hemolytic Transfusion Reactions

A variety of settings can lead to red cell hemolysis in transfusion recipients[4,5] (Table 14.4). Many of these are not immunologic. The most dangerous immunologic complication of transfusion is an ABO-incompatible hemolytic transfusion reaction.[3,6,7] About 41% of transfusion fatalities reported to the U.S. Food and Drug Administration are caused by ABO-incompatible transfusions.[3] Approximately 16 patients per year die from fatal ABO-incompatible transfusions, giving an apparent incidence of 1 in 200,000 patients transfused.

ABO-incompatible hemolytic transfusion reactions are very dangerous because the patient has preformed ABO antibodies that often are IgM and bind complement, causing activation of the complement system with associated systemic manifestations and leading to red cell lysis. However, the nature and severity of the symptoms do not correlate with the severity or ultimate outcome of a hemolytic transfusion reaction.[7,8] Some patients may experience a severe reaction after only 20 mL of ABO-incompatible red cells, while others may tolerate an entire unit with no unusual signs or symptoms. The reaction may begin almost immediately upon beginning the transfusion or up to several hours after transfusion. The signs and symptoms that may accompany a hemolytic transfusion reaction include fever, chills, flushing, low back pain, hypotension, dyspnea, abdominal pain, vomiting, diarrhea, chest pain, and unexpected bleeding. In one study of 47 patients with hemolytic reactions, the most common signs and symptoms were fever with or without chills (40%), chest pain (12%), and hypotension (12%) (Table 14.5).[7]

Table 14.3 Estimated frequencies per units transfused* for adverse effects of blood transfusion

Adverse effect	De Christopher	Walker
Immune-Mediated Adverse Effects		
Acute hemolytic reaction		25,000
Death	500,000–800,000	NS†
Occurrence caused by ABO incompatibility	6,000–33,000	NS
Delayed hemolytic reaction		
Hemolytic reaction	4,000	2,500
Serologic reaction	183	NS
Febrile nonhemolytic transfusion reaction	200	200
Alloimmunization to WBC or platelets	100	10
Allergic transfusion reactions	333	1,000
Transfusion-related acute lung injury	5,000	10,000
Acute anaphylaxis	20,000–50,000	150,000
Posttransfusion purpura	Rare to very uncommon	Rare
Transfusion-associated GVHD	Unknown	Rare
Transfusion-induced immunosuppression	Unknown	Unknown
Red blood cell alloimmunization	NS	100
Cytomegalovirus seroconversion	NS	14
EBV seroconversion	NS	200
Non–Immune-Mediated Effects		
Circulatory overload	100–300	10,000
Transfusion-associated sepsis (bacteria)	435–12,500	Rare
Mechanically hemolyzed unit	Infrequent	NS
Thermally hemolyzed unit	Infrequent	NS
Cold-induced thrombopathy	Infrequent	NS
Osmotically hemolyzed unit	Infrequent	NS
Other storage lesions		
Electrolyte imbalance (K^+, Mg^{2+})	Uncommon	Unknown
Citrate toxicity	Uncommon	Unknown
Transfusion hemosiderosis	Uncommon	Unknown

Source: Data summarized from Walker RH. Special report: transfusion risks. Am J Clin Pathol 1987;88:374 and from De Christopher P, Anderson R. Risks of transfusion and organ and tissue transplantation. Pathology Patterns. Am J Clin Pathol 1997;107(Suppl 1):57.
*Estimates depend largely on the actual frequencies (which are variable in given studies), the detection rates, and the reporting of suspected cases.
†NS, not stated.

Most of the signs and symptoms of a hemolytic transfusion reaction have been thought to be caused by complement activation. Several activated components of the complement system, especially C3a and C5a, are vasoactive and cause the release of serotonin and histamine from mast cells, possibly accounting for the hypotension that often occurs. During the past few years, a new line of research has brought new concepts to the pathophysiology of red cell hemolysis.

In general, IgM red cell antibodies activate complement and IgG antibodies do not; the signs and symptoms of a hemolytic transfusion reaction to either type of antibody may be similar. The most common of these are fever, chills, hypotension, dyspnea, nau-

Table 14.4 Causes of red cell hemolysis associated with red cell transfusions

Red cell antibody in recipient
Red cell antibody in transfused plasma
Large volumes of aged red cells
Addition of drugs or intravenous solutions to donor unit
Bacterial contamination of red cell unit
Red cell enzyme deficiency in the donor
Excessive warming of donor unit
Erroneous freezing of donor unit
Trauma to red cells from extracorporeal instruments

Source: McCullough J. Transfusion medicine. In: Handin RI, Lux SE, Stossel TP, eds. Blood: Principles and practice of hematology. Philadelphia: J.B. Lippincott Company, 1995:1991.

sea, vomiting, and malaise.[7] For IgM-type antibody-antigen reactions, the pathophysiology may result from activation of complement.[9] However, this would not account for the symptoms in IgG-type hemolysis. As a unifying hypothesis, Davenport and associates[10] have proposed that several cytokines are important biological modifications in hemolytic transfusion reactions. In initial studies, they demonstrated increase in IL-1, IL-6, IL-8, and tumor necrosis factor (TNF) in an in vitro system of IgG-mediated hemolysis. IL-1 may be a key mediator since it causes fever, neutrophil and endothelial cell activation, and increased expression of IL-1 itself, IL-8, IL-6, TNF, complement, tissue factor, and plasminogen activator inhibitor.[10] TNF has a similar biological effect. Subsequent studies by this group have added more data to establish the role of IL-1 in hemolysis due to IgG antibodies.[11]

In a separate series of studies, Davenport and associates have shown that cytokines also play a key role in ABO-incompatible hemolysis. IL-8, which activates neutrophils,

Table 14.5 Signs and symptoms of a hemolytic transfusion reaction

Fever	47.5%
Fever and chills	40%
Chest pain	15%
Hypotension	15%
Nausea	5%
Flushing	5%
Dyspnea	5%
Hemoglobinuria	2.5%

Source: Pineda AA, Brzica SM, Taswell HF. Hemolytic transfusion reaction: recent experience in a large blood bank. Mayo Clin Proc 1978;53:378.

is increased in an in vitro ABO hemolysis assay,[12] as is TNF.[13] Thus, it appears that substantial cytokine production occurs in response to red cell incompatibility.[13] This could be somewhat like a final common pathway for both the IgM- and IgG-incompatible systems. Another common feature is that the cytokine production appears to be lacking if complement is inactivated. Thus, binding of complement to the red cell surface is probably a major factor in initiating cytokine production.

Coagulopathy is also often part of a hemolytic transfusion reaction, especially those due to IgM antibodies. The coagulation system may be activated in several ways: antigen-antibody complexes activate Hageman factor (XII), which in turn activates the coagulation system; red cell stroma contain thromboplastic substances that activate the coagulation system; activation of platelets releases platelet factor 3, which activates the coagulation system; hypotension leads to tissue hypoxia, causing release of tissue factors, which in turn activates the coagulation system. Thus, through one or more of these mechanisms, patients with a severe hemolytic transfusion reaction may develop a coagulopathy and/or disseminated intravascular coagulation. Recent studies have suggested an additional possibility. As studies of the role of cytokines in hemolytic transfusion reactions have continued, additional studies have investigated their potential role in coagulopathy. Procoagulant activity is induced in monocytes by endotoxin, TNF, and C3. In an in vitro assay of ABO incompatibility, procoagulant activity was generated and it was hypothesized that this could contribute to the disseminated intravascular coagulopathy that develops with ABO-incompatible hemolysis.[14]

Hemolytic transfusion reactions also may cause oliguria and renal failure. The exact cause of this is not known, but several mechanisms may be involved. These are (a) activated Hageman factor (XII) promotes the release of bradykinin, which causes vasoconstriction and hypotension; and (b) disseminated intravascular coagulopathy causes the formation of microthrombi. These events in combination cause a reduced renal blood flow and renal damage.

There is a classic pattern of alteration in laboratory tests in a hemolytic transfusion reaction (Figure 14.1). In any series of cases, the incidence of abnormalities in different tests cannot be easily related to this pattern because patients will be studied at different periods after the onset of hemolysis. Nevertheless, one study illustrates the kind of laboratory abnormalities seen in practice. Pineda et al.[7] found that in most patients who experienced an acute hemolytic transfusion reaction there was hemoglobinemia and/or hemoglobinuria, reduced serum haptoglobin, positive direct antiglobulin test, elevated bilirubin, and unexpected red cell antibody (Table 14.6). Thus, in general, laboratory testing should be quite helpful in diagnosing hemolysis, and the red cell serologic studies have a high likelihood of detecting the antibody involved.

Delayed Hemolytic Transfusion Reaction

A delayed hemolytic transfusion reaction occurs in a patient in whom no red cell antibody was detected at the time of compatibility testing but who experiences accelerated destruction of the transfused red cells after an interval during which an immune response to the transfused red cells occurs. The interval after transfusion may be as little as 24 hours or up to about 1 week. A delayed hemolytic transfusion reaction (DHTR)

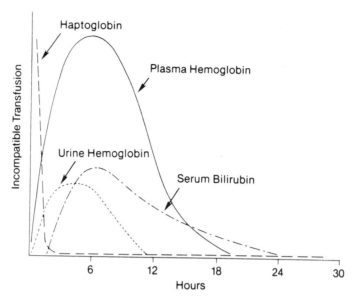

Figure 14.1 Time relationship of pigmentary changes in serum following hemolytic transfusion reaction (not to scale). *(Reproduced with permission from Complications of transfusion. In: Huestis DW, Bove JR, Case J, eds. Practical Blood Transfusion, 4th ed. Boston: Little, Brown and Company, 1988:251.)*

may be symptomatic or nonsymptomatic. When symptomatic, the most common symptom is a decrease in hemoglobin after transfusion,[15] and this is the way most DHTRs are identified. Other signs or symptoms of a hemolytic transfusion reaction such as fever, elevated bilirubin, or reduced urine output can occur, but these are not common. The DHTR can also be recognized by finding a red cell antibody in a subsequent blood specimen and initiating a serologic investigation that reveals a positive direct antiglobulin test and the red cell antibody in an eluate of the patient's red cells. This situation has been called a delayed serologic transfusion reaction (DSTR) to distinguish it from a situation in which there is a clinical effect of the process. A DHTR or DSTR occurs about once in 1,900 units transfused.[15] The DSTRs occur more frequently than DHTRs at a ratio of about 2 to 1.[15] A DHTR can create substantial clinical difficulties because the most common sign—falling hemoglobin—can imply many other important problems. For instance, a search for occult bleeding might be undertaken or the DHTR can appear as a sickle crisis,[16] cause renal failure,[17] or masquerade as autoimmune hemolytic anemia.[18]

Because of the time involved for antibody formation in primary immunization, DHTRs usually occur in patients who have previously been immunized to red cell antigens. Thus, DHTRs usually occur in women (immunized during a previous pregnancy) or previously transfused males. The antibodies involved are most commonly Rh such as E or c, but also Kell, Fy[a], Jk[a], and many others.[15] The sensitivity of the antibody screening test in the patient is very important in preventing DHTRs,[19] since an insensitive method will miss weak antibodies and allow a DHTR to occur. Thus, the best strategy for preventing a DHTR is use of an effective antibody screening method. Treatment

**Table 14.6 Laboratory test abnormalities
in patients experiencing a hemolytic
transfusion reaction**

Hemoglobinemia or hemoglobinuria	87%
Positive direct antiglobulin test	87%
Reduced haptoglobin	87%
Unexpected red cell antibody	85%
Elevated bilirubin	80%
Urine hemosiderin	49%
Methemalbumin	0%

Source: Pineda AA, Brzica SM, Taswell HF. Hemolytic transfusion reaction: recent experience in a large blood bank. Mayo Clin Proc 1978;53:378.

of a DHTR depends on the severity of the symptoms. A falling hemoglobin level can be managed by transfusion of red cells negative for the offending antigen. More severe symptoms of hemolysis are treated as for any hemolytic transfusion reaction even though they may be occurring several days after the transfusion.

Febrile Nonhemolytic Transfusion Reactions

Febrile nonhemolytic transfusion (FNHT) reactions occur in association with about 0.5 to 1.0% of transfusions. It has been believed that they are caused by leukocyte antibodies present in the patients that react with leukocytes present in the transfused components.[20,21] The severity of the reaction is directly related to the number of leukocytes in the blood component.[22] However, many patients who experience an FNHT reaction do not possess leukocyte antibodies, and the presence of a leukocyte antibody does not always predict a reaction.[23–26] Patients' sera may contain HLA antibodies or antibodies to granulocytes or platelets.[24,27] Thus, although leukocyte antibodies may play a key role in FNHT reactions, other factors are probably involved. Cytokines are good candidates for this (see below).

These leukocyte reactions do not cause red blood cell hemolysis but can be extremely uncomfortable for the patient and are potentially fatal. Symptoms such as chills, fever, headache, malaise, nausea, vomiting, and chest or back pain may persist for up to 8 hours[21,26] and seem to be caused by immune damage to donor granulocytes. Thus, it is not surprising that these febrile/leukocyte reactions can be prevented by removing leukocytes from the blood components.[21,23,24,26,28] This can be done in several different ways (see Chapter 11). Many FNHT reactions can also be prevented by the administration of antipyretics such as acetaminophen. However, the routine use of either leukocyte-depleted blood components or antipyretics after a first FNHT reaction is not recommended, because there is only a 12% likelihood that a patient will experience a reaction to the following transfusions.[28] Thus, the use of antipyretics or leukocyte-poor red cells should be reserved for patients who have experienced two or more reactions. The increasing use of leukocyte-depleted blood components for a variety of

conditions (see Chapters 11 and 12) is probably reducing the incidence of FNHT, and the clinical situation with these kinds of reactions can be expected to decline over the next few years as the trend to leukodepletion increases.

Allergic Reactions

Allergic reactions are probably the most frequent kind of reaction, occurring after 1% to 2% of transfusions. Allergic reactions involve hives only with no other symptoms. Allergic reactions are more likely to occur from red cells that have been stored longer.[29] As described below, cytokines accumulate in stored blood unless it is depleted of leukocytes, and so cytokines might be involved in allergic reactions. In addition, histamine levels increase during storage of red cell units containing leukocytes,[29] and plasma histamine levels were higher in patients experiencing anaphylactoid reactions compared with other types of reactions.[29] These data and those described below for reactions to platelet transfusions suggest that leukocytes in stored blood components produce cytokines and vasoactive substances that play a key role in transfusion reactions.

Allergic reactions are the only situation in which the patient can be given an antihistamine, and after 15 to 30 minutes the transfusion can be restarted. It may be that as more is learned about the role of cytokines in transfusion reactions, this practice will be discontinued.

Pulmonary Reactions—Transfusion-Related Acute Lung Injury

A very severe type of transfusion reaction is the acute, sometimes fatal, pulmonary reaction that has been termed transfusion-related acute lung injury (TRALI).[30–32] TRALI begins within 4 hours of initiating the transfusion and consists of fever, hypotension, tachypnea, and dyspnea, with diffuse pulmonary infiltrates on x-ray and the general clinical presentation of noncardiogenic pulmonary edema. It is not clear how commonly TRALI occurs. Although only about 25 cases have been reported,[30] TRALI has been estimated to occur once in 4,500 transfusions.[30,31] TRALI may be more common than this because of underreporting and failure to recognize more mild cases.[30,33]

Leukocyte antibodies have been thought to be the inciting cause of TRALI, as they are found in almost 90% of cases.[30] Many of the leukocyte antibodies have been HLA but some have been granulocyte-specific. Most TRALI type reactions seem to involve transfusion of leukocyte antibodies in the donor unit that react with the patient's leukocytes. This was first described in 1957, when Brittingham reported that transfusion of 50 mL of whole blood containing a leukoagglutinating antibody caused fever, vomiting, diarrhea, chills, dyspnea, tachycardia, hypotension, cyanosis, pulmonary infiltrates, and leukopenia.[21] Although the pathophysiology of these reactions is not completely understood, it has been thought that transfused leukocyte antibody may react with leukocytes activating complement, causing adherence of granulocytes to pulmonary endothelium with release of proteolytic enzymes and toxic oxygen metabolites, which cause further endothelial damage. However, leukocyte antibodies are not present in all cases of TRALI, and the variation in the type of antibody and its presence in either the

donor or recipient suggest that there are other factors involved. Because of the apparent central role of neutrophils, Ambruso and colleagues in Denver have investigated the possibility that other causes of neutrophil activation may be involved. Recently, they showed that at the time of TRALI, lipids with neutrophil priming activity increased.[33] They suggested that two events are necessary for TRALI to occur: first a phenomenon causing general adherence of neutrophils to pulmonary endothelium, then neutrophil activation leading to pulmonary endothelial damage. The initial adherence to endothelium is caused by the underlying disease process, and then the neutrophil-priming lipids in the transfused blood component cause activation and endothelial damage.[33] In some patients transfused leukocyte antibodies could also participate in this process. This is an intriguing potential explanation for the complexities of TRALI. At present there are no practical methods to prevent these reactions. It has been suggested that blood from multiparous donors should not be used to produce plasma-containing components, although this has not been put into practice. The prompt recognition and treatment of TRALI is essential.

Anaphylactic Reactions

Patients who are IgA deficient and have anti-IgA antibodies may experience an anaphylactic reaction if they receive blood components containing IgA.[34] These reactions may be dramatic and rapidly fatal. The treatment is the same as for any anaphylactic reaction. The reactions can be prevented by using red cells or platelet concentrates washed to remove plasma IgA and by using plasma components prepared from IgA-deficient donors. Although such donors are not readily available, most blood banks have access to blood components from IgA-deficient donors through rare donor registries. Many community blood centers have screened donors for IgA and have a small registry of local IgA-deficient donors.

Some anaphylactoid reactions may be related to cytokines.[29]

Reactions to Platelet Transfusions

Patients with platelet or HLA antibodies may have febrile nonhemolytic reactions, probably caused by leukocytes contained in the platelet concentrates. The reactions usually involve chills and fever, but platelets may be trapped in the pulmonary capillaries, causing dyspnea and pulmonary edema. These febrile nonhemolytic reactions occur following 5% to 30% of platelet transfusions.[35] The reactions have been thought to be caused by antibodies to leukocytes and have been considered similar to febrile nonhemolytic reactions from units of red cells. However, the reactions sometimes occur in nontransfused males and are more common when stored platelet are used.[35] Heddle et al.[35] believed that this suggested that some bioactive substance other than leukocyte antibodies might be involved. They separated platelet concentrates into the plasma and the platelets and transfused each portion. The plasma component was more likely than the platelets to cause a reaction. The reactions were correlated with the concentrations of IL-1 and IL-6 in the plasma, and the concentrations of these cytokines increased during storage of the platelets. Thus, this landmark study established that

many (if not most) reactions to platelet transfusion are the result of cytokines, not antigen-antibody reactions. These authors subsequently demonstrated that removal of the leukocytes soon after collection of the blood prevented the accumulation of cytokines in the platelet concentrate and avoided platelet transfusion reactions.[36] Removal of leukocytes at the time of transfusion does not decrease the incidence of platelet transfusion reactions.[37]

Allergic reactions may also occur with platelet transfusions. In one study, the IL-6 levels in platelet concentrates were correlated with allergic reactions,[38] suggesting that cytokines might be involved in allergic as well as febrile reactions.

Recently, hypotensive reactions to platelet transfusions have been reported.[39] It is not clear if these are a new form of reaction or have become more recognized. It is possible that they are the result of activation of bradykinin by leukoreduction filters and the bradykinin is not inactivated in patients taking angiotensin-converting enzyme inhibitors for hypertension.[40]

Reactions to Granulocyte Transfusions

Transfusion reactions are common following granulocyte transfusions.[41] In some series almost all transfusions were associated with fever and chills—some so severe that meperidine was used to control the rigors. Many of these reactions are probably caused by the physiologic activity of the large dose of leukocytes being administered to infected neutropenic patients. Some of the reactions are also probably attributable to leukocyte antibodies that form commonly in these patients (see below). Since granulocyte concentrates do not undergo a leukocyte crossmatch, leukocyte incompatibility may be present in many granulocyte transfusions. In the past, some reactions might have been caused by damaged cells, because the reactions were more common with the administration of granulocytes collected by filtration leukapheresis, a procedure known to damage the granulocytes (see Chapters 7 and 11).

SIGNS, SYMPTOMS, AND MANAGEMENT OF A TRANSFUSION REACTION

Signs and Symptoms of a Transfusion Reaction

The most common signs and symptoms are chills, fever, and urticaria. It is not possible to predict the cause or ultimate severity of a transfusion reaction from the presenting signs and symptoms. Therefore, all patients who exhibit signs or symptoms during or within several hours after transfusion should be managed initially as if a transfusion reaction were occurring. The monitoring and nursing care that should be provided to patients receiving a transfusion are described in Chapter 13. Because the signs and symptoms of different kinds of transfusion reactions vary widely, it is difficult to accurately define the type of reaction that is occurring. Nevertheless, it is necessary to manage the specific clinical problems present. Symptoms more likely to be associated with different kinds of transfusion reactions are presented in Table 14.7.

Table 14.7 Symptoms related to different transfusion reactions

Type of reaction	Associated symptoms
Acute hemolytic reaction	Restlessness
	Anxiety
	Severe chill
	Rapid temperature increase
	Headache
	Pleuritic pain
	Lumbar or thigh pain
	Hemoglobinuria
	Nausea
	Vomiting
	Pulse rate increase
	Blood pressure increase
	Oliguria
	Feeling of impending doom
Febrile (leukocyte) reaction	Chill
	Temperature increase greater than 1°C
	Nausea
	Muscle aching
Allergic reaction	Rash
	Hives
	Facial swelling
	Respiratory distress
Cardiac overload or acute respiratory distress syndrome	Sudden dyspnea
	Cyanosis
	Cough
	Frothy sputum
	Blood pressure increase
	Distended neck veins
	Central venous pressure increase

Initial Steps in the Management of a Transfusion Reaction

When a transfusion reaction is suspected, the steps listed in Table 14.8 should be taken. The transfusion should be stopped immediately to avoid transfusing additional blood. However, the needle should be left in the vein to maintain a route for administration of medications or fluids. If the patient goes into shock, it may be difficult and time consuming to restart another intravenous route. Infusion of normal saline should be begun through the intravenous line. Vital signs should be obtained, including temperature, pulse, respiratory rate, and blood pressure. A brief physical examination should be carried out, including auscultation of the lungs and heart, inspection of the skin for hives, and inspection of the patient for signs of abnormal bleeding. A new blood sample should be obtained for repeat red blood cell compatibility testing and inspection of the plasma for evidence of hemolysis. A urine sample should be obtained if the patient can void, and a chest x-ray should be performed if pulmonary symptoms are prominent. At

Table 14.8 Steps to take when a transfusion reaction occurs

1. Stop the transfusion immediately
2. Leave the needle in the vein and begin infusing normal saline
3. Obtain vital signs of temperature, pulse, respiratory rate, and blood pressure
4. Begin oxygen administration if pulmonary symptoms are prominent
5. Carry out a brief physical examination; auscultate the lungs and heart; inspect the skin for hives; inspect the patient for signs of abnormal bleeding
6. Obtain a new blood sample for repeat red blood cell compatibility testing and inspection of the plasma for evidence of hemolysis
7. Obtain a urine sample if the patient can void
8. Obtain a chest x-ray if pulmonary symptoms are prominent
9. Make a preliminary assessment of the situation
10. Begin definitive treatment based on initial assessment

this point it is possible to make a preliminary assessment of the situation to decide if more specific treatment is needed. If during the performance of these steps the patient's condition deteriorates, specific measures should be taken to deal with the problems.

Initial Treatment of a Transfusion Reaction

Respiratory problems may require epinephrine, nasal oxygen, and/or incubation. Hypotension should be treated with infusions of crystalloid. Red or pink plasma or serum suggesting hemolysis necessitates accurate monitoring of urine flow. If necessary, the patient should be catheterized. If there is evidence of oliguria, mannitol should be added to maintain urine volume at approximately 100 mL/hour. If the patient demonstrates only hives, he or she can be given diphenhydramine 50 mg intramuscularly and the transfusion restarted slowly after about 15 minutes.

IMMUNOLOGIC COMPLICATIONS OF TRANSFUSION RESULTING IN IMMUNE MODULATION

Immunization to Blood Group Antigens

As a result of exposure to blood, patients may form antibodies to red cells; lymphocyte, granulocyte, or platelet surface antigens; or plasma proteins. The likelihood of antibody formation depends on the immunogenicity of the antigen and the ability of the individual to mount an antibody response. Each kind of antibody can cause a particular clinical problem later if the patient requires subsequent transfusions or organ or tissue grafts, or becomes pregnant (Table 14.9).

Alloimmunization to red cells Walker[1] estimated that 1 in 100 patients becomes alloimmunized to red cell antigens; however, the source of data to support this estimate was not provided. In an active follow-up study of patients undergoing elective surgery, Redman et al.[42] found newly formed red cell antibodies in 8.3% of patients. The patients received an average of three units of red cells, and the antibodies developed within 2 to 24 weeks. Many antibodies were detected initially only with enzyme-treated

Table 14.9 Kinds of clinical problems caused by immunization after blood transfusion

Antibody target	Possible clinical problem
Red cells	Hemolytic reactions Difficulty locating compatible blood if transfusion needed Hemolytic disease of the newborn
Lymphocytes (HLA)	Febrile reaction Difficulty locating compatible organ if transplant needed Poor response to platelet transfusion
Granulocytes	Febrile reaction Acute pulmonary reaction Poor response to granulocyte transfusions Alloimmune neonatal neutropenia
Platelets	Poor response to platelet transfusions Alloimmune neonatal thrombocytopenia Posttransfusion purpura
Plasma proteins	Allergic reaction Anaphylactic reaction (IgA)

Source: McCullough J. Transfusion medicine. In: Handin RI, Lux SE, Stossel TP, eds. Blood: Principles and practice of hematology. Philadelphia: J.B. Lippincott Company, 1995:1993.

test red cells, but most became active in the antihuman globulin phase. Most (76%) of the antibodies had Rh specificity. The likelihood of developing an antibody was similar for males (8.2%) and females (8.6%).

Alloimmunization affecting platelet transfusion Alloimmunization to platelets or leukocytes that occurs during pregnancy or transfusion can cause a poor response to platelet transfusion (see Chapter 11). This is a very major problem in platelet transfusion and can be considered a complication of transfusion. Platelet refractoriness occurs in about 20% of multitransfused patients.[43] Strategies are being implemented to prevent the development of refractoriness. These include the use of single-donor platelets[44] and leukodepleted blood components,[45–51] and UV irradiation of the blood components.[43,52–55]

Alloimmunization following granulocyte transfusion The rate of alloimmunization from granulocyte transfusions or the leukocyte content of platelet or red cell transfusions ranges from 12% to 88%.[56] This may be manifested as either HLA or granulocyte-specific antibodies. These antibodies interfere with intravascular survival and tissue localization of transfused granulocytes and thus are clinically very significant[57] (see Chapter 11).

Transfusion-Associated Graft versus Host Disease

Transfusion-associated graft versus host disease (GVHD) is caused by viable lymphocytes contained in the blood components.[58-76] This is discussed extensively in Chapters 11 and 12. In patients who are severely immunocompromised, transfused lymphocytes proliferate, causing a syndrome characterized by fever, liver dysfunction, skin rash, diarrhea, and marrow hypoplasia. The syndrome begins less than 30 days following transfusions and is fatal in approximately 90% of patients.[77] The cellular mechanisms involved in transfusion-associated GVHD are assumed to be similar to those in GVHD due to allogeneic bone marrow.[77] Recently GVHD has been reported in immunocompetent patients. It appears that they develop GVHD after receiving blood from a donor who is homozygous for one of the recipient's HLA haplotypes, and thus the donor's leukocytes are not recognized as foreign and are not destroyed.[73,75,76] Transfusion-associated GVHD can be prevented by irradiating the blood components prior to transfusion (see Chapter 11). Proper control of the irradiation device is essential.

Alteration of Graft Survival

Blood transfusion has two opposite effects on allograft success depending on the particular allograft. In 1973, Opelz and Terasaki[78] demonstrated that transfusion to patients awaiting a kidney transplant resulted in a better outcome of transplantation than occurred in nontransfused patients. This enhancing effect of transfusion was also seen in living related transplants.[78,79] Thus, an immunologically beneficial effect of transfusion was demonstrated. This effect is no longer apparent today because of the improvements in kidney transplant management, but the biological principle has been established.

In contrast, transfusion has a detrimental effect on the outcome of marrow transplantation. The presence of HLA antibodies is associated with marrow graft rejection,[80] and pretransplant transfusions are associated with reduced patient and graft survival.[81,82] Thus, for marrow transplantation the biological effect is the opposite of that seen with kidney grafts. The mechanism in marrow transplants seems to be a rather straightforward alloimmunization that causes rejection of the transplanted material. However, the pathophysiological mechanism that provides the opposite effect for kidney grafts remains unknown. This demonstration of a reduced immune response may be relevant to the growing concerns that transfusion may render the recipient more susceptible to infection or recurrence of malignancy (see below).

Increased Susceptibility to Recurrence of Malignancy

In mice, transfusion of allogeneic blood before infusion of tumor cells accelerates tumor growth and promotes metastasis.[83] This effect can be reduced by the transfusion of blood depleted of leukocytes.[83] A follow-up study by the same group showed that this reduction in the tumor promotion effect of transfusion was not achieved if the leukocytes were removed from the blood after it had been stored.[84] Blajchman[85] has suggested that leukocyte products generated during storage can promote tumor growth and the effect is mediated by a cytokine. Other animal studies indicate that blood trans-

fusion can induce tolerance in a transplant setting and that this effect is not present if the leukocytes are removed. Based on animal studies, the proposed mechanisms of the immunomodulatory effect of blood transfusion include clonal deletion, active suppression, and host anergy.[85]

Vamvakis[86] summarized 60 different clinical studies of the effect of transfusion on cancer recurrence and found that 28 of these studies concluded that transfusion was associated with an increased likelihood of cancer recurrence. Rather than cite a few of the studies here, the reader is referred to Vamvakis'[86] summary for all 60 references. The crude data summary showed a significantly increased relative risk of recurrence for all cancers studied except breast cancer. However, Vamvakis concluded that the data did not establish whether the differences were due to a true transfusion effect or confounding variables. The three most recent studies reached different conclusions. Busch et al.[87] found that the relative rate of recurrence of colorectal cancer was about two times higher in patients receiving transfusions than in nontransfused patients. There were no differences between patients who received allogeneic blood and those who received autologous blood. Heiss et al.[88] also reported a deleterious effect of transfusion in colorectal cancer, but Houbiers[89] did not find an effect. Thus, we are currently in a situation in which there are studies showing conflicting results and no good way of developing a controlled randomized clinical trial.[90] As stated by Blumberg and Heal,[91] "Perhaps the strongest scientific evidence that the transfusion immunomodulation theory may be relevant to human cancer is that the majority of animal experimental studies demonstrate a deleterious effect of allogeneic transfusions on cancer growth or metastasis." If this effect of transfusion is real, the clinical impact will be substantial. Blumberg estimates that the number of excess cancer deaths annually in the United States could be about 16,000 per million units of blood transfused.[85] If this effect can be prevented by depleting the blood of leukocytes, this will be a simple way to prevent a major transfusion complication.

Increased Susceptibility to Infection

In addition to the possible role the immunomodulatory effect of blood transfusion has on cancer, blood transfusion may also influence infection. The posttransfusion immunomodulation might lead to an increased susceptibility to infection. Several studies have reported such an effect. Of the recently reported studies, three[90,92,93] showed an adverse effect of transfusion on postoperative infection, while others did not.[89,94] In another recent study of patients undergoing surgery for colorectal cancer, Vamvakis[95] found a 14% increased risk of postoperative infection when he used the confounding factors used in other studies but no increased risk when he adjusted for additional variables. He suggested that the effects reported by others might be the result of incomplete consideration of the variables that confound the situation.[95] Thus, as in the case of cancer recurrence, we are left with conflicting data from human studies but solid data from animal studies indicating that transfusion can cause an increase in postoperative infections, but little likelihood that a true controlled trial comparing transfusion with no transfusion can be done. It seems that the conclusions of Blumberg apply to infection

as well as to cancer recurrence. If the effect of transfusion on postoperative infection is real, this will have a substantial clinical impact. Blumberg estimates that for an infection rate of 15%, half of which is due to transfusion, an average of three units of blood per patient, and a mortality rate of 0.5% for postoperative infections, there would be 125 deaths per million units of blood transfused.[85] As with the effect on cancer recurrence, if the transfusion effect on infection is true and can be prevented by depleting the blood of leukocytes, this will be a very major step in improving blood safety.

NONIMMUNOLOGIC COMPLICATIONS OF BLOOD TRANSFUSION

Hypothermia

Red cells are stored in the refrigerator, and if the transfusion is begun very soon after the unit is removed from the refrigerator the patient will receive blood that is only slightly above 4°C. Transfusion of large volumes of cold blood is associated with cardiac arrhythmias and increased mortality.[96,97] Transfusion of cold blood does not cause a clinical problem if the transfusion is being administered over 1 hour or at a flow rate in an adult of about 5 mL per minute or less. This flow represents about 1% of the normal 5,000 mL per minute cardiac output, and the transfused cold blood is effectively mixed with the patient's body-temperature blood. If the transfusion is given rapidly, such as in massive transfusion or during cardiac surgery where blood may be transfused in large volumes near the coronary circulation, it is advisable to warm the blood[98] (also see Chapter 13).

Citrate Toxicity

Whole blood is collected into citrate anticoagulant and so one of the potential complications of transfusion is citrate toxicity. Citrate toxicity manifests itself as hypocalcemia with symptoms of muscle paresthesias, twitching, anxiety, and, in more severe situations, seizures and cardiac arrhythmia.[99,100] Citrate toxicity is discussed in considerable detail in relation to apheresis (Chapter 7) because of the continuous flow of citrate back to the donor during apheresis. Those studies have established that rates of citrate administration of 1 mg/kg/minute are well tolerated.[99,100] These rates are rarely encountered in the transfusion of red cell, plasma, or platelet concentrates. In the preparation of red cells, most of the plasma is removed and the cells are resuspended in additive preservative solutions. Thus, most of the citrate anticoagulant has been removed and travels with the plasma and platelet concentrate. However, it is rare for large volumes of those components to be transfused rapidly over a long period; thus the dose of citrate administered is not sufficient to cause citrate toxicity. Citrate toxicity is a greater concern in the transfusion of neonates, wherein even though the volume of blood administered is small, it may amount to a massive transfusion in relation to the patient's blood volume. Thus, it is customary to administer supplemental calcium during exchange transfusion.

Bleeding Tendency

Since red cells are almost pure red cells suspended in the additive preservative solution, red cell transfusion does not provide coagulation factor replacement. Transfusion of blood that does not contain coagulation factors theoretically might lead to a bleeding tendency due to depletion of coagulation factors. This occurs in massive transfusion[101] and usually involves a depletion of platelets[102,103] rather than bleeding due to depletion of coagulation factors (see Chapter 12). Unfortunately, there seems to be little relation between the degree of bleeding and the level of coagulation factors,[102,104] and routine coagulation tests may not be very helpful in elucidating the cause of the bleeding.[102,105] Many blood banks have predetermined schemes for replacement of coagulation factors or platelets after certain volumes of blood have been used, although some authors do not believe these schemes are clinically helpful.[103,106,107]

Electrolyte and Acid-Base Imbalance

Electrolyte imbalance was thought to be more of a potential problem than has developed in practice. Theoretical concerns are that the patient might develop elevated potassium or ammonia levels or acidosis because of the composition of the stored red cells (see Chapter 5). This complication would be most likely to occur during massive transfusion (see Chapter 12), but fluid replacement strategies and overall management techniques for these patients have almost eliminated this as a problem. Electrolyte imbalance is also a concern in the transfusion of very small patients such as neonates, in whom even small volumes of red cells constitute a massive transfusion (see Chapter 12). Modern techniques now make it possible to avoid this potential complication.

Circulatory Overload

When whole blood was commonly used, circulatory overload was not uncommon. With the conversion to red cells, the additional unnecessary plasma has been eliminated from most transfusions, and this has almost eliminated circulatory overload. Certainly some patients who have very compromised cardiac function, or those with massive blood loss or fluid shifts in whom it is difficult to maintain a proper blood volume, may experience this complication.

Iron Overload

Patients who receive chronic transfusion therapy may become overloaded with iron and develop iatrogenic hemochromatosis (see Chapter 12). Iron chelators, supertransfusion, and neocytes have been used, but this problem remains a serious potential complication.

Embolism

In the early days of transfusion therapy, emboli of rubber plugs (from the needles passing through the rubber stoppers of the glass bottles), pieces of intravenous tubing, and other particulate matter and air occurred. As the techniques of transfusion improved and

modern equipment was developed, these complications have almost disappeared. Occasionally a piece of a catheter may dislodge, but this is really a complication of the vascular access device being used. Air embolism is still a theoretical complication of blood cell separators used for apheresis (see Chapters 7 and 19), but this is a donor complication and is not considered a complication of transfusion. During the 1970s and 1980s, concern developed that the microaggregates that form in stored red cells might act as microemboli, and at one time these were thought to be involved in adult respiratory distress syndrome (ARDS).[108,109] Microaggregate filters were developed to prevent this problem. However, the relationship between microaggregates and ARDS was never clearly established, and microaggregate filters are not widely used today.[108] One reason for this is the trend to use leukodepleted components for patients in whom contaminating leukocytes are thought to pose a problem (see Chapter 11). This avoids the development of microaggregates if the leukocytes are removed soon after the blood is collected.

REFERENCES

1. Walker RH. Special report: transfusion risks. Am J Clin Pathol 1987;88:374.
2. De Christopher P, Anderson R. Risks of transfusion and organ and tissue transplantation. Pathology Patterns. Am J Clin Pathol 1997;107(Suppl 1):57.
3. Sazama K. 355 reports of transfusion-associated deaths. Transfusion 1990;30:583.
4. DeCesare WR, Bove JR, Ebaugh FG Jr. The mechanism of the effect of iso- and hyperosmolar dextrose-saline solutions on in vivo survival of human erythrocytes. Transfusion 1964;4:237.
5. Ryden SE, Oberman HA. Compatibility of common intravenous solutions with CPD blood. Transfusion 1975;15:250.
6. Linden JF, Tourault MA, Scribner CL. Decrease in frequency of transfusion fatalities. Transfusion 1997;37:243–244.
7. Pineda AA, Brzica SM, Taswell HF. Hemolytic transfusion reaction: recent experience in a large blood bank. Mayo Clin Proc 1978;53:378.
8. Honing CL, Bove JR. Transfusion-associated fatalities: review of Bureau of Biologics reports, 1976–1978. Transfusion 1980;20:653.
9. Goldfinger D. Acute hemolytic transfusion reactions—a fresh look at pathogenesis and considerations regarding therapy. Transfusion 1997;2:85–98.
10. Davenport RD, Burdick M, Moore SA, Kunkel SL. Cytokine production in IgG-mediated red cell incompatibility. Transfusion 1993;33:19–24.
11. Davenport RD, Burdick MD, Strieter RM, Kunkel SL. In vitro production of interleukin-1 receptor antagonist in IgG-mediated red cell incompatibility. Transfusion 1994;34:297–303.
12. Davenport RD, Strieter RM, Standiford TJ, Kunkel SL. Interleukin-8 production in red blood cell incompatibility. Blood 1990;76:2439–2442.
13. Davenport RD, Strieter RM, Kunkel SL. Red cell ABO incompatibility and production of tumour necrosis factor-alpha. Br J Haematol 1991;78:540–544.
14. Davenport RD, Polak TJ, Kunkel SL. White cell-associated procoagulant activity induced by ABO incompatibility. Transfusion 1994;34:943–949.
15. Vamvakis EC, Pineda AA, Reisner R, Santrach PJ, Moore SB. The differentiation of delayed hemolytic and delayed serologic transfusion reactions: incidence and predictors of hemolysis. Transfusion 1995;35:26–32.
16. Diamond WJ, Brown FL, Bitterman P, et al. Delayed hemolytic transfusion reaction presenting as sickle-cell crisis. Ann Intern Med 1980;93:231–233.
17. Meltz DJ, Bertles JF, David DS, de Ciutiis AC. Delayed hemolytic transfusion reaction with renal failure. Lancet 1971;1:1348–1349.

18. Croucher BE, Crookston MC, Crookston JH. Delayed haemolytic transfusion reactions simulating autoimmune haemolytic anemia. Vox Sang 1967;12:32–42.

19. Moore SB, Taswell HF, Pineda AA, Sonnenberg CL. Delayed hemolytic transfusion reactions—evidence of the need for an improved pretransfusion compatibility test. Am J Clin Pathol 1980;74:94–97.

20. McCullough J, Clay ME, Press C, Kline W. Granulocyte Serology: A clinical and laboratory guide. Chicago: ASPC Press, 1988:83–112.

21. Brittingham TE, Chaplin H. Febrile transfusion reactions caused by sensitivity to donor leukocytes and platelets. JAMA 1957;165:819.

22. Perkins HA, Payne R, Ferguson J, et al. Nonhemolytic febrile transfusion reactions: quantitative effects of blood components with emphasis on isoantigenic incompatibility of leukocytes. Vox Sang 1966;11:578.

23. Heinrich D, Mueller-Eckhard C, Stier W. The specificity of leukocyte and platelet alloantibodies in sera of patients with nonhemolytic transfusion reactions. Vox Sang 1973;25:442–456.

24. Thulstrup H. The influence of leukocyte and thrombocyte incompatibility on non-haemolytic transfusion reactions. II. A prospective study. Vox Sang 1971;21:434–442.

25. Kevy SV, Schmidt PJ, McGinnis MH, Workman WG. Febrile, nonhemolytic transfusion reactions and the limited role of leukoagglutinins in their etiology. Transfusion 1962;2:7–16.

26. de Rie MA, van der Plas-van Dalen CM, Engelfriet CP, von dem Borne AEGKr. The serology of febrile transfusion reactions. Vox Sang 1985;49:126–134.

27. Payne R, Rolfs MR. Further observations on leukoagglutinin transfusion reactions—with special reference to leukoagglutinin transfusion reactions in women. Am J Med 1960;29:449–458.

28. Menitove JE, McElligott MC, Aster RH. Febrile transfusion reaction: what blood component should be given next. Vox Sang 1982;42:318.

29. Frewin DB, Jonsson JR, Frewin CR, et al. Influence of blood storage time and plasma histamine levels on the pattern of transfusion reactions. Vox Sang 1989;56:243–246.

30. Popovsky MA, Chaplin HC, Moore SB. Transfusion-related acute lung injury: a neglected, serious complication of hemotherapy. Transfusion 1992;32:589.

31. Popovsky MA, Abel MD, Moore SB. Transfusion-related acute lung injury associated with passive transfer of antileukocyte antibodies. Am Rev Respir Dis 1983;128:185–189.

32. Popovsky MA, Moore SB. Diagnostic and pathogenetic considerations in transfusion-related acute lung injury. Transfusion 1985;25:573–577.

33. Silliman CC, Paterson AJ, Dickey WO, et al. The association of biologically active lipids with the development of transfusion-related acute lung injury: a retrospective study. Transfusion 1997;37:719–726.

34. Vyas GN, Holmdahl L, Perkins HA, Fudenberg HH. Serologic specificity of human anti-IgA and its significance in transfusion. Blood 1969;34:573.

35. Heddle NM, Klama L, Singer J, et al. The role of the plasma from platelet concentrates in transfusion reactions. N Engl J Med 1994;331:625–628.

36. Heddle NM, Blajchman MA. The leukodepletion of cellular blood products in the prevention of HLA-alloimmunization and refractoriness to allogeneic platelet transfusions. Blood 1995;85:603–606.

37. Goodnough LT, Riddell J, Lazarus H, et al. Prevalence of platelet transfusion reactions before and after implementation of leukocyte-depleted platelet concentrates by filtration. Vox Sang 1993;65:103–107.

38. Muylle L, Wouters E, Peetermans ME. Febrile reactions to platelet transfusion: the effect of increased interleukin 6 levels in concentrates prepared by the platelet-rich plasma method. Transfusion 1996;36:886–890.

39. Hume HA, Popovsky MA, Benson K, et al. Hypotensive reactions: a previously uncharacterized complication of platelet transfusion? Transfusion 1996;36:904–909.

40. Fried MR, Eastlund T, Christie B, Mullin GT, Key NS. Hypotensive reactions to white cell-reduced plasma in a patient undergoing angiotensin-converting enzyme inhibitor therapy. Transfusion 1996;36:900–903.

41. McCullough J. Leukapheresis and granulocyte transfusion. CRC Crit Rev Clin Lab Sci 1979;10:275.

42. Redman M, Regan F, Contreras M. A prospective study of the incidence of red cell allo-immunisation following transfusion. Vox Sang 1996;71:216–220.

43. TRAP Trial Study Group. A randomized trial evaluating leukocyte-reduction and UV-B irradiation of platelets to prevent alloimmune platelet refractoriness. N Engl J Med 1997 (in press).

44. Gmur J, von Felten A, Osterwalder B, et al. Delayed alloimmunization using random single donor platelet transfusions: a prospective study in thrombocytopenic patients with acute leukemia. Blood 1983;62:473.
45. Williamson LM, Wimperis JZ, Williamson P, et al. Bedside filtration of blood products in the prevention of HLA alloimmunization—a prospective randomized study. Blood 1994;83:3028–35.
46. Sintnicolaas K, van Marwijk Kooy M, van Prooijen HC, et al. Leukocyte depletion of random single-donor platelet transfusions does not prevent secondary human leukocyte antigen-alloimmunization and refractoriness: a randomized prospective study. Blood 1995;85:824–828.
47. Sniecinski I, O'Donnell MR, Nowicki B, Hill LR. Prevention of refractoriness and HLA-alloimmunization using filtered blood products. Blood 1988;71:1402–1407.
48. Novotny VMJ, van Doorn R, Witvliet MD, et al. Occurrence of allogeneic HLA and non-HLA antibodies after transfusion of prestorage filtered platelets and red blood cells: a prospective study. Blood 1995;85:1736–1741.
49. Andreu G, Dewailly J, Leberre C, et al. Prevention of HLA immunization with leukocyte-poor packed red cells and platelet concentrates obtained by filtration. Blood 1988;72:964–969.
50. Saarinen UM, Kekomaki R, Siimes MA, Myllyla G. Effective prophylaxis against platelet refractoriness in multitransfused patients by use of leukocyte-free blood components. Blood 1990;75:512–517.
51. van Marwijk Kooy M, van Prooijen HC, Moes M, et al. Use of leukocyte-depleted platelet concentrates for the prevention of refractoriness and primary HLA alloimmunization: a prospective, randomized trial. Blood 1991;77:201–205.
52. Deeg JH. Transfusions with a tan—prevention of allosensitization by ultraviolet irradiation. Transfusion 1989;29:450–455.
53. Capon SM, Sacher RA, Deeg JH. Effective ultraviolet irradiation of platelet concentrates in teflon bags. Transfusion 1990;30:678–681.
54. Kahn RA, Duffy BF, Rodey GG. Ultraviolet irradiation of platelet concentrate abrogates lymphocyte activation with affecting platelet function in vitro. Transfusion 1985;25:547–550.
55. Deeg HJ, Aprile J, Graham TC, Appelbaum FR, Storb R. Ultraviolet irradiation of blood prevents transfusion-induced sensitization and marrow graft rejection in dogs. Blood 1986;87:537–539.
56. Stroncek DF, Leonard K, Eiber G, Malech HL, Gallin JJ, Seitman SF. Alloimmunization after granulocyte transfusions. Transfusion 1996;36:1009–1015.
57. McCullough J, Clay M, Hurd D, Richards K, Ludvigsen C, Forstrom L. Effect of leukocyte antibodies and HLA matching on the intravascular recovery, survival and tissue localization of 111-indium granulocytes. Blood 1986;677:522–528.
58. Parkman R, Mosier D, Umansky I, et al. Graft-versus-host disease after intrauterine and exchange transfusions for hemolytic disease of the newborn. N Engl J Med 1974;290:359.
59. Bohm N, Kleine W, Enzel U. Graft-versus-host disease in two newborns after repeated blood transfusions because of Rhesus incompatibility. Beitr Pathol 1977;160:381.
60. Douglas SD, Fudenberg HH. Graft versus host reaction in Wiskott-Aldrich syndrome: antemortem diagnosis of human GVH in an immunologic deficiency disease. Vox Sang 1969;16:172.
61. Weiden PL, Zuckerman N, Hansen JA, et al. Fatal graft-versus-host disease in a patient with lymphoblastic leukemia following normal granulocyte transfusions. Blood 1981;57:328.
62. Siimes MA, Koskimies S. Chronic graft-versus-host disease after blood transfusions confirmed by incompatible HLA antigens in bone marrow. Lancet 1982;1:42.
63. Lowenthal RM, Menon C, Challis DR. Graft-versus-host disease in consecutive patients with acute myeloid leukemia treated with blood cells from normal donors. Aust NZ J Med J 1981;11:179.
64. Schmidmeier W, Feil W, Gebhart W, et al. Fatal graft-versus host reaction following granulocyte transfusions. Blut 1982;45:115.
65. Cohen D, Weinstein H, Mihm M, Yankee R. Nonfatal graft-versus-host disease occurring after transfusion with leukocytes and platelets obtained from normal donors. Blood 1979;53:1053.
66. von Fliedner V, Higby DJ, Kim U. Graft-versus-host reaction following blood transfusion. Am J Med 1982;72:951.
67. Woods WG, Lubin BH. Fatal graft versus host disease following a blood transfusion in a child with neuroblastoma. Pediatrics 1981;67:217.
68. Ford JM, Lucey JJ, Cullen MH, et al. Fatal graft-versus-host disease following transfusion of granulocytes from normal donors. Lancet 1976;2:1167.

69. Schwarzenberg L, Mathe G, Amiel JL, et al. Study of factors determining the usefulness and complications of leukocyte transfusions. Am J Med 1967;43:206.

70. Hathaway WE, Githens JH, Blackburn WR, et al. Aplastic anemia, histiocytosis and erythrodermia in immunologically deficient children: probable human runt disease. N Engl J Med 1965;271:953.

71. Park BH, Good RA, Gate J, et al. Fatal graft-versus-host reaction following transfusion of allogeneic blood and plasma in infants with combined immunodeficiency disease. Transplant Proc 1974;6:385.

72. Dinsmore RE, Straus DJ, Pollack MS, et al. Fatal graft-versus-host disease following blood transfusion in Hodgkin's disease documented by HLA typing. Blood 1980;55:831.

73. Thaler M, Shamiss A, Orgad S, et al. The role of blood from HLA-homozygous donors in fatal transfusion-associated graft-versus-host disease after open-heart surgery. N Engl J Med 1989;321:25.

74. Sheehan T, McLaren KM, Brettle R, Parker AC. Transfusion-induced graft-versus-host disease in pregnancy. Clin Lab Haematol 1987;9:205.

75. Arsura EL, Bertelle A, Minkowitz S, Cunningham JN, Crob D. Transfusion-associated graft-versus-host disease in a presumed immunocompetent patient. Arch Intern Med 1988;148:1941.

76. Otsuka S, Kunieda K, Hirose M, et al. Fatal erythroderma (suspected graft-versus-host disease) after cholecystectomy. Transfusion 1989;29:544–548.

77. Leitman SF, Holland PV. Irradiation of blood products: indications and guidelines. Transfusion 1985;25:293.

78. Opelz G, Sengar DPS, Mickey MR, et al. Effect of blood transfusions on subsequent kidney transplants. Transplant Proc 1973;5:253.

79. Opelz G, Terasaki PI. Improvement of kidney-graft survival with increased numbers of blood transfusions. N Engl J Med 1978;299:799.

80. Storb R, Prentice RL, Thomas ED. Marrow transplantation for treatment of aplastic anemia: an analysis of factors associated with graft rejection. N Engl J Med 1977;296:61.

81. Storb R, Thomas ED, Buckner CD, et al. Marrow transplantation in 30 "untransfused" patients with severe aplastic anemia. Ann Intern Med 1980;92:30.

82. Champlin RE, Horowitz MM, van Bekkum DW, et al. Graft failure following bone marrow transplantation for severe aplastic anemia: risk factors and treatment results. Blood 1989;73:606.

83. Blajchman MA, Bardossy L, Carmen R, Sastry A, Singal DP. Allogeneic blood transfusion-induced enhancement of tumor growth: two animal models showing amelioration by leukodepletion and passive transfer using spleen cells. Blood 1993;81:1880–1882.

84. Bordin JO, Bardossy L, Blajchman MA. Growth enhancement of established tumors by allogeneic blood transfusion in experimental animals and its amelioration by leukodepletion: the importance of the timing of the leukodepletion. Blood 1994;84:344–348.

85. Dzik S, Blajchman MA, Blumberg N, Kirkley SA, Heal JM, Wood K. Current research on the immunomodulatory effect of allogeneic blood transfusion. Vox Sang 1996;700:187–194.

86. Vamvakis EC. Perioperative blood transfusion and cancer recurrence: meta-analysis for explanation. Transfusion 1995;34:760–768.

87. Busch ORC, Hop WCJ, Hoynck van Papendrecht MAW, et al. Blood transfusions and prognosis in colorectal cancer. N Engl J Med 1993;328:1372–1376.

88. Heiss MM, Mempel W, Delanoff C, et al. Blood transfusion-modulated tumor recurrence: first results of a randomized study of autologous versus allogeneic blood transfusion in colorectal cancer surgery. J Clin Oncol 1994;12:1859–1867.

89. Houbiers JG, Brand A, van de Watering LM, et al. Randomised controlled trial comparing transfusion of leucocyte-depleted or buffy-coat-depleted blood in surgery for colorectal cancer. Lancet 1994;344:573–578.

90. Jensen LS, Andersen AJ, Christiansen PM, et al. Postoperative infection and natural killer cell function following blood transfusion in patients undergoing elective colorectal surgery. Br J Surg 1992;79:513–516.

91. Blumberg N, Heal JM. Immunomodulation by blood transfusion: an evolving scientific and clinical challenge. Am J Med 1996;101:299–308.

92. Heiss MM, Mempel W, Jauch KW, et al. Beneficial effect of autologous blood transfusion on infectious complications after colorectal cancer surgery. Lancet 1993;342:1328–1333.

93. Houbiers JG, van de Velde CJ, van de Watering LM, et al. Transfusion of red cells is associated with increased incidence of bacterial infection after colorectal surgery: a prospective study. Transfusion 1997;37:1226–1234.

94. Busch OR, Hop WC, Marquet RL, Jeekel J. Autologous blood and infections after colorectal surgery. Letter. Lancet 1994;343:668 (discussion, 668–669).

95. Vamvakis EC. Transfusion-associated cancer recurrence and postoperative infection: meta-analysis of randomized, controlled clinical trials. Transfusion 1996;36:175–186.

96. Boyan CP. Cold or warmed blood for massive transfusions. Ann Surg 1964;160:282–286.

97. Boyan CP, Howland WS. Cardiac arrest and temperature of bank blood. JAMA 1963;183:58–60.

98. Iserson KV, Huestis DW. Blood warming: current applications and techniques. Transfusion 1991;31:558–571.

99. Olson PR, Cox C, McCullough J. Laboratory and clinical effects on the infusion of ACD solution during plateletpheresis. Vox Sang 1977;33:79–87.

100. Szymanski IO. Ionized calcium during plateletpheresis. Transfusion 1978;18:701–708.

101. Faringer PD, Mullins RJ, Johnson RL, Trunkey DD. Blood component supplementation during massive transfusion of AS-1 red cells in trauma patients. J Trauma 1993;34:481–488.

102. Counts RB, Haisch C, Simon TL, Maxwell NG, Heimbach DM, Carrico CJ. Hemostasis in massively transfused trauma patients. Ann Surg 1979;190:91.

103. Mannucci PM, Federici AB, Sirchia G. Hemostasis testing during massive blood replacement: a study of 172 cases. Vox Sang 1982;42:113.

104. Martin D, Lucas C, Ledgerwood A, et al. Fresh-frozen plasma supplement to massive red blood cell transfusion. Ann Surg 1985;202:505.

105. Wilson RF, Dulchavsky SA, Soullier G, Beckman B. Problems with 20 or more blood transfusions in 24 hours. Am Surg 1987;53:410.

106. Reed RL, Ciavarella D, Heimbach, DM, et al. Prophylactic platelet administration during massive transfusion. Ann Surg 1986;203:40.

107. Martin DJ, Lucas CE, Ledgerwood AM, et al. Fresh frozen plasma supplement to massive red blood cell transfusion. Ann Surg 1985;202:505.

108. Snyder EL, Bookbinder M. Role of microaggregate blood filtration in clinical medicine. Transfusion 1983;23:460–470.

109. Wenz B. Microaggregate blood filtration and the febrile transfusion reaction: a comparative study. Transfusion 1983;23:95–98.

TRANSFUSION-TRANSMITTED DISEASES

During the past decade great interest and concern have developed about the safety of the nation's blood supply.[1] This has been driven primarily by the public's fear of AIDS. The result has been a great change in the nature of transfusion practice, in the regulation of blood banks, and in the organization and operation of blood collection organizations.[1,2]

There are several strategies that can be used to reduce the risks of transfusion (Table 15.1). These strategies are discussed more fully throughout this book. The use of blood can be reduced either by changing the indications or by using pharmacologic substitutes. The number of donor exposures can be reduced by new transfusion strategies. Very active research programs are under way to develop and implement blood substitutes or methods of inactivating viruses and bacteria in blood components.

In addition to these approaches, blood banks have implemented many changes to increase blood safety (Table 15.2). Major changes have been made in the selection of blood donors. Eligibility criteria have been changed to reflect the understanding of behavior that places potential donors at risk of transmitting disease. The number of donor screening questions has increased by about 30%, and the nature of the questions has changed to become quite specific. Laboratory testing of donated blood has also undergone extensive change. For most of the first 50 years of blood banking, blood underwent one or two tests (first for syphilis; later, also for hepatitis B antigen). With the introduction of the test for human immunodeficiency virus (HIV), six additional tests were implemented. The impact of this can be illustrated by test activity of the American Red Cross (ARC) Blood Service. During the last 5 years of the 1980s the ARC carried out about 95 million more transmissible disease tests than during the first half of the decade (Fig. 15.1). These steps have been extremely effective in reducing

Table 15.1 Strategies to reduce disease transmission

Improve donor selection
Improve transmissible disease testing
Reduce donor exposure
  Autologous blood
  Directed donors
  Limited-donor programs
Decrease blood use
  Change indications for transfusion
  Pharmacologic stimulation or substitution
Modify the blood component
Inactivate viruses and bacteria
Use blood substitutes

the risks of blood transfusion—today the blood supply is safer than ever (Table 15.3).[3–5] This chapter discusses the risks of transfusion and the approaches being taken to minimize those risks.

SYPHILIS

Transmission of syphilis by blood transfusion was common in the early days of blood transfusion, but now it is extremely rare. The treponeme survives in refrigerated blood for 48 to 96 hours.[6] Thus, syphilis can be transmitted from refrigerated components stored only a few days or from platelet concentrates stored at room temperature.[7,8] All blood donors are tested for syphilis; however, this is not a very effective method of preventing transfusion-transmitted syphilis in the United States. Serologic tests for syphilis are negative in 50% or more at the time of spirochetemia in persons with primary syphilis. In the mid 1980s it was recommended that syphilis testing be abandoned, but the test was retained as a surrogate marker for sexually transmitted diseases because of the possibility that this would identify donors at risk for transmitting HIV. This did not prove to be so,[8] but in the absence of laboratory data establishing that fresh blood components or those stored at room temperature are not infectious, the test requirement was retained.[8] With the present general concern regarding the safety of the blood supply, it is unlikely that the requirement for routine syphilis testing will be eliminated in the absence of good laboratory data to support the decision.

Table 15.2 Methods of reducing the infectivity of the blood supply

Recruitment health criteria
Medical history
Physical examination
Donor deferral registry
Laboratory tests
Donor callback
Confidential unit exclusion

Table 15.3 Estimates of transfusion-transmitted diseases in the United States. One case of each disease would be expected following the number of units of blood shown.

	Lackritz	Sloand	Williams	Total U.S. Cases*
Hepatitis C		3,300	103,000	117
Hepatitis B		50,000	63,000	190
HTLV-I/II		69,272	641,000	19
HIV	450,000–660,000	40,000–400,000	493,000	27
HBV and HCV			34,000	353

Source: Lackritz EM, Satten GA, Aberle-Grasse J, et al. Estimated risk of transmission of the human immunodeficiency virus by screened blood in the United States. NEJM 1995;333:1721–1725; Sloand EM, Pitt E, Klein HG. Safety of the blood supply. JAMA 1995;274:1368–1373; and Williams AE, Thomson RA, Schreiber GB, et al. Estimates of infectious disease risk factors in US blood donors. JAMA 1997;277:967–972.
*Calculated from Schreiber GB, Busch MP, Kleinman SH. The risk of transfusion-transmitted viral infections. N Engl J Med 1996; 334:1685–90.

HEPATITIS

Posttransfusion hepatitis is the most common disease transmitted by blood transfusion. Posttransfusion hepatitis can be caused by hepatitis A virus, hepatitis B virus, hepatitis C virus, cytomegalovirus, or Epstein-Barr virus or may be defined as non-A, non-B, non-C, which means hepatitis due to none of the agents listed above. Estimates of the frequency of posttransfusion hepatitis are complicated, because this depends on the blood donor population and when the studies were done. There was a substantial reduction in the incidence of posttransfusion hepatitis in the United States in the early 1970s because of the conversion from paid to volunteer donors; this also occurred in other countries such as Japan, where there was a decrease in posttransfusion hepatitis from 50.9% in 1963 and 1964 to 16.2% between 1968 and 1972.[9] Prospective studies involv-

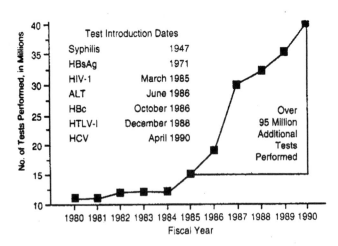

Figure 15.1 Number of transmissible-disease screening tests carried out by the American Red Cross Blood Service during the 1980s. Data represent activity for each fiscal year, beginning July 1, 1980.
Source: McCullough J. The nation's changing blood supply system. JAMA 1993;269:2239.

ing the period from 1974 to 1981 showed rates of posttransfusion hepatitis ranging from 5.9% to 21% of patients.[10] Some of these studies involved patients who received many units of blood, and most studies defined hepatitis as abnormal liver functions without regard to clinical signs or symptoms.

Posttransfusion hepatitis is a major health problem. Based on the estimated number of persons transfused in the United States annually and the proportion of those who survive the illness that necessitated the transfusion, it is estimated that 120,000 cases of posttransfusion hepatitis occur annually.[11]

Hepatitis A

Hepatitis A usually has a short period of viremia that occurs for about 7 days before the onset of acute symptoms. Although about 10% of patients may have a relapsing course for up to 1 year, hepatitis A generally does not involve a carrier state, and thus there is no chronic viremia. Although posttransfusion hepatitis A is rare, it can occur if a donor is unaware of the hepatitis A exposure and donates blood during the few days of viremia before symptoms develop.[12,13] However, because of the absence of hepatitis A antibody at the time of viremia, the lack of a practical test for the hepatitis A virus itself, and the rarity of posttransfusion hepatitis A, laboratory testing of blood donors for hepatitis A is not done. Thus, in evaluating a patient with suspected posttransfusion hepatitis, hepatitis A should be considered but as a very remote possibility.

Hepatitis B

Hepatitis B transmission requires that the virus penetrate the skin and enter the recipient's tissues. Thus, it is transmitted primarily by the parenteral route. Until a few years ago, blood transfusion was an important method of spread of hepatitis B and hepatitis B was a major complication of transfusion. This is also a result of the biology of hepatitis B virus infection. The most common response to infection with the hepatitis B virus is asymptomatic (Fig. 15.2). If the individual does develop symptoms, viremia and HBsAg positivity occur 2 to 6 weeks before the onset of symptoms; thus, an infectious

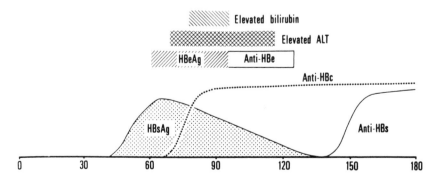

Figure 15.2 Serologic and biochemical events in acute hepatitis B.
Source: Dodd RY. Hepatitis. In: Petz LD, Swisher SN, Kleiman S, et al (eds). Clinical Practice of Transfusion Medicine. 3rd ed. 1996; 847–873 (Fig. 38-1).

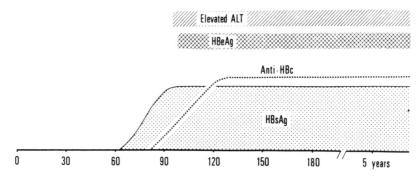

Figure 15.3 Serologic and biochemical events in chronic hepatitis B/HBsAG carrier state.
Source: Dodd RY. Hepatitis. In: Petz LD, Swisher SN, Kleinman S, et al (eds). Clinical Practice of Transfusion Medicine. 3rd ed. 1996; 847–873 (Fig. 38-2).

but apparently healthy individual may meet all of the donor medical history and laboratory testing criteria and donate a unit of infectious blood. Individuals who develop symptomatic hepatitis B virus infection would be screened out from subsequent blood donations on the basis of their medical history. About 90% of acute hepatitis B virus infections clinically resolve, the virus disappears, and the individual becomes HBsAg negative. Antibody to the hepatitis B virus (anti-HBs) develops in almost all (80% to 90%) of these individuals. However, in about 10% of patients, chronic hepatitis B virus infection develops, the virus persists, and the individual remains HBsAg positive (Fig. 15.3). If any of these individuals have experienced a subclinical (asymptomatic) initial infection, they would pass the medical history, but their blood should be found to be infectious by the HBsAg testing done prior to the release of blood for transfusion.

In the past, hepatitis B was an important complication of blood transfusion.[14,15] The adoption of routine screening of blood donors for hepatitis B surface antigen reduced the incidence of posttransfusion hepatitis B. However, data defining the extent of this reduction in the United States are not available because studies were not done throughout the introduction of routine hepatitis B testing and because the donor population has also changed. In Japan, the introduction of increasingly sophisticated screening tests for hepatitis B has reduced the incidence of posttransfusion hepatitis B from 8.3% to less than 0.01%.[9] Recently, in the United States hepatitis B has represented only approximately 10% of all posttransfusion hepatitis. The reasons for this continued small number of cases of posttransfusion hepatitis B are not well understood. In 1987, routine screening of blood donors' antibody to the hepatitis B core antigen (anti-HBc) was introduced in an effort to reduce the transmission of non-A, non-B hepatitis. However, an additional benefit of this screening is the possible further reduction or virtual elimination of the remaining cases of transfusion-transmitted hepatitis B.[16–18]

Non-A, Non-B Hepatitis and Surrogate Testing

Non-A, non-B hepatitis has been a diagnosis of exclusion, referring to hepatitis not caused by the agents described above. The disease does have some general characteris-

tics, however. There are two forms: one is similar to hepatitis A in that it has an epidemic person-to-person spread, while the second form resembles hepatitis B in that it is sporadic and usually related to parenteral exposure.

There has been considerable debate as to whether non-A, non-B hepatitis has a major long-term health impact. Of patients with posttransfusion hepatitis, 50% to 70% had liver function abnormalities for 1 to 3 years.[11,19] Of those who underwent liver biopsy, 90% had either chronic active or chronic persistent hepatitis or cirrhosis. It now appears that non-A, non-B hepatitis leads to cirrhosis or chronic hepatitis.

In 1986, blood banks in the United States instituted routine testing of donors for alanine aminotransferase (ALT) and hepatitis B core antibody (HBc) as a way of reducing posttransfusion non-A, non-B hepatitis. The use of these tests—which are not specific for non-A, non-B hepatitis—has been controversial. In 1981, data from the transfusion-transmitted virus study showed that there was an association between elevated ALT and posttransfusion non-A, non-B hepatitis[15] and that excluding blood with an elevated ALT level would reduce posttransfusion non-A, non-B hepatitis by 30%. A similar study at the National Institutes of Health gave a similar result.[20] However, neither study was randomized and blood with elevated ALT was not excluded from use; thus, the effect on reduction in posttransfusion non-A, non-B hepatitis was a calculated projection, not an actual observation. ALT as a screening test for blood donors is helpful in only a general way, because eliminating blood with an elevated ALT level would not eliminate about 70% of posttransfusion hepatitis; also, about 70% of donors with elevated ALT are not implicated in posttransfusion hepatitis.

Later the transfusion-transmitted virus study data were analyzed to determine whether there was also an association between anti-HBc and posttransfusion non-A, non-B hepatitis.[16] This and National Institutes of Health data[20] showed that posttransfusion non-A, non-B hepatitis was more than twice as frequent in recipients of anti-HBc–positive blood compared with anti-HBc–negative blood. It was projected that eliminating blood that was anti-HBc positive would eliminate about 40% of posttransfusion hepatitis. The ALT and anti-HBc tests have very little overlap in the individuals who are positive and so seem to identify two different groups of potentially infectious donors.

One study prospectively analyzed the effect of ALT and anti-HBc testing of donated blood in reducing posttransfusion hepatitis.[21] In Canada, surrogate testing was not implemented. This provided an opportunity to evaluate the testing. From 1988 to 1992, 4,588 patients who received allogeneic blood were enrolled in a study in which they received blood from which units that tested positive for either surrogate marker (ALT or anti-HBc) were either withheld or not withheld. Withholding blood that tested positive for one or both markers decreased posttransfusion hepatitis by 40%.[21] Since this study took place during the time that hepatitis C virus (HCV) testing was implemented, it was possible to determine the effect of surrogate testing on hepatitis C as well as on non-A, non-B, non-C hepatitis. Most of the benefit of surrogate testing was in the reduction of hepatitis C before testing for anti-HCV was introduced. After the introduction of anti-HCV testing, the difference in posttransfusion hepatitis between the two groups of patients was not significant.[21] The availability of the anti-HCV test has eliminated the effectiveness of the ALT testing, and a recent consensus conference

sponsored by the National Institutes of Health (NIH) concluded that ALT testing is not useful in reducing posttransfusion hepatitis.[8] Its use has been discontinued by most, if not all, blood banks. Anti-HBc testing of donated blood is continuing, however, because of the possibility that it might detect a few donors who are infectious for hepatitis B but have a negative HBsAg test.[8]

Hepatitis C

In 1989, an RNA virus similar in classification to a togavirus[22] was identified and termed hepatitis C because it appears to account for most posttransfusion non-A, non-B hepatitis.[23] Anti-HCV was found in six of seven human sera that caused non-A, non-B hepatitis in chimpanzees and in donor units from nine of ten patients with posttransfusion non-A, non-B hepatitis.[22] About 80% of patients with posttransfusion non-A, non-B hepatitis in Italy and Japan and 15 of 15 patients in the United States[22] had anti-HCV.[23] The identification of the virus has made it possible to determine the long-range effect of this disease. Acute hepatitis C is usually mild, with up to 80% of patients being asymptomatic.[24] However, the long-term effects are more serious, because the virus tends to be persistent and develop into chronic liver disease.[24,25] Many patients cope with the chronic liver disease quite well,[26] while a few have a more rapid course.[24]

Anti-HCV has been found in 0.68% of French[27] and 0.87% of Italian blood donors[28] and a similar proportion of donors in the United States. A donor screening test for anti-HCV was introduced in 1992. Most donors who are anti-HCV positive have chronic hepatitis C regardless of their ALT levels[29,30] Anti-HCV–positive donors are more likely to be male, to be older, to have less than a high school education, to be of black race or Hispanic ethnicity, to be a first-time blood donor, and to have been the recipient of a transfusion.[31]

The impact of testing donors for anti-HCV is enormous.[32] It is estimated that the first-generation test prevented about 40,000 cases of posttransfusion hepatitis per year in the United States, and the newer version of the test, an additional 10,000 to 13,000.[24] The availability of a specific test for hepatitis C has had an effect on surrogate testing for non-A, non-B hepatitis. About half of individuals with antibodies to hepatitis C virus are also anti-HBc positive and 33% have an elevated ALT. Thus, now that the long-awaited screening test for the non-A, non-B (hepatitis C) virus is available, it is possible to discontinue ALT and anti-HBc testing—although anti-HBc is being retained because it might detect a few donors infectious for hepatitis B.[8]

Hepatitis G

Despite the discovery of the hepatitis C virus and the implementation of screening of donated blood for this virus, some patients with posttransfusion hepatitis test negative for the known hepatitis viruses.[33,34] This led to studies identifying a new RNA virus in the plasma of some of these patients. The virus has been termed hepatitis G. There is a rather high rate of hepatitis G carriers (detected using polymerase chain reaction techniques) in the normal donor population, with rates ranging from 1% to 4%.[34] Hepatitis G RNA is found in some but not all patients with posttransfusion hepatitis who test negative for other hepatitis viruses, and it is clear that the virus is transmitted by transfusion.[33,35] It is

not clear whether the hepatitis G virus can be found in hepatocytes or whether it replicates in the liver.[34] Since hepatitis G does not seem to complicate coexisting hepatitis B or C or make liver disease worse, there is some question about the role of this virus in liver disease. It has even been suggested that the designation "hepatitis" virus was premature, and definition of the biological effect of this virus must await further molecular and epidemiologic studies. At present there is no plan to screen blood donors for the virus. There is no practical test and no established role in disease transmission.

HIV INFECTION AND AIDS

Acquired immune deficiency syndrome (AIDS) first came to the attention of the medical community and the public in 1981 as an unusual fatal wasting disease of unknown etiology. In the United States, the disease appeared to be limited to sexually active male homosexuals, injecting drug users, migrants from Haiti, and hemophiliacs exposed to clotting factor concentrates. It soon became apparent that the disease had the characteristics of a blood-borne viral disease, and speculation arose that it could be transmitted by blood transfusion. The possibility of transfusion-transmitted AIDS was strengthened in 1982 with the report of hemophiliacs with *Pneumocystis carinii* pneumonia and an apparently new syndrome similar to that occurring in homosexual men.[36] Later that year the occurrence of the syndrome in a child who had received a transfusion from a donor who later developed AIDS[37] further linked transfusion to AIDS. First epidemiologic evidence,[38] then more clear and extensive clinical and laboratory evidence established that AIDS is caused by the HIV-1 retrovirus and can be transmitted by blood transfusion. A number of studies have shown that HIV-1 infection can be transmitted by blood transfusion.[38–43] With the identification of HIV as the causative agent, it is now believed that worldwide as many as 18 million people have been infected with the virus,[44] although a very small proportion of these individuals have been infected through blood transfusion.

Because HIV was almost entirely limited to the risk groups described above in the United States, it was possible to substantially reduce the infectivity of the blood supply through donor education and selective questioning to defer members of these risk groups. In 1983, blood banks altered their medical screening practices to defer potential donors from AIDS risk groups such as sexually active homosexual males and Haitian immigrants. Another AIDS high-risk group, intravenous drug abusers, were already not acceptable donors. These steps were extremely effective in reducing the infectivity of the blood supply. For instance, in the San Francisco Bay area, the changes in donor eligibility criteria reduced the infectivity of blood by about 90% before the introduction of the laboratory test for the HIV virus (Fig. 15.4).[45]

In late 1984 the HIV-1 virus was shown to be the cause of AIDS, and in May 1985 routine testing of all donated blood for anti-HIV-1 was begun. With the introduction of screening of blood for HIV, transfusion transmission of the disease has been almost eliminated. Although there has been great concern about transfusion-transmitted HIV, transfusion accounts for less than 2% of all AIDS cases in the United States.[44] Only about 35 cases of transfusion-transmitted HIV have been identified after the implementation of screening in 1985.[44]

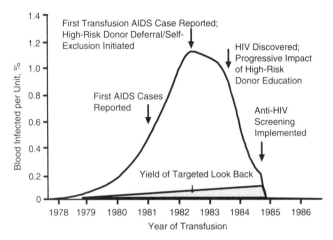

Figure 15.4 Impact of different donor screening procedures on the estimated infectivity of blood by the human immunodeficiency virus (HIV) in San Francisco, CA. Yield of targeted look back refers to detection of HIV cases by identifying recipients of previous blood donations from donors newly found to test positive for HIV. AIDS indicates acquired immunodeficiency syndrome. (Adapted with permission from Transfusion 1991;31:655–661.) Busch MP, Young MJ, Samson SJ, et al. Risk of human immunodeficiency virus (HIV) transmission by blood transfusions before the implementation of HIV-1 antibody screening. Transfusion 1991;31:4.

HIV-1 is a retrovirus and the proviral DNA is integrated into the host DNA, thus conferring permanent infection. Development of antibodies does not result in eradication of the virus but does signify previous infection and probable present infectivity. Although rare exceptions have been reported,[46,47] once present, anti-HIV persists until the individual becomes symptomatic. The specific practices used by blood banks in the medical history and laboratory testing of donors are described in Chapters 4 and 8. Thus, the test for HIV-1 antibody is used to detect infectious donated blood.

HIV-1 Antibody Tests

The HIV-1 antibody test is an excellent test. The specificity of a test is the probability that the test will be negative when the infection is not present. In a study of more than 67,000 blood donors in Atlanta, the HIV-1 antibody test had a test specificity of 99.82%.[48] In a separate study,[49] 630,190 units of blood from an estimated 290,110 donors were tested for HIV-1 antibody. No false-positive results were obtained, and with a 95% confidence interval, no more than four false-positive tests would have been expected in this low-risk population of Minnesota blood donors. In this study, the estimated test specificity was 99.9994%. In widespread clinical use the HIV antibody test has generally been shown to detect HIV antibody in 98% to 100% of AIDS patients and to give a negative test result in approximately 99.8% of individuals who have not been infected with HIV. Although the specificity and sensitivity of the HIV antibody tests is excellent, the predictive value of a positive HIV antibody test in blood donors is low because of the low prevalence of HIV infection in that population. In a population with a known prevalence of the virus for a test with a known sensitivity and specificity, the

positive predictive value varies with the prevalence of the virus in the population. Thus, the predictive value of the HIV-1 antibody test will be slightly different in different parts of the United States where the prevalence of HIV in blood donors is different.

When a blood donor is found to be anti-HIV positive on initial testing, the test is repeated in duplicate. If at least one of the subsequent tests is also positive, the donor unit is said to be repeatably reactive, and that unit is discarded. Units that are not positive on the repeat test (and thus not repeatably reactive) are suitable for transfusion. The blood sample from all repeatably reactive donors is then tested using the Western blot method, which identifies antibodies directed against the individual structural polypeptides of HIV.[50] The viral proteins included in the Western blot are the p24 gag protein, the p31 pol protein, and the gp41 and/or gp120/160 env glycoproteins (see Chapter 8). The criteria for a positive test include antibodies to at least two of the proteins. A number of other patterns of reactivity with different bands may be observed. These are usually classified as indeterminate. The implications of these indeterminate Western blot results for the significance of infection by HIV or the future health of the individual are not known at present. Little is known about the frequency of loss of antibody, but this is probably rare in asymptomatic individuals.[46,47] A few individuals with an indeterminate pattern of reactivity on the Western blot may show conversion to a clearly positive pattern in blood samples obtained a few weeks later. Most individuals do not show any change in the pattern of reactivity of their serum. This is thought to indicate that they are not infected.[51,52] Although the impact on the individual's future health is not known, it has been proposed that they could be reinstated as blood donors.[53,54]

Risk of Acquiring HIV Infection from Transfusion of Anti-HIV-1–Positive Blood

The risk of acquiring HIV infection following transfusion with anti-HIV-1–positive blood has been estimated to be as high as 70% to 91%.[55,56] It has been estimated that prior to the introduction of HIV-1 antibody testing in May 1985, approximately 12,000 patients were infected with HIV-1 by transfusion.[57,58] The incubation period between transmission-transmitted HIV-1 infection and the development of AIDS is difficult to determine, but it may be from 4.5 to 14.2 years.[59]

Risk of Acquiring HIV by Transfusion of Anti-HIV–Negative Blood (Window Phase)

The interval between infection and the development of antibody to the infecting virus is known as the "window phase." Because the test for HIV detects anti-HIV, there is a window phase during which the individual is infectious but does not have a positive screening test for anti-HIV. Thus, despite testing for HIV, transmission of the virus could still occur from blood donated during the window phase or by asymptomatic individuals who carry the virus but have lost the antibody. Two reports described disturbingly long window periods of 31 and 35 months,[60,61] and in other reports HIV was recovered from the lymphocytes of high-risk individuals who did not have anti-

HIV.[47,62] However, experience does not substantiate this long window phase. Instead it appears that the window phase during which HIV-1 infection can be transmitted by anti-HIV–negative donors between infection and the appearance of antibody is about 6 weeks or 45 days.[63–65] However, this type of transmission occurs very rarely. The present risk of acquiring HIV infection through blood transfusion is extremely low. The risk will depend on the prevalence of HIV infection in the community and thus in the donor population from which the unit of blood was obtained. Therefore, it is difficult to apply a single figure to the entire United States. Estimates of the risk of acquiring HIV from a unit of blood that has been tested and found to be negative for HIV antibody range from 1 in 33,000 units[66,66a] to 1 in 40,000,[67] 1 in 60,000,[68] 1 in 68,000,[69] and 1 in 200,000 units.[10,58] The changes in these numbers represent the improvement in testing. The most recent estimates are that 1 in about 440,000 units of blood that tests negative for HIV might transmit the infection.[4,5] Extrapolating the latter estimate would project that about 27 persons might become infected with HIV annually by transfusion of donated blood that was negative for HIV antibodies.

Approaches to Reducing the Window Phase

Since the virus should be present during the window phase prior to the development of antibody and since HIV antigen has been detected in some patients prior to their becoming HIV antibody positive, it has been suggested that HIV antigen screening of blood donors may be an effective way of reducing or eliminating transmission of infection by blood donated during the window phase. Two large studies involving approximately 500,000 donors each did not identify any donors whose serum contained HIV antigen but no HIV antibody.[70,71] Based on these studies it appeared that HIV antigen testing would not be helpful. However, because of the occurrence of cases of infection due to donation during the window phase[64,65] and the commitment of the U.S. Food and Drug Administration (FDA) to do everything possible to avoid window phase transmission,[72] routine blood donor screening has been advised by the FDA and implemented by blood banks.

Other approaches to reducing the window phase include (a) the use of tests in which the antigens used in the antibody test are produced by recombinant DNA techniques and (b) the use of the polymerase chain reaction or other methods to amplify DNA or RNA sequences, thus making it possible to detect minute amounts of proviral DNA. The FDA has formally stated a desire to shift testing for infectious disease to direct identification of the offending organism and is committed to facilitate the development of such tests.[72] It is projected that such tests will be available by about the year 2000.[72] In the meantime, continued emphasis must be placed on the medical history process used to identify blood donors who might be at risk of transmitting HIV infection. In addition, public education and education of potential blood donors continue to be essential in order to encourage high-risk individuals not to donate blood.

Effect of Transfusion on AIDS

Blood transfusion appears to be associated with a short survival in patients with AIDS.[73] In vitro, allogeneic leukocytes activate HIV-infected cells and increase viral

expression.[74] At present, a large-scale clinical trial, the Viral Activation Transfusion Study VATS, is under way in the United States to determine whether transfusion exacerbates the HIV infection and has an overall detrimental effect to patients.

OTHER TRANSFUSION-TRANSMITTED VIRUSES

Although HIV and hepatitis are the agents of most concern, several other infectious diseases can be transmited by transfusion (Table 15.4).

Cytomegalovirus

Cytomegalovirus (CMV) is a herpesvirus that is common in the general population. In healthy individuals infection with CMV usually causes few or no symptoms. CMV can be transmitted by blood transfusion to both immunocompetent and immunodeficient patients (see Chapters 11 and 12 for extensive discussion). The earliest indications that CMV might be transmitted by blood transfusion were the observation of a mononucleosis-like syndrome that occurred several weeks after open heart surgery in immunocompetent patients. This became known as postperfusion or postpump syndrome. The heterophil-negative cases were shown to be caused by CMV[75] and the heterophil-positive cases, by Epstein-Barr virus.[75,76] Most of the immunocompetent patients who acquired transfusion-transmitted CMV were asymptomatic; in contrast, CMV can be a serious viral pathogen in patients with either congenital or acquired immunodeficiency. Thus, posttransfusion CMV infection can range from asymptomatic with development of CMV antibody (in patients who are immunocompetent) to an infectious mononucleosis–like syndrome to severe, even fatal, generalized CMV infection.[77–93]

Table 15.4 Other transfusion-transmitted disease of potential concern

Agent	Disease
Parvovirus	RBC aplasia
Trypanosoma	Chagas' disease
Plasmodium malariae	Malaria
Babesia	Babesiosis
Borrelia	Lyme disease
Prions	Creutzfeldt-Jakob disease
Epstein-Barr virus	Mononucleosis
	Lymph malignancy
Yersinia	Sepsis
HHV-6	Roseola; other?
Cytomegalovirus*	CMV disease
Leishmania**	Leishmaniasis

*For immunodeficient patients only.
**Temporary following Gulf War.

The incidence of CMV antibodies in blood donors ranges from 30% to 80%. Healthy individuals who pass all the medical screening requirements for blood donation may harbor CMV and transmit the virus via their donated blood components to susceptible patients. The CMV remains latent in the leukocytes of many infected healthy individuals, but efforts to isolate the virus have been unsuccessful.[94] Thus, there is no practical laboratory test to determine which patients previously infected with CMV but presently healthy enough to donate blood may transmit the virus. Since most previously infected persons have CMV antibodies, the presence of antibodies is used as a screening test. However, of these individuals only 2% to 12% have blood that may be capable of transmitting the virus.[95] A suggestion that individuals with IgM anti-CMV are more likely to transmit the virus than those with IgG anti-CMV has not been substantiated. Since the virus resides in the leukocytes, blood components depleted of leukocytes may have a reduced or even absent risk of transmitting CMV infection. Plasma components (fresh frozen plasma, liquid plasma, and cryoprecipitate) contain few leukocytes, and it does not appear that these components transmit CMV infection. Recent studies have also shown that removal of the leukocytes from cellular components, such as red cells or platelet concentrates, eliminated transfusion-transmitted CMV infection.[88,89,96] Frozen deglycerolized red cells contain only about 1% to 5% of the original leukocytes and do not appear to transmit CMV infection,[97] although washed red cells may transmit CMV.[98]

To summarize, the approaches that have been used to prevent transfusion-transmitted CMV infection include use of CMV antibody–negative blood products, use of leukocyte-depleted blood products, administration of acyclovir prophylactically,[99] administration of CMV immune globulin,[100] and administration of intravenous immunoglobulin.[87] The effectiveness of preventing transfusion-transmitted CMV in the specific situations in which CMV infection is a clinical problem is described in Chapters 11 and 12. Because it has been established that leukocyte depletion is effective in preventing CMV transmission (see Chapters 11 and 12), this is becoming the most common approach.

Human T-Lymphotrophic Virus I AND II (HTLV-I/II)

Adult T-cell leukemia (ATL) was first recognized in Japan in the mid-1970s. Later the disease was shown to be caused by the HTLV virus, and this became the first retrovirus shown to cause malignancy in humans.[101] In ATL there is peripheral lymphadenopathy, hepatosplenomegaly, skin lesions, abdominal pain, diarrhea, and abnormal pulmonary findings on chest x-ray. ATL disease is not very amenable to therapy. The HTLV-2 virus is associated with a form of myelopathy and is referred to as HTLV-associated myelopathy or tropical spastic paraparesis (TSP).[101]

The virus and the ATL disease are endemic in Japan, the Caribbean Islands, parts of Central Asia, and Melanesia and also among the Australian aborigines. The virus can be transmitted vertically to newborns by maternal breast milk and also can be spread by parenteral and sexual routes.[102–105] Approximately two-thirds of initially reactive donor blood samples fail to react on subsequent testing, and only about 10% of the repeatably reactive samples can later be shown to be infectious.[106,107] Thus, a very large proportion

of donors whose blood is initially reactive for anti-HTLV are not infectious but are nevertheless notified that they have a positive screening test result. Of those donors with a true positive test for HTLV-I/II who are carriers, there is approximately a 1% to 5% chance of developing ATL during a 70-year life span if early deaths from other diseases are not considered. Another 2% may develop TSP 5 to 10 years later.[106]

No cases of transfusion-transmitted adult T-cell leukemia or TSP have been identified. However, transmission of the virus by blood transfusion does occur.[108] Approximately 60% of seronegative recipients developed anti-HTLV-I after transfusion of cellular blood products containing anti-HTLV-I.[102–104,108] In the United States, anti-HTLV-I is found almost exclusively in intravenous drug abusers or in persons from areas endemic for HTLV-I. The incidence of anti-HTLV-I in blood donors is 0.025%.[109] Because of the potential for disease transmission, routine testing of all donated blood for anti-HTLV-I was initiated in the United States in December 1988. This has been done in the hope of avoiding the potential problem of transfusion-transmitted ALT or TSP.

Parvovirus

The parvovirus B19 has been implicated as a cause of aplastic anemia.[110,111] This virus has been transmitted by blood transfusion.[112,113] Parvovirus is a common infection in children. Infected individuals may be asymptomatic or have a mild febrile illness. Infections apparently are infrequent in adults. The prevalence of parvovirus in blood donors is estimated to be between 1 in 3,300 to 1 in 50,000.[114] This, combined with the brief period of viremia, makes transmission of parvovirus by blood transfusion rare. However, because large numbers of units of plasma are used to produce derivatives, it is possible that parvovirus could contaminate derivatives. No parvovirus DNA was detected in 17 batches of albumin;[114] however, it appears that parvovirus may be contained in coagulation factor concentrates.[115,116]

Epstein-Barr Virus

Epstein-Barr virus is the cause of heterophil-positive mononucleosis. Following infection with Epstein-Barr virus, there is lifelong carrier state, and most adults have been infected. Epstein-Barr virus can be transmitted by transfusion[117,118] and is one of the causes of the "postperfusion" syndrome—a viral-like illness occurring after transfusion of fresh blood during open heart surgery. Transfusion-transmitted Epstein-Barr virus has not been a major clinical problem, although it can be transmitted to organ recipients.[119]

TRANSFUSION-TRANSMITTED BACTERIAL INFECTIONS

It has been known for years that a small percentage of units of whole blood contain viable bacteria. Transmission of bacterial infection was a major problem in the early days of blood transfusion;[120–124] however, improvements in blood containers, the development of the closed system for producing blood components, and storage at refriger-

ator temperatures were thought to have virtually eliminated this problem. However, with the storage of platelets for 7 days at room temperature, the problem of bacterial contamination and transfusion transmission resurfaced.[125–128] As a result, it was necessary to reduce the storage time of platelets to 5 days. After this, the issue of bacterial contamination seemed to disappear. However, during the past few years, concern about transfusion-transmitted infection have been renewed once again, because cases of transfusion-transmitted bacterial infection seem to be increasing. The scope of the problem of bacterial contamination of blood components is difficult to ascertain. In Canada and the United States, the rate of contaminated platelets is estimated to be between 0.04% and 0.1%.[129] The number of deaths due to contaminated blood components reported to the FDA between 1986 and 1991 was twice as great as the number reported in the previous 10 years.[129] Over half of the deaths were due to contaminated units of red cells, with platelet contamination being somewhat more common than plasma contamination. Of the contaminated red cells, half are caused by *Yersinia enterocolitica.*[129]

There are two general types of concerns: bacterial contamination of platelet concentrates stored at room temperature and transmission of bacteria, especially *Y. enterocolitica,* from red cells stored at refrigerator temperatures.[130] For either of these situations, the sources of potential contamination include the donor's blood, the skin at the venipuncture site, and the environment such as air, equipment, water, and the phlebotomist.[130] The type of organism involved can provide a clue about the source. For instance, *Staphylococcus epidermidis* is among the normal skin flora and suggests contamination from the venipuncture site, whereas *Pseudomonas* suggests water or equipment contamination. The growth pattern of the particular organism is another consideration. Most patients can clear a rather large number of organisms; for instance, 10^4 coagulase-negative staphylococci. The nature of the blood component may also be important. Contamination is apparently more common from pooled units of platelets from whole blood than from single-donor platelets collected by apheresis and from platelets stored for longer periods.[125–129] The issue of contaminated platelet concentrates is also made more complicated by the differences in rates of contamination observed in different institutions. This has caused some to believe that this is a very serious problem, while others contend that they rarely encounter these kinds of reactions in patients.

The contamination of red cell units with cold-growing organisms is rare and does not seem to have increased lately. However, there does seem to be an increase in contamination of red cell units with *Y. enterocolitica.*[130–135] *Y. enterocolitica* can grow at temperatures below 37°C and in a calcium-free medium, thus making it more suitable for proliferation in refrigerated anticoagulated blood. There is a rather long lag phase of growth, and this is consistent with the observation that most units contaminated with *Y. enterocolitica* have been stored 20 days or longer.[129,130] Although the organism loses some of its virulence during growth, the endotoxins produced can have a severe clinical effect. *Y. enterocolitica* infection in normal, healthy individuals is often asymptomatic or may be associated with mild gastrointestinal symptoms. Questioning donors about gastrointestinal symptoms in the preceding 30 days is not an effective method of preventing the collection of blood from donors who might have circulating organisms,

because only about 50% of infected donors recall any symptoms and 11% of otherwise healthy suitable donors do report minor symptoms. Another strategy considered was to take advantage of the lag phase of growth and reduce the allowable storage period of red cells to 21 days. However, it was feared that this would create major difficulties in the management of the red cell inventory, and so this was not pursued.

Several systems have been suggested to prevent transfusion of contaminated blood components. Yomtovian carried out a surveillance system using Gram staining.[136] Other proposals include routine leukocyte depletion, the limulus lysate assay for endotoxin, automated culture systems, antigen detection systems, immunologic methods, and nucleic acid probes. Kim et al.[137] showed that red cells contaminated with *Y. enterocolitica* have a noticeably different color and can be identified visually. None of these methods is currently used routinely and effectively. Thus, bacterial contamination of blood components continues to be an infrequent but potentially serious complication of transfusion.

TRANSFUSION-TRANSMITTED PARASITIC DISEASES

Transfusion transmission of some parasites such as malaria have been known for years, and donor selection procedures are designed to identify potentially infectious donors. However, during the past few years a few cases of transfusion transmission of other parasitic diseases have been reported. As these diseases become more widespread[138] there is a growing need to develop strategies to deal with this situation. There are no easy solutions. Many of the diseases have local or regional areas of prevalence, but as people move it may not be practical to limit donor selection procedures to those areas. In addition, there may not be suitable tests available for large-scale donor screening. Thus, approaches to dealing with these parasitic diseases—especially tick-borne diseases—will probably undergo considerable development during the next few years.

Malaria

Transmission of malaria by transfusion is possible but so rare in North America that few physicians have seen a case. All four species of *Plasmodium* can survive in refrigerated blood and have caused transfusion-transmitted malaria, although most cases involve *Plasmodium malariae*.[139] Malaria has been transmitted by platelet transfusion as well as by red cells, and malarial parasites have been found in platelets of infected individuals. Thus, periodic spiking fever in a patient who has recently received a transfusion could be due to malaria, but this would be very unlikely.

Donors who might transmit malaria are screened out by medical history. *Plasmodium falciparum* and *Plasmodium vivax* produce symptoms within 6 months of infection. Thus, travelers returning from areas where malaria is endemic are deferred for 6 months unless they took antimalarial prophylaxis, in which case they are deferred for 3 years. *Plasmodium malariae* infection may be asymptomatic for years, and so the present screening procedures would not defer such donors. However, the risk is extremely

small, and adjustment of present donor criteria is not warranted. Laboratory testing of donors for malaria is not practical or cost-effective in the United States.

Chagas' Disease

Trypanosoma cruzi, a parasite, is endemic in many parts of Central and South America, but only a few rare cases of infection in the United States have been reported. The organism causes Chagas' disease, in which patients may develop megacolon, megaesophagus, and heart failure. Once an individual is infected, it appears that lifelong parasitemia results. Many patients with chronic *T. cruzi* infection may be asymptomatic and thus could pass the blood donor medical questions. The organisms can survive in refrigerated blood and can be transmitted by transfusion.[140] However, cases of transfusion-transmitted Chagas' disease are extremely rare in the United States.[141,142] It is estimated that up to 100,000 infected Latin American immigrants live in the United States. In the Los Angeles area, which has a large Latin American population, about 1 in 1,000 donors has antibodies to *T. cruzi.*[143] Thus, transfusion-transmitted *T. cruzi* infection could potentially develop into a larger problem than it seems at present. To prepare for this, efforts are under way to develop improved antibody detection tests. A questionnaire designed to identify donors at risk combined with antibody testing indicates that a substantial portion of at-risk Los Angeles donors have antibodies, and the use of an antibody test could reduce or eliminate the potential of transfusion-transmitted *T. cruzi.*[144] In some endemic areas of Central and South America, donated blood is screened for *T. cruzi.*

Babesiosis

Babesia microti and *Babesia bovis* are protozoans that occasionally infect humans by tick bites. The protozoan causes an acute illness of fever, malaise, and sometimes hemolytic anemia; however, many infected individuals are asymptomatic. Thus, *B. microti* can be transmitted by blood donated by asymptomatic infected donors.[145] The ticks are prevalent in the Northeast, mid-Atlantic, and upper Midwest. There is no suitable laboratory screening test. Some blood banks defer individuals from heavily tick-infested areas during the summer months.

Lyme Disease

Borrelia burgdorferi, a spirochete that is transmitted by ticks to humans, causes an acute illness of fever, malaise, and an erythematous annular spreading skin lesion followed by a chronic phase characterized by neurologic and/or cardiac symptoms with or without arthritis. However, in up to 40% of persons the infection is asymptomatic.[146] The spirochetes survive in stored blood for up to 45 days.[147] Thus, transmission of *B. burgdorferi* by transfusion is theoretically possible, but this has not been reported. Although a serologic test is available, it is not a suitable laboratory test for donor screening and the widespread prevalence of the tick makes it impractical to defer donors from endemic areas.[146]

CURRENT ISSUES IN TRANSFUSION-TRANSMITTED DISEASES

Creutzfeldt-Jacob Disease

Reports from England of the possible association of a variant of Creutzfeldt-Jacob disease (CJD) with ingestion of beef from cows affected with "mad cow disease"[148] raised the question of whether the variant of CJD could be transmitted by blood transfusion. CJD is a rare neurological disorder thought to be associated with a transmissible agent.[149–151] The agent may be an abnormally configured host protein called a prion. However, since the exact cause or causative agent of CJD is not known, there is no laboratory test to identify the infectious agent if one exists. Prions are highly resistant to inactivation with methods currently used in the production of plasma derivatives. Thus, even one unit of plasma contaminated with the CJD agent could render a large lot of plasma derivatives infectious.

CJD has been transmitted by dura, corneas, and pituitary growth hormone from CJD patients and EEG electrodes used on CJD patients.[148] There is no evidence of blood-borne transmission and no evidence of a recent "outbreak" of CJD in the United States.[152] However, during the past few years several instances have been recognized in which a blood donor subsequently developed CJD. One donor had given 90 times over 35 years. In response to this developing situation, the FDA formed a special panel on spongiform encephalopathies, and several policies were formed regarding use of blood components and plasma derivatives from donors subsequently found to have CJD. At present, when a blood bank learns of a donor who has CJD, all components remaining in inventory must be recovered. A lookback is initiated for all previous components from that donor, and all derivatives manufactured from the donor's plasma are placed in quarantine. This has led to donors being questioned to determine whether there is a family history of CJD and to the discontinuation of use for fractionation of plasma from donors over 50 years of age. Some transfusion medicine professionals and policy makers believe that handling of possible transfusion-transmitted CJD is excessively conservative and is not based on rational thinking. Others believe that these actions are appropriate given the public's fears of transfusion and the perception that the transfusion medicine community did not act as aggressively as it should have in the early days of the AIDS epidemic. Whether CJD will prove to be a threat to the blood supply and blood safety remains to be learned.

Other Diseases

Theoretically, any disease in which microbes circulate in the blood and survive for a few days in stored blood components could be transmitted by transfusion. This is even more of a potential if the initial disease is often asymptomatic or if a carrier state develops often. The diseases of most concern for transmission by blood transfusion have been discussed above. A few other diseases that are almost never transmitted by transfusions in the United States are toxoplasmosis, leishmaniasis, microfilaremia, and African trypanosomiasis. There is concern, however, that emerging pathogens, the mobility of people, and continued immigration can alter the situation with transfusion-transmitted diseases.[8]

Introduction of New Tests

As new transfusion-transmitted diseases are recognized or as transfusion transmission of presently known diseases becomes a greater factor, the issue of how to minimize disease transmission continues to be crucial. As should be apparent from discussions in this chapter and in Chapters 3, 4, 8, and 10, it is not so simple as merely adding another screening test. Several of the chapters cited emphasize that blood safety depends on many strategies, not just the laboratory test. The example of the effect of donor history in reducing the infectivity of the blood in San Francisco is an excellent one, as well as the reduction in posttransfusion hepatitis from the change to volunteer instead of paid donors. In considering testing, some of the diseases may be regional in nature, but with the mobility of the population, regional screening practices may not be suitable. However, this probably means that the screening tests will be very inefficient in many parts of the United States where the disease is not endemic. There are many factors about the infectious agent and the disease that can be taken into consideration when making a decision about a screening test (Table 15.5). Factors such as the prevalence of the disease, the infectivity of the agent, the status of the epidemic, and the likelihood of a carrier state are examples. In addition, the severity of the disease and the availability of treatment might be considered. However, when all of the scientific discussion is completed, there are the issues of social policy and the public expectations of their blood supply. Recently a report from the National Academy of Sciences[153] has been critical of the handling of the early days of the AIDS epidemic, although this report has been criticized as using hindsight and being inaccurate.[154] Nevertheless, the message from the public is that they expect the transfusion medicine community to take steps to achieve the maximum possible safety. The recent addition of HIV antigen testing is a good

Table 15.5 Issues in considering new transfusion-transmissible disease screening tests

"Because it's there"
Prevalence of agent in general population
Geographic distribution of agent
Value of medical history
Known high-risk groups
Infectivity of agent
Likelihood of disease
Nature of disease
Availability of therapy for disease
Quality of screening test
Availability of confirmatory test
Status of epidemic (stable; increasing)
Asymptomatic chronic phase
Potential for secondary spread
Cost

Source: Dodd RY. Scaling the heights. Transfusion 1995;35:186–187.

example. To what extent should cost-effectiveness be a consideration in improving blood safety? In the past, policy makers and politicians have shown little tolerance for failure to take steps that would decrease risks to their constituents, regardless of the cost. A more rational approach has been sought by many and has been publicly advocated by at least two thoughtful, knowledgeable transfusion medicine professionals.[34,155] However, the decision-making process is still a complex one with no easily discernible structure for these decisions. Perhaps the newly formed Advisory Committee on Blood Safety and Availability of the U.S. Department of Health and Human Services can be helpful, but the effectiveness of this group remains to be determined.

REFERENCES

1. McCullough J. The nation's changing blood supply system. JAMA 1993;269:2239–2245.
2. McCullough J. The continuing evolution of the nation's blood supply system. Am J Clin Pathol 1996;105:689–695.
3. Dodd RY. The risk of transfusion-transmitted infection. N Engl J Med 1992;327:419. Editorial.
4. Schreiber GB, Busch MP, Kleinman SH. The risk of transfusion-transmitted viral infections. N Engl J Med 1996;334:1685–1690.
5. Lackritz EM, Satten GA, Aberle-Grasse J, et al. Estimated risk of transmission of the human immunodeficiency virus by screened blood in the United States. N Engl J Med 1995;333:1721–1725.
6. Turner TB, Diseker TH. Duration of infectivity of Treponema pallidum in citrated blood stored under conditions obtained in blood banks. Bull Johns Hopkins Hosp 1941;68:269.
7. Chambers RW, Foley HT, Schmidt PJ. Transmission of syphilis by fresh blood components. Transfusion 1969;9:32.
8. NIH Consensus Development Panel on Infectious Disease Testing for Blood Transfusions. Infectious disease testing for blood transfusion. JAMA 1995;274:1374–1379.
9. Nishioka K. Transfusion-transmitted HBV and HCV. Vox Sang 1996;70:4–8.
10. Bove JR. Transfusion-associated hepatitis and AIDS: what is the risk? N Engl J Med 1987;317:242.
11. Alter HJ. You'll wonder where the yellow went: a 15-year retrospective of posttransfusion hepatitis. In: Moore SB, ed. Transfusion-transmitted viral diseases. Arlington, VA: American Association of Blood Banks, 1987:53.
12. Hollinger FB, Khan NC, Oefinger PA, et al. Posttransfusion hepatitis type A. JAMA 1983;250:2313.
13. Noble RC, Kane MA, Reeves SA, Roeckel I. Posttransfusion hepatitis A in a neonatal intensive care unit. JAMA 1984;252:2711.
14. Alter HJ, Holland PV, Purcell RH, et al. Posttransfusion hepatitis after exclusion of commercial and hepatitis-B antigen-positive donors. Ann Intern Med 1972;77:691.
15. Aach RD, Szmuness W, Mosley JW. Serum alanine aminotransferase of donors in relation to the risk of non-A, non-B hepatitis in recipients. N Engl J Med 1981;304:989.
16. Stevens CE, Aach RD, Hollinger FB. Hepatitis B virus antibody in blood donors and the occurrence of non-A, non-B hepatitis in transfusion recipients: an analysis of the transfusion-transmitted viruses study. Ann Intern Med 1984;101:733.
17. Koziol DE, Holland PV, Alling DW, et al. Antibody to hepatitis B core antigen as a paradoxical marker for non-A, non-B hepatitis agents in donated blood. Ann Intern Med 1986;104:488.
18. Stevens CE, Taylor PE, Liu P. Hepatitis B virus infection: epidemiology and immunoprophylaxis. In: Moore SB, ed. Transfusion-Transmitted Viral Diseases. Arlington, VA: American Association of Blood Banks, 1987:1.
19. Dienstag JL. Non-A, non-B hepatitis: I. Recognition, epidemiology, and clinical features. Gastroenterology 1983;85:439.
20. Alter HJ, Purcell RH, Holland PV, Alling DW, Koziol DE. Donor transaminase and recipient hepatitis: impact on blood transfusion services. JAMA 1981;246:630.

21. Blajchman MA, Bull SB, Feinman SV. Post-transfusion hepatitis: impact of non-A, non-B hepatitis surrogate tests. Lancet 1995;345:21–25.
22. Choo QL, Kuo G, Weiner AJ, et al. Isolation of a cDNA derived from a blood-borne non-A, non-B viral hepatitis genome. Science 1989;244:359.
23. Alter HJ, Purcell RH, Shih JW, et al. Detection of antibody to hepatitis C virus in prospectively followed transfusion recipients with acute and chronic non-A, non-B hepatitis. N Engl J Med 1989;321:1494.
24. Alter HJ. To C or not to C: these are the questions. Blood 1995;85:1681–1695.
25. Tong MJ, El-Farra NS, Reikes AR, Co RL. Clinical outcomes after transfusion-associated hepatitis C. N Engl J Med 1995;332:1463–1466.
26. Seeff LB, Buskell-Bales Z, Wright EC, et al. Long-term mortality after transfusion-associated non-A, non-B hepatitis. N Engl J Med 1992;327:1906.
27. Janot C, Courouce AM, Maniez M. Antibodies to hepatitis C virus in French blood donors. Lancet 1989;2:796.
28. Sirchia G, Bellobuono A, Giovanetti A, Marconi M. Antibodies to hepatitis C virus in Italian blood donors. Lancet 1989;2:797.
29. Shakil AO, Conry-Cantilena C, Alter HJ, et al. Volunteer blood donors with antibody to hepatitis C virus: clinical, biochemical, virologic, and histologic features. Ann Intern Med 1995;123:330–237.
30. Rossini A, Gazzola GB, Ravaggi A, et al. Long-term follow-up of an infectivity in blood donors with hepatitis C antibodies and persistently normal alanine aminotransferase levels. Transfusion 1995;35:108–111.
31. Murphy EL, Bryzman S, Williams AE, et al. Demographic determinants of hepatitis C virus seroprevalence among blood donors. JAMA 1996;275:995–1000.
32. Donahue JG, Munoz A, Ness PM, et al. The declining risk of post-transfusion hepatitis C virus infection. N Engl J Med 1992;327:369.
33. Alter HJ, Nakatsuji Y, Melpolder J, et al. The incidence of transfusion-associated hepatitis G virus infection and its relation to liver disease. N Engl J Med 1997;336:747–754.
34. Alter HJ. G-pers creepers, where'd you get those papers? A reassessment of the literature on the hepatitis G virus. Transfusion 1997;37:569–572.
35. Yoshikawa A, Fukuda S, Itoh K, et al. Infection with hepatitis G virus and its strain variant, the GB agent (GBV-C), among blood donors in Japan. Transfusion 1997;27:657–663.
36. Centers for Disease Control. Pneumocystis carinii pneumonia among persons with hemophilia A. MMWR 1982;31:365.
37. Centers for Disease Control. Possible transfusion-associated acquired immune deficiency syndrome (AIDS): California. MMWR 1982;31:652.
38. Curran JW, Lawrence DN, Jaffe HW, et al. Acquired immunodeficiency syndrome (AIDS) associated with transfusions. N Engl J Med 1984;310:69.
39. Peterman TA, Jaffe HW, Feorino PM, et al. Transfusion-associated acquired immunodeficiency syndrome in the United States. JAMA 1985;254:2913.
40. Jaffe HW, Sarngadharan MG, DeVico AL, et al. Infection with HTLV-III/LAV and transfusion-associated acquired immunodeficiency syndrome: serologic evidence of an association. JAMA 1985;254:770.
41. Feorino PM, Kalyanaraman VS, Haverkos HW, et al. Lymphadenopathy associated virus infection of a blood donor-recipient pair with acquired immunodeficiency syndrome. Science 1984;225:69.
42. Feorino PM, Jaffe HW, Palmer E, et al. Transfusion-associated acquired immunodeficiency syndrome: evidence for persistent infection in blood donors. N Engl J Med 1985;312:1293.
43. Lange JMA, van den Berg H, Dooren LJ, et al. HTLV-III/LAV infection in nine children infected by a single plasma donor: clinical outcome and recognition patterns of viral proteins. J Infect Dis 1986;154:171.
44. Dodd RY. Transfusion transmitted HIV. Vox Sang 1996;70:1–3.
45. Busch MP, Young MJ, Samson SJ, et al. Risk of human immunodeficiency virus (HIV) transmission by blood transfusions before the implementation of HIV-1 antibody screening. Transfusion 1991;31:4.
46. Farzadegan H, Polis MA, Wolinsky SM, et al. Loss of human immunodeficiency virus type 1 (HIV-1) antibodies with evidence of viral infection in asymptomatic homosexual men. Ann Intern Med 1988;108:785.

47. Salahuddin SZ, Markham PD, Redfield RR, et al. HTLV-III in symptom-free seronegative persons. Lancet 1984;2:1418.

48. Ward JW, Grindon AJ, Feorino PM, et al. Laboratory and epidemiologic evaluation of an enzyme immunoassay for antibodies to HTLV-III. JAMA 1986;256:357.

49. MacDonald KL, Jackson JB, Bowman RJ, et al. Performance characteristics of serologic tests for human immunodeficiency virus type 1 (HIV-1) antibody among Minnesota blood donors. Ann Intern Med 1989;110:617.

50. The Consortium for Retrovirus Serology Standardization. Serological diagnosis of human immunodeficiency virus infection by Western blot testing. JAMA 1988;260:674.

51. Eble BE, Busch MP, Khayam-Bashi H, et al. Resolution of infection status of HIV- seroindeterminate and high-risk seronegative individuals using PCR and virus-culture: absence of persistent silent HIV-1 infection in a high-prevalence area. Transfusion 1992;32:503.

52. Jackson JB. Human immunodeficiency virus (HIV)-indeterminate Western blots and latent HIV infection. Transfusion 1992;32:497.

53. Sayre KR, Dodd RY, Tegtmeier G, Layug L, Alexander SS, Busch MP. False-positive human immunodeficiency virus type 1 Western blot tests in noninfected blood donors. Transfusion 1996;36:45–52.

54. Busch MP, Kleinman SH, Williams AE, et al. Frequency of human immunodeficiency virus (HIV) infection among contemporary anti-HIV-1 and anti-HIV-1/2 supplemental test-indeterminate blood donors. Transfusion 1996;36:37–44.

55. Menitove JE. Status of recipients of blood from donors subsequently found to have an antibody to HIV. N Engl J Med 1986;315:1095.

56. Donegan E, Transfusion Safety Study Group. Serum antibody positivity in recipients of anti-HIV positive blood. Transfusion 1986;26:576.

57. Centers for Disease Control. Human immunodeficiency virus infection in transfusion recipients and their family members. MMWR 1987;36:137.

58. Peterman TA, Lui KJ, Lawrence DN, Allen JR. Estimating the risks of transfusions-associated acquired immune deficiency syndrome and human immunodeficiency virus infection. Transfusion 1987;27:371.

59. Lui KJ, Lawrence DN, Morgan WM, et al. A model-based approach for estimating the mean incubation period of transfusion-associated acquired immunodeficiency syndrome. Proc Natl Acad Sci USA 1986;83:3051.

60. Ranki A, Valle SL, Krohm M, et al. Long latency precedes overt seroconversion in sexually transmitted human-immunodeficiency-virus infection. Lancet 1987;2:589.

61. Imagawa DT, Lee MH, Wolinsky SM, et al. Human immunodeficiency virus type 1 infection in homosexual men who remain seronegative for prolonged periods. N Engl J Med 1989;320:1458.

62. Mayer KH, Stoddard AM, McCusker J, et al. Human T-lymphotropic virus type III in high-risk, antibody-negative homosexual men. Ann Intern Med 1986;104:194.

63. Dodd RY. The risk of transfusion-transmitted infection. N Engl J Med 1992;327:419. Editorial.

64. Irani MS, Dudley AW, Lucco LJ. Case of HIV-1 transmission by antigen-positive, antibody negative blood. N Engl J Med 1991;325:1174–115. Letter.

65. Roberts CS, Longfield JN, Platte RC, et al. Transfusion-associated human immunodeficiency virus type 1 from screened antibody-negative blood donors. Arch Pathol Lab Med 1994;118:1188–1192.

66. Cohen ND, Munoz A, Reitz BA, et al. Transmission of retroviruses by transfusion of screened blood in patients undergoing cardiac surgery. N Engl J Med 1989;320:1172.

66a. Ward JW, Holmberg SD, Allen JR, et al. Transfusion of human immunodeficiency virus (HIV) by blood transfusions screened as negative for HIV antibody. N Engl J Med 1988;318:473.

67. Busch MP, Bernard EE, Khayam-Bashi H, et al. Evaluation of screened blood donation from human immunodeficiency virus type I infection by culture and DNA amplification of pooled cells. N Engl J Med 1991;325:1.

68. Donahue JG, Nelson KE, Munoz A, et al. Transmission of HIV by transfusion of screened blood. N Engl J Med 1990;323:1709.

69. Kleinman S, Secord K. Risk of human immunodeficiency virus (HIV) transmission by anti-HIV negative blood: estimates using the lookback methodology. Transfusion 1988;28:499.

70. Busch MP, Taylor PE, Lenes BA, et al. Screening of selected male blood donors for p24 antigen of human immunodeficiency type 1. Transfusion Safety Study Group. N Engl J Med 1990;323:1308–1312.

71. Alter HJ, Epstein JS, Swenson SG, et al. Prevalence of human immunodeficiency virus type 1 p24 antigen in US blood donors—an assessment of the efficacy of testing in donor screening. HIV-antigen study group. N Engl J Med 1990;323:1312–137.

72. Hewlett IK, Epstein JS. Food and Drug Administration conference on the feasibility of genetic technology to close the HIV window in donor screening. Transfusion 1997;37:346–351.

73. Vamvakas E, Kaplan HS. Early transfusion and length of survival in acquired immune deficiency syndrome: experience with a population receiving medical care at a public hospital. Transfusion 1993;33:111–118.

74. Busch MP, Lee TH, Heitman J. Allogeneic leukocytes but not therapeutic blood elements induce reactivation and dissemination of latent human immunodeficiency virus type I infection: implication for transfusion support of infected patients. Blood 1992;80:2128–2135.

75. Tegtmeier GE. Transfusion-transmitted cytomegalovirus infections: significance and control. Vox Sang 1986;51:22.

76. Gerber P, Walsh JH, Rosenblum EN. Association of EB-virus infection with the post-perfusion syndrome. Lancet 1969;1:593.

77. Yaeger AS, Grumet FC, Hafleigh EB, et al. Prevention of transfusion-acquired cytomegalovirus infections in newborn infants. J Pediatr 1981;98:281.

78. Stagno S, Pass RF, Dworsky ME, et al. Congenital cytomegalovirus infection: the relative importance of primary and recurrent maternal infection. N Engl J Med 1982;306:945.

79. Adler SP. Neonatal cytomegalovirus infections due to blood. CRC Crit Rev Clin Lab Sci 1985;23:1.

80. Tegtmeier GE. Cytomegalovirus and blood transfusion. In: Dodd RY, Barker LF, eds. Infection, immunity, and blood transfusion. New York: Alan R Liss, 1985;182:175.

81. Glenn J. Cytomegalovirus infection following renal transplantation. Rev Infect Dis 1981;3:1151.

82. Rubin RH, Tolkoff-Rubin NE, Oliver D, et al. Multicenter seroepidemiologic study of the impact of cytomegalovirus infection on renal transplantation. Transplantation 1985;40:243.

83. Chou S. Acquisition of donor strains of cytomegalovirus by renal-transplant recipients. N Engl J Med 1986;314:1418.

84. Miller W, Flynn P, McCullough J, et al. Cytomegalovirus infection after bone marrow transplantation: an association with acute graft-vs-host disease. Blood 1986;67:1162.

85. Bowden RA, Sayers M, Flournoy N, et al. Cytomegalovirus immune globulin and seronegative blood products prevent primary cytomegalovirus infection after marrow transplantation. N Engl J Med 1986;314:1006.

86. Miller WJ, McCullough J, Balfour HH, et al. Prevention of cytomegalovirus infection following bone marrow transplantation: a randomized trial of blood product screening. Bone Marrow Transplant 1991;7:227–234.

87. Winston DJ, Ho WG, Lin C, et al. Intravenous immunoglobulin for modification of cytomegalovirus infections associated with bone marrow transplantation. Am J Med 1984;76:128.

88. Gilbert GL, Hudson IL, Hayes JJ. Prevention of transfusion-acquired cytomegalovirus infection in infants by blood filtration to remove leucocytes. Lancet 1989;1:1228.

89. Murphy MF, Grint PCA, Hardiman AE, Lister TA, Waters AH. Use of leukocyte-poor blood components to prevent primary cytomegalovirus (CMV) infection in patients with acute leukemia. Br J Haematol 1988;70:253.

90. Preiksaitis JK, Rosno S, Grumet C, Merigan TC. Infections due to herpesviruses in cardiac transplant recipients: role of the donor heart and immunosuppressive therapy. J Infect Dis 1983;147:1974.

91. Rakela J, Wiesner RH, Taswell HF, et al. Incidence of cytomegalovirus infection and its relationship to donor-recipient serologic status in liver transplantation. Transplant Proc 1987;19:2399.

92. Preiksaitis JK, Grumet FC, Smith WK, Merigan TC. Transfusion-acquired cytomegalovirus infections in cardiac surgery patients. J Med Virol 1985;15:283.

93. Adler SP, Baggett J, McVoy M. Transfusion-associated cytomegalovirus infections in seropositive cardiac surgery patients. Lancet 1985;2(8458)743–747.

94. Jackson JB, Orr HT, McCullough JJ, Jordan MC. Failure to detect human cytomegalovirus DNA in IgM-seropositive blood donors by spot hybridization. J Infect Dis 1987;156:1013.

95. Adler SP. Transfusion-associated cytomegalovirus infections. Rev Infect Dis 1983;5:977.

96. Bowden RA, Slichter SJ, Sayers M, Weisdorf D, Cays M, Schoch G, Banaji M, Haake R, Welk K, Fisher L, McCullough J, Miller W. A comparison of filtered leukocyte-reduced and cytomegalovirus (CMV) seronegative blood products for the prevention of transfusion-associated CMV infection after marrow transplant. Blood 1995; 86:3598–3603.

97. Brady MT, Milam JD, Anderson DC, et al. Use of deglycerolized red blood cells to prevent posttransfusion infection with cytomegalovirus in neonates. J Infect Dis 1984;150:334.

98. Luban NLC, Williams AE, MacDonald MG, et al. Low incidence of acquired cytomegalovirus infection in neonates transfused with washed red blood cells. Am J Dis Child 1987;141:4161.

99. Meyers JD, Reed EC, Shepp DH, et al. Acyclovir for prevention of cytomegalovirus infection and disease after allogeneic marrow transplantation. N Engl J Med 1988;38:70.

100. Meyers JD, Leszczynski J, Zaia JA, et al. Prevention of cytomegalovirus infection by cytomegalovirus immune globulin after marrow transplantation. Ann Intern Med 1983;98:442.

101. Hollsberg P, Hafler DA. Pathogenesis of diseases induced by human lymphotropic virus type I infection. N Engl J Med 1993;328;1173–1182.

102. Shih JWK, Lee HH, Falchek M, et al. Transfusion-transmitted HTLV-I/II infection in patients undergoing open-heart surgery. Blood 1990;75:5466–5469.

103. Okochi K, Sato H, Hinuma Y. A retrospective study on transmission of adult T-cell leukemia virus by blood transfusion: seroconversion in recipients. Vox Sang 1984;46:245–253.

104. Donegan E, Busch MP, Galleshaw JA, et al. Transfusion of blood components from a donor with human T-lymphotropic virus type II (HTLV-II) infection. Ann Intern Med 1990;113:555–556.

105. Murphy EL, Figueroa JP, Gibbs WN, et al. Sexual transmission of human T-lymphotropic virus type I (HTLV-I). Ann Intern Med 1989;111:555–560.

106. Holland PV. Notification and counseling of blood donors. Vox Sang 1996;70:46–49.

107. Busch MP, Laycock M, Kleinman SH, et al. Accuracy of supplementary serologic testing for human T-lymphotropic virus types I and II in US blood donors. Blood 1994;83:1143–1148.

108. Okochi K, Sato H. Adult T-cell leukemia virus, blood donors and transfusion: experience in Japan. Prog Clin Biol Res 1985;182:245.

109. Williams AE, Fang CT, Slamon DJ, et al. Seroprevalence and epidemiologic correlates of HTLV-1 infection in U.S. blood donors. Science 1988;240:643.

110. Serjeant GR, Mason K, Topley JM, et al. Outbreak of aplastic crisis in sickle cell anemia associated with parvovirus-like agent. Lancet 1981;2:595.

111. Harris JW. Parvovirus B19 for the hematologist. Am J Hematol 1992;39:119–130.

112. Mortimer PP, Luban NL, Kelleher JF, Cohen BJ. Transmission of serum parvovirus-like agent by clotting factor concentrates. Lancet 1983;2:482.

113. Zanell A, Rossi F, Cesana C, et al. Transfusion-transmitted human parvovirus B19 infection in a thalassemic patients. Transfusion 1995;35:769–772.

114. Lefrere JJ, Mariotti M, de la Croix I, et al. Albumin batches and B19 parvovirus DNA. Transfusion 1995;35:389–391.

115. Williams MD, Cohen BJ, Beddall AC, Pasi KJ, Mortimer PP, Hill FGH. Transmission of human parvovirus B19 by coagulation factor concentrates. Vox Sang 1990;58:177–181.

116. Ragni MV, Koch WC, Jordan JA. Parvovirus B19 infection in patients with hemophilia. Transfusion 1996;36:238–241.

117. Gerber P, Walsh JH, Rosenblum EN, Parcell RH. Association of EB-virus infection with the post-perfusion syndrome. Lancet 1969;1:593.

118. Henle W, Henle G, Scriba M, et al. Antibody responses to the Epstein-Barr virus and cytomegalovirus after open-heart and other surgery. N Engl J Med 1970;282:1068.

119. Alfieri C, Tanner J, Carpentier L, et al. Epstein-Barr virus transmission from a blood donor to an organ transplant recipient with recovery of the same virus strain from the recipient's blood and oropharynx. Blood 1996;87:812–817.

120. Braude AI, Carey FJ, Siemienski J. Studies of bacterial transfusion reactions from refrigerated blood: the properties of cold growing bacteria. J Clin Invest 1955;34:311.

121. Braude AI. Transfusion reactions from contaminated blood—their recognition and treatment. N Engl J Med 1958;258:1289–1293.

122. Braude AI, Sanford JP, Bartlett JE, Mallery OT. Effects and clinical significance of bacterial contaminants in transfused blood. J Lab Clin Med 1952;39:902–916.

123. Stevens A, Legg JS, Henry S, et al. Fatal transfusion reactions from contamination of stored blood by cold growing bacteria. Ann Intern Med 1953;39:1228.

124. Pittman M. A study of bacteria implicated in transfusion reactions and of bacteria isolated from blood products. J Lab Clin Med 1953;42:273–287.

125. Heal JM, Singal S, Sardisco E, Mayer T. Bacterial proliferation in platelet concentrates. Transfusion 1986;26:388–390.

125a. Braine HG, Kickler TS, Charache P, et al. Bacterial sepsis secondary to platelet transfusion: an adverse effect of extended storage at room temperature. Transfusion 1986;26:391.

126. Morrow JF, Braine HG, Kickler TS, Ness PM, Dick JD, Fuller AK. Septic reactions to platelet transfusions—a persistent problem. JAMA 1991;266:555–558.

127. Buchholz DH, Young VM, Friedman NR, et al. Bacterial proliferation in platelet products stored at room temperature. N Engl J Med 1971;285:429–433.

128. Anderson KC, Lew MA, Gorgone BC. Transfusion-related sepsis after prolonged platelet storage. Am J Med 1986;81:405–411.

129. Klein HG, Dodd RY, Ness PM, Fratantoni JA, Nemo GJ. Current status of microbial contamination of blood components: summary of a conference. Transfusion 1997;37:95–101.

130. Sazama K. Bacteria in blood for transfusion—a review. Arch Pathol Lab Med 1994;118:350–365.

131. Stenhouse MAE, Milner LV. Yersinia enterocolitica: a hazard in blood transfusion. Transfusion 1982;222:396–398.

132. Wright DC, Selss IF, Vinton KJ, Pierce RN. Fatal Yersinia enterocolitica sepsis after blood transfusion. Arch Pathol Lab Med 1985;109:1040–1042.

133. Bufill JA, Ritch PS. Yersinia enterocolitica serotype 0:3 sepsis after blood transfusion. N Engl J Med 1989;320:810.

134. Tipple MA, Bland LA, Murphy JJ, et al. Sepsis associated with transfusion of red cells contaminated with Yersinia enterocolitica. Transfusion 1990;30:207–213.

135. Red blood cell transfusions contaminated with Yersinia enterocolitica—US, 1991–1996, and initiation of a national study to detect bacteria-associated transfusion reactions. MMWR 1997;46:553–555.

136. Yomtovian R, Lazarus HM, Goodnough LT, et al. A prospective microbiologic surveillance program to detect and prevent transfusion of bacterially contaminated platelets. Transfusion 1993;33:902–909.

137. Kim DM, Brecher ME, Bland LA, et al. Visual identification of bacterially contaminated red cells. Transfusion 1992;32:221–225.

138. Fishbein DB, Dennis D. Tick-borne diseases—a growing risk. N Engl J Med 1995;333:452–453.

139. Bruce-Chwatt LJ. Transfusion-associated parasitic infections. In: Dodd RY, Barker LF, eds. Infection, Immunity and Blood Transfusion. New York: Alan R Liss, 1985:101.

140. Schmunis GA. Chagas' disease and blood transfusion. In: Dodd RY, Barker LF, eds. Infection, Immunity and Blood Transfusion. New York: Alan R Liss, 1985:127.

141. Grant IH, Gold JWM, Wittner M, et al. Transfusion-associated acute Chagas disease acquired in the United States. Ann Intern Med 1989;111:849–851.

142. Cimo PL, Luper WE, Scouros MA. Transfusion-associated Chagas' disease in Texas: report of a case. Tex Med 1993;89:48–50.

143. Galel S, Kirchhoff LV. Risk factors for Trypanosoma cruzi infection in California blood donors. Transfusion 1996;36:227–231.

144. Shulman IA, Appleman MD, Saxena S, Hiti AL, Kirchhoff LV. Specific antibodies to Trypanosoma cruzi among blood donors in Los Angeles, California. Transfusion 1997;37:727–731.

145. Smith RP, Evans AT, Popovsky M, et al. Transfusion-acquired babesiosis and failure of antibiotic treatment. JAMA 1986;256:2726.

146. Aoki SK, Holland PV. Lyme disease: another transfusion risk? Transfusion 1989;29:646.

147. Badon SJ, Fister RD, Cable RG. Survival of Borrelia burgdorferi in blood products. Transfusion 1989;29:581.

148. Centers for Disease Control. World Health Organization consultation on public health issues related to bovine spongiform encephalopathy and the emergence of a new variety of Creutzfeldt-Jakob disease. MMWR 1996;45:295–303.

149. Manuelidis L. The dimensions of Creutzfeldt-Jakob disease. Transfusion 1994;34:915–928.
150. DeArmond SJ, Prusiner SB. Etiology and pathogenesis of prion diseases. Am J Pathol 1995;146:785–811.
151. Mestel R. Putting prions to the test. Science 1996;273:184–189.
152. Centers for Disease Control. Surveillance for Creutzfeldt-Jakob disease—United States. MMWR 1996;45:665–668.
153. Leveton LB, Sox HC, Stoto MA, eds. HIV and the Blood Supply. Washington, DC: National Academy Press, 1995:25–55.
154. Zuck TF, Eyster ME. Blood safety decisions, 1982 to 1986: perceptions and misconceptions. Transfusion 1996;36:928–931.
155. Dodd RY. Scaling the heights. Transfusion 1995;35:186–187.

THE HLA SYSTEM IN TRANSFUSION MEDICINE

Yoon Choo

THE HLA SYSTEM

The HLA system was first investigated in the 1950s by Dausset, Payne, and van Rood,[1] who studied leukocyte-agglutinating antibodies as possible causes for autoimmune diseases and febrile transfusion reaction. Leukoagglutinins were observed in sera from multiparous women and previously transfused patients. The first HLA antigen defined by a leukoagglutinin called MAC was later renamed HLA-A2.

Graft rejection was found to be associated with the development of antibodies against allogeneic leukocytes. The genetic loci involved in the rejection of foreign tissues are known as the major histocompatibility complex (MHC), and highly polymorphic cell surface molecules are encoded by the MHC. The human MHC has been called the HLA (human leukocyte antigen) system because these antigens were first identified and characterized using alloantibodies against leukocytes.

The HLA system has been best known as transplantation antigens, but the primary biological role of HLA molecules is in the regulation of immune response.[2]

Genomic Organization of the Human MHC

The human MHC maps to the short arm of chromosome 6 (6p21) and spans approximately 3,800 kilobases of DNA.[3] The human MHC can be divided into three regions. The class I region is located at the telomeric end of the complex, the class II region at the centromeric end, and the class III region in the center.

The class I region consists of the classical genes *HLA-A, HLA-B,* and *HLA-C* and the nonclassical genes or pseudogenes *HLA-E, HLA-F, HLA-G, HLA-H, HLA-J, HLA-K,* and *HLA-L.*[4] The *HLA-A, HLA-B,* and *HLA-C* loci encode the heavy chains of class I

antigens. Some of the nonclassical class I genes may be expressed with limited polymorphism, and their functions are unknown at this time.

The class II region consists of a series of subregions, each containing *A* and/or *B* genes encoding α and β chains, respectively.[4] The *DR, DQ,* and *DP* subregions encode the major expressed products of the class II region. The *DR* gene family consists of a single *DRA* gene and nine *DRB* genes (*DRB1* to *DRB9*). Different HLA haplotypes contain particular numbers of *DRB* loci. The *DRB1, DRB3, DRB4,* and *DRB5* loci are usually expressed, and the other *DRB* loci are pseudogenes. The *DRA* locus encodes an invariable α chain and it binds various β chains. DR antigen specificities (i.e., DR1 to DR18) are determined by the polymorphic DRβ1 chains encoded *DRB1* alleles. The *DQ* and *DP* families each have one expressed gene for α and β chains and a second pair of genes that may not be functional. The *DQA1* and *DQB1* gene products associate to form the DQ molecule, and the *DPA1* and *DPB1* products form DP molecules. The expression and functional role of the *DNA, DOB, DMA,* and *DMB* regions are unknown at this time.

The class III region does not encode HLA molecules but contains genes for complement components (C2, C4, factor B), 21-hydroxylase, and tumor necrosis factors (TNFs).[3]

HLA Haplotypes

HLA genes are closely linked and the entire MHC is inherited as an HLA haplotype in a mendelian fashion from each parent. Recombination within the HLA system occurs with a frequency less than 1%, and it appears to occur most frequently between the *DQ* and *DP* loci. The segregation of HLA haplotypes within a family can only be assigned by family studies. Two siblings have a 25% chance of being genotypically HLA identical, a 50% chance of being HLA haploidentical (sharing one haplotype), and a 25% chance that they share no HLA haplotypes.

Possible combinations of antigens from different HLA loci on an HLA haplotype are enormous, but some HLA haplotypes are found more frequently than expected by chance in certain populations. This phenomenon is called the linkage disequilibrium. For example, A1, B8, DR3 is the most common HLA haplotype, with a frequency of 5% among Caucasians.

The distribution and frequency of HLA antigens vary greatly among different ethnic groups. It has been postulated that this diversity of HLA polymorphism was derived and evolved by unique selective pressure in different geographic areas. This could be related to the role of the HLA molecule in the presentation of significant infectious agents in the different areas of the world.

Tissue Expression of HLA

HLA class I molecules are expressed on the surface of almost all nucleated cells. They can also be found on red blood cells and platelets. Class I molecules on the red cell surface likely derive from endogenous synthesis by erythroid precursor cells and also from adsorption of soluble antigen present in plasma. The Bg serological specificities in

immunohematology represent various anti-HLA antibodies (see Chapter 9). HLA class I molecules present on the platelet surface probably derive from megakaryocytes and also from adsorption from plasma.

Class II molecules are expressed on B lymphocytes, antigen-presenting cells (monocytes, macrophages, and dendritic cells), and activated T lymphocytes.

Structure and Polymorphism of HLA Molecules

Class I molecules consist of glycosylated heavy chains of 44,000 to 45,000 daltons (44 to 45 kDa) encoded by the HLA genes and a noncovalently bound extracellular 12 kDa β_2- microglobulin $(\beta_2 m)$[5] (Fig. 16.1). Human $\beta_2 m$ is invariant and is encoded by a non-MHC gene. The class I heavy chain has three extracellular domains (α_1, α_2, and α_3), a transmembrane region, and an intracytoplasmic domain. Each extracellular domain comprises about 90 amino acids. The α_1 and α_2 domains contain variable amino acid sequences, and these domains determine the serologic specificities of the HLA class I antigens. Three dimensional structures of the extracellular portion of several HLA class I molecules have been revealed by x-ray crystallography[6] (Fig. 16.2). The heavy chain α_1 and α_2 domains form a unique structure consisting of a platform of eight antiparallel β strands and two antiparallel α-helices on top of the platform (Fig. 16**b**). A groove is formed by the two α-helices and the β-pleated floor, and this is the binding site for processed peptide antigen[2]. The class I peptide binding groove accommodates a processed peptide of 8 to 10 (predominantly nonamers) amino acid residues.[7,8] The α_3 and $\beta_2 m$ domains form immunoglobulin constant domain-like folds (Fig. 16.2**a**).

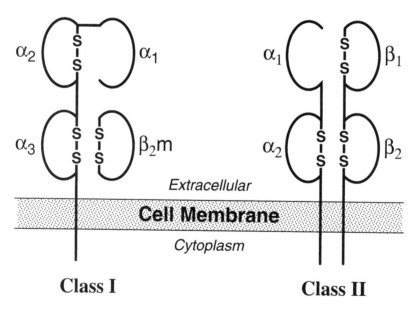

Figure 16.1 Schematic diagram of HLA class I and class II molecules. The class I molecule consists of a heavy chain and a light chain β_2-microglobulin. The class II molecule is a heterodimer consisting of α and β chains. Disulfide bonds are denoted by -s-s-.

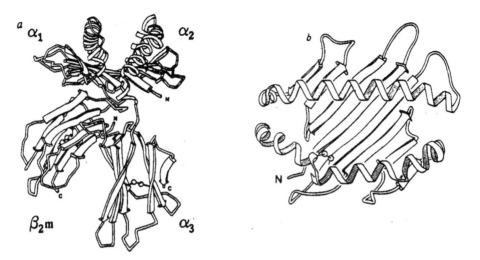

Figure 16.2 Schematic representation of the structure of HLA-A2 molecule. **a,** Extracellular domains of HLA-A2. The polymorphic α_1 and α_2 domains are located at the top and the membrane proximal immunoglobulin-like domains ($\alpha3$ and β_2m) at the bottom. **b,** The domains α_1 and α_2 form a platform with a single eight-stranded β-pleated sheet (shown as thick arrows), covered by two α-helices (represented as helical ribbons). Disulfide bonds are indicated as two connected spheres. N, amino terminus. *(From Bjorkman PJ, Saper MA, Samraoui B, et al. The structure of the human class I histocompatibility antigen, HLA-A2. Nature 1987;329:506–512.)*

The products of the class II genes *DR, DQ,* and *DP* are heterodimers of two non-covalently associated glycosylated polypeptide chains: α (30 to 34 kDa) and β (26 to 29 kDa) (Fig. 16.1). The difference in molecular weights of the α and β chains is primarily due to different glycosylation. The α and β chains are transmembrane and they have the same overall structures. An extracellular portion composed of two domains (α_1 and α_2, or β_1 and β_2) is anchored on the membrane by a short transmembrane region and a cytoplasmic domain. The three-dimensional structure of the HLA-DR molecule is similar to that of the class I molecule.[9] The α_1 and β_1 domains form an antigen-binding groove. The class II groove is more open so that longer peptides (12 amino acids or longer) can be accommodated.[10] The α_2 and β_2 domains are similar to immunoglobulin constant domains.

The HLA system is known to be the most polymorphic in humans. The HLA polymorphism is not evenly spread throughout the molecule but is concentrated in particular regions. The amino acid variation in class I heavy chains is clustered in several regions of the α_1 and α_2 domains.[5] In class II molecules, the extent of variation varies in the subregion and the polypeptide chain. Most polymorphisms occur in the first amino terminal domain of *DRB1, DQB1,* and *DPB1* gene products. Most of the polymorphic positions in the class I and class II molecules are clustered in the antigen-binding groove.[2] Amino acid variations in these positions change the fine shape ("pockets") of the groove and thus the peptide-binding specificity of HLA molecules.[11] This is the structural basis for the binding specificity between HLA molecules and peptides that in turn determines the immune response.

Immunologic Role of HLA Molecules: Peptide Presentation

T cells recognize processed peptides on the cell surface. Zinkernagel and Dougherty demonstrated in 1974 that T lymphocytes must have the same MHC molecules as the antigen-presenting cell to induce immune response.[12] The phenomenon that peptides are bound to MHC molecules and these complexes are recognized on the cell surface by the T-cell receptor is called the MHC restriction. During the T-cell maturation in the thymus, T lymphocytes are educated and selected to recognize the self MHC molecules, and thereafter MHC molecules play a role as determinants of immune response.

The peptide-binding specificities of HLA molecules are determined by a relatively limited number of amino acid residues located in the peptide-binding pockets.[13] Fine structure of these pockets changes depending on the nature of the amino acids within the groove. Different HLA molecules show characteristic amino acid residue patterns in the bound peptides.[11] Amino acid residues that are commonly found at a particular position of the peptides are thought to act as peptide's anchoring residues in the peptide-binding groove.

The nature and source of peptides that will bind to class I or class II molecules are different.[10,14] Class I-restricted T cells recognize endogenous antigens synthesized within the target cell, whereas class II-restricted T cells recognize exogenously derived antigens. Antigen processing involves degrading of the antigen into peptide fragments.[15,16] Cellular or virus-induced proteins are processed by the cytoplasmic proteasome complex. Proteasomes are multi-subunit proteinase complexes, and two genes (*LMP2* and *LMP7*) encoding components of the proteasomes are located within the class II region.[3] The resulting peptide fragments are transported into the endoplasmic reticulum (ER), and this process is mediated by the transmembrane peptide transporters. Two genes (*TAP1* and *TAP2*) located within the class III region encode members of the ATP-binding cassette (ABC) transmembrane transporter of antigen peptide (TAP). The ABC superfamily proteins transport peptides across cellular membranes in an ATP-dependent manner. Within the ER, peptides associate with newly synthesized class I molecules. The antigen-binding groove of class I molecules is closed at both ends and the optimal size of peptides appears to be usually nonamers (nine amino acids). The peptide-bound class I molecules are transported to the cell surface via the Golgi apparatus, and the complex is recognized by the T-cell receptor of CD8+ lymphocytes.

Class II expression is mainly restricted to the antigen-presenting cells (APCs), including B cells, monocytes/macrophages, dendritic cells, and Langerhans cells. Specialized APCs are capable of stimulating T-cell division. Class II molecules on the APC surface present exogenously derived antigens to CD4+ helper T cells.[16] Newly synthesized class II αβ heterodimer chains are complexed to a 31 kDa polypeptide called the invariant I (Ii) chain in the ER. The Ii chain is encoded by a non-MHC gene and prevents binding of the αβ heterodimers to peptides present in the ER. The class II αβ-Ii complex is transported through the Golgi complex to an acidic endosomal compartment, where the Ii chain is released. This dissociation of Ii from the αβ heterodimer permits binding of peptides into the peptide-binding groove. Class II molecules are presenting antigens originated from an exogenous source. Extracellular exogenous proteins are endocytosed and undergo degradation in the acidic endosomal compartment.

Class II molecules accommodate relatively longer peptides, usually 12 or longer, because both ends of their peptide-binding grooves are open.[17] After class II molecule-peptide complex is transported to the APC surface, the complex is recognized by the T-cell receptor of CD4+ lymphocytes.

There are two forms of T-cell receptor (TCR): polypeptide heterodimers composed of disulfide-linked subunits of either αβ or γδ[18,19] The αβ TCR is present on more than 95% of peripheral blood T cells. The TCR molecule is associated on the cell surface with a complex of polypeptides, CD3. The amino acid sequence variability of the TCR resides in the amino terminal domains of the α and β chains. This domain is encoded by rearranging V, D, and J gene segments. During the recognition process between TCR and HLA-peptide complex, accessory molecules on T lymphocytes are enhancing the interaction between T lymphocytes and HLA molecules. The CD4 molecule interacts with a class II molecule on the APC, and the CD8 molecule interacts with a class I heavy chain on the target cells.

CLINICAL HLA TYPING

Laboratories involved in clinical HLA typing have been called by various names: HLA laboratory, tissue typing laboratory, histocompatibility laboratory, or clinical immuno-genetics laboratory. HLA testing in the transplant workup includes HLA typing of the recipient and the donor, screening and identification of preformed HLA antibodies in the recipient, and detection of antibodies of the recipient that are reactive with lymphocytes of a prospective donor (crossmatch).

Serologic Typing of HLA Antigens

The complement-mediated microlymphocytotoxicity technique[20,21] has been used as the standard for serologic typing of HLA class I and class II antigens. HLA typing sera are mainly obtained from multiparous alloimmunized women, and their HLA specificities are determined against a panel of cells with known HLA antigens. Some mono-clonal antibody reagents are also used.

Peripheral blood lymphocytes (PBLs) express HLA class I antigens and are used for the serologic typing of HLA-A, HLA-B, and HLA-C. HLA class II typing is done with isolated B lymphocytes because these cells express class II molecules. PBLs are commonly isolated by density-gradient separation; various techniques are available to isolate B lymphocytes, including monoclonal antibody-coated magnetic beads. HLA typing is performed in multiwell plastic trays with each well containing a serum of known HLA specificities. Lymphocytes are placed in the well and incubated, and com-plement is added to mediate the lysis of antibody-bound cells. The common source of complement is rabbit. Cell lysis can be detected by eosin staining or, more recently, by fluorescence dye staining.

When a serum shows reactivity with only one antigen, the antibody is called mono-specific and the antigen specificity is called private. Some antibody molecules can be

reactive with two or more distinct antigens if the antigens share a same or similar antigenic determinant. Antigenic determinants shared by two or more antigens are called public specificities. Since the HLA polymorphism is formed by a patchwork of variable sequences shared by different antigens,[5] public specificities are commonly encountered. Cross-reactivity is observed when a number of antigens share an antigenic determinant. A cluster of antigens sharing antigenic determinants are called a cross-reactive group (CREG).

Formal assignments of serologically defined antigens are given by the World Health Organization HLA Nomenclature Committee, which is responsible for the nomenclature of the HLA system.[4] HLA antigens are designated alphabetically by the locus and numerically by the order of assignment. HLA-C antigens are given the designation Cw to avoid confusion with complement components. HLA alleles are designated by the locus followed by an asterisk, a two-digit number corresponding to the antigen specificity, and the assigned allele number. For example, *HLA-A*0210* represents the tenth assigned allele within the serologically defined HLA-A2 antigen family.

Molecular Typing of HLA Alleles

Recent studies of the HLA system using monoclonal antibodies, electrophoretic gel analysis, cellular assay, and molecular techniques have revealed that the extent of HLA polymorphism is far higher than previously known antigen specificities (Table 16.1). Serologically undistinguishable variants or subtypes of HLA class I antigens were identified, and it was demonstrated that these variants are different from the wild type by a few (one to five) amino acids, but these can be recognized by alloreactive or MHC-restricted T lymphocytes.[22,23] Clinical molecular typing has been developed to distinguish serologically undistinguishable but functionally discrete HLA alleles.

Molecular HLA typing of class II genes began in the mid-1980s. The first technique used was a restriction fragment length polymorphism (RFLP) Southern blotting analysis. RFLP analysis is based on DNA sequence polymorphism that can be detected by restriction endonucleases recognizing and cutting specific DNA sequences. The lim-

Table 16.1 Numbers of recognized private antigen specificities and alleles

Locus	Antigen specificities	Alleles
HLA-A	24	82
HLA-B	55	174
HLA-C	9	38
HLA-DR*	17	165
Total	105	459

*Private antigen specificities, DR1–DR18, determined by *DRB1* alleles.

itation in the RFLP analysis is that the number of restriction sites recognized by a given enzyme is limited in the gene, and thus only a few selected sequence polymorphisms are detected. Furthermore, detected DNA polymorphism may reside in the coding region or noncoding region, and the polymorphism in the latter region is not relevant. RFLP analysis is no longer used for clinical typing.

The polymerase chain reaction (PCR) using thermostable DNA polymerase, called *Taq* I polymerase, became available to amplify and study HLA genes.[24] Synthetic oligonucleotide primers were designed to initiate DNA amplification of specific HLA genes. Resulting PCR products have been sequenced, and the accumulated data established the HLA allele sequence database. PCR-based clinical HLA typing was first developed using sequence-specific oligonucleotide probe (SSOP) methods.[25] The hypervariable exon 2 sequences encoding the first amino terminal domains of the *DRB1, DQB1,* and *DPB1* genes are amplified from genomic DNA by PCR reaction. Based on the HLA sequence database, a panel of synthetic oligonucleotide sequences corresponding to variable regions of the gene are designed and used as SSOP in hybridization with the amplified PCR products. Alternatively, polymorphic DNA sequences can be used as amplification primers, and in this case only alleles containing sequences complementary to these primers will anneal to the primers and amplification will proceed. This strategy of DNA typing is called the sequence-specific primer (SSP) method, and it detects sequence polymorphism at given areas by the presence of a particular amplified DNA fragment.

The development of molecular HLA class I typing has been much behind that of class II. The class I polymorphism is located in the two domains of α_1 and α_2, and there are many more polymorphic sequences than in class II. These differences make it more challenging to develop typing strategies for class I.

There are different levels of resolution in molecular HLA typing. High-resolution DNA typing usually means the typing of HLA at the allele level. Low-resolution DNA typing indicates that the results given are equivalent to either private or public antigen specificities. Intermediate- or medium-resolution typing may be defined as equivalent to private antigen specificities. At present, high-resolution DR typing is routinely used to support unrelated donor marrow transplantation.[26]

Cellular Typing

The mixed lymphocyte culture (MLC) test is performed by mixing peripheral blood mononuclear cells from two individuals in vitro and observing cellular proliferation.[27] HLA class II disparity between individuals is responsible for the stimulation of lymphocytes. The one-way MLC test is performed by mixing responder T cells with irradiated stimulator cells. After 5 or 6 days, response of the responder's cells is indicated by increased DNA synthesis, usually by measuring incorporation of tritiated thymidine into the DNA. Reactive MLC results indicate HLA-D region incompatibility. The MLC technique has also been used to type cellularly defined HLA-D specificities using HLA-D region homozygous typing cells as stimulators. These cellular typing techniques for class II region compatibility have now been replaced by the high-resolution class II allele typing in the clinical laboratory.[28]

Cell-mediated lympholysis or cytotoxic T lymphocyte assay can demonstrate the in vitro killing effect of sensitized T lymphocytes against allogeneic cells. The cytotoxic effect mainly represents HLA class I disparity. The target lymphocytes are radiolabeled with ^{51}Cr, and the cytotoxic effect is measured by the release of ^{51}Cr after culture of the two lymphocyte populations. This assay was once tried in an attempt to predict the risk of acute graft versus host disease (GVHD) in marrow transplantation,[29] but its clinical use has not been proved.

HLA Antibody Screening and Lymphocyte Crossmatch

Preformed HLA antibodies can be detected by testing the patient's serum against a panel of lymphocytes with known HLA specificities. The complement-mediated microlymphocytotoxicity technique has been the standard, but the anti-human globulin method provides higher sensitivity.[30] This test is called HLA antibody screening and the results are expressed as the percentage of the panel cells that are reactive; this is called the panel reactive antibody percentage (%PRA). For instance, if 10 of 40 different panel cells are reactive with a serum, the PRA is 25%. With a panel of well-selected cells representing various HLA antigens, antibody specificities can be assigned. This information is particularly important for the prospective organ transplant recipient to predict the chance of finding a compatible or crossmatch-negative cadaver donor and to avoid specific mismatched HLA antigens in the donor. When a potential donor becomes available, a final donor crossmatch is performed between the recipient's serum and the donor's lymphocytes to determine the compatibility. The positive crossmatch results are predictive of the risk of graft rejection.[31]

In recent years, a lymphocyte crossmatch using flow cytometry has been developed and used clinically.[32] This technique presumably offers higher sensitivity, but it remains to be determined whether flow cytometric crossmatching would be more predictive of allograft rejection with higher specificity.

THE HUMAN MINOR HISTOCOMPATIBILITY ANTIGENS

Minor histocompatibility antigens are processed peptides naturally derived from normal cellular proteins that associate with HLA molecules.[33] Minor histocompatibility antigens are inherited and have allelic forms. The number of minor histocompatibility loci is probably high, and the extent of polymorphism for each locus is not known. Minor histocompatibility antigens have been defined by both class I and class II MHC-restricted T cells. Examples include the male-specific H-Y antigen and a series of HA antigens.

Non-HLA minor histocompatibility antigens may affect the outcome of solid organ and marrow transplants.[34] Minor histocompatibility antigen disparity may be associated with GVHD in HLA-identical transplants (e.g., H-Y antigen in a male recipient and a female donor who has been immunized by pregnancy). Whether minor histocompatibility antigen disparity can have an impact as a risk factor for graft rejection or GVHD might depend on the tissue-specific expression of proteins, the frequency of allelic

forms, and the immunogenicity of peptides. Some minor histocompatibility antigens show restricted tissue distribution for expression.[33]

THE HLA SYSTEM AND TRANSPLANTATION

HLA-A, HLA-B, and HLA-DR are currently known as major transplantation antigens. The role of HLA-C and other class II antigens remains to be further studied.

Both T-cell and B-cell (antibody) immune responses are important in graft rejection.[35] T lymphocytes recognize donor-derived peptides in association with the HLA molecules on the graft.[36] The graft may present different allelic forms of the minor histocompatibility antigens, and the donor's HLA molecules may present a different set of peptides to the recipient's T-cells. CD4+ T helper cells are activated by APCs carrying HLA class II molecules. The APCs from either the donor or the recipient can activate the recipient's T-cells. The donor's APCs present in the graft cause the "direct" activation of the recipient's T helper cells. The recipient's APCs can acquire alloantigens that are shed from the graft, process into peptides, and present to T helper cells to cause the "indirect" activation. Direct activation has a more important role in inducing rejection. Various lymphokines are involved in the rejection response: interleukin (IL)-2, IL-4, IL-5, IL-6, interferon-γ, and tumor necrosis factor β.[35]

Antibodies to the graft fix complement and cause damage to the vascular endothelium, resulting in hemorrhage, platelet aggregation, and thrombosis. Hyperacute rejection occurs in patients who already have antibodies specific to a graft. Antibodies against ABO blood group and preformed HLA antibodies induce this rejection. HLA alloimmunization can be induced by blood transfusions, pregnancies, or failed transplants. Hyperacute rejection can be avoided in most cases by ABO-identical or compatible transplantation and by performing lymphocyte crossmatching.[31] Acute rejection is primarily the result of T cell-mediated response. Chronic rejection may be due to antibody and cell-mediated responses.

Solid Organ Transplantation

Solid organs can be donated by cadaveric donors, living related donors, or living unrelated donors. Cadaveric donors are brain dead but are maintained hemodynamically stable until the time of organ harvest. Living unrelated donors and most related donors are for kidneys. About one-third of transplanted kidneys nationwide are from living related donors: siblings, parents, or grown-up children. Other organs from living related donors are lung (segmentectomy or lobectomy), pancreas (hemipancreatectomy), liver (segmentectomy), or small intestine. Transplant success can be measured by several factors: rejection, graft survival, half-life of transplanted organ, and patient survival.

The United Network for Organ Sharing (UNOS) administers organ procurement and allocation and monitors national policies for transplantation.[37] Evaluation of potential donors is done by taking the donor's history and performing a physical examination and laboratory testing for infectious disease markers, organ function, and HLA typing

with samples of peripheral blood, lymph nodes, or spleen. There are general and organ-specific criteria for the acceptance of donors,[38] and the final decision on the suitability of donor organs is made by the transplantation programs. Local or regional organ procurement organizations are responsible for acquiring and allocating solid organs. Increasing numbers of patients are waiting for cadaveric organs, and the national waiting list on the UNOS as of June 1997 exceeds 50,000.[39] The UNOS has developed separate allocation policies for different types of solid organ.[38]

All potential transplant candidates are registered with the UNOS. Each patient is HLA typed and evaluated for various clinical conditions, and each individual is given a numeric score. When a cadaver becomes available, HLA typing is performed, and the results are compared with those of the waiting patients on the national list. When a six-antigen matched patient is identified, the kidney is offered to that patient. Cases of no mismatched HLA antigens in the rejection direction (donors homozygous for HLA antigens) are considered the same as a six-antigen match. This policy has been implemented based on clinical experience showing the best transplant results in these categories.[40] When there is no such "perfect" match, the kidneys are usually offered to patients with the highest score within the local organ procurement area. The UNOS algorithm for allocating kidneys takes into account the waiting time, the degree of HLA matching between donor and recipient, HLA alloimmunization, and age. Prepubertal patients and those with high HLA alloimmunization (80% or higher PRA) are given preference. Prospective HLA matching is done only for kidneys and pancreas. Allocation of livers and hearts is based primarily on medical urgency and waiting time. Pretransplantation crossmatching is requested by the transplantation program. Other factors influencing the allocation of organs include the preservation time and the size of the organ.[38] Organ preservation is important to prevent significant ischemic changes. Organs are allocated first within the area, then within the UNOS region, and finally at the national level. The complex system of solid organ procurement and allocation was developed to increase the supply of organs and ensure their equitable distribution under conditions of limited donor organ supply.[37]

In solid organ transplantation, blood group ABO system is the most important major histocompatibility antigen.[41] Preexisting anti-A and anti-B antibodies cause hyperacute rejection because ABO antigens are expressed on endothelial cells. Kidney transplantation is performed only from ABO-identical or compatible donors. Preformed HLA antibodies also cause hyperacute rejection.[31] The problem of hyperacute rejection can be predicted by a positive donor lymphocyte crossmatch and can be prevented when transplantation is performed from a donor whose lymphocytes are not reactive with recipient's serum. The presence in the recipient of preformed HLA antibodies reactive with a donor's lymphocytes is a contraindication to kidney transplantation. Even though transplant candidates awaiting a heart or a liver are screened for HLA antibodies, prospective lymphocyte crossmatching with a donor is not universally performed for these patients because of the urgent need of organs and the uncertain benefits of a cross-match-negative donor.[31]

The benefits of HLA matching are well established in renal transplantation. There is a clear relationship between the degree of HLA matching and kidney graft survival

in transplants from living related donors.[42] Better results are obtained from an HLA-identical sibling donor than with HLA-haploidentical parents, siblings, or children. Kidney transplantation from a living unrelated donor, usually a spouse, shows graft survival superior to cadaveric transplantation (except for six-antigen match) despite a greater degree of HLA mismatch.[43] These favorable results are probably the result of shorter ischemic time and less renal damage.

The influence of HLA matching on the survival of liver and thoracic organs is yet uncertain, even though there is some evidence that the outcome of heart transplantation may be influenced by the degree of HLA matching.

Immunomodulatory effect of transfusion   Red cell transfusions had been given to end-stage renal failure patients with chronic anemia. In spite of a risk of developing alloimmunization against HLA, some transfused patients had better allograft survival.[44] The beneficial effect of pretransplant blood transfusion was the basis for the implementation of a protocol of donor-specific transfusion (DST) prior to renal transplantation from a living related donor in an attempt to induce tolerance while waiting for a transplant. DST for living related donor transplants resulted in better outcomes, especially when the donor and recipient shared at least one HLA haplotype or one DR antigen.[45] The beneficial effect of pretransplant blood transfusion has also been documented in patients receiving transfusions from random donors.

DST carries a risk of sensitization of the patients, and some do develop antibodies against HLA antigens and thus cannot receive the planned transplant because of the risk of hyperacute rejection. Since cyclosporine was introduced as an immunosuppressive drug, it significantly increased graft survival and now no significant differences are found in the graft survival rates between the transfused and nontransfused recipients of cadaveric kidneys. The use of recombinant human erythropoietin reduced or eliminated the need for red cell transfusion, and as a result, the primary HLA sensitization in uremic patients has diminished (see Chapter 17).

Immunomodulatory mechanisms of transfusion are not clearly understood, but the effect could be due to multiple factors (see Chapter 14). Probably leukocytes contained in the red cell components are involved in the transfusion effects. Possible mechanisms include induction or activation of suppressor cells, induction of anergy, selective activation of TH2 cells, enhancing antibodies (blocking recognition of specific donor antigens), negative selection of nonimmune responders, provision of soluble HLA antigen, and clonal deletion.[46]

Recently, donor bone marrow infusion at the time of cadaveric organ transplantation has been tried to facilitate hematopoietic microchimerism and tolerance.[47] It is not known whether this may predispose the recipient to develop GVHD in certain cases of one-way HLA match.

Allogeneic Bone Marrow Transplantation

Allogeneic marrow transplantation is used to treat hematologic malignancy, severe aplastic anemia, congenital severe immunodeficiencies, and selected inherited meta-

bolic diseases.[48] The source of hematopoietic stem cells has traditionally been bone marrow, but recent alternatives are mobilized peripheral blood stem or progenitor cells and umbilical cord blood.

ABO blood group incompatibility is not a clinically significant barrier to stem cell transplantation (see Chapter 12). The HLA system is the major histocompatibility antigen in stem cell transplants. HLA-A, HLA-B, and HLA-DR are considered for HLA matching, and the degree of HLA matching is predictive of the clinical outcome.[49] HLA mismatch between a recipient and a marrow donor represents a risk factor not only for graft rejection or failure but also for acute GVHD because immunocompetent donor T-cells are introduced to the recipient, who is in a highly immunosuppressed state. T-cell depletion of donor marrow results in lower incidence of acute GVHD[50] but higher incidence of graft failure, graft rejection, and later complication of Epstein-Barr virus-associated lymphoproliferative disorders.[51,52]

The rate of graft rejection or failure is especially higher in patients with severe aplastic anemia because these patients are frequently alloimmunized by multiple blood transfusions and their preconditioning regimen is less intensive than that for leukemia.[53]

The best compatible stem cells are from an identical twin and a genotypically HLA-identical sibling. An HLA-identical sibling is found in approximately 30% of patients. For those who do not have a matched sibling, an alternative related family member who is HLA haploidentical and partially mismatched for the nonshared HLA haplotypes may serve as a donor, but these transplants have a higher risk of developing acute GVHD and graft rejection or failure.[49]

When an HLA-matched or partially mismatched acceptable related donor is not available, phenotypically matched unrelated donors can be considered.[54] The National Marrow Donor Program (NMDP) was founded in the United States in 1987 to establish a volunteer marrow donor registry[55] and to serve as a source of HLA-matched unrelated marrow donors.[56] The chance of finding an HLA-matched unrelated donor depends on the patient's HLA phenotype.[57] Since there is high diversity of HLA polymorphism among different race groups, there is a different chance of finding a match within different race groups. Volunteer donors were initially HLA-A, B typed at the time of registration, and HLA-A, B matched selected donors for a patient are further HLA-DR typed. The NMDP registry now contains more than 2.8 million donors, and more than one-third of them have been HLA-DR typed. The NMDP has coordinated more than 5,900 unrelated marrow donations. There are also international marrow donor registries in other countries, and most of these registries share their donors.

HLA-matched unrelated donor transplants are associated with an increased incidence of acute GVHD compared to HLA-matched sibling transplants. Such an increase may result partly from mismatch in untested HLA alleles or from non-HLA minor histocompatibility antigens. For this reason, *HLA-DRB1* allele typing is strongly recommended for phenotypically matched unrelated donor transplants.[26] It has been shown that about 20% of HLA-A, B, DR antigen matched patient-unrelated donor pairs are indeed mismatched for *DRB1* alleles, and a *DRB1* allele mismatch results in a higher incidence of acute GVHD.

Transfusion practice in stem cell transplantation   Transfusion from blood relatives should be avoided for a patient who is a candidate for a stem cell transplant. The minor histocompatibility antigens are inherited independently of the MHC region, and thus any transfusions from blood relatives could lead to an exposure to possibly relevant antigens.

Tissue Transplantation

HLA disparity is a barrier to skin allografting. Human skin allograft is usually rejected by the recipient, but these allografts provide temporary coverage until sufficient auto-graft skin is available.[58] HLA does not seem to play a major role in the clinical trans-plantation of freeze-dried and frozen bone, corneas, and human heart valves.

THE HLA SYSTEM IN TRANSFUSION THERAPY

The HLA system can cause adverse immunologic effects in transfusion therapy. These effects are primarily mediated by "passenger" donor leukocytes contained in the cellular blood components. HLA antibodies can be induced from previous alloimmunization episodes and can cause platelet immune refractoriness, febrile transfusion reaction, and transfusion-related acute lung injury.

HLA Alloimmunization

Primary HLA alloimmunization by blood transfusion is caused by the leukocytes in the cellular blood products.[59] Multiparous women are frequently alloimmunized to HLA. HLA antibodies found in alloimmunized patients are usually broadly reactive. It is more common to find broadly specific antibodies instead of multiple antibodies of private specificities in patients with high PRA. HLA antibodies may disappear with time.

The incidence of HLA alloimmunization following transfusions can vary with the patient's diagnosis and therapy.[60] HLA antibodies can be detected in 25% to 30% of transfused leukemic patients and can be present in as high as 80% of aplastic anemia patients. Leukemic patients are usually transfused while receiving intensive chemotherapy, which induces immunosuppression and this reduces the incidence of transfusion-induced alloimmunization. Severe aplastic anemia patients who had received blood transfusions have a higher incidence of graft rejection following marrow transplantations.[61]

Leukocyte reduction to less than 5×10^6 can prevent or reduce the development of primary HLA alloimmunization.[62] Leukoreduction can be achieved for platelets and red blood cell components by the use of third-generation leukocyte reduction filters (see Chapters 12, 13 and 14). Leukoreduced platelet products can be specially collected from certain models of apheresis equipment (see Chapter 7). The incidence of HLA alloimmunization, however, is not decreased or delayed by the leukocyte reduction filtration in patients with previous pregnancies.[63] It appears that the secondary HLA immune response cannot be prevented by the degree of leukocyte reduction currently available.

Refractoriness to Platelet Transfusion

Platelet transfusions are given to prevent or stop microvascular bleeding in patients with thrombocytopenia or platelet dysfunction. Prophylactic platelet transfusion is usually indicated to maintain the platelet count higher than 10 or 20×10^9/L to prevent serious spontaneous hemorrhage (see Chapter 11). Every platelet transfusion should be followed by a clinical evaluation (changes in the status of bleeding) and platelet counts. Ideally platelet count monitoring should be done immediately before the transfusion, 10 minutes to 1 hour after the transfusion (measuring peak recovery after splenic pooling), and 24 hours later (representing survival of transfused platelets). Because the number of platelets per unit varies, accurate calculation of expected posttransfusion increments is impossible. A clinically useful crude estimate of expected 1-hour posttransfusion platelet count is an increment of 50,000/μL when the usual dose of one platelet concentrate per 10 kg of body weight or one platelet apheresis product in an average-sized adult is given.

Platelet refractoriness is a consistently inadequate response to platelet transfusions (see Chapter 11). There are immune and nonimmune causes for poor posttransfusion increments.[64,65] The major nonimmune adverse factors are fever, splenomegaly/hypersplenism, antibiotics (amphotericin B, vancomycin, ciprofloxacin), disseminated intravascular coagulation, infection/sepsis, marrow transplantation, venoocclusive disease, and bleeding at the time of transfusion. Practically, platelet immune refractoriness can be suspected if the 1 hour posttransfusion platelet recovery is less than 20% of expected platelet recovery and there are no known nonimmune adverse factors.

HLA class I antigens are expressed on platelets (see Chapter 9) and the development of antibodies to HLA or platelet-specific antigens can cause immune destruction of platelets, resulting in a refractoriness to random-donor platelet transfusions. Definite diagnosis of platelet immune refractoriness is confirmed if antibodies against HLA or platelet-specific antigens are detected, the platelet increment is unsatisfactory, and nonimmune causes of platelet refractoriness are ruled out. When patients are suspected for immune refractoriness, HLA antibody screening is done. Platelet-specific antibodies should be considered in all patients who are refractory to HLA-matched platelets. Platelet-specific and HLA antibodies can be distinguished in platelet assays.[66] Most patients are immunized to HLA, and immunization to platelet-specific antigens is much less frequent.

Once the clinical and laboratory diagnosis of immune refractoriness is made, the use of special platelet products is indicated (see Chapter 11). Most patients who are refractory to random donor platelets because of HLA antibodies respond to HLA-matched platelets.[64] Some regional blood centers maintain large pools of HLA-A, B typed volunteer platelet apheresis donors. Patients with common HLA types will have a higher chance of receiving platelets from HLA-matched donors. For many recipients who require frequent platelet transfusions, it is not possible to find enough perfectly matched donors. Constraints of time and donor availability can also be problematic. It usually takes at least 2 days to recruit donors, collect platelets, and complete infectious disease marker studies. HLA-matched siblings or HLA-haploidentical family members can donate platelets by apheresis, but to prevent alloimmunization to minor his-

tocompatibility antigens, these donors should not support patients who are candidates for a stem cell transplant. If the specificity of the patient's antibodies can be determined, donors who are negative for corresponding HLA antigens can be selected. Crossmatching the patient's serum against donor lymphocytes can also be used to identify compatible donors. Community blood donors who are mismatched with the patients for cross-reactive HLA antigens can also be tried, but most of the benefit derives from platelets well matched for HLA.[67] Transfusions of closely HLA-matched platelets to refractory patients are not always effective.

A number of techniques have been tried to detect platelet antibodies, but most of them have not been practical for large-scale routine use.[68] Platelet crossmatching using a solid-phase red cell adherence technique has been developed.[69,70] This technique will detect platelet antibodies against HLA class I and platelet-specific antigens. Collected single-donor platelet apheresis units are crossmatched with the patient's serum, and crossmatch-compatible units are identified. The efficacy of crossmatched platelets may not be as good as perfectly HLA-matched platelets, but this approach appears to be effective in some patients.[67]

Other approaches to the management of platelet refractoriness include use of ABO-identical platelets, fresh platelets, corticosteroids, intravenous immunoglobulin, plasma exchange, staphylococcal protein A column immunoadsorption, and removal of HLA antigens by acid treatment (see Chapter 11). In the near future, thrombopoietin or recombinant human megakaryocyte growth and development factor may shorten the thrombocytopenic period and increase the platelet counts in patients undergoing chemotherapy (see Chapter 17).

Since primary HLA alloimmunization caused by platelet transfusion is induced by contaminating leukocytes,[59] this potential problem can be prevented or delayed by the use of the third-generation leukoreduction filter.[63] In patients with previous pregnancies, leukocyte reduction does not reduce the incidence of platelet refractoriness and HLA antibodies. Most previously pregnant patients appear to develop HLA antibodies by a secondary immune response during transfusion therapy. Platelets per se, soluble HLA antigens, microparticles, or leukocyte fragments escaping leukocyte filtration may be able to induce a secondary HLA immune response.[63] Prevention of alloimmunization would be highly desirable at least for some selected patients who have not been previously immunized by transfusion or pregnancy and are expected to need long-term platelet transfusions.[71]

Ultraviolet B (UVB) (wavelength 280 to 320 nm) irradiation can reduce primary HLA alloimmunization.[72] UVB irradiation interferes with the function of APC, thus preventing the alloantigen presentation to the recipient's T helper cells. It is not known whether UVB irradiation can prevent a secondary HLA immune response.

Transfusion-Associated Graft versus Host Disease

When functionally competent allogeneic T lymphocytes are transfused into an individual who is severely immunocompromised, these T lymphocytes are not removed and mount an immune attack against the recipient's cells, causing transfusion-associated graft versus host disease (TA-GVHD) (see Chapter 11). TA-GVHD is not common and

typically occurs in patients with congenital or acquired immunodeficiencies or immunosuppression that affects lymphocytes .

TA-GVHD has also been reported in patients without apparent evidence of immunodeficiency or immunosuppression.[73] The majority of these studied cases involved a blood donor who was homozygous for one or more HLA loci for which the recipient was heterozygous for the same antigen and a different one.[74] This relationship can be called a one-way HLA mismatch in the GVHD direction and a one-way HLA match in the rejection direction. As a result, the donor's cells will not be recognized as foreign by the recipient's lymphocytes, while the donor's lymphocytes will recognize foreign HLA antigens present in the recipient. Other risk factors that appear to predispose to TA-GVHD in immunocompetent patients possibly include fresh blood, family-directed donation, and Japanese heritage, although the latter two factors probably reflect the HLA homozygous donor.[73] Many affected patients received transfusions of freshly donated cellular blood products. Fresh blood contains larger numbers of viable and presumably competent lymphocytes than stored blood. The minimum number of viable donor lymphocytes required to mediate TA-GVHD is unknown. The one-way match more likely occurs when an HLA haplotype is shared by a donor and a recipient (HLA haploidentical), such as in directed donation from blood relatives and among populations with relatively homogeneous HLA phenotypes.[74] The latter possibility may account for the observation that more cases of TA-GVHD have been reported among Japanese patients.

The clinical features of TA-GVHD are similar to those of GVHD following a marrow transplant; i.e., fever, skin rash, diarrhea, and abnormal liver function. TA-GVHD is further characterized by prominent pancytopenia due to marrow aplasia. Demonstration of donor-derived lymphocytes in the circulation of a patient with characteristic clinical findings is diagnostic for TA-GVHD. The presence of donor lymphocytes can be tested by conventional or DNA-based HLA typing, by cytogenetic analysis if donor and patient are of different sexes, and by other molecular techniques. The demonstration of donor-derived lymphohematopoietic cells in a transfusion recipient is not diagnostic of TA-GVHD per se, because donor lymphocytes can be detected in the recipient's circulation a few days after transfusion.

There is no effective treatment for TA-GVHD, and most affected patients die within 3 weeks from complications of infections and hemorrhage. Rare survivors may develop chronic GVHD.

The primary emphasis in TA-GVHD is prevention.[75] Gamma irradiation of cellular blood products with 25 Gy is the effective way of inactivating donor lymphocytes (see Chapter 11). Sources of gamma irradiation in the blood bank laboratory are ^{137}Cs and ^{60}Co. Irradiation is indicated for susceptible patients with various conditions—e.g., congenital immunodeficiencies, hematopoietic stem cell transplants (both allogeneic and autologous), hematologic malignancies or lymphoproliferative diseases undergoing chemotherapy—and for patients receiving intrauterine transfusion, HLA-matched platelets, or blood components donated from a blood relative. Solid organ transplant recipients and patients undergoing cytotoxic chemotherapy and radiation therapy for solid tumors probably do not require irradiated blood products.[76] GVHD can occur following transplantation of solid organs, but this is more likely mediated by passenger

T lymphocytes present in the transplanted organ than by blood transfusions. TA-GVHD has not been observed in patients with acquired immunodeficiency syndrome.

Gamma irradiation inactivates lymphocytes, but platelets and granulocytes are not functionally impaired by the dose used. Red blood cells sustain detectable damage, and the storage time for irradiated red cells is limited to 28 days. Extracellular potassium levels are significantly elevated in red blood cells with storage.

UVB irradiation may become an alternative way to inactivate lymphocytes in blood components. UVB irradiation has a potential of preventing both TA-GVHD and HLA alloimmunization.[72] Reduction of lymphocytes from blood products using the currently available leukoreduction filter is not effective in preventing TA-GVHD.

Febrile Nonhemolytic Transfusion Reaction

Febrile nonhemolytic transfusion reaction (FNHTR) is defined as a temperature rise of more than 1°C or 2°F during or shortly after the transfusion (see Chapter 14). Fever can be accompanied by chills, and chills in the absence of fever can be considered as a minor febrile reaction. Fever and chills are the most common reactions, observed in up to 5% of transfused patients.

FNHTR is caused by either an interaction between the recipient's antileukocyte antibodies (usually anti-HLA and less commonly neutrophil-specific) and donor leukocytes contained in the blood components or pyrogenic cytokines present in the blood components. Alloimmunization to leukocytes occurs commonly in previously pregnant or multiply transfused patients, and they are at higher risk of developing the reaction. A number of cytokines—TNF-α, IL-1β, IL-6, and IL-8—are released from leukocytes during the storage of platelets at room temperature, and these cytokines have pyrogenic effects.[77,78] FNHTR is frequently associated with transfusions of platelets stored for more than 3 days (see Chapter 14). Febrile reactions to platelet transfusions may be associated with alloimmunization and poor posttransfusion platelet recoveries.

Repeated FNHTR occurs in approximately 15% of transfusions, and thus preventive measures are usually not considered for patients with a first reaction. Premedication with acetaminophen can prevent or minimize FNHTR. Leukoreduction to a level of 5×10^8 or less in RBC components prevents most FNHTR. Leukoreduction of stored platelets is not effective to prevent a febrile reaction, but prestorage leukoreduced platelets have reduced cytokine release during storage and less frequently cause FNHTR.[79] Fresh platelet products with lower amounts of pyrogenic cytokines can be an alternative for patients with repeated febrile reactions. Slower infusion of blood products can be helpful in minimizing the reaction. FNHTR is treated with acetaminophen; severe shaking chills are treated with meperidine.

Granulocyte Transfusion

Granulocyte transfusions are discussed in Chapter 11. Granulocyte concentrates contain other white blood cells and significant numbers of platelets and RBCs. Granulocyte products contain high numbers of lymphocytes and thus should be irradiated to prevent TA-GVHD. Because of the significant amounts of RBCs, granulocytes should be

obtained from an ABO-compatible donor, and red cell crossmatch should be tested with the recipient's serum. Cytomegalovirus (CMV) seronegative donors are preferred to prevent transfusion-transmitted CMV infection for neonates and patients at risk of developing serious CMV disease.

There is no effective pretransfusion compatibility test for granulocytes. HLA matching or lymphocyte crossmatch is recommended if the patient is known to be alloimmunized, because alloantibodies limit the effectiveness of granulocyte transfusion and can cause a severe febrile transfusion reaction.[80] Granulocyte transfusion can induce alloimmunization, which in turn will decrease future transfusion effectiveness.

Transfusion-Related Acute Lung Injury

Cardiogenic pulmonary edema associated with transfusions is most frequently caused by heart failure secondary to hypervolemia, especially in very young or old patients. Transfusion-related acute lung injury (TRALI) is a rare complication of transfusion resulting in noncardiogenic pulmonary edema.[81,82] TRALI is characterized by acute respiratory distress, bilateral pulmonary edema, and severe hypoxemia. Fever and hypotension may be present. Chest x-ray reveals bilateral pulmonary infiltrates (see also Chapter 14).

TRALI is caused by HLA antibodies or leukoagglutinins that react with leukocytes.[81] The antigen-antibody reaction probably activates complement, resulting in neutrophil aggregation and sequestration in the lung. The release of neutrophil granules leads to pulmonary vascular damage and extravasation of fluid into the alveoli and interstitium. Implicated antibodies are usually found in the plasma of blood components,[81] and these were probably induced by previous transfusions or pregnancies in the donor. Demonstration of the HLA specificity of the donor's antibody against the patient's HLA antigens is direct evidence for TRALI. Less commonly, implicated antibodies are found in the recipient.

When respiratory distress occurs, transfusion is stopped and respiratory support with oxygen is provided. Most patients have resolution of their symptoms within 12 to 24 hours, and the bilateral pulmonary infiltrates clear within a few days. Leukocyte reduction can be effective to prevent TRALI when the recipient is found to have antibodies, but it is not helpful if the antibodies are from plasma of the blood donor. All blood donors implicated with a TRALI case should be deferred from the preparation of plasma-containing blood products.

Neonatal Alloimmune Thrombocytopenia

Fetal and neonatal alloimmune thrombocytopenia (NAIT) develop as a result of maternal sensitization to paternally inherited platelet antigens in the fetus.[83] Antiplatelet IgG antibodies cross the placenta and cause fetal immune thrombocytopenia. About half of cases involve the first child. The most commonly involved platelet antigen is HPA-1a (Pl^{A1}), which is expressed on the platelet glycoprotein IIIa.[83] Platelet-specific antigens are generally weak immunogens, and genetic factors may influence whether HPA-1a-negative women will develop anti-HPA-1a antibodies. Individuals with certain HLA

haplotypes with *DR3* or *DRB3*0101* allele are more likely to develop antibodies against HPA-1a antigen.[84]

Traditionally, it has been thought that NAIT was caused only by antibodies against platelet-specific antigens. However, it appears that HLA antibodies may occasionally be involved[85] (see Chapter 12).

HLA-Disease Association

Certain diseases, especially of autoimmune nature, are associated more frequently with particular HLA types.[86] The association level, however, varies among diseases and there is a lack of a strong concordance between the HLA phenotype and the disease. The exact mechanism underlying the HLA-disease association is not known, and other genetic and environmental factors may play roles as well.

The most prominent associations are ankylosing spondylitis with HLA-B27, narcolepsy with HLA-DR15, and celiac disease with HLA-DQ2. The HLA-A1, B8, DR3 haplotype is frequently involved in autoimmune disorders. Rheumatoid arthritis is associated with a particular sequence of the amino acid positions 66 to 75 in the DRβ1 chain that is common to the major subtypes of DR4 and DR1. Type I diabetes mellitus is associated with DR3/4 heterozygotes, and the absence of asparagine at position 57 on the DQβ1 chain appears to render susceptibility to this disease.

Primary or hereditary hemochromatosis is one of the most common inherited diseases manifested by an increased absorption of dietary iron, resulting in excess iron deposition in the liver, heart, and endocrine organs and finally organ failure. This disease is determined by an autosomal recessive gene, and up to 10% of the population are heterozygous (carriers) and 0.5% homozygous. The unidentified disease gene has been known to be closely linked to the HLA-A locus, especially on the HLA-A3 haplotype.[87] This HLA haplotype linkage has been clinically used to identify which siblings of the affected proband inherited the disease genes based on the HLA haplotype segregation in the family. Siblings who inherited two HLA haplotypes identical to the affected proband will be homozygous for the disease gene.[88] The identification of homozygous siblings allows monitoring of the iron status and initiation of phlebotomy therapy to prevent iron overload. Recently HLA-H was suggested as a strong candidate gene for hemochromatosis.[89] HLA-H is a nonclassical class I gene located approximately 6 megabases telomeric to the HLA-A locus. One amino acid substitution, cysteine to tyrosine, at position 282 in a highly conserved region of the HLA-H gene product appears to be clearly associated with hemochromatosis. The underlying mechanism is not understood, and other genetic and environmental factors may affect the severity of iron overload, but HLA-H DNA typing may become the test of choice to detect the homozygosity and heterozygosity for the gene.

Parentage HLA Testing

In paternity testing, genetic markers of a child, biological mother, and alleged father are compared to determine exclusion or nonexclusion of the alleged father.

There are some advantages of using HLA types in parentage testing. The HLA system is inherited in a mendelian manner and is extensively polymorphic; its recombination rate is low; mutation has not been observed in family studies; and antigen frequencies are known for many different ethnic groups. HLA-A and HLA-B antigens provide a higher probability of exclusion than HLA-DR antigens because of the larger number of antigens at the class I loci. The HLA system, however, does not provide a high exclusion probability when the case involves a paternal HLA haplotype that is common in the particular ethnic group. Molecular techniques using Southern blotting and PCR are gaining popularity,[90] and there is decreasing use of HLA typing for paternity testing.

CONCLUSION AND SUMMARY

The human major histocompatibility complex HLA is located on the short arm of chromosome 6. It is known to be the most polymorphic genetic system in humans. The biological role of the HLA class I and class II molecules is to present processed peptide antigens and thus determine the immune response. The HLA system is clinically important as transplantation antigens, and HLA alloimmunization causes various problems in transfusion therapy. Molecular HLA typing has been evolving to provide class II allele matching in marrow transplantation, but this high-level resolution is not required in solid organ transplantation. The HLA system has been associated with certain diseases, but its underlying mechanisms are not yet fully explained.

REFERENCES

1. Terasaki PI, Dausset J, Payne R, et al. History of HLA: Ten recollections. Los Angeles: UCLA Tissue Typing Laboratory, 1990.
2. Bjorkman PJ, Samraoui B, Bennett WS, et al. The foreign antigen binding site and T-cell recognition regions of class I histocompatibility antigens. Nature 1987;329:512–515.
3. Powis SH, Trowsdale J. Human major histocompatibility complex genes. Behring Inst Mitt 1994;94:17–25.
4. Bodmer JG, Marsh SGE, Albert ED, et al. Nomenclature for factors of the HLA system, 1996. Hum Immunol 1997;53:98–128.
5. Bjorkman PJ, Parham P. Structure, function and diversity of class I major histocompatibility complex molecules. Annu Rev Biochem 1990;59:253–288.
6. Bjorman PJ, Saper MA, Samraoui B, et al. The structure of the human class I histocompatibility antigen, HLA-A2. Nature 1987;329:506–512.
7. Madden DR, Gorga JC, Strominger, Wiley DC. The structure of HLA-B27 reveals nonamer self-peptides bound in an extended conformation. Nature 1991;353:321–325.
8. Jardetzky TS, Lane WS, Robinson RA, Madden DR, Wiley DC. Identification of self peptides bound to purified HLA-B27. Nature 1991;353:326–329.
9. Brown JH, Jardetzky TS, Gorga JC, et al. Three-dimensional structure of the human class II histocompatibility antigen HLA-DR1. Nature 1993;364:33–39.
10. Engelhard VH. Structure of peptides associated with class I and class II MHC molecules. Annu Rev Immunol 1994;12:181–207.

11. Falk K, Rotzschke O, Stevanovic S, Jung G, Rammensee HG. Allele-specific motifs revealed by sequencing of self-peptides eluted from MHC molecules. Nature 1991;351:190–196.

12. Zinkernagel RM, Doherty PC. Restriction of in vitro T cell mediated cytotoxicity in lymphocytic choriomeningitis within a syngeneic or semiallogeneic system. Nature 1974;248:701–702.

13. Garratt TPJ, Saper MA, Bjorkman PJ, Strominger JL, Wiley DC. Specificity pockets for the side chains of peptide antigens in HLA-w68. Nature 1989;342:692–696.

14. Stern LJ, Wiley DC. Antigenic peptide binding by class I and class II histocompatibility proteins. Structure 1994;2:245–251.

15. Germain RN, Margulies DH. The biochemistry and cell biology of antigen processing and presentation. Annu Rev Immunol 1993;11:403–450.

16. Cresswell P. Assembly, transport, and function of MHC class II molecules. Annu Rev Immunol 1994;12:259–293.

17. Stern LJ, Wiley DC. Antigenic peptide binding by class I and class II histocompatibility proteins—the recent determination of the structure of a class II MHC molecule complexed to a specific peptide reveals both similarities and differences with peptide binding by class I MHC. Structure 1994;2:245–251.

18. Clevers H, Alarcon B, Wileman T, Terhorst C. The T-cell receptor/CD3 complex: a dynamic protein ensemble. Annu Rev Immunol 1988;6:629–662.

19. Hass W, Pereira P, Tonegawa S. Gamma/delta cells. Annu Rev Immunol 1993;11:637–685.

20. Terasaki PI, McLelland JP. Microdroplet assay of human serum cytotoxins. Nature 1964;294:998–1000.

21. Amos DB, Baskin H, Boyle W, MacQueen M, Tiilikaineen A. A simple microcytotoxicity test. Transplantation 1969;7:220–222.

22. Choo SY, St. John T, Orr HT, et al. Molecular analysis of the variant alloantigen HLA- B27d (HLA-B*2703) identifies a unique single amino acid substitution. Hum Immunol 1988;21:209–219.

23. Choo SY, Fan LA, Hansen JA. Allelic variations clustered in the antigen binding sites of HLA-Bw62 molecules. Immunogenetics 1993;37:108–113.

24. White TJ, Arnheim N, Erlich HA. The polymerase chain reaction. Trends Genet 1989;5:185–189.

25. Bugawan TL, Begovich AB, Erlich HA. Rapid HLA-DPB typing using enzymatically amplified DNA and radioactive sequence-specific oligonucleotide probes. Immunogenetics 1990;32:231–241.

26. Petersdorf EW, Longton GM, Anasetti C, et al. The significance of HLA-DRB1 matching on clinical outcome after HLA-A, B, DR identical unrelated donor marrow transplantation. Blood 1995;86:1606–1613.

27. Hirschhorn K, Bach F, Kolodny RL, et al. Immune response and mitosis in human peripheral blood lymphocytes in vitro. Science 1963;142:1185–1187.

28. Mickelson EM, Guthrie LA, Etzioni R, Anasetti C, Martin PJ, Hansen JA. Role of the mixed lymphocyte culture (MLC) reaction in marrow donor selection: matching for transplants from related haploidentical donors. Tissue Antigens 1994;44:83–92.

29. Kaminski E, Sharrock C, Hows J, et al. Frequency analysis of cytotoxic T lymphocyte precursors—possible relevance to HLA-matched unrelated donor marrow transplantation. Bone Marrow Transplant 1988;3:149–165.

30. Johnson AH, Rossen RD, Butler WT. Detection of allo-antibodies using a sensitive antiglobulin microcytotoxcity test: identification of low levels of preformed antibodies in accelerated allograft rejection. Tissue Antigens 1972;2:215–255.

31. Wang-Rodriguez J, Rearden A. Effect of crossmatching on outcome in organ transplantation. Crit Rev Clin Lab Sci 1995;32:345–376.

32. Thistlewaite JR, Buckingham MM, Stuart JK, et al. T cell immunofluorescence flow cytometry crossmatch results in cadaver donor renal transplantation. Transplant Proc 1987;19:722–724.

33. Goulmy E. Human minor histocompatibility antigens. Curr Opin Immunol 1996;8:75–81.

34. Goulmy E, Schipper R, Pool J, et al. Mismatches of minor histocompatibility antigen between HLA-identical donors and recipients and the development of graft-versus-host disease after bone marrow transplantation. N Engl J Med 1996;334:281–285.

35. Krams SM, Ascher NL, Martinez OM. New immunologic insights into mechanisms of allograft rejection. Gastroenterol Clin North Am 1993;22:381–340.

36. Auchincloss H, Sultan H. Antigen processing and presentation in transplantation. Curr Opin Immunol 1996;8:681–687.

37. Hauptman PJ, O'Connor KJ. Procurement and allocation of solid organs for transplantation. N Engl J Med 1997;336:422–431.
38. Phillips MG, Malinin G. Donor evaluation for organ and tissue procurement. In: Phillips MG, ed. Organ Procurement, Preservation, and Distribution in Transplantation, 2nd ed. Richmond, VA: United Network for Organ Sharing, 1996.
39. The UNOS Bulletin. 1997;2(6).
40. Takemoto S, Terasaki PI, Cecka JM, et al. Survival of nationally shared, HLA-matched kidney transplants from cadaveric donors. N Engl J Med 1992;327:834–839.
41. Starzl T, Marchioro TL, Holmes JH, et al. Renal homografts in patients with major donor-recipient blood group incompatibilities. Surgery 1964;55:195–200.
42. Terasaki PI, Cho Y, Takemoto S, Cecka M, Gjertson D. Twenty-year follow-up on the effect of HLA matching on kidney transplant survival and prediction of future twenty-year survival. Transplant Proc 1996;28:1144–1145.
43. Terasaki PI, Cecka JM, Gjertson DW, et al. High survival rates of kidney transplants from spousal and living unrelated donors. N Engl J Med 1995;333:333–336.
44. Opelz G, Sengar DPS, Mickey MR, et al. Effect of blood transfusions on subsequent kidney transplants. Transplant Proc 1973;5:253.
45. Lagaaij EL, Hennemann IPH, Ruigrok M, et al. Effect of one HLA-DR antigen matched and completely HLA-DR mismatched blood transfusions on survival of heart and kidney allograft. N Engl J Med 1984;321:701.
46. Claas FH, de Koster HS, Lagaaij EL, van Rood JJ. A molecular mechanism of T cell downregulation by blood transfusion. Exp Nephrol 1993;1:134–138.
47. Brennan DC, Mohanakumar T, Flye MW. Donor-specific transfusion and donor bone marrow infusion in renal transplantation tolerance: a review of efficacy and mechanisms. Am J Kidney Dis 1995;26:701–715.
48. Thomas ED, Storb R, Clift RA, et al. Bone marrow transplantation. N Engl J Med 1975;292:895–902.
49. Beatty PG, Lift RA, Mickelsen EM, et al. Marrow transplantation from related donors other than HLA-identical siblings. N Engl J Med 1984;313:765–771.
50. Martin PJ, Hansen JA, Torok-Storb B, et al. Effects of treating marrow with a CD3- specific immunotoxin for prevention of acute graft-versus-host disease. Bone Marrow Transplant 1988;3:437–444.
51. Kernan NA. Graft failure following transplantation of T cell depleted marrow. In: Burakoff SJ, Deeg HJ, Ferrara J, Atkinson K, eds. Graft-vs-Host Disease: Immunology, Pathophysiology and Treatment. New York: Marcel Dekker, 1990:557–568.
52. Zutter MM, Martin PJ, Sale GE, et al. Epstein-Barr virus lymphoproliferation after bone marrow trans-plantation. Blood 1988;72:520–529.
53. Storb R, Thomas ED, Buckner CD, et al. Allogeneic marrow grafting for treatment of aplastic anemia. Blood 1974;43:157–180.
54. Beatty PG. Hansen JA, Longton GM, et al. Marrow transplantation from HLA-matched unrelated donors for treatment of hematologic malignancies. Transplantation 1991;51:443–447.
55. Stroncek D, Bartsch G, Perkins HA, Randall BL, Hansen JA, McCullough J. The National Marrow Donor Program. Transfusion 1993;33:466–467.
56. Stroncek DF, Holland PV, Bartsch G, et al. Experiences of the first 493 unrelated marrow donors in the National Marrow Donor Program. Blood 1993;81:1940–1946.
57. Beatty PG, Dahlberg S, Mickelson EM, et al. Probability of finding HLA-matched unrelated marrow donors. Transplantation 1988;45:714.
58. Choo SY, Eastlund T. Tissue transplantation and HLA typing. Tissue and Cell Report 1996;2:3–4.
59. Claas FHJ, Smeenk FTJ, Schmidt R, et al. Alloimmunization against the MHC antigens after platelet transfusions is due to contaminating leukocytes in the platelets. Exp Hematol 1981;9:84–89.
60. Abou-Elella AA, Camarillo TA, Allen MB, et al. Low incidence of red cell and HLA antibody formation by bone marrow transplant patients. Transfusion 1995;335:931–935.
61. Storb R, Thomas ED, Buckner DC, et al. Marrow transplantation for aplastic anemia. Semin Hematol 1984;21:27–35.

62. van Marwijk-Kooy M, van Prooijen HC, Moes M. Use of leukocyte-depleted platelet concentrates for the prevention of refractoriness and primary HLA alloimmunization: a prospective, randomized trial. Blood 1991;77:201–205.

63. Sintnicolaas K, van Marwijk Kooij M, van Prooijen HC, et al. Leukocyte depletion of random single-donor platelet transfusions does not prevent secondary human leukocyte antigen-alloimmunization and refractoriness: a randomized prospective study. Blood 1995;85:824–828.

64. McFarland JG, Anderson AJ, Slichter SJ. Factors influencing the transfusion response to HLA-selected apheresis donor platelets in patients refractory to random platelet concentrates. Br J Haematol 1989;73:380–386.

65. Doughty HA, Murphy MF, Metcalfe P, Rohatiner AZ, Lister TA, Waters AH. Relative importance of immune and non-immune causes of platelet refractoriness. Vox Sang 1994;66:200–205.

66. Pulkrabek SM. Platelet antibodies. Clin Lab Med 1996;16:817–835.

67. Moroff G, Garratty G, Heal JM, et al. Selection of platelets for refractory patients by HLA matching and prospective crossmatching. Transfusion 1992;32:633–640.

68. McGrath K, Holdsworth R, Veale M, Bishop J, Wolf M. Detection of HLA antibodies by platelet cross-matching techniques. Transfusion 1988;28:214–216.

69. Rachel JM, Summers TC, Sinor LT, Plapp FV. Use of a solid phase red blood cell adherence method for pretransfusion platelet compatibility testing. Am J Clin Pathol 1988;90:63–68.

70. Friedberg RC, Donnelly SF, Mintz PD. Independent roles for platelet crossmatching and HLA in the selection of platelets for alloimmunized patients. Transfusion 1994;34:215–220.

71. Lane TA, Anderson KC, Goodnough LT, et al. Leukocyte reduction in blood component therapy. Ann Intern Med 1992;117:151–162.

72. Kao KJ. Effects of leukocyte depletion and UVB irradiation on alloantigenicity of major histocompatibility complex antigens in platelet concentrates: a comparative study. Blood 1992;80:2931–2937.

73. Petz LD, Calhous L, Yam P, et al. Transfusion-associated graft-versus-host disease in immunocompetent patients: report of a fatal case associated with transfusion of blood from a second-degree relative, and a survey of predisposing factors. Transfusion 1993;33:742–750.

74. Shivdasani RA, Anderson KC. HLA homozygosity and shared HLA haplotypes in the development of transfusion-associated graft-versus-host disease. Leuk Lymphoma 1994;15:227–234.

75. Davey RJ. Transfusion-associated graft-versus-host disease and the irradiation of blood components. Immunol Invest 1995;24:431–434.

76. Anonymous. Guidelines on gamma irradiation of blood components for the prevention of transfusion-associated graft-versus-host disease. BCSH Blood Transfusion Task Force. Transfus Med 1996;6:261–271.

77. Muylle L, Wouters E, De Bock R, Peetermans ME. Transfusion reactions to platelet concentrates: the effect of the storage time of the concentrate. Transfusion Med 1992;2:289–293.

78. Muylle L, Joos M, Wouters E, De Bock R, Peetermans ME. Increased tumor necrosis factor α (TNFα), interleukin-1, and interleukin-6 (IL-6) levels in the plasma of stored platelet concentrates; relationship between TNFα and IL-6 levels and febrile transfusion reactions. Transfusion 1993;33:195–199.

79. Muylle L, Peetermans ME. Effect of prestorage leukocyte removal on the cytokine levels in stored platelet concentrates. Vox Sang 1994;66:14–17.

80. Goldstein JM, Eyre JH, Terasaki PI, et al. Leukocyte transfusions: role of leukocyte alloantibodies in determining transfusion response. Transfusion 1971;11:19–24.

81. Popovsky MA, Abel MD, Moore SB. Transfusion-related acute lung injury associated with passive transfer of antileukocyte antibodies. Am Rev Respir Dis 1983;128:185–189.

82. Popovsky MA, Moore SB. Diagnostic and pathogenetic considerations in transfusion- related acute lung injury. Transfusion 1985;25:573–577.

83. Deaver JE, Leppert PC, Zaroulis CG. Neonatal alloimmune thrombocytopenic purpura. Am J Perinatol 1986;3:127–131.

84. Valentin N, Vergrcht A, Bignon J, et al. HLA-DR52a is involved in alloimmunization against PlA1 antigen. Hum Immunol 1990;27:73–79.

85. Sternbach MS, Malette M, Nadon F, Guevin RM. Severe alloimmune neonatal thrombocytopenia due to specific HLA antibodies. Curr Stud Hematol Blood Transfus 1986;52:97–103.

86. Fauchet R, Genetet N, Simon M, Bourel M. HLA determinants in idiopathic hemochromatosis. Tissue Antigens 1979;14:10–14.

87. Thorsby E. HLA associated diseases. Hum Immunol 1997;53:1–11.

88. Simon M, Yaouanq J, Fauchet R, Le Gall JY, Brissot P, Bourel M. Genetics of hemochromatosis: HLA association and mode of inheritance. Ann NY Acad Sci 1988;526:11–22.

89. Feder JN, Gnirke A, Thomas W, et al. A novel MHC class I-like gene is mutated in patients with hereditary haemochromatosis. Nat Genet 1996;13:399–408.

90. Pena SD, Chakraborty R. Paternity testing in the DNA era. Trends Genet 1994;10:204–209.

HEMATOPOIETIC GROWTH FACTORS IN TRANSFUSION MEDICINE

The increased understanding of hematopoiesis and the identification of the molecules that influence hematopoiesis (Table 17.1) have enabled spectacular advances in hematology. The availability of hematopoietic growth factors on a large scale for in vivo and in vitro use has also opened a new era in transfusion medicine.[1-4] This chapter focuses on the influence of these growth factors on hematopoiesis in vivo and, thus, the impact of growth factors on transfusion therapy. Chapter 18 describes the use of hematopoietic growth factors in vitro to produce new kinds of blood components for novel therapies.

ERYTHROPOIETIN

Description and Pharmacology

Erythropoietin (EPO) was the first hematopoietic growth factor identified. The EPO gene is located on chromosome 7. EPO is a glycoprotein with a molecular weight of 34,000 daltons. It is produced primarily in the kidney in adults and has a very narrow spectrum of activity because it reacts only with surface receptors found primarily on erythroid cells.[5] EPO is also an unusual growth factor in that it behaves like a hormone[6] because it is synthesized in response to hypoxia. EPO stimulates erythroid proliferation and differentiation, and the plasma level of EPO appears to increase at hemoglobin levels of 10.5 g/dL or less.[7] EPO is found widely throughout the evolutionary tree, and therefore EPO produced in many animals is almost identical to human EPO. As a result, immunization to EPO of other species does not occur in humans, and this conveniently avoids the development of refractoriness to EPO therapy.

Table 17.1 Hematopoietic growth factors

Factor	Major target cell
Erythropoietin	Erythrocyte precursors
G-CSF	Granulocytes, monocytes
GM-CSF	Granulocytes, monocytes, eosinophils, basophils, megakaryocytes, erythrocytes
M-CSF (CSF-1)	Monocytes
IL-3 (Multi-CSF)	Granulocytes, monocytes, eosinophils, basophils, erythrocytes, megakaryocytes, multipotential progenitor cells
c-kit ligand	Synergizes with multiple factors to simulate (stem-cell factor) proliferation and differentiation in multiple lineages, pre-B cells
IL-1a and b	Fibroblasts, stem cells
IL-2 (T-cell growth factor)	T cells, activated B cells
IL-4	B and T cells, myeloid cofactor
IL-5	B cells and eosinophils
IL-6	B cells, myeloma cells, megakaryocytes, granulocytes, monocytes, multipotential progenitor cells
IL-7	Pre-B and T lymphocytes, megakaryocytes
IL-9	Helper T cells and erythroid progenitors
IL-11	B cells, megakaryocytes, mast cells
IL-12	Helper T cells, natural killer cells

Source: Cottler-Fox M, Klein HG. Transfusion support of hematology and oncology patients—the role of recombinant hematopoietic growth factors. Arch Pathol Lab Med 1994;118:417–420.

Abbreviations: G-CSF, granulocyte colony-stimulating factor; GM-CSF, granulocyte-macrophage CSF; M-CSF, monocyte CSF; IL, interleukin.

It seems likely that erythropoietin will be used and may be of some value in other forms of anemia, even those not caused by erythropoietin deficiency. Thus, the potential exists to manage many anemic patients with erythropoietin alone or with some combined strategy of erythropoietin plus red cell replacement in which the red cell transfusion requirement is substantially reduced. EPO is also being studied for its potential value in increasing autologous blood donation or reducing the homologous blood requirements of patients undergoing elective surgery. This exciting new drug has already drastically altered red cell transfusion practices and has the potential to be used in more situations and further influence transfusion therapy.[8] Recent recommended guidelines for use of these EPO are presented in Table 17.2.

Chronic Renal Failure

EPO was initially used clinically in situations of anemia with low erythropoietin levels. The major group of these patients were those with chronic renal failure. EPO therapy

Table 17.2 Guidelines for EPO therapy

I. Currently approved indications
    A. Anemia* of chronic renal failure (creatinine $\geq$ 1.8 mg%)
    B. Anemia with human immunodeficiency virus infection, in patients undergoing treatment with AZT
    C. Anemia in cancer patients undergoing chemotherapy

II. Indications under investigation
    A. Anemia of chronic disease, including rheumatoid arthritis and cancer
    B. Donation of blood for autologous use
    C. Surgical blood loss
    D. Bone marrow transplantation
    E. Anemia of prematurity
    F. Myelodysplastic syndromes
    G. Sickle cell anemia

III. Current contraindications
    A. Patients in whom therapy will result in polycythemia
    B. Patients with uncontrolled hypertension

Source: Goodnough LT, Anderson KC, Kurtz S, et al. Indications and guidelines for the use of hematopoietic growth factors. Transfusion 1993;33:944–959.
*Anemia is defined as reduced RBC volume, for which a blood transfusion is anticipated or needed.

results in an increase in reticulocyte count in about 10 days and increases in hematocrit and hemoglobin in 2 to 6 weeks. EPO is extremely effective in elevating the hemoglobin and reducing or eliminating the need for transfusion in patients with end-stage renal disease.[9,10] This treatment has drastically altered the state of these patients, greatly improving their stamina and quality of life.[11] EPO is now a standard part of the treatment of patients with chronic renal failure, and it has been estimated that this has eliminated the use of 250,000 to 500,000 units of red cells annually in the United States.[1,12] The usual dose of EPO is 50 to 100 units/kg, three times weekly.[2]

Anemia of Chronic Disease

In the anemia of chronic disease, there may be marrow suppression due to the disease itself or the therapy being administered, or there may be decreased synthesis of EPO.[13] In these patients, often the EPO levels are lower than expected from the degree of anemia. These patients use a substantial amount of blood. For instance, it has been estimated that cancer patients use approximately 200,000 units of red cells annually.[1] Thus, strategies to reduce this need would have an important effect on the nation's blood supply. Controlled trials of EPO have shown a reduction in blood use in cancer patients.[1,13] Reductions of 32% to 85% in blood use have been reported.[13] In general, patients with the lowest EPO levels respond the most, and EPO is not recommended for patients with anemia of chronic disease whose EPO levels are normal or elevated. EPO therapy has also been shown to elevate the hemoglobin in patients with rheumatoid arthritis, but there was not a concomitant improvement in activity levels or well being.[14] The major use of EPO in these patients may be in preparation for elective surgery (see below). Patients with chronic anemia associated with inflammatory bowel disease also experi-

enced increases in hemoglobin when receiving EPO.[15] Thus, there are various situations in which the anemia of chronic disease includes low EPO levels or levels inappropriate for the degree of anemia and in which EPO may be of benefit. Current experience is too limited to draw more specific conclusions.

Acquired Immune Deficiency Syndrome

Many patients with acquired immune deficiency syndrome (AIDS) are anemic because of the drugs used to treat the HIV infection, marrow suppression associated with the HIV infection, superinfections due to the immunosuppression, and the drugs used to treat the superinfections. In AIDS patients, EPO levels are lower than might be expected for the degree of anemia present. In patients receiving zidovudine therapy, EPO treatment increases their hemoglobin concentration and reduces the red cell transfusion requirements.[16] EPO is not effective in AIDS patients who have normal or elevated EPO levels.

Anemia of Prematurity

Premature infants are usually anemic because there is diminished EPO production and iatrogenic blood loss due to laboratory testing (see Chapter 12). However, there is some uncertainty whether the response to EPO is normal[17] or impaired.[18] It appears that EPO is helpful in these patients, especially those with a birth weight under 1.3 kg.[19,20]

Autologous Blood Donors

The use of EPO to stimulate erythropoiesis to increase the amount of blood that autologous donors can provide for their surgery is described more fully in Chapter 6.

Perioperative Situations

Some patients planning elective surgery are anemic and thus are not eligible to donate autologous blood. There has been considerable interest in using EPO in the perioperative period to increase the patient's hemoglobin concentration before surgery and to establish more vigorous erythropoiesis at the time of surgery, thus potentially reducing perioperative transfusion requirements. Few careful controlled studies have been carried out, and in general, this remains an interesting idea whose value is not established. However, in the situation of patients with rheumatoid arthritis, treatment with EPO before surgery results in an increased hemoglobin level at the time of surgery and reduced need for blood in the perioperative period.[21]

Bone Marrow Transplantation

EPO therapy is being attempted in patients undergoing bone marrow transplantation in hopes of shortening the time to erythroid engraftment. It is not clear at present whether EPO will be effective when used in this way. EPO has been used to stimulate erythro-

poiesis in allogeneic marrow donors, and in one case this enabled the patient to receive all red cell transfusions from only the marrow donor.[22]

Patients Who Refuse Blood Transfusion

EPO can be used to increase the hemoglobin level in anemic patients who refuse red cell transfusion but who require elective surgery.[23] EPO can also be used to speed recovery from anemia in patients who experience acute blood loss but refuse transfusion.

GRANULOCYTE COLONY-STIMULATING FACTOR

Description and Pharmacology

Granulocyte colony-stimulating factor (G-CSF) is a 19,000-dalton protein produced by monocytes, fibroblasts, and endothelial cells.[24] The gene encoding for G-CSF is located on chromosome 17. G-CSF exerts its action by binding to a specific receptor on neutrophil precursors, the gene for which is located on chromosome 1.[25] Following administration of a single dose of G-CSF to humans, plasma levels increase in about 2 to 8 hours and there is a half clearance time of 3 to 4 hours.[24] G-CSF increases myeloid production and maturation, thus increasing the size of the myeloid pool, but there is no change in the survival of myeloid cells in the circulation.[25,26] The neutrophil count begins to increase within a few hours, reaches its maximum at about 12 hours, and gradually returns to baseline by about 2 to 3 days.[24] The degree of increase in the granulocyte count is related to the dose of G-CSF and the duration of treatment.[24,27] G-CSF also has effects on the in vitro function of granulocytes. These effects include increases in phagocytosis, bactericidal capacity, chemotaxis, and antibody-dependent cell-mediated cytotoxicity.[24,25]

Myeloid growth factors are being used in an increasing number of clinical situations (Table 17.3).

Neutropenia Due to Marrow Suppression

Most of the use of myeloid growth factors in myelosuppression has involved granulocyte-macrophage colony-stimulating factor (GM-CSF). A few clinical trials of G-CSF in cancer patients have shown reductions in the period of chemotherapy-induced leukopenia, the number of infectious episodes during neutropenia, the number of febrile episodes, the number of days of treatment with intravenous antibiotics, and the number of days of hospitalization.[2,3,25,28,29] Thus, G-CSF is used in conjunction with chemotherapy in many types of malignancy. G-CSF has also been used in patients undergoing bone marrow transplantation. There is a reduction in time to neutrophil engraftment, infections, and days of hospitalization in patients undergoing autologous transplants.[3,25,30] In a randomized controlled trial, autologous G-CSF mobilized peripheral blood stem cells (PBSCs) were compared with autologous marrow transplants.[31] PBSC

Table 17.3 Guidelines for myeloid recombinant growth factor therapy

Currently approved indications:

GM-CSF to accelerate myeloid recovery in patients with non-Hodgkin's lymphoma, acute lymphoblastic leukemia, and Hodgkin's disease who are undergoing autologous BMT

G-CSF to decrease the incidence of infection, as manifested by febrile neutropenia, in patients with nonmyeloid malignancies receiving myelosuppressive anticancer drugs that are associated with a significant incidence of severe neutropenia with fever

Indications under investigation:

To accelerate myeloid recovery in patients with myelodysplastic syndrome, AIDS, marrow graft failure, PBSC transplantation, congenital agranulocytosis, or malignancies not mentioned above

Current contraindications:

GM-CSF in patients with excessive leukemia myeloid blasts in the bone marrow or peripheral blood (>10%); known hypersensitivity to GM-CSF, yeast-derived products, or any component of the product

G-CSF in patients with known hypersensitivity to *E. coli*-derived proteins

Source: Goodnough LT, Anderson KC, Kurtz S, et al. Indications and guidelines for the use of hematopoietic growth factors. Transfusion 1993;33:944–959.

transplants resulted in shortened periods of thrombocytopenia, neutropenia, and hospitalization and were more cost-effective. The effects of G-CSF in allogeneic transplants have not been established.

Although the use of G-CSF in these marrow suppression situations may have a major impact on the morbidity and mortality of these procedures, it probably will not greatly alter transfusion therapy in the near future, since leukocyte replacement is not widely practiced. However, reducing the incidence or the severity of infection could modify transfusion therapy if sepsis and disseminated intravascular coagulopathy are avoided, with resulting decline in the use of platelets and fresh frozen plasma. Some studies in patients undergoing marrow transplantation have suggested that the use of platelet transfusions might be decreased in those receiving G-CSF.[25]

Chronic Benign Neutropenia

G-CSF increases the granulocyte count in patients with severe chronic benign agranulocytosis.[25,32] This is associated with decreases in preexisting infections, new infections, and use of intravenous antibiotics. The long-term effects of G-CSF treatment in these patients is a subject of great interest because of the concern that long-term therapy with growth factors might increase the likelihood of the development of myeloid malignancy.[33]

AIDS

AIDS patients may be neutropenic because of the disease, the chemotherapeutic agents, or infections and the chronic disease state. A few studies have suggested that G-CSF may be beneficial in the neutropenia of AIDS.[25]

Aplastic Anemia

The overall value of G-CSF in aplastic anemia is not established. G-CSF has been administered to a few patients with aplastic anemia with mixed results.[2, 25] Some patients experienced an increase in granulocyte count, while others did not. This is not surprising, since aplastic anemia is a disease of marrow failure, and there is often little response to administration of growth factors.[25]

Stem Cell Mobilization in Normal Donors

Hematopoietic stem cells circulate in the peripheral blood[34] and can be collected using standard apheresis procedures (see Chapter 7). The number of stem cells usually circulating is very small but increases as a rebound after chemotherapy. This situation was used to advantage, and the techniques for collection and initial experiences with the collection and transfusion/transplantation of PBSCs were developed in autologous donor-patients. Most of these studies involved cytotoxic chemotherapy only, but a few also included administration of G-CSF.[25,35,36] There has been hesitation to use PBSCs for allogeneic transplantation because of the large number of T lymphocytes contained in the PBSC concentrates. Also, since normal donors would not be undergoing chemotherapy, the number of PBSCs that can be obtained is not adequate for transplantation. However, G-CSF can be used to increase the level of circulating stem cells, and recent transplant experience indicates that the T-lymphocyte content of PBSCs may not be as serious a problem as was initially believed. In the first patient to undergo transplantation using allogeneic PBSCs, there was successful early engraftment but also early death.[37] Subsequently, quite a few allogeneic transplants have been successfully accomplished using PBSCs.[36,38–41] It is clear that this form of transplantation is successful. A number of issues remain, however, such as the nature and extent of graft versus host disease that will occur and the desirability of processing the PBSC concentrate either to positively select CD34+ cells or to deplete T lymphocytes. Although these issues remain to be resolved, there is considerable interest in developing policies and procedures for the collection of PBSCs from allogeneic normal donors, especially those unrelated to the patient, since this could replace the collection of marrow and the attendant risks.

A considerable amount of information is now available about the effects of G-CSF on normal donors.[24,25,27] In normal donors, G–CSF causes an increase in circulating CD34+ cells beginning at about 3 days and reaching a peak after 5 to 6 days (Fig. 17.1). The increase is dose dependent, and the levels of CD34+ cells begin to decline by about day 8, even if G-CSF is continued (Fig. 17.2). With the levels of circulating CD34+ cells achieved, a cytapheresis procedure produces approximately 12 to 140 $\times$ 10^9 mononuclear cells and 70 to 1658 $\times$ 10^6 CD34+ cells.[42] Approximately 50% of cytapheresis procedures yield a dose of CD34+ cells adequate to transplant a 75-kg recipient, and two procedures provide an adequate cell dose in 90% of cases.[42] The procedures for stem cell collection and the composition of the stem cell concentrate are described in detailed in Chapter 7. It is clear that a dose of PBSCs adequate to transplant most patients can be obtained from G–CSF-stimulated normal donors,[24,42,43] and this is a cost-effective approach to stem cell transplantation.[31]

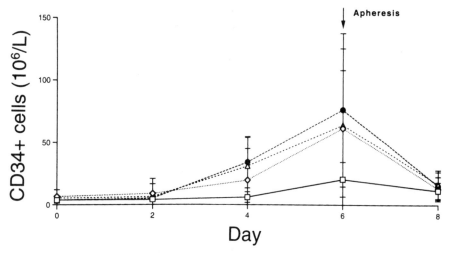

Figure 17.1 The number of CD34+ cells in donors given 5 days of G-CSF. The subjects were given 2 (–□–) (*n* = 5), 5 (···◊···) (*n* = 16), 7.5 (- -△- -) (*n* = 27), or 10 (–●–) (*n* = 21) μg /kg per day, and PBSCs were collected on day 6. (*Reproduced with permission from Stroncek DF, Clay ME, Petzoldt ML, et al. Treatment of normal individuals with granulocyte-colony-stimulating factor: donor experiences and the effects on peripheral blood CD34+ cell counts and on the collection of peripheral blood stem cells. Transfusion 1996;36:601–610.*)

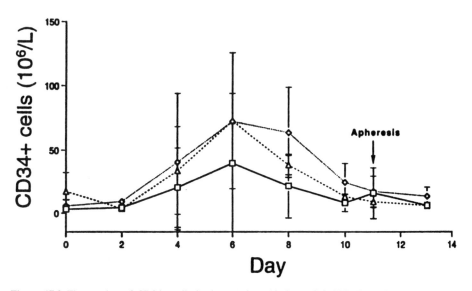

Figure 17.2 The number of CD34+ cells in donors given 10 days of G-CSF. The subjects were given 2 (–□–) (*n* = 6), 5 (···◊···) (*n* = 7), or 7.5 (- -△- -) (*n* = 2) μg/kg per day, and PBSCs were collected on day 11. (*Reproduced with permission from Stroncek DF, Clay ME, Petzoldt ML, et al. Treatment of normal individuals with granulocyte-colony-stimulating factor: donor experiences and the effects on peripheral blood CD34+ cell counts and on the collection of peripheral blood stem cells. Transfusion 1996;36:601–610.*)

The next issue then is the safety of this procedure in normal donors. Fortunately, a considerable amount of information is available to answer this issue. Most normal donors who receive G-CSF experience side effects.[27] The most common are headache, myalgia, bone pain, and flu-like symptoms (Table 17.4). These side effects are more severe in females and in donors receiving higher doses of G-CSF.[27] There are also some biochemical and electrolyte changes (Table 17.5), but these are not clinically significant. The changes include increased alkaline phosphatase, ALT, LDH, and sodium and decreased glucose, potassium, bilirubin and BUN.[27] Following cytapheresis for the collection of stem cells, there is a 36% decrease in platelet count and a rebound to levels above baseline at about 2 weeks,[27] followed by return to baseline by 1 month[44] (Fig. 17.3). The decrease in platelet count is greater than can be accounted for by the number of platelets collected in the stem cell concentrate,[27] suggesting an effect of G-CSF on megakaryopoiesis. The neutrophil levels, which are elevated at the time of cytapheresis, decrease immediately but do not return to baseline until about 2 weeks.[27]

The long-term effects of G-CSF on normal donors are still being studied. The major concern is whether the stimulation of hematopoiesis by G-CSF might lead to hematopoietic malignancy in individuals somehow predisposed to this. One case of hematopoietic malignancy has occurred in a patient receiving long-term G-CSF,[33] but at present there

Table 17.4 Experiences of people given G-CSF for 5 or 10 days

	All donors	
	N	%
Bone pain	85	83
Headache	40	39
Body aches	23	23
Fatigue	14	14
Nausea and/or vomiting	12	12
Redness, swelling, or warmth at the injection site	7	7
Feeling hot and/or having night sweats	7	7
Trouble sleeping	4	4
Skin pain and/or itching	2	2
Enlarged and/or painful lymph nodes		
Arthralgias	2	2
Shortness of breath	2	2
Irritability	1	1
Feeling dazed	1	1
Feeling foggy-headed	1	1
Skin rash	1	1
Took acetaminophen or ibuprofen	1	1

Source: Stroncek DF, Clay ME, Petzoldt ML, et al. Treatment of normal individuals with granulocyte-colony-stimulating factor: donor experiences and the effects on peripheral blood CD34+ cell counts and on the collection of peripheral blood stem cells. Transfusion 1996;36: 601–610.

Table 17.5 Serum chemistries in people given G-CSF for 5 days*

Test	Day 6
Sodium (mmol/L)	142 ± 2**
Potassium (mmol/L)	37 ± 0.4**
Chloride (mmol/L)	102 ± 3
Bicarbonate (mmol/L)	27 ± 3
BUN (mg/dL)	10 ± 3
Creatinine (mg/dL)	1.0 ± 0.2
Glucose (mg/dL)	103 ± 12
Alkaline phosphatase (U/L)	179 ± 43**
ALT (U/L)	38 ± 21†
Bilirubin (mg/dL)	0.4 ± 0.2**
Calcium (mg/dL)	9.4 ± 0.4
γ-Glutamyl transferase (U/L)	31 ± 17
LDH (U/L)	1307 ± 363**

Source: Stroncek DF, Clay ME, Petzoldt ML, et al. Treatment of normal individuals with granulocyte-colony-stimulating factor: donor experiences and the effects on peripheral blood CD34+ cell counts and on the collection of peripheral blood stem cells. Transfusion 1996;36:601–610.
*Values represent the mean ± 1 SD.
**When compared to Day 0, $P < 0.01$.
†When compared to Day 0, $P < 0.05$.

is no indication that a short course of G-CSF as is given to PBSC donors poses a long-term risk to normal donors. Blood counts in normal donors are unchanged from baseline 12 months after an initial exposure to G-CSF and PBSC donation,[44] and the PBSC yield from a second donation 1 year later is similar to the original donation.[44] Thus, these initial follow-up studies do not indicate any long-term adverse effects of G-CSF.

G–CSF-mobilized PBSCs collected from normal donors are rapidly assuming an important role in hematopoietic transplantation, and it seems likely that this general activity will continue (see also Chapters 7 and 18). The additional significance of the acquisition of stem cells by apheresis is that this is the second major use of a strategy to stimulate donors to produce a blood component. The stimulation of normal donors was used originally when corticosteroids were administered to granulocyte donors. However, this never gained widespread use because granulocyte transfusions did not become widely used. The availability of hematopoietic growth factors likely will launch a new era in donor stimulation and a new, larger-scale strategy for the mobilization of cells for new therapeutic uses.

Granulocyte Mobilization in Normal Donors

G-CSF has been used to increase the level of circulating granulocytes in normal donors. This makes it possible to increase the yield of granulocytes collected by leukapheresis for granulocyte transfusion. Bensinger et al.[45] were able to increase the donor's granu-

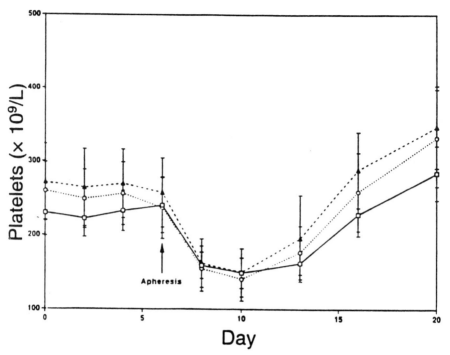

Figure 17.3 Peripheral blood platelet counts in healthy people who were given G-CSF for 5 days (days 1–5) and donated PBSCs (day 6, *arrow*). Donors were given 5 (–□–) (*n* = 9), 7.5 (- -▲- -) (*n* = 31), or 10 (··○··) (*n* = 20)μg/kg per day of G-CSF. Values represent mean ±1 SD. *(Reproduced with permission from Stroncek DF, Clay ME, Smith J, Ilstrup S, Oldham F, McCullough J. Changes in blood counts after the administration of peripheral blood stem cells from healthy donors. Transfusion 1996;36:596–600.)*

locyte levels by an average of tenfold to 29,600, which resulted in collection of approximately 10^4 granulocytes for transfusion. In another study, G-CSF alone increased the granulocyte count to about 25,000 at 12 hours, but when combined with dexamethasone the granulocyte count increased to 35,000 (300μg of G-CSF) or 45,000 (600 μg of G-CSF).[46] The use of G-CSF in these situations resulting in a much larger dose of granulocytes may lead to renewed interest in granulocyte transfusions (see Chapter 11).

GRANULOCYTE-MACROPHAGE COLONY-STIMULATING FACTOR

Description and Pharmacology

GM-CSF is a protein composed of 127 amino acids with a molecular weight of 14,000 to 35,000 daltons. The gene has been localized to the long arm of chromosome 5. GM-CSF promotes the growth not only of the granulocyte lineage but also of monocytes and, under certain conditions, erythroid and megakaryocytic precursors.[1, 2] The level of circulating granulocytes increases soon after administration of GM-CSF and returns to

normal about 3 days after discontinuing the drug. GM-CSF, like other growth factors, affects cell function as well as production. The following effects have been reported:[1,2] increased chemotaxis, oxidative metabolism, antibody-dependent cell-mediated cytotoxicity (ADCC) by neutrophils, increased ADCC by monocytes, and decreased production of natural killer (NK) cells.

Bone Marrow Transplantation

In marrow transplant patients, GM-CSF may be administered after the transplant to shorten the period of cytopenia or before transplant to help mobilize progenitors to be transplanted. In patients undergoing autologous transplantation for various diseases, GM-CSF therapy is associated with a shorter period of neutropenia, fewer days with fever, and a shorter hospital stay.[1,2,47–49] Similar data are emerging for allogeneic transplants.[50] Some studies have shown an effect of reducing the duration of thrombocytopenia, but others have not, and it remains undetermined whether GM-CSF has an effect of platelet recovery, bleeding, and platelet transfusion requirements. There may be an indirect impact on platelet transfusion by reducing the incidence of infection, resulting in a general improvement in the patient's status. The ability of G-CSF and GM-CSF to mobilize PBSCs is similar.[42] However, mobilization of peripheral blood cells in normal donors using growth factors has involved G-CSF but not GM-CSF because of the more severe side effects of GM-CSF.

AIDS

GM-CSF has been used with some success to increase the neutrophil count in AIDS patients.[1]

Solid Tumors

GM-CSF has been used alone or with other cytokines as a strategy to reduce the duration and severity of chemotherapy-induced myelosuppression. There is accelerated marrow recovery in many situations.[1–3] As with marrow transplantation, it is not clear whether there is a megakaryocytic response with a reduced need for platelet transfusions.

THROMBOPOIETIN

Description and Pharmacology

The identification and clinical use of a platelet growth factor should have a major impact on transfusion medicine. Platelet transfusions have increased more rapidly than those of other blood components[51] and currently constitute a very large part of the activity of most large blood banks. The ability to shorten the duration of thrombocytopenia, reduce the risk of hemorrhage, and reduce the need for platelet transfusion has a very great potential benefit. This would affect many patients with chemotherapy-induced thrombocytopenia.

Nearly 40 years ago, it was hypothesized that there is a humoral substance that causes an increase in the size, ploidy, and number of marrow megakaryocytes, resulting in increased circulating platelet levels. Each day adults produce 1×10^{11} platelets, but this may increase up to tenfold when demand increases. The plasma from thrombocytopenic patients could stimulate megakaryopoiesis.

This suggests that thrombocytopenic patients produce a specific substance that promotes platelet production. The pathway[52] to identification of this substance, termed thrombopoietin, became more specific in the mid-1980s with a description of the murine retrovirus myeloproliferative leukemia virus (MPLV). This virus was shown to cause a proliferation of hematopoietic progenitors with cell lines of multiple hematopoietic lineages arising. The responsible viral oncogene and corresponding cellular protooncogene were later cloned, and the receptor that these genes coded was named c-*mpl*. Following identification of the c-*mpl* receptor, several groups purified and cloned the *mpl* ligand.[53–57] This *mpl* ligand was found to increase megakaryocyte size and ploidy and behave as thrombopoietin was expected. The *mpl* receptor is found on CD34+ cells, megakaryocytes, and platelets, and *mpl* ligand promotes cell division and the differentiation of cells into megakaryocytes and platelets.

Thrombopoietin is a 38,000-dalton protein that is glycosylated to form a 90,000-dalton active protein.[52] The 322-amino acid protein has two domains, one with erythropoietic-like activity. In vitro this domain provides the thrombopoietic activity, but in vivo this domain has a very short half-life.[52] This has led to the development of two different agents now under clinical evaluation. One is the full thrombopoietin molecule and the other is the erythropoietin-like domain coupled with polyethylene glycol to provide stability in vivo. The former agent is called thrombopoietin, and the latter PEG megakaryocyte growth and development factor (MGDF). The site of production of thrombopoietic activity is the liver and kidneys, with minor amounts produced in the bone marrow, spleen, testes, muscle, and brain. Thrombopoietin causes an increase in the number, size, and ploidy of megakaryocytes and speeds the maturation of megakaryocytes into platelets.[52] Platelets produced in response to MGDF have normal function in vitro (as evidenced by aggregometry), normal ATP release, and no indication of activation or increased reactivity.[52,58]

Thrombocytopenia due to Marrow Suppression

In patients with advanced cancer, administration of MGDF increases the platelet count beginning at about day 6 and peaking at about day 12.[59] The platelet response is dose dependent and is significantly greater than the controls. Increases of 51% to 584% were achieved in one study, and the average platelet count remained above 450,000/μL for 21 days.[59] In a separate study of cancer patients receiving chemotherapy, administration of MGDF decreased the degree of thrombocytopenia (188,000/μL versus 111,000/μL in controls) and shortened the period of thrombocytopenia (14 days versus 21 days in controls).[60] To summarize, the initial data indicate that administration of thrombopoietin elevates the nadir platelet count and shortens the duration of thrombocytopenia after chemotherapy.[61] This is a remarkable achievement, given that the gene was cloned only about 3 years ago and clinical results are becoming available.

Stimulation of Megakaryopoiesis in Normal Platelet Donors

MGDF can be administered to normal plateletpheresis donors to increase the level of circulating platelets and thus the yield of platelets following plateletpheresis. Studies to determine the safety and effectiveness of this approach are just beginning at this writing. If the use of MGDF for this purpose is successful, it will have a major impact on platelet production and transfusion.

MGDF could be used to enable the collection of two to four times more platelets than are currently obtained. If platelet transfusion continued using the present customary dose, these new concentrates containing large numbers of platelets could be split into several concentrates, thus significantly lowering the cost of single-donor platelets. Alternatively, the high dose concentrates could be used as a single transfusion, providing a larger increase in platelet count and possibly prolonging the interval between transfusions and reducing the number of donor exposures.

Present Status of MGDF and Thrombopoietin

The use of platelet growth factors could shorten the period of cytopenia and reduce the need for platelet transfusions. The use of myeloid growth factors to shorten the period of neutropenia and reduce infections could also reduce the need for platelet and cryoprecipitate or fresh frozen plasma transfusion by reducing sepsis and disseminated intravascular coagulation (DIC). These strategies could substantially reduce the need for platelets and coagulation factor components. However, as the complications of infection and hemorrhage are reduced and the overall safety of the therapy is improved, this decreased component use by individual patients could be counterbalanced by an overall increase in the number of patients being treated or by escalation in the extent of therapy given. Thus, the total demand for these components could remain unchanged or even increase. The availability of these growth factors then may not decrease blood component use but instead may make therapies more readily available to more patients.

IN VITRO USES OF HEMATOPOIETIC GROWTH FACTORS IN TRANSFUSION MEDICINE

In addition to the use of hematopoietic growth factors in vivo as described in this chapter, many growth factors are being used in vitro. The uses are primarily to stimulate the proliferation or maturation of hematopoietic cells in culture systems to produce larger numbers of the desired cells. Examples of these in vitro uses of growth factors are expansion of myeloid cells, expansion of CD34 (stem) cells, generation of lymphokine activated killer (LAK) cells or activated NK cells, production of cells with specific cytotoxicity against Epstein-Barr virus or cytomegalovirus, or expansion of cells during transduction for gene therapy. These activities are described more completely in Chapter 18.

REFERENCES

1. Miller YM, Klein HG. Growth factors and their impact on transfusion medicine. Vox Sang 1996;71:196–204.
2. Goodnough LT, Anderson KC, Kurtz S, et al. Indications and guidelines for the use of hematopoietic growth factors. Transfusion 1993;33:944–959.
3. Vose JM, Armitage JO. Clinical applications of hematopoietic growth factors. J Clin Oncol 1995;13:1023–1035.
4. Cottler-Fox M, Klein HG. Transfusion support of hematology and oncology patients—the role of recombinant hematopoietic growth factors. Arch Pathol Lab Med 1994;118:417–420.
5. d'Andrea AD, Lodish HF, Wong GG. Expression cloning of the murine erythropoietin receptor. Cell 1989;57:277–285.
6. Spivak JL. Recombinant human erythropoietin and its role in transfusion medicine. Transfusion 1994;34:1–4.
7. Kickler TS, Spivak JL. Effect of repeated whole blood donations on serum immunoreactive erythropoietin levels in autologous donors. JAMA 1988;260:65–67.
8. Goodnough LT, Monk TG, Andriole GL. Erythropoietin therapy. N Engl J Med 1997;336:933–938.
9. Eschbach JW, Abdulhadi MH, Browne JK, et al. Recombinant human erythropoietin in anemic patients with end-stage renal disease: results of a phase III multicenter clinical trial. Ann Intern Med 1989;111:992–1000.
10. Winearls CG, Oliver DO, Pippard MJ, et al. Effect of human erythropoietin derived from recombinant DNA on the anaemia of patients maintained by chronic haemodialysis. Lancet 1986;2:1175–1178.
11. Evans R, Rader B, Manninen D. Cooperative multicenter EPO clinical trial group: the quality of life of hemodialysis recipients treated with recombinant human erythropoietin. JAMA 1990;263:825–830.
12. Eschbach JW, Egrie JC, Downing MR, Browne JK, Adamson JW. Correction of the anemia of end-stage renal disease with recombinant human erythropoietin. N Engl J Med 1987;316:73.
13. Spivak JL. Recombinant human erythropoietin and the anemia of cancer. Blood 1994;84:997–1004.
14. Pincus T, Olsen NJ, Russell IJ, et al. Multicenter study of recombinant human erythropoietin in correction of anemia in rheumatoid arthritis. Am J Med 1990;89:161–168.
15. Schreiber S, Howaldt S, Schnoor M, et al. Recombinant erythropoietin for the treatment of anemia in inflammatory bowel disease. N Engl J Med 1996;334:619–623.
16. Henry D, Beall G, Benson C, et al. Recombinant human erythropoietin in the treatment of anemia associated with human immunodeficiency virus (HIV) infection and zidovudine therapy: overview of four clinical trials. Ann Intern Med 1992;117:739–748.
17. Shannon KM, Naylor GS, Torkildson JC, et al. Circulating erythroid progenitors in the anemia of prematurity. N Engl J Med 1987;317:728–33.
18. Brown MS, Garcia JF, Phibbs RH, et al. Decreased response of plasma immunoreactive erythropoietin to "available oxygen" in anemia of prematurity. J Pediatr 1984;105:793.
19. Messer J, Haddad J, Donato L, et al. Early treatment of premature infants with recombinant human erythropoietin. Pediatrics 1993;92:519–523.
20. Strauss RG. Erythropoietin in the pathogenesis and treatment of neonatal anemia. Transfusion 1995;35:68–73.
21. Fullerton DA, Campbell DN, Whitman GJ. Use of human recombinant erythropoietin to correct severe preoperative anemia. Ann Thorac Surg 1991;51:825–826.
22. Mitus AJ, Antin JH, Rutherford CJ, McGarigle CJ, Goldberg MA. Use of recombinant human erythropoietin in allogeneic bone marrow transplant donor/recipient pairs. Blood 1994;83:1952–1957.
23. Gaudiani VA, Mason HDW. Preoperative erythropoietin in Jehovah's Witnesses who require cardiac procedures. Ann Thorac Surg 1991;41:823–824.
24. Anderlini P, Przepiorka D, Champlin R, Korbling M. Biologic and clinical effects of granulocyte colony-stimulating factor in normal individuals. Blood 1996;88:2819–2825.
25. Welte K, Gabrilove J, Bronchud MH, Platzer E, Morstyn G. Filgrastim (r-metHuG-CSF): the first 10 years. Blood 1996;88:1907–1929.

26. Price TH, Chatta GS, Dale DC. Effect of recombinant granulocyte colony-stimulating factor on neutrophil kinetics in normal young and elderly humans. Blood 1996;88:335–340.

27. Stroncek DF, Clay ME, Petzoldt ML, et al. Treatment of normal individuals with granulocyte-colony-stimulating factor: donor experiences and the effects on peripheral blood CD34+ cell counts and on the collection of peripheral blood stem cells. Transfusion 1996;36:601–610.

28. Pettengell R, Gurney H, Radford JA, et al. Granulocyte colony-stimulating factor to prevent dose-limiting neutropenia in non-Hodgkin's lymphoma: a randomized controlled trial. Blood 1992;80:1430–1436.

29. Crawford J, Ozer H, Stoller R, et al. Reduction by granulocyte colony-stimulating factor of fever and neutropenia induced by chemotherapy in patients with small-cell lung cancer. N Engl J Med 1991;325: 164–170.

30. Linch DC, Scarffe H, Proctor S, et al. A randomized vehicle controlled dose finding study of glycosylated recombinant human granulocyte colony-stimulating factor after bone marrow transplantation. Bone Marrow Transplant 1993;11:307–311.

31. Hartmann O, Corroller AG, Blaise D, et al. Peripheral blood stem cell and bone marrow transplantation for solid tumors and lymphomas: hematologic recovery and costs—a randomized, controlled study. Ann Intern Med 1997;126:600–607.

32. Bonilla MA, Gillio AP, Ruggeiro M, et al. Effects of recombinant human granulocyte colony-stimulating factor on neutropenia in patients with congenital agranulocytosis. N Engl J Med 1989;320:11574–11580.

33. Wong W, Williams D, Slovak ML, et al. Terminal acute myelogenous leukemia in a patient with congenital agranulocytosis. Am J Hematol 1993;43:133–138.

34. Lasky LC. Hematopoietic reconstitution using progenitors recovered from blood. Transfusion 1989; 29:552.

35. Pettengell R, Morgenstern GR, Woll PJ, et al. Peripheral blood progenitor cell transplantation in lymphoma and leukemia using a single apheresis. Transfusion 1993;82:3770–3777.

36. Bensinger WI, Weaver CH, Appelbaum FR. Transplantation of allogeneic peripheral blood stem cells mobilized by recombinant human granulocyte colony-stimulating factor. Blood 1995;85:1655–1658.

37. Kessinger A, Smith DM, Strandjord SE, et al. Allogeneic transplantation of blood-derived, T cell-depleted hemopoietic stem cells after myeloablative treatment in a patient with acute lymphoblastic leukemia. Bone Marrow Transplantation 1989;4:643–646.

38. Korbling M, Huh YO, Durett A, et al. Allogeneic blood stem cell transplantation: peripheralization and yield of donor-derived primitive hematopoietic progenitor cells (CD34+ Th-1dim) and lymphoid subsets, and possible predictors of engraftment and graft-versus-host disease. Blood 1995;86:2842–2848.

39. Weaver CH, Buckner CD, Longin K. Syngeneic transplantation with peripheral blood mononuclear cells collected after the administration of recombinant human granulocyte colony-stimulating factor. Blood 1993;82:1981–1984.

40. Bensinger WI, Clift RA, Anasetti C, et al. Transplantation of allogeneic peripheral blood stem cells mobilized by recombinant human granulocyte colony stimulating factor. Stem Cells 1996;14:90–105.

41. Bensinger WI, Buckner CD, Shannon-Dorcy K, et al. Transplantation of allogeneic CD34+ peripheral blood stem cells in patients with advanced hematologic malignancy. Blood 1996;88:4132–4138.

42. Stroncek DF, Clay ME, Smith J, et al. Composition of peripheral blood progenitor cell components collected from healthy donors. Transfusion 1997;37:411–417.

43. Lane TA, Law P, Maruyama M, et al. Harvesting and enrichment of hematopoietic progenitor cells mobilized into the peripheral blood of normal donors by granulocyte-macrophage colony-stimulating factor (GM-CSF) or G-CSF: potential role in allogeneic marrow transplantation. Blood 1995;85:275–282.

44. Stroncek DF, Clay ME, Herr G, et al. Comparison of G-CSF mobilization and collection of blood stem cells twice from the same person. Transfusion 1997;37:304–308.

45. Bensinger WI, Price TH, Dale DC, et al. The effects of daily recombinant human granulocyte-colony-stimulating factor administration on normal granulocyte donors undergoing leukapheresis. Blood 1993;81:1883–1888.

46. Liles WC, Huang JE, Llewellyn C, SenGupta D, Price TH, Dale DC. A comparative trial of granulocyte-colony-stimulating factor and dexamethasone, separately and in combination, for the mobilization of neutrophils in the peripheral blood of normal volunteers. Transfusion 1997;37:182–187.

47. Brandt SJ, Peters WP, Atwater SK, et al. Effect of recombinant human granulocyte-macrophage colony-stimulating factor on hematopoietic reconstitution after high-dose chemotherapy and autologous bone marrow transplantation. N Engl J Med 1988;318:869–876.

48. Bishop MR, Anderson JR, Jackson JD, et al. High-dose therapy and peripheral blood progenitor cell transplantation: effects of recombinant human granulocyte-macrophage colony-stimulating factor on the autograft. Blood 1994;83:610–616.

49. Nemunaitis J, Rabinowe SN, Singer JW, et al. Recombinant granulocyte-macrophage colony-stimulating factor after autologous bone marrow transplantation for lymphoid cancer. N Engl J Med 1991;324: 1773–1778.

50. Nemunaitis J, Anasetti C, Storb R, et al. Phase II trial of recombinant human granulocyte-macrophage colony-stimulating factor in patients undergoing allogeneic bone marrow transplantation from unrelated donors. Blood1992;79:2572–2577.

51. Wallace EL, Churchill WH, Surgenor DM, An J, Cho G, McGurk S, Murphy L. Collection and transfusion of blood and blood components in the United States, 1992. Transfusion 1995;35:802–812.

52. Kuter DJ. Thrombopoietin: biology, clinical applications, role in the donor setting. J Clin Apheresis 1996;11:149–159.

53. de Sauvage FJ, Hass PE, Spencer SD, et al. Stimulation of megakaryocytopoiesis and thrombopoiesis by the c-Mpl ligand. Nature 1994;369:533.

54. Bartley TD, Bogenberger J, Hunt P, et al. Identification and cloning of a megakaryocyte growth and development factor that is a ligand for the cytokine receptor Mpl. Cell 1994;77:1117.

55. Lok S, Kaushansky K, Holly RD, et al. Cloning and expression of murine thrombopoietin cDNA and stimulation of platelet production in vivo. Nature 1994;369:565.

56. Kato T, Iwamatsu A, Shimada Y, et al. Purification and characterization of thrombopoietin derived from thrombocytopenic rat plasma. Blood 1994;84:329a.

57. Kuter DJ, Beeler DL, Rosenberg RD. The purification of megapoietin: a physiological regulator of megakaryocyte growth and platelet production. Proc Natl Acad Sci USA 1994;91:11104–11108.

58. O'Malley CJ, Rasko JEJ, Basser RL, et al. Administration of pegylated recombinant human megakaryocyte growth and development factor to humans stimulates the production of functional platelets that show no evidence of in vivo activation. Blood 1996;88:3288–3298.

59. Basser RL, Rasko JEJ, Klarke K, et al. Thrombopoietic effects of pegylated recombinant human megakaryocyte growth and development factor (PEG-rHUMGDF) in patients with advanced cancer. Lancet 1996;348:1279–1281.

60. Fanucchi M, Glaspy J, Crawford J, et al. Effects of polyethylene glycol-conjugated recombinant human megakaryocyte growth and development factor on platelet counts after chemotherapy for lung cancer. N Engl J Med 1997;336:404–409.

61. Kaushansky K. Thrombopoietin: platelets on demand? Ann Intern Med 1997;126:731–733.

CELLULAR ENGINEERING FOR THE PRODUCTION OF NEW BLOOD COMPONENTS

PRESENT GENERATIONS OF BLOOD COMPONENTS

Blood component therapy as it was developed in the 1960s is based on maximizing the use of a standard "unit" of whole blood. The volume of the unit is fixed at 450 mL $\pm 10\%$, and the blood is separated into several components (see Chapter 5). The volume and amount of cells or protein in each component is limited by the volume of the original unit of whole blood. In addition, the cells are in their physiologic state as they are normally in the circulation and are present in the components in the same approximate ratios as in whole blood. This approach to the preparation of blood components has been extremely successful and has made possible the sophisticated hematotherapy used today. This could be considered the first generation of blood component therapy. To overcome the limitations of the content of a standard unit of whole blood, techniques were developed to process larger volumes of donor blood, extracting only some of the components and returning the remainder to the donor. These cytapheresis procedures made it possible to obtain larger amounts of a particular blood component than would be present in an ordinary unit of whole blood. This can be considered the second generation of blood component production and therapy. Platelet concentrates obtained by plateletpheresis are the best example of this second generation of blood components. Now, a third generation of component therapy is forming.

Developments in the understanding of hematopoiesis, the identification of hematopoietic growth factors and cytokines, and advances in technology for cell separation and culture are being combined to create innovative ways to manipulate blood cells in the laboratory to create new kinds of blood components for new therapeutic

uses.[1] It is now possible to create unique therapeutic blood products in the laboratory that cannot be obtained directly from donors. In addition, new materials are becoming available that allow stimulation of normal donors for the collection of new blood components. Many of these new components involve the use of hematopoietic stem cells for transplantation, but stem cells may be used for other purposes such as gene therapy, and there are other applications of this new cellular therapy that do not involve transplantation (Table 18.1). These new components include hematopoietic stem cells for transplantation, cells for gene therapy, cells for adoptive immunotherapy for malignancy or immunologic diseases, and the production of blood cells in vitro.

DEVELOPMENT AND PRODUCTION OF NEW BLOOD COMPONENTS

The development of new components to provide novel cellular therapies involves four general activities: (*a*) basic research involving the development of novel culture techniques, cell isolation techniques, growth factors, cytokines, monoclonal antibodies, or improved understanding of cell growth characteristics; (*b*) methods development and application involving scaling up the research procedures so they can be carried out on an operational basis with proper safety, cell handling, quality control, documentation, and conformance with regulatory requirements; (*c*) production of the new components using state-of-the-art technology and quality systems; and (*d*) clinical trials and patient therapy in which the "production" versions of the research developments are used on a scale that makes possible decisions about their overall value in patient care. The basic research involves the development of novel culture techniques and cell isolation techniques; isolation of new growth factors, cytokines, or monoclonal antibodies; and improvement in the understanding of cell growth characteristics. The methods devel-

Table 18.1 Types of applications for which new blood components are being developed

Hematopoietic stem cell transplantation
Gene therapy
    Inherited diseases
    Malignant diseases
Adoptive immunotherapy
    Malignant diseases
    Immunologic diseases
Production of blood cells for transfusion
    Lymphokine activated killer cells
    Activated natural killer cells
    Lymphocytes for gene therapy
    Myeloid concentrates

opment and translational research involves adapting the research method's practical operational mode on a scale to prepare cellular components for clinical use. This also involves development of procedures for cell handling, quality control, safety, and conformance with regulatory requirements (Table 18.2). The production activity is the actual preparation of components as part of a clinical trial. This requires conformance to standard operating procedures, quality control, possibly the development of material for an investigational new drug application, and conformance with those ongoing requirements. A close interaction with those carrying out the clinical investigations is essential. The clinical trials activity is well known and involves the use of these new therapeutic agents on a scale that makes possible decisions about their role in medical care.

The skills and facilities needed for each of these four activities in the development of a new cell therapy are unique. A close working relationship and the integration of these activities are essential for a potential new cell therapy to move effectively from a concept through basic research into production and through clinical trials. The basic research and clinical trials activities are familiar; however, the complexity of the method scaleup and production activity is not well understood. The development of new techniques for isolating certain cell populations or manipulating the cells in vitro to produce the novel cell preparation is carried out in research laboratories, usually with small numbers of cells or small volumes of a cell suspension. These research techniques must then be scaled up and adapted into a practical operational method to produce cells for human use. This begins with procedures to collect the large numbers of cells needed for the

Table 18.2 Activities involved in the production of new blood components by cellular engineering

1. Quality control and quality assurance
2. Complete documentation of all steps of procedure, reagents used, staff qualifications, equipment validation, and process validation
3. Interaction with manufacturers of reagents and equipment to obtain proper licensure and approval for use
4. Interaction with the U.S. Food and Drug Administration (FDA)
5. Development of appropriate manufacturing information for investigational new drug (IND) submission
6. Producing cells using producers that comply with FDA good manufacturing practices (GMPs)
7. Conducting activities in a facility that meets the FDA expectations for good laboratory practices and good manufacturing practices
8. Conducting a regulatory affairs program that meets the FDA expectations
9. Expertise in handling blood components
10. Expertise in the separation of blood into its different cellular components
11. Preservation of blood cells
12. Safety programs for laboratory personnel
13. Development or application of new technology such as special containers, cell separators, cell harvesters, culture systems, etc.
14. Data handling
15. Specimen identification

final product. The cells of interest may need to be isolated from the heterogeneous starting mixture, but the scale of this selection step may pose substantial difficulties. The cells may then be activated or expanded using culture techniques in vitro. Genes may be inserted to prepare the cells for gene therapy and any of these various cell suspensions may require preservation for short or long periods. All of these methods must result in a cell suspension with the desired properties but accomplished efficiently, at minimum cost, maintaining safety of the cell suspension and laboratory personnel, and in a manner enabling the treatment of many patients simultaneously. Almost always, the original research technique must be modified in some way because it does not lend itself to a "production" technology.

HEMATOPOIETIC PROGENITOR AND STEM CELLS AS A BLOOD COMPONENT

Increasing Variety of Sources of Stem Cells and Processing Methods

The variety of these new components is almost exploding because of the dramatic increase in the number and variety of sources of cells and the increasing types of processing procedures. For many years, almost the only source of cells was marrow and this was usually from a relative of the patient. Beginning in the mid-1980s, with the use of unrelated marrow donors, the variety began to increase. The current sources of hematopoietic stem cells include bone marrow, peripheral blood, and umbilical cord blood obtained from matched siblings, partially matched relatives, the patient himself or herself, unrelated volunteers, and, most recently, umbilical cord blood from unrelated volunteer mothers (Table 18.3).

These hematopoietic progenitor cells are subjected to an increased variety of processes or manipulations (Table 18.4). These include volume reduction, RBC depletion, T-cell depletion, positive stem cell (CD34+) selection, purging marrow of malignant cells, buffy coat preparation, freezing and storing, and transduction (inserting genes

Table 18.3 Increasing variety of hematopoietic stem cells used as source material

Marrow
    Sibling
    Patient
    Partially matched relative
    Unrelated volunteer
Peripheral blood stem cells
    Patient
    Unrelated volunteer
Umbilical cord blood
    Sibling
    Unrelated volunteer

**Table 18.4 Examples of methods used
to process hematopoietic stem cells**

Volume reduction
RBC depletion
    Bone marrow
    Cord blood
T-cell depletion of bone marrow
    Elutriation
    Immunotoxin
    Antibody-complement
Positive stem cell (CD34+) selection
    Magnetic beads
    Antibody-coated flasks
    Antibody-coated columns
Purging marrow of malignant cells
    Immunotoxins
    4-Hydroxycyclophosphamide
    Antibody-complement
Buffy coat preparation
Freezing and storing
    Bone marrow
    Peripheral blood stem cells
    Cord blood
Transduction—genes using viral vectors
    Peripheral blood lymphocytes
    Bone marrow stem cells
    Peripheral blood stem cells
    Cord blood stem cells

using viral vectors). Many of these procedures are performed on either marrow, peripheral blood, or cord blood. This combination of cell sources and manipulative procedures has led to a greatly increased variety of final products being used for transplantation.[2] In addition, several other types of new cellular therapy such as gene therapy and adoptive immunotherapy are in the different stages of development, and some are already undergoing clinical trials.

Cell Depletion

The first marrow cellular manipulation procedure was the depletion of red cells to avoid hemolysis when the marrow was ABO incompatible with the recipient (see Chapter 12). This was done in plastic bags using sedimenting agents such as hydroxyethyl starch and ordinary blood component handling techniques.[3–7] Techniques involving the use of blood cell separators were available.[4–6] Because of the nature of the component being manipulated, the procedure seemed far from ordinary, however. Currently, red cell depletion is carried out if the donor red cells are incompatible with the patient's antibody. This approach may be used not only for ABO incompatibility but for any clinically significant red cell incompatibility in which the patient has a red cell antibody

and the donor is positive for the corresponding antigen. Since many of the marrow processing techniques involve treating mononuclear cell suspensions, a common initial marrow processing step is the preparation of a mononuclear cell concentrate. This also serves as a red cell depletion step. Several semiautomated devices originally developed for aphereses can be used for marrow processing. These include the Fenwal CS-3000, the Cobe Spectra, and the IBM 2991.[8]

One of the severe complications of marrow transplantation is graft versus host disease (GVHD) caused by donor lymphocytes. A major strategy to reduce GVHD has been the depletion of marrow T lymphocytes. A large number of different methods have been used, and these will not be reviewed comprehensively here. The basic approaches have been the use of T-cell rosetting, monoclonal antibodies plus complement,[9] immunotoxins,[10] and physical separation by elutriation.[11] The general experience with these methods is that T-cell depletion seems to reduce GVHD but is also associated with a higher rate of graft failure. The balance of improved results from the reduction in GVHD against the problems of graft failure are difficult to determine. A major clinical trial sponsored by the National Institutes of Health to compare the different T-cell depletion methods is currently under way.

Another type of cell depletion process is that attempting to remove tumor cells from marrow being used for autologous transplantation in patients with solid tumors. Carcinoma of the breast is the most common example of this situation. The marrow is collected when the patient is in remission and there is thought to be no marrow involvement. Methods used for depleting any residual tumor cells include monoclonal antibodies plus complement or immunotoxins, immunomagnetic bead separation using monoclonal antibodies, or cytotoxicity using pharmacologic agents such as 4-hydroxycyclophosphamide.[12] The process has been termed "purging" because several approaches other than tumor cell depletion have been used. These include molecular or genetic processes, cytokine activation of immune effector cells, and positive selection of stem cells using magnetic beads, cell sorting, and adherence to antibody-coated flasks.[12] These different strategies result in a slightly different blood component. Removal or destruction of tumor cells leaves a more heterogeneous mixture of cells in the component the patient receives compared to methods that positively select stem cells. This is another example of the growing diversity of these new cellular blood components.

Positive Selection

Several methods are now available to positively select stem cells for marrow, peripheral blood, or cord blood. All of them involve the use of anti-CD34 reagent to isolate CD34+ cells. The methods include magnetic beads coated with monoclonal antibody against the CD34 antigen, flasks coated with monoclonal antibody against the CD34 antigen, and anti-CD34 in combination with an avidin-biotin column. The CD34 selection steps are carried out as part of many different processes such as isolation of CD34+ cells from peripheral blood for transplantation, isolation of CD34+ cells as starting material for subsequent ex vivo expansion, isolation of CD34+ cells as part of T-cell depletion protocols, and many more. It is likely that positive selection of CD34+ cells will become the common first step in manipulating most stem cell components. The one major drawback is that other cells contained in the original cell suspension may have

clinical biological importance. The dynamics and optimum concentrations or mixtures of various cell populations necessary for different clinical strategies is not well understood, and thus some combination of positive selection steps may be necessary.

Expansion

Hematopoietic growth factors can be used in ex vivo culture systems to increase the number of cells and thus produce a component in the laboratory that is not obtainable directly from a donor. Different combinations of growth factors have been used to stimulate myeloid precursor expansion ex vivo, but in general it appears that after about 14 days of culture a 20- to 60-fold increase in myeloid progenitors can be achieved.[13,14] This then is a new cellular component produced in the laboratory and composed of some primitive progenitors and many partially differentiated myeloid progenitors. The component might be used as an adjunct in bone marrow transplantation. Studies in mice indicate an accelerated hematopoietic reconstitution[15] following transfusion of such components. Even if this cellular component does not cause accelerated permanent engraftment, it could supplement the transplant by providing a source of myeloid cells during the initial period of neutropenia following transplantation. This might in turn lead to a reduction in infections and related morbidity.

Lymphoid Cells

It has been possible for years to maintain or expand lymphocytes in culture. The availability of hematopoietic growth factors and new devices or containers have improved these culture systems. The lymphocyte culture/expansion procedures are done to produce large numbers of cells for immunotherapy. Because of the variety and extent of these activities, they are described under Adoptive Immunotherapy below. Lymphocyte expansion is also carried out as part of gene therapy, and those activities are described below under Gene Therapy.

Megakaryocytes and Platelets

The most recent initiatives in ex vivo cell expansion involve the use of megakaryocyte growth and development factor to stimulate megakaryopoiesis. Just as granulocyte colony-stimulating factor (G-CSF) and other growth factor combinations can be used to increase the number of myeloid cells in vitro, megakaryocyte growth and development factor (MGDF) has been used in in vitro culture systems to increase the number of megakaryocyte progenitors by 7 to 14 times and eliminate the need for platelet transfusions in two of four patients.[16] This work is at a very early stage, and its success and ultimate clinical value remain to be established.

New Donor-Related Strategies: Peripheral Blood Stem Cells

Hematopoietic progenitor cells circulate in the peripheral blood, although in relatively smaller numbers than in the bone marrow. Although peripheral blood stem cells (PBSCs) can be obtained from the peripheral blood by apheresis, multiple procedures

have been necessary to obtain enough cells for transplantation. One approach to reducing the number of procedures necessary is large-volume leukapheresis, in which 15 or more liters of donor blood are processed to increase the number of PBSCs obtained.[17] Another approach is to increase the level of circulating PBSCs by administering the growth factors G-CSF or granulocyte-macrophage colony-stimulating factor (GM-CSF). The initial experience with this approach was obtained in patients receiving chemotherapy. In recent studies of normal subjects, the administration of G-CSF causes an increase in the percentage of CD34+ K cells from 0.05% before treatment to about 1.5% after 5 days.[18–20] This results in a yield of about 4.5×10^8 CD34+ cells from a single apheresis.[18] The usual dose of CD34+ cells considered suitable for transplantation is about 2.5 to 5×10^6/kg or about 2×10^8 for a 70-kg person. Thus, one such apheresis concentrate might be adequate for a transplant, as has been shown for autologous transplants.[21] The side effects of G-CSF administration in normal donors include bone pain, headache, and flu-like symptoms but are manageable with analgesics.[18] The relatively high content of T lymphocytes has been thought to preclude the use of PBSCs for allogeneic transplants, but quite a few have now been done successfully.[16,22–27] If this proves to be effective on a large scale, use of PBSCs for allogeneic transplantation would eliminate marrow collection in the operating suite, along with the attendant risks of anesthesia and the marrow collection process. Thus, the new hematopoietic progenitor component for allogeneic stem cell transplantation could become PBSCs.

CORD BLOOD BANKING AND TRANSPLANTATION

Bone marrow transplantation is an effective and successful form of therapy that is being used to treat an increasing number of diseases in an increasing number of institutions.[28] Matching a donor and recipient is so complex that for many years transplantation was considered feasible only between HLA-matched siblings. A few patients without HLA-matched siblings could receive an autologous transplant or one from a partially HLA-matched relative. However, donors still were available for only about 40% of patients.[29] During the last several years, it has been established that transplantation can be successful using marrow from properly matched unrelated individuals.[30] However, graft failure and GVHD remain substantial issues in successful bone marrow transplantation (BMT). Therefore, there has been considerable interest in alternative sources of marrow cells that might reduce or eliminate these problems and increase the availability of transplantation for patients who lack HLA-identical siblings.

Pluripotent hematopoietic stem cells are abundant in human umbilical cord blood.[31,32] Successful hematopoietic reconstitution has been accomplished using cord blood stem cells (CBSCs).[33–36] To date, many of these transplants have been done using HLA-matched sibling donor CBSCs; however, a large number have also been done using blood from donors with two or three HLA antigens mismatched with the recipient. The apparent ease of engraftment and lack of GVHD suggest that CBSCs might have advantages over bone marrow for use in a wider variety of situations, especially for transplants between unrelated individuals. Cord blood has the potential advantages over marrow of

being free of contamination with latent viruses (cytomegalovirus, Epstein-Barr virus) and having a low number of GVHD-producing T lymphocytes.[31,32,37]

To carry out larger clinical trials to establish the role of cord blood cells in transplantation, it is necessary to establish "banks" of stored CBSCs. At present, this is being accomplished through a group of contracts sponsored by the National Heart, Lung, and Blood Institute. However, there are many issues that must be resolved, specific procedures to be developed, and requirements to be defined as these banks are established[38,39] (Table 18.5).

Blood banks are organizations with experience and expertise in the medical assessment and laboratory testing of normal donors, blood cell preservation, transportation of blood components, matching of donor and recipient, the operation of unrelated volunteer marrow donor programs, and blood collection. In addition, many blood banks already have programs for processing bone marrow and thus are experienced in procedures similar to those used for handling and preserving CBSCs. Therefore, it is appropriate to draw upon the strengths and experience of traditional blood banking, along with more recent experiences with marrow and cord blood transplantation, to develop the requirements and procedures to operate a cord blood bank and to consider cord blood as a new blood component.[1,38,40]

Obtaining Consent

There is considerable debate about when consent should be obtained. This has a practical impact on the operation of the bank as well as ethical importance.[39] Written consent should be obtained from the mother authorizing placement of the cord blood in the

Table 18.5 Issues to be considered in developing cord blood banks

Informational material provided
Obtaining consent
Determination of the suitability of cord blood for placement in an allogeneic bank
    Donor medical history
    Donor laboratory testing for infectious diseases
    Laboratory testing for genetic diseases
    Contamination of CBSCs with maternal blood
Cord blood collection and preservation
    Collection
    Containers for cord blood
    Anticoagulant for short-term storage
    Short-term storage conditions
    Freezing and long-term storage
Red cell depletion or other processing
Histocompatibility testing
Transplant-related testing specimens
Data, information, and labeling
Transportation conditions
Cord blood testing for suitability for transplantation
Confidentiality

bank and using the blood for transplantation. Preferably the consent would be obtained during prenatal care prior to delivery. Informational material about cord blood banking could be made available through obstetricians and in hospital obstetrical units. Unfortunately, there are many women who receive little or no prenatal care. Thus, alternatively, the cord blood could be collected and consent obtained from the mother after delivery. Consent of the father is not necessary. In addition to obtaining consent for placing the CBSCs in a bank, consent must be obtained for testing the CBSCs and testing the mother for transmissible diseases.

Determination of the Suitability of Cord Blood for Placement in an Allogeneic Bank

It is necessary to define the steps necessary to ensure that cord blood stem cells placed in a bank will be as safe as possible and will provide long-term normal hematopoiesis after transplantation. This can be accomplished by a combination of a medical history and laboratory tests.[40,41] The medical history and laboratory tests used for allogeneic blood donors can be used as a model since they address the issues of maximum safety and normal blood cell function. In marrow transplantation, in addition to minimal transmissible disease risk, the cells must provide a long-term proliferative potential of normal cells. Thus, the medical history and laboratory tests must ensure the absence of hematopoietic stem cell defects. Blood donor requirements include those designed to protect the safety of the recipient and those to protect the safety of the donor. The requirements that protect the safety of the recipient should be used, while those that protect the safety of the donor can be modified because of the different donation situation under which cord blood is obtained. In addition, a history of inherited diseases in the mother's and father's families and some unique criteria relating to the pregnancy and delivery are also included.

Currently, donor laboratory testing is carried out on blood of the infant and the mother. In any disease involving viremia in the mother, there is the potential that the virus can cross the placenta. Examples are varicella, cytomegalovirus, hepatitis B, and human immunodeficiency virus. Thus, when the mother is viremic, there is a possibility that umbilical cord blood may also be viremic. However, since IgG antibodies cross the placenta, transmissible disease tests that detect these antibodies may be falsely reactive on cord blood because of maternal antibody but not necessarily reflecting infection in the infant. The tests are the same as those currently done for blood donors, since that group of tests is selected for the same reasons as testing of cord blood, namely to minimize the risk of transmitting an infectious disease. If a test is positive, the mother and proper public health authorities must be notified so that early treatment can be initiated; if indicated, steps should be taken to minimize the transmission of disease to contacts of the infant or mother. The possibility of testing the cord blood for genetic diseases is a complex one that is currently unresolved. Umbilical cord blood contains some maternal blood cells, and these could cause GVHD in the transplant recipient. However, in the absence of additional data, routine testing for contaminating maternal blood is not recommended.[32,41]

Cord Blood Collection and Preservation

Although the cord blood could be collected in the delivery room immediately after the cord is clamped and while the placenta remains in the uterus, the blood is usually collected after delivery. The placenta is taken to a nearby laboratory, where the umbilical vein is cannulated and the cord blood is drained and collected into a plastic bag system such as those used to collect whole blood.[41,42] Both acid-citrate-dextrose (ACD) and citrate-phosphate-dextrose (CPD) have been used successfully as anticoagulants.[31,42]

Storage Conditions for Cord Blood

The cord blood usually will not be frozen immediately after collection, since deliveries occur at all hours and in locations removed from the cell processing laboratory. Thus, it is necessary to specify the maximum period between collection and freezing of the cord blood. Lasky et al.[43] showed that the number of bone marrow progenitors was well maintained for 24 to 36 hours when stored in a blood bank refrigerator. In specific studies of cord blood, Broxmeyer et al.[31] reported that cord blood could be stored at 4°C for at least 24 hours without significant decrease in mononuclear cells or hematopoietic progenitors. Thus, it seems that initially a collection and banking system could be established in which the cord blood could remain unfrozen for up to 24 hours after collection.

Bone marrow stem cells are frozen and preserved using dimethyl sulfoxide and controlled-rate freezing. This same method can also be used to freeze cord blood stem cells.[42] Although the long-term storage conditions for cord blood are not established, the present recommendation is that using controlled-rate freezing and the cryoprotectant 10% DMSO, CBSCs could be stored in liquid nitrogen (approximately −185°C) for up to 5 years.

Red Cell Depletion or Other Processing

It is desirable to purify the CBSCs by removing red cells to avoid hemolysis in cases of donor-recipient ABO incompatibility and to reduce the volume of cord blood that must be stored. Reducing the volume of stored material may reduce the costs of storage and reduces the volume of DMSO transfused, and thus should reduce the frequency and severity of reactions. It appears that an RBC depletion step can be accomplished successfully, and it is recommended that this be done to remove red cells prior to freezing. In the future, it may be that a procedure for the positive selection of CD34 cells will also provide the desired RBC depletion, but such data have not been reported yet.

Other Issues

There are several other issues that determine the nature of the operations of the cord blood bank.[40,41] These include histocompatibility testing, the nature of the transplant-related testing specimens necessary, the data and information to be retained and measures

to ensure its confidentiality, the labeling requirements for the cord blood units, the transportation conditions, and the nature of tests to determine that the cord blood is suitable for transplantation.

ADOPTIVE IMMUNOTHERAPY

Adoptive immunotherapy refers to the strategy of altering the patient's immune function using the patient's own or allogeneic mononuclear cells, usually lymphocytes, that are treated in vitro to expand their number or activate the desired function. Adoptive immunotherapy has been used to treat malignancy, or diseases with altered immunity such as acquired immune deficiency syndrome (AIDS), or autoimmune diseases.

Lymphokine-Activated Killer Cells

The discovery that T-cell growth factor, later renamed interleukin-2 (IL-2), caused the production of cells with antitumor effect led to a substantial amount of work using lymphokine-activated killer (LAK) cells clinically. When adoptive immunotherapy has been used to treat malignancies, first the patient's lymphocytes are collected by apheresis, then the peripheral blood lymphocytes are cultured with IL-2, and the resulting cell suspension is composed predominantly of natural killer (NK) cells as well as some other T cells. These lymphokine-activated killer cells or other cells with anticancer activity are transfused to the original cell donor along with the infusion of IL-2. Encouraging response rates of approximately 20% have been observed in renal cell carcinoma, melanoma, colorectal carcinoma, and non-Hodgkin's lymphoma[44] in patients with advanced metastatic disease. There is serious toxicity associated with this therapy, generally thought to be due to the IL-2. In addition, the administration of IL-2 alone provides some clinical benefit; as a result, the specific benefit from the LAK cells themselves is not established. Efforts to refine and improve this therapy have continued, and it seems likely that more trials of lymphocytes with some form of activated anticancer activity will occur.

Tumor-Infiltrating Lymphocytes

Tumor-infiltrating lymphocytes (TILs) are lymphocytes isolated from resected tumors and cultured with IL-2. They are thought to be tumor-sensitized lymphocytes and thus to have antitumor activity. TILs differ from LAK cells in that TILs apparently recognize the specific tumor, are a combination of CD4 and CD8 cells, have antitumor activity even in the absence of IL-2, and appear to have considerably more potential than LAK cells in lysing tumor cells. In one trial of 50 patients with metastatic melanoma, a 38% overall clinical response was achieved.[45] Apparently some work with TILs has continued at the National Institutes of Health; however, the clinical role of these cells has not been established.

Peripheral Blood Mononuclear Cells: Graft versus Leukemia Effect

Clinical studies, particularly in chronic myelogenous leukemia (CML), have suggested that there is an immunologic graft versus leukemia effect provided by peripheral blood mononuclear cells.[46–53] It is now clear that transfusion of allogeneic mononuclear cells from the original bone marrow donors destroys the CML cells. Despite the rather large number of T cells transfused (approximately 11 ($\times$ 10^8/kg), the acute GVHD is more mild than expected. It also appears that there is some graft versus leukemia effect in acute myelogenous leukemia (AML) and acute lymphocytic leukemia (ALL). Thus, lymphocytes collected by apheresis from the marrow donor are transfused as a mononuclear cell concentrate—a new blood component.

Epstein-Barr Virus Lymphoproliferative Disorders

Posttransplant Epstein-Barr virus (EBV)-induced lymphoproliferative disorder can be successfully treated by transfusions of lymphocytes obtained from the original bone marrow donor.[54] Approximately 1 $\times$ 10^6 T cells per kilogram are transfused. T-lymphocyte clones with cytotoxicity against EBV-specific proteins can be isolated from patients with Hodgkin's disease, forming the basis of potential immunotherapy in EBV-positive Hodgkin's disease patients.[55] Similarly, immunity against cytomegalovirus can be restored by the transfusion of clones of T cells from the marrow donor.[56] The ability to select these specific clones, combined with the techniques for in vitro expansion, have laid the groundwork for exciting clinical possibilities for immunotherapy.[57] Thus, lymphocytes collected by apheresis from the marrow donor or the patient can be manipulated in the laboratory to create a new blood component with a new transfusion strategy.

HIV Infection and AIDS

Because the complications of AIDS are caused by decreased cellular immunity, lymphocyte transfusions might be used to treat this condition. Although a few attempts have been made, lymphocyte transfusion has not yet been established as being helpful in the management of HIV-infected patients.

Autoimmune Diseases

Type I diabetes mellitus, rheumatoid arthritis, systemic lupus erythematosus, scleroderma, and multiple sclerosis all result in decreased suppressor T-cell activity. In type I diabetes, the anti-beta cytotoxicity appears to be due to lymphocyte-mediated cellular cytotoxicity. A few type I diabetes mellitus patients have been treated with lymphocyte transfusions, but experience is very limited and a clinical benefit of this approach has not been established.[44] It is exciting to speculate that type I diabetes mellitus and other autoimmune disorders might be amenable to transfusion therapy using suppressor T cells.

Recurrent Spontaneous Abortions

Some patients may experience recurrent spontaneous abortion because of immunologic factors. It has been postulated that a successful pregnancy depends on maternal recognition of paternal alloantigens followed by suppression of reactivity against cross-reactive antigens in the trophoblast.[58] This may be due to high NK cell activity, because reduction of NK activity improves the likelihood of maintaining a successful pregnancy. Immunization of women with paternal mononuclear cells reduces the rate of spontaneous abortion in these patients.[59]

GENE THERAPY

Inherited Diseases

Treating inherited disease by inserting a normal copy of the defective gene into the patient's own cells—gene therapy—is now a reality. The cells used for therapy have for the most part been blood cells. Although there are several methods for introducing genes into cells, genes for therapy are inserted into cells using retroviral vectors. The vector is produced in a "batch" large enough to accommodate the planned clinical trial, quality control testing is carried out, and the vector is stored in aliquots suitable for use in the trial. The approaches currently being used involving blood cells can be thought of as either transfusion or transplantation gene therapy.

In transfusion gene therapy, lymphocytes are collected by apheresis. Cells are isolated, placed in culture (usually along with cytokines), and cultured (possibly involving media changes); then the culture medium is removed and the cells are made ready for transfusion. Some final processing may be necessary, and the cells may be used immediately or frozen for later use. The gene may be inserted either before or after culture, depending on the specific situation. Regardless of when the vector is inserted, there are several cell processing steps involved. In the first gene therapy accomplished, this general strategy was used to treat two patients with adenosine deaminase deficiency.[60] This new blood component provided temporary therapy as the long-lived lymphocytes containing the new gene produced the needed enzyme. This transfusion gene therapy involves standard blood collection techniques but creates a new function for the cells by adding the normal gene in the laboratory. Thus, these new blood cellular products can also be considered new components.

Insertion of genes into hematopoietic progenitor cells has the potential for permanent cure of the disease, but in animal studies it is difficult to obtain a high percentage of transduced cells and to maintain stable gene expression after the cells are transplanted. The starting material might be marrow, cord blood, or peripheral blood progenitors. Isolation of the primitive cells of interest, followed by some type of culture technique for gene insertion and probably a final processing step, will be necessary. The cells may be used immediately or stored for later transplantation. A variety of devices, reagents, and culture conditions exist for this process, but the optimum complete procedure to produce the ideal final component for the most part has not been established.

Malignant Disease

Another form of gene therapy is being developed as a potential treatment for cancer. By inserting genes such as tumor necrosis factor, interleukin-2, or others into tumor cells, it is possible to increase the immune recognition of the tumor and thus deliver toxic agents directly to the tumor.[61] In separate studies, a marker gene was inserted into lymphocytes to determine the survival of the activated anticancer cells.[61] Whether peripheral blood cells will be used as part of this anticancer gene therapy—thus becoming another blood component—remains to be determined.

GRANULOCYTES FOR TRANSFUSION

G-CSF has also been given to normal donors to increase the peripheral granulocyte count to improve the yield of granulocytes for transfusion. Depending on the dose schedule, the granulocyte count increases to between 20,000 and 40,000/μL after several days of G-CSF treatment,[18,19,62,63] and this has resulted in a sixfold increase in the number of granulocytes in concentrates collected for transfusion.[62] Using G-CSF-stimulated normal donors, it is possible to obtain granulocyte concentrates containing about 4×10^{10} granulocytes. More recently, use of the corticosteroid dexamethasone has been combined with G-CSF to provide even higher granulocyte levels in the donor.[63] This very substantial dose of granulocytes could lead to a renewed interest in using granulocyte transfusions for the treatment of refractory infections.

REGULATION OF CELL PROCESSING

The Code of Federal Regulations (CFR) defines a biological product as one containing some organic constituent derived from whole blood, plasma, or serum.[64] These biological materials are regulated under U.S. Food and Drug Administration (FDA) law. The FDA has also stated its intention to regulate somatic cell therapy.[65] The FDA considers that somatic cell therapy products are autologous or allogeneic cells that "have been propagated, expanded, selected, pharmacologically-treated, or otherwise altered in biological characteristics ex vivo to be administered to humans and applicable to the prevention, treatment, cure, diagnosis, or mitigation of disease."[65] Such somatic cell biological products are "subject to establishment and product licensure to ensure product safety, purity, and potency."[65] Clinical trials involving FDA-regulated products must be conducted under an investigational new drug (IND) application.

The FDA has clearly stated[65] that the following kinds of cells will be subject to FDA licensure: (*a*) "autologous or allogeneic lymphocytes activated and expanded ex vivo . . ."; (*b*) "encapsulated autologous allogeneic or xenogeneic cells intended to secrete a bioactive factor . . ."; (*c*) "autologous or allogeneic somatic cells . . ."; (*d*) "cultured cell lines . . ."; and (*e*) "autologous or allogeneic bone marrow transplants using expanded or activated bone marrow cells." Cells for which FDA approval is not currently required include "minimally manipulated or purged bone marrow transplants . . . including . . . allogeneic bone marrow transplantation employing ex vivo T-cell purging with a monoclonal antibody approved for such purging, autologous bone marrow transplantation

employing ex vivo tumor cell purging by an approved agent, and autologous bone marrow transplantation employing bone marrow enriched for stem cells by immuno adherence." More recently, the FDA definition of minimal manipulation as applied to hematopoietic cell processing includes cell separation, cryopreservation, and freezing.[66] The extent of regulation of cell processing will be based on whether the cells are (a) more than minimally manipulated, (b) used for their normal homologous function, (c) combined with noncell or nontissue products, or (d) used to provide a metabolic function.[66]

Thus, it is clear that the collection and processing of marrow or blood cells for the development of novel cellular therapies is an FDA-regulated function. The FDA will expect this activity to be carried out in conformance with their regulations regarding the manufacture of biological or pharmaceutical products. The major issue that will continue to evolve with experience will be to redefine the procedures that will be subject to extensive regulation. Most cell-processing procedures are used in the equivalent of phase I or II clinical trials. Many cell-processing procedures will never become routinely used on a scale that would warrant licensure. However, if the procedures involve more than minimal manipulation, they will probably have to be done under an IND application. Many of these procedures will also involve devices or reagents that will be under IND applications or investigational device exemptions (IDEs). Thus, there will be extensive regulatory requirements and involvement in cell-processing programs. The reagents will have to be produced in appropriate facilities in a manner suitable for human (not laboratory) use; the starting material (marrow, blood cells) will have to be obtained in accordance with proper medical and laboratory screening procedures and to be processed in a properly controlled facility using containers and reagents intended for human use.

Cord blood stem cells are also regulated by the FDA. These cells are mentioned along with marrow and peripheral blood as sources of stem cells in the FDA description of the regulatory approach for cells undergoing more than minimal processing or being used for unrelated allogeneic transplants.[66] However, it appears that an IND application will be required for cord blood even for related-donor transplants including all of the appropriate consents, record keeping, and approval mechanisms. This means that even "local" CBSC banks would be regulated by the FDA.

QUALITY ASSURANCE AND GOOD MANUFACTURING PRACTICES FOR CELLULAR ENGINEERING

Because of the dramatic increase in the complexity and diversity of the new cellular products, the FDA regulation of the components, and the production and use of the components under IND applications, it has become essential to develop effective quality assurance programs for cell processing.

Despite the developmental and evolving nature of cellular engineering, it is possible to develop quality assurance systems that are supportive of and consistent with these laboratory activities. The general issues and approaches to quality assurance programs in transfusion medicine are described in the Appendix. The major components of a quality assurance program are the adherence to good manufacturing practices (GMPs)

Table 18.6 Good manufacturing practices as defined in Code of Federal Regulations

General
Organizational
Buildings and facilities
Equipment
Production and process controls
Finished product controls
Laboratory controls
Records and reports

Source: McCullough J. Quality assurance and good manufacturing practices for processing hematopoietic progenitor cells. J Hematother 1995;4:493–501.

(Table 18.6) and the development and use of critical control points. When a pharmaceutical or biological agent has been licensed and is being produced commercially on a large scale, the GMPs are extensive, the facilities are complex, and quality assurance systems are comprehensive. At the present relatively immature stage of somatic cell processing, no product is near licensure for large-scale use. Instead, the products are used in small numbers as part of experimental therapeutic programs and clinical trials.

The quality assurance and GMP process is intended to provide for the safety, purity, and potency of the product.[64,67,68] These are essential qualities of somatic cell products even during phase I or II trials. It is important to ensure that the product is as safe as possible, does not contain any unintended materials (chemicals, infectious agents, cells), and does contain the desired amount of the therapeutic agent (cells). In this way, investigators can more easily determine the cause of any unexpected adverse effects, and the therapeutic benefit (or lack thereof) of the product can be attributed to the therapeutic strategy, not a failure in the product potency. Thus, it is important to design GMPs that are appropriate to somatic cell processing so that the products will be as standard as possible to maximize the likelihood that the therapeutic outcome—including any adverse effects—can be clearly related to the product.

There are eight parts or components of good manufacturing practices as defined in the Code of Federal Regulations (Table 18.2). The GMPs describe the organization and requirements for personnel responsible for different aspects of the operation; the buildings, equipment, and facilities necessary for different aspects of the operation; the production and process control requirements; requirements for controlling and releasing the finished product; laboratory controls; and the records and reports that should be maintained.

A quality control program for any biological agent should include control of the biological source, the production process, and the final product. The laboratory must have a complete, up-to-date, written procedure manual readily available and understood by the staff. The staff must have the skills necessary to carry out their tasks, training programs must be in place, and there must be evidence that personnel are proficient at these tasks. Ideally, standardized work sheets should be completed as the cord blood is processed, and they should be designed in a step-by-step style or format. The labora-

tory should also establish a mechanism to ensure that all necessary data are recorded and that the data meet preset criteria. There should be a mechanism to carry out structured calculation or formulas in a worksheet format, including a system to double-check all calculations. The data describing the final product and tests at intermediate steps should be recorded. The identity of all personnel who are involved in the procedures must be recorded. The conditions of storage must be recorded, and any deviations documented and explained.

After frozen storage, the hematopoietic stem cell component must be prepared for transfusion. Important considerations at this stage include the rate of thawing, post-thaw storage temperature and duration, and the method of transfusion. Procedures must be in place for all of these steps. A report containing pertinent information about CBSCs administered should be included in the patient's chart.

The equipment that would be part of a stem cell processing facility include laminar air flow hoods, centrifuges, programmable freezers, storage containers for frozen stem cells, alarms, liquid nitrogen supply, refrigerators/freezers for storage of reagents and media, water baths, and CO_2 incubators. Procedures for testing each piece of equipment must be established, the frequency of such tests described, and acceptable limits set.

The development and application of GMPs to progenitor cell processing must take into account the variety and continually evolving nature of the procedures. Progenitor cell processing procedures currently in use may involve one or more variations of methods for volume reduction, red cell depletion, T-cell depletion of bone marrow, positive selection of stem cells (CD34+), purging marrow of malignant cells, preparing buffy coats, freezing and storing cells, and transduction of cells inserting genes using viral vectors. There may be several variations of these methods, and each may be carried out on marrow, peripheral blood, or cord blood. Thus, the GMPs must take this variety into account.

Because these somatic cell, hematopoietic progenitor, and gene therapy products are still quite developmental and undergo change based on research developments, the GMPs should reflect the developing, evolving nature of somatic cell processing. In other words, GMPs as applied to progenitor and somatic cell processing are not necessarily the same as GMPs as applied to the manufacture of a well-established pharmaceutical.

REFERENCES

1. McCullough J. The new generation of blood components (Editorial). Transfusion 1995;35:374–377.
2. Sobocinski KA, Horowitz MM, Rowlings PA, et al. Bone marrow transplantation—1994: A report from the International Bone Marrow Transplant Registry and the North American Autologous Bone Marrow Transplant Registry. J Hematother 1994;3:95–102.
3. Lasky L, Warkentin P, Ramsay N, Kersey J, McGlave P, McCullough J. Hemotherapy in patients undergoing blood group incompatible bone marrow transfusion. Transfusion 1983;23:277–285.
4. McCullough J, Lasky LC, Warkentin PI. Role of the blood bank in bone marrow transplantation. In: Advances in Immunobiology: Blood cell antigens and bone marrow transplantation. New York: Alan R. Liss, Inc., 1984:379–412.
5. McCullough J. The role of the blood bank in transplantation. Arch Pathol Lab Med 1991;115:1195–1200.
6. Sniecinski IJ, Oien L, Petz LD, Blume KG. Immunohematologic consequences of major ABO-mismatched bone marrow transplantation. Transplantation 1988;45:530–534.

7. Warkentin PI, Hilden JM, Kersey JH, Ramsay NKC, McCullough J. Transplantation of major ABO-incompatible bone marrow depleted of red cells by hydroxyethyl starch. Vox Sang 1985;48:89–104.

8. Areman EM, Spitzer T, Sacher RA. Automated processing of human bone marrow can result in a population of mononuclear cells capable of achieving engraftment following transplantation. Transfusion 1991;31:724–730.

9. Filipovich AH, Ramsay NKC, Warkentin PI, McGlave PB, Goldstein G, Kersey JH. Pretreatment of donor bone marrow with monoclonal antibody OKT3 for prevention of acute graft-versus-host disease in allogeneic histocompatible bone-marrow transplantation. Lancet 1982;1266–1269.

10. Vallera DA, Ash RC, Kersey JH, et al. Anti-T-cell reagents for human bone marrow transplantation: ricin linked to three monoclonal antibodies. Science 1983;222:512–515.

11. Wagner JE, Santos GW, Noga SJ, et al. Bone marrow graft engineering by counterflow centrifugal elutriation: results of a phase I-II clinical trial. Blood 1990;75:1370–1377.

12. Champlin R. Purging: the separation of normal from malignant cells for autologous transplantation. Transfusion 1996;36:910–918.

13. Koller MR, Emerson SG, Palsson BO. Large-scale expansion of human stem and progenitor cells from bone marrow mononuclear cells in continuous perfusion cultures. Blood 1993;82:378–384.

14. Haylock DN, To LB, Dowse TL, Juttner CA, Simmons PJ. Ex vivo expansion and maturation of peripheral blood CD34+ cells into the myeloid lineage. Blood 1992;80:1405–1412.

15. Muench MO, Firpo MT, Moore MAS. Bone marrow transplantation with interleukin-1 plus kit-ligand ex vivo expanding bone marrow accelerates hematopoietic reconstitution in mice without the loss of stem cell lineage and proliferative potential. Blood 1993;81:3463–3473.

16. Bertolini F, Battaglia M, Pedrazzoli P, et al. Megakaryocytic progenitors can be generated ex vivo and safely administered to autologous peripheral blood progenitor cell transplant recipients. Blood 1997;89:2679–2688.

17. Hillyer CE, Lackey DA, Hart KK, Stempora LL, Bray RA, Bender JG, Donnenberg AD. CD34+ progenitors and colony-forming units—granulocyte macrophage are recruited during large-volume leukapheresis and concentrated by counterflow centrifugal elutriation. Transfusion 1993;33:316–321.

18. Stroncek DF, Clay ME, Petzoldt ML, Smith J, Jaszcz W, Oldham FB, McCullough J. Treatment of normal individuals with granulocyte-colony-stimulating factor: donor experiences and the effects on peripheral blood CD34+ cell counts and on the collection of peripheral blood stem cells. Transfusion 1996;36:601–610.

19. Stroncek DF, Clay ME, Smith J, Ilstrup S, Oldham F, McCullough J. Changes in blood counts following the administration of G-CSF and the collection of peripheral blood stem cells from healthy donors. Transfusion 1996;36:596–600.

20. Lane TA, Law P, Maruyama M, et al. Harvesting and enrichment of hematopoietic progenitor cells mobilized into the peripheral blood of normal donors by granulocyte-macrophage colony-stimulating factor (GM-CSF) or G-CSF: potential role in allogeneic marrow transplantation. Blood 1995;85:275–282.

21. Pettengell R, Morgenstern GR, Woll PJ, et al. Peripheral blood progenitor cell transplantation in lymphoma and leukemia using a single apheresis. Blood 1993;82:3770–3777.

22. Bensinger WI, Clift RA, Anasetti C, et al. Transplantation of allogeneic peripheral blood stem cells mobilized by recombinant human granulocyte colony stimulating factor. Stem Cells 1996;14:90–105.

23. Goldman J. Peripheral blood stem cells for allografting. Blood 1995;85:1413–1415.

24. Korbling M, Huh YO, Durett A, et al. Allogeneic blood stem cell transplantation: peripheralization and yield of donor-derived primitive hematopoietic progenitor cells (CD34+ Th-1dim) and lymphoid subsets, and possible predictors of engraftment and graft-versus-host disease. Blood 1995;86:2842–2848.

25. Schmitz N, Dreger P, Suttorp M, et al. Primary transplantation of allogeneic peripheral blood progenitor cells mobilized by filgrastim (granulocyte colony-stimulating factor). Blood 1995;86:1666–1672.

26. Korbling M, Przepiorka D, Gajewski J, et al. With first successful allogeneic transplantations of apheresis-derived hematopoietic progenitor cells reported, can the recruitment of volunteer matched, unrelated stem cell donors be expanded substantially? Blood 1995;86:1235–1239.

27. Weaver CH, Buckner CD, Longin K. Syngeneic transplantation with peripheral blood mononuclear cells collected after the administration of recombinant human granulocyte colony-stimulating factor. Blood 1993;82:1981–1984.

28. Bortin MM, Horowitz MM, Rimm AA. Increasing utilization of allogeneic bone marrow transplantation. Ann Intern Med 1992;116:505–512.

29. O'Reilly RJ. Allogeneic bone marrow transplantation: current status and future directions. Blood 1983;62:941–964.

30. Kernan NA, Bartsch G, Ash RC, et al. Analysis of 462 transplantations from unrelated donors facilitated by the national marrow donor program. N Engl J Med 1993;328:593–602.

31. Broxmeyer HE, Douglas GW, Hangoc G, et al. Human umbilical cord blood as a potential source of transplantable hematopoietic stem/progenitor cells. Proc Natl Acad Sci USA 1989;86:3828–3832.

32. Broxmeyer HE, Kurtzberg J, Gluckman E, et al. Umbilical cord blood hematopoietic stem and repopulating cells in human clinical transplantation. Blood Cells 1991;17:313–329.

33. Gluckman E, Broxmeyer HE, Auerbach AD, et al. Hematopoietic reconstitution in a patient with Fanconi's anemia by means of umbilical cord blood from an HLA-identical sibling. N Engl J Med 1989;321:1174–1178.

34. Wagner JE, Broxmeyer HE, Byrd RL, et al. Transplantation of umbilical cord blood after myeloablative therapy: analysis of engraftment. Blood 1992;79:1874.

35. Kurtzberg J, Laughlin M, Graham ML, et al. Placental blood as a source of hematopoietic stem cells for transplantation into unrelated recipients. N Engl J Med 1996;335:157–166.

36. Wagner JE, Rosenthal J, Sweetman R, et al. Successful transplantation of HLA-matched and HLA-mismatched umbilical cord blood from unrelated donors: analysis of engraftment and acute graft-versus-host disease. Blood 1996;88:795–802.

37. Wagner JE. Umbilical cord blood stem cell transplantation. Am J Pediatr Hematol Oncol 1993;15(2):169–174.

38. Silberstein LE, Jefferies L. Placental-blood banking—a new frontier in transfusion medicine. N Engl J Med 1996;335:199–200.

39. Sugarman J, Reisner EG, Durtzberg J. Ethical aspects of banking placental blood for transplantation. JAMA 1995;274:1783–1785

40. McCullough J, Clay ME, Fautsch S, Noreen H, Segall M, Perry E, Stroncek D. Proposed policies and procedures for the establishment of a cord blood bank. Blood Cells 1995; 20:609–626.

41. Rubinstein P, Rosenfeld RE, Adamson JW, Stevens CE. Stored placental blood for unrelated bone marrow reconstitution. Blood 1993;81:1679–1690.

42. Wagner WE, Broxmeyer HE, Cooper S. Umbilical cord and placental blood hematopoietic stem cells: collection, cryopreservation, and storage. J Hematother 1992;1:167–173.

43. Lasky LC, McCullough J, Zanjani ED. Liquid storage of unseparated human bone marrow: evaluation of hematopoietic progenitors by clonal assay. Transfusion 1986;26:331–334.

44. Lee JH, Klein H. Mononuclear cell adoptive immunotherapy. Hematology/Oncology Clinics of North America - Transfusion Medicine 1994;8:1203–1221.

45. Rosenberg SA, Packard BS, Aebersold PM, et al. Use of tumor-infiltrating lymphocytes and interleukin-2 in the immunotherapy of patients with metastatic melanoma, special report. N Engl J Med 1988;319:1676–1680.

46. Baer BMAM, Schattenberg A, Mensink EJBM, et al. Donor leukocyte infusions for chronic myeloid leukemia after allogeneic bone marrow transplantation. J Clin Oncol 1993;11:513.

47. Gale RP, Champlin RE. How does bone-marrow transplantation cure leukaemia? Lancet 1984;2:28.

48. Horowitz MM, Gale RP, Sondel PM, et al. Graft-versus-leukemia reactions after bone marrow transplantation. Blood 1990;75:555.

49. Weiden PL, Flournoy N, Sanders JE, et al. Anti-leukemic effect of graft-versus-host disease contributes to improved survival after allogeneic marrow transplantation. Transplant Proc 1981;13:248.

50. Weiden PL, Sullivan K, Flournoy J, et al. The Seattle Marrow Transplant Team: antileukemic effect of chronic graft-versus-host disease. Contribution to improved survival after allogeneic marrow transplantation. N Engl J Med 1981;304:1529.

51. van Rhee F, Lin F, Cullis JO, et al. Relapse of chronic myeloid leukemia after allogeneic bone marrow transplant: The case for giving donor leukocyte transfusions before the onset of hematologic relapse. Blood 1994;83:3377–3383.

52. Kolb HJ, Mittermuller J, Clemm CH. Donor leukocyte transfusions for treatment of recurrent chronic myelogenous leukemia in marrow transplant patients. Blood 1990;76:2462.

53. Porter D, Roth M, McGarigle C, Ferrara J, Antin J. Adoptive immunotherapy induces molecular remission in relapsed CML following allogeneic bone marrow transplantation (BMT). Proc Am Soc Clin Oncol 1993;12:303.
54. Papadopoulos EB, Ladanyi M, Emanuel D, et al. Infusions of donor leukocytes to treat Epstein-Barr virus-associated lymphoproliferative disorders after allogeneic bone marrow transplantation. N Engl J Med 1994;330;1185–1191.
55. Sing AP, Ambinder RF, Hong DJ. Isolation of Epstein-Barr virus (EBV)-specific cytotoxic T lymphocytes that lyse Reed-Sternberg cells: implications for immune-mediated therapy of EBV+ Hodgkin's disease. Blood 1997;89:1978–1986.
56. Walter EA, Greenberg PD, Gilbert MJ. Reconstitution of cellular immunity against cytomegalovirus in recipients of allogeneic bone marrow by transfer of T-cell clones from the donor. N Engl J Med 1995;333:1038–1044.
57. Riddell SR, Watanabe KS, Goodrich JM, et al. Restoration of viral immunity in immunodeficient humans by the adoptive transfer of T cell clones. Science 1992;257:238–240.
58. McIntyre JA, Faulk WP, Nichols-Johnson VR, Taylor CG. Immunologic testing and immunotherapy in recurrent spontaneous abortion. Obstet Gynecol 1986;67:169–175.
59. Smith JB, Cowchock FS, Lata JA, Hankinson TB. The number of cells used for immunotherapy of repeated spontaneous abortion influences pregnancy outcome. J Reprod Immunol 1992;22:217–224.
60. Blaese RM, Anderson WF, Culver KW. The ADA human gene therapy clinical protocol. Hum Gene Ther 1990;1:327–362.
61. Rosenberg SA. Gene therapy for cancer. JAMA 1992;268:2416–2419.
62. Bensinger WI, Price TH, Dale DC. The effects of daily recombinant human granulocyte colony-stimulating factor administration on normal granulocyte donors undergoing leukapheresis. Blood 1993;81:1883–1888.
63. Liles WC, Huang JE, Llewellyn C, SenGupta D, Price TH, Dale DC. A comparative trial of granulocyte-colony-stimulating factor and dexamethasone, separately and in combination, for the mobilization of neutrophils in the peripheral blood of normal volunteers. Transfusion 1997;37:182–187.
64. Code of Federal Regulations, part 606, subparts a–i.
65. Kessler DA, Siegel JP, Noguchi PD, Zoon KC, Feiden KL, Woodcock J. Regulation of somatic-cell therapy and gene therapy by the Food and Drug Administration. N Engl J Med 1993;329:1169–1173.
66. A proposed approach to the regulation of cellular and tissue-based products. Rockville, MD: U.S. Food and Drug Administration, February 28, 1997.
67. Callery MF, Nevalainen DE, Kirst TM. Quality systems and total process control in blood banking. Transfusion 1994;34:899–906.
68. Guidelines for Quality Assurance in Blood Establishments. Docket No. 91N-0450. Rockville, MD: U.S. Food and Drug Administration, July 11, 1995.

THERAPEUTIC APHERESIS

Much of the original impetus to develop apheresis techniques was for the removal of excess unwanted materials from patients (see Chapters 1 and 7). Work at the National Cancer Institute on the development of the IBM Blood Cell Separator was initiated to create an instrument that would remove an accumulation of leukocytes from a child with leukemia. Since those initial developmental efforts, the primary use of apheresis has shifted to the collection of blood components or plasma from normal donors. However, the pathophysiology or symptoms of some diseases are due to the excessive accumulation of blood cells or plasma constituents. In these situations, blood cell separators ordinarily used to collect blood components by apheresis from normal donors can also be used therapeutically. Plasma, granulocytes, lymphocytes, platelets, or red cells can be removed selectively from patients.

The organization and operation of a therapeutic apheresis program is complex. An example of the kinds of issues that must be included are provided in guidelines developed by the American Society for Apheresis.[1] These include the physician staff and their qualifications, nonphysician staff and their qualifications and responsibilities, the facilities, written procedures, equipment, records, quality assurance program, and safety procedures.

There are no data summarizing the therapeutic apheresis activity in the United States. It has been estimated that between 20,000 and 30,000 procedures are done annually,[2] but it is difficult to know the trends. Some information is available from other countries. In Canada, the Canadian Apheresis Study Group is composed of representatives of 17 major medical centers and probably provides the best available idea of therapeutic apheresis activities on a national basis. The group has collected information on more than 58,000 procedures and reports that they are performed at a rate of about 6,000 per year, or 23 procedures for each 100,000 of the population.[3] Between 1981 and

1991, the diseases treated with therapeutic apheresis shifted from being predominantly hematologic to predominantly neurologic diseases, primarily because of the use of therapeutic plasma exchange (TPE) for the treatment of Guillain-Barré disease.[3] The number of procedures done for collagen vascular diseases also decreased. A national registry in the former East Germany from 1987 to 1989 included data on 1,945 procedures in 419 patients, probably representing about 80% of the therapeutic apheresis activity in that country.[4] Renal and neurologic diseases were the ones most commonly treated. This preponderance of neurologic diseases among those treated by apheresis is probably also true in the United States.

CLINICAL USES OF PLASMA EXCHANGE

Plasma exchange, the most common form of therapeutic apheresis, is used in a wide variety of diseases[5–7] (Table 19.1). The diseases in which plasma exchange is used can be categorized by the type of disease (hematologic, neurologic, etc.) or the type of material being removed (IgG antibodies, IgM antibodies, immune complexes, excess accumulation of normal substances, or to replace normal constituents). Many of the diseases in which plasma exchange is used are quite well understood, the constituent being removed is known, and good clinical studies have been reported establishing the value of plasma exchange therapy. In other situations, the pathophysiology of the disease is poorly understood and there may not be specific laboratory measurements of a known pathologic agent that can be correlated with improvement in laboratory values and the patient's clinical condition following plasma exchange. As a result, there have not been careful controlled trials of plasma exchange in many of these diseases; and since many of these patients experience fluctuations or spontaneous improvements, the exact benefits of plasma exchange are difficult to document.

Neurologic Diseases

It is estimated that half of the 20,000 to 30,000 plasma exchange procedures performed in the United States are done to treat neurologic diseases.[5] Thus, neurologic diseases probably account for the largest group of plasma exchange procedures. Plasma exchange is recommended as part the treatment of several diseases. Usually plasma exchange is carried out as a course of treatment involving six procedures in about 2 weeks. For some situations, such as Guillain-Barré syndrome and Goodpasture's syndrome, we believe more intensive therapy is helpful. For other diseases a more prolonged course has been used.

Guillain-Barré syndrome   Plasma exchange shortens the duration of motor weakness, reduces the hospital stay, and reduces the period of ventilation dependence in patients who can breathe on their own at the time treatment is initiated but subsequently require ventilatory assistance.[2,8,9] Plasma exchange therapy is more effective if (*a*) it is performed early in the disease, (*b*) it is applied to rapidly progressive disease, and (*c*) there is an absence of other general contraindications such as infection, cardiac arrhyth-

Table 19.1 Indications for therapeutic apheresis generally accepted for reimbursement by third-party payors

Plasma Exchange

IgG
  Myasthenia gravis
  Eaton-Lambert syndrome
  Goodpasture's syndrome
  Myeloma with renal failure
  Guillain-Barré syndrome
  Hemophilia with factor VIII inhibitor
  Chronic inflammatory demyelinating polyradiculopathy
IgM
  Waldenström's macroglobulinemia
  Cryoglobulinemia
  Hyperviscosity
Immune complex
  Glomerulonephritis, rapidly progressive
  Rheumatoid vasculitis
Metabolic
  Refsum's disease
  Hyperlipoproteinemia, familial
  Cholestasis—intractable pruritus
Unknown
  Thrombotic thrombocytopenic purpura
  Thyroid storm
  Scleroderma, refractory
  Polymyositis, refractory

Cytapheresis

Acute leukemia—debulking
Hairy-cell leukemia—maintenance
Thrombocytosis, symptomatic
Chronic myelogenous leukemia, acute symptoms

Red Cell Exchange

Sickle cell disease

Source: Adapted from McCullough J. Transfusion medicine. In: Handin RI, Lux SE, Stossel TP, eds. Blood: Principles and practice of hematology. Philadelphia: J.B. Lippincott Company, 1995;1998.

mia, myocardial insufficiency, or coagulation disorders.[10] Personal experience suggests that plasma exchange is more effective if used very early; therefore, therapy should be initiated within 12 hours of recognizing the problem and should be continued daily for several days. Some authors[10] also recommend that patients be started on high-dose corticosteroids to prevent a rebound antibody formation following plasma exchange. An analysis of prognostic factors suggests that low-amplitude muscle action potential, advanced age, longer time from the onset of disease, and increased need for ventilatory

support are correlated with poorer outcome of plasma exchange.[11] A more recent study[12] suggests that intravenous immune globulin is as effective as plasma exchange. If this claim is substantiated, the role of plasma exchange in the treatment of Guillain-Barré syndrome may change in the future.

Myasthenia gravis IgG-type antibodies to the acetylcholine receptor are an important part of the pathogenesis of myasthenia gravis. Plasma exchange has been used to lower the level of these antibodies.[13,14] There are many anecdotal reports of clinical improvement following plasma exchange in patients with myasthenia gravis.[2] However, no controlled trial of plasma exchange in this situation has ever been carried out. It appears that plasma exchange results in improvement in about two-thirds of patients, usually within 1 to 3 days of the start of the therapy.[15] Therefore, plasma exchange is recommended but only in certain specific situations of myasthenia gravis such as in the early stage before other treatments have become effective, in a crisis, or in chronic cases as an adjunct to other forms of immunosuppressive therapy.[2,15]

Multiple sclerosis The pathogenesis of multiple sclerosis is not known, but immunologic processes play an important role. Therefore, there has been interest in the use of plasma exchange to alter the humoral immunity in these patients. One clinical trial comparing plasma exchange with sham exchange found improvement in 28 of 45 patients in the plasma exchange arm.[16] There are few results from other structured trials. Because most patients with multiple sclerosis have a gradual downhill course but survive for 25 years, the Consensus Conference[2] concluded that "a treatment as uncomfortable, time-consuming, and expensive as plasma exchange is unlikely to be appropriate." It was also believed that plasma exchange would not be effective for patients who have already developed substantial neurologic damage. Thus, the use of plasma exchange might be beneficial in the approximately 5% of patients who develop a malignant course with severe disability in about 5 years.[2] However, currently plasma exchange is not recommended as a part of the therapy for multiple sclerosis.[2, 15, 17–19]

Eaton-Lambert syndrome Eaton-Lambert syndrome is a rare disorder that resembles myasthenia gravis. It is probably caused by an antibody to calcium channels in the myoneural junction. Because of the immunologic pathogenesis of the disease and a few individual reports suggesting that patients are improved by plasma exchange, plasma exchange is recommended as a part of the treatment of Eaton-Lambert syndrome.[2,20]

Chronic inflammatory demyelinating polyradiculoneuropathy One controlled study comparing plasma exchange with sham apheresis demonstrated a benefit for plasma exchange in this disease. However, the Consensus Conference considered that the overall benefit was probable rather than proven.[2] About one-third of the patients in the trial showed an improvement. Plasma exchange is used as part of the treatment of this disease if it is unresponsive to other forms of therapy.

Paraproteinemias Neurologic impairment can occur in patients with paraproteinemias. Reduction of the level of the paraproteins by chemotherapy or plasma exchange

may improve the neurologic symptoms,[21] but large-scale studies and extensive data to support this are not available. Thus, plasma exchange can be used as a part of the treatment strategy in these diseases, but data are not available to establish its value.

Amyotrophic lateral sclerosis   The cause of amyotrophic lateral sclerosis (ALS) is not known, and plasma exchange has not been shown to be of benefit in treating this disease.

Renal Diseases

Goodpasture's syndrome   Goodpasture's syndrome is a rapidly progressive syndrome in which renal damage is caused by antiglomerular basement membrane antibodies. Plasma exchange has been effective in slowing or reversing the renal and pulmonary damage.[22–24] Plasma exchange seems to be more helpful if it is instituted early in the course of disease. If pulmonary hemorrhage is present, we consider this to be a situation requiring urgent therapy and would institute plasma exchange within about 12 hours. If renal function is deteriorating, plasma exchange can be done in conjunction with hemodialysis. We would carry out plasma exchange frequently, almost daily for the first few days, on the rationale that early aggressive therapy is the most likely to be beneficial.

Rapidly progressive glomerulonephritis   This is a condition sometimes associated with antinucleophil cytoplasmic antibodies or immune complexes in which the causative antigen is not known. The role of plasma exchange in this situation is not clear. Plasma exchange may be more beneficial in patients with antinuclear cytoplasmic antibodies and is sometimes used as initial therapy in combination with immunosuppressive drugs.[25,26]

Multiple myeloma   Although multiple myeloma is a hematologic disease, renal damage occurs in a high proportion of patients, and survival is short once renal failure occurs. Light chains are thought to play a major role in the renal damage. Several studies have reported that plasma exchange is effective in removing light chains and improving renal function.[27–29] A controlled trial of plasma exchange in patients with renal failure due to myeloma was rather dramatic, with 13 of 15 plasma exchange patients recovering renal function compared with only two of 11 in the control group.[30] The 1-year survival was 66% in the plasma exchange group and 28% in the control group. Thus, plasma exchange, along with diuresis and chemotherapy, may be helpful in the management of renal damage in multiple myeloma.

Hematologic Diseases

Thrombotic thrombocytopenic purpura   Thrombotic thrombocytopenic purpura (TTP), a disease of unknown etiology, carried a very high mortality rate until the 1970s when treatment began to include plasma exchange. This in addition to probably better

overall care resulted in a dramatic improvement in survival to 70% to 80%.[26] Because the pathogenesis of TTP is not known, the exact physiologic role of plasma exchange is also not known. Exchange transfusions had been shown to be effective in a few cases as early as the 1950s,[31] and this led to interest in giving plasma transfusion because of the "consumptive" nature of TTP.[32,33] Both of these strategies were effective, and this led to the use of larger volumes of plasma instead of whole blood exchange or simple plasma transfusion, and plasma exchange was shown to be very effective.[34,35]

Although the pathophysiology of TTP is still not known, there is some evidence that von Willebrand factor high–molecular weight multimers are involved. Since von Willebrand factor is essential for binding of platelets to endothelium, there is reason to believe that alterations in these multimers could alter platelet-endothelial interactions. Therefore, the possibility of depleting high–molecular weight multimers was considered. This can be done by using the supernatant from cryoprecipitate, because the von Willebrand factor high-molecular weight multimers are found in the cryoprecipitate. An initial trial of plasma exchange using cryoprecipitate-poor plasma was effective.[36] A larger study from the Canadian Apheresis Group substantiated the effectiveness of cryoprecipitate-poor plasma.[37]

Plasma exchange is a major part of the therapy of TTP. It should be initiated early in the disease and continued daily if necessary to increase the platelet count. Either fresh frozen or cryoprecipitate-poor plasma can be used initially. If the patient fails to respond, the other form of plasma should be used. When the disease appears to have stabilized, the frequency of plasma exchange can be reduced gradually—for instance, to every other day. Some patients may require multiple plasma exchange to maintain their platelet count. One man was treated with more than 150 plasma exchanges over 2 years before he ultimately resolved his disease; he has remained symptom free for several years.

Cryoglobulinemia Cryoglobulinemia with symptoms due to abnormal IgM can be treated with plasma exchange. Neurologic or renal complications or Raynaud's phenomenon have been improved by plasma exchange.[38,39] Because IgM is primarily intravascular, plasma exchange is very effective in lowering the levels. The underlying disease must be treated, but plasma exchange can be very helpful in dealing with acute problems caused by the cryoglobulins.

Cold agglutinin disease The symptoms and hemolysis associated with high levels of cold agglutinins can be improved acutely with plasma exchange.[40] As with cryoglobulinemia, the underlying disease must be treated, but plasma exchange is an effective strategy to reduce the level of IgM antibody and reduce the hemolysis.[40]

Hyperviscosity syndrome Hyperviscosity syndrome is usually caused by IgM-type immunoglobulins, and plasma exchange is very effective in lowering IgM, reducing (improving) viscosity, and relieving symptoms. Plasma exchange can be a valuable part of the acute treatment of hyperviscosity while measures such as chemotherapy take effect.

Collagen Vascular Diseases

Rheumatoid arthritis   Rheumatoid arthritis is a chronic autoimmune inflammatory disease of unknown etiology. Because the immunologic alterations are thought to be important in the pathogenesis of the disease, some treatment has involved removing lymphocytes, plasma, or both. Initial studies suggested that a course of lymphoplasma-pheresis over about 3 months caused clinical improvement that lasted 3 to 4 months after therapy was stopped.[41] A later small controlled trial involving sham apheresis also demonstrated reductions in circulating immune complexes, rheumatoid factor, and joint swelling and improvement in clinical function.[42] An accompanying editorial[43] advised caution in interpreting the results and especially in applying this to the general treatment of rheumatoid arthritis. A subsequent controlled trial involving sham apheresis or plasma exchange but no lymphocyte removal did not show a clinical benefit.[44] Patients in the groups receiving plasma exchange and sham apheresis improved equally, suggesting a placebo effect. Several laboratory measures improved, but these changes were not associated with improvements in clinical measures. In the absence of very substantial data defining a clear benefit for plasma exchange in some phase of rheumatoid arthritis, this has not become a part of therapy and is not recommended at present.[45]

Other Miscellaneous Diseases

Pemphigus   IgG autoantibodies directed against intracellular bridges and skin basement membrane may be involved in the pathophysiology of pemphigus. High-dose corticosteroids are effective treatment in most patients, but this therapy requires several weeks to become effective. Plasma exchange has been used in the early acute stage of the disease or for maintenance in patients who respond poorly to corticosteroids. Individual case reports and series have shown a reduction in the IgG autoantibodies and a clinical benefit from plasma exchange.[46] A controlled trial did not show a benefit, and there was no reduction in autoantibody level. Thus, although the data are not conclusive, plasma exchange may be used in the early stages of pemphigus or for patients who fail to respond to steroids.

AIDS-related idiopathic thrombocytopenic purpura   Although plasma exchange has not been used successfully in idiopathic thrombocytopenic purpura (ITP), it has occasionally been helpful in AIDS-related ITP when combined with intravenous immunoglobulin.[47] This was attempted because of the desire to avoid immunosuppressive therapies such as corticosteroids or splenectomy in these patients. However, plasma exchange has not been generally used in this situation. Several reports of the use of the staphylococcal protein A column also appeared promising (see below), but this also has not gained much use.

Rejection of transplanted organs   Occasionally plasma exchange has been used as an adjunct to other strategies to treat acute rejection of transplanted organs.[48,49] Although it appeared that plasma exchange might have been helpful in the multifaceted

approach to the rejection episodes, this has not become a commonly used part of anti-rejection therapy. It seems likely that physical removal of the antibody is not a practical way to overcome the rate of antibody production.

Although ABO incompatibility has been thought to preclude transplantation of kidneys, some ABO-incompatible kidney transplants have been attempted during the past few years. Plasma exchange was used to reduce the level of circulating ABO antibody; however, this was only modestly effective, and transplantation of ABO-incompatible kidneys has not become practical.

Preparation for liver transplantation   Patients awaiting liver transplantation may have coagulopathy or other metabolic complications due to the liver disease. Plasma exchange can be used to stabilize and maintain these patients while they await a donor organ.

PLASMA EXCHANGE

Vascular Access for Plasma Exchange

Vascular access for plasma exchange may be via peripheral veins or by venous catheters. Peripheral venous access is preferable because there are additional complications associated with the use of venous catheters. Plasma exchange can usually be initiated using antecubital veins, as illustrated by the observation that only 4% of patients were ineligible for one randomized trial because of inadequate peripheral venous access.[50] Unfortunately, venous catheters are often necessary because peripheral veins are too small or are inadequate for the multiple venipunctures necessary for several plasma exchanges. In one study, central venous lines were placed in 72% of patients, an arteriovenous fistula or shunt in 17%; peripheral veins were suitable in only 11%.[4] In another summary of 381 procedures in 68 patients with neurologic diseases,[51] antecubital veins were used in 30% of procedures. In a third report of 363 procedures in 46 patients with neurologic diseases, antecubital veins were used successfully in 50% of procedures.[52] If a catheter is necessary, the apheresis personnel should discuss the venous access needs with the patient's primary physician so that the optimum catheter can be selected. Some considerations are (*a*) the number of therapeutic apheresis procedures expected, (*b*) other treatments that might require venous access, (*c*) the expected duration of treatment, (*d*) whether or not the patient will remain in the hospital, and (*d*) the availability of family members to assist with catheter care if the patient will be out of the hospital.[53] The types of catheters that have been used most commonly for plasma exchange include Hickman, Quinton-Mahurkar, and triple lumen. The Quinton-Mahurkar catheters may be placed in the jugular, subclavian, or femoral veins. In one study,[52] the complication rate was lower with Quinton-Mahurkar catheters than with the other two. The Quinton-Mahurkar catheter has a double lumen, and the outflow and inflow holes at the tip are separated to minimize recirculation.[53] If catheters are to be used, they must have sufficient rigidity so they do not collapse when negative pressure for blood removal is applied. The Quinton-Mahurkar catheter is made of

temperature-sensitive material that is rigid during insertion but softens as the temperature increases inside the vein after insertion. It is not advisable to position the return flow from a catheter near the right atrium endocardium because of the possibility that the replacement solution might create an irritable focus and result in cardiac arrhythmia.

Techniques of Plasma Exchange

In plasma exchange using blood cell separators, the whole blood enters the instrument, where most of the red cells, leukocytes, and platelets are separated from the cell-poor plasma. This plasma is diverted into a waste bag and is replaced with one or more of several available solutions.[54] These include fresh frozen plasma, albumin, and saline. For plasma exchange using the COBE Spectra, the instrument is set up and primed according to the manufacturer's instructions for plasma exchange. The single-stage channel filler and TPE tubing set are used. Transfer packs are attached to collect the plasma being removed. The alarms should be tested at least once each day. The patient's gender, height, and weight are entered into the instrument control panel. The microprocessor in the instrument will calculate the estimated total blood volume from the data entered. Then the patient's hematocrit, type of replacement fluid, and desired fluid balance are entered. The screen will display the estimated volume of plasma to be removed, volume of replacement fluid, volume of anticoagulant, and procedure time. The instrument is then connected to the venous access and return lines, and saline drips keep each line open. If heparin is to be administered, it is given at this time and the procedure is initiated after a 5-minute wait for the heparin to take effect. The operator confirms the values for volumes to be removed and replaced and, if correct, activates the instrument. Anticoagulation may be accomplished with ACD-A, heparinized saline, heparinized ACD-A, or other locally selected solutions. The inlet flow value is set using the key pads. Depending on the anticoagulant, the inlet flow to anticoagulant ratio is selected and the inlet flow rate adjusted to reflect this. If changes in the inlet flow rate are desired, these can be made during the procedure by using the key pad. When the desired plasma volume has been exchanged, the procedure is terminated by pressing the change mode and rinseback instructions on the key pad. The control panel provides instructions for completing the termination of the procedure. The lines can then be disconnected from the patient. The plasma removed must be discarded as biohazardous waste.

The volume of plasma to be exchanged is usually based on the estimated plasma volume of the patient. Because there is continuous mixing in the patient of replacement solution and patient's plasma, the relationship between the fraction of the unwanted compound remaining and the proportion of the patient's plasma volume exchanged is exponential (Fig. 19.1). After exchange equal to the patient's plasma volume, the unwanted component will be reduced to approximately 35% of the initial value. Exchanging 2 times the patient's plasma volume further reduces the unwanted component only to approximately 15% of the initial value. Because of this diminishing effectiveness, we usually try to exchange about 1.5 times the patient's plasma volume. Depending on the size of the patient, this procedure may last between 4 and 6 hours. It does not appear that a rebound overshoot in antibody levels occurs after plasma exchange.[55,56] Usually plasma exchange therapy involves several exchanges over a

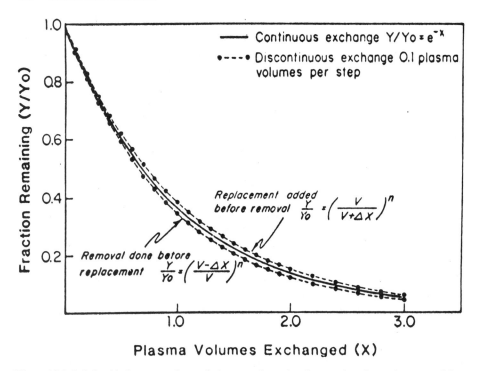

Figure 19.1. Relationship between volume of plasma exchanged and proportion of constituent remaining. *(Source: Chopek M, McCullough J. Therapeutic plasma exchange. Lab Med 1981;12:745–753.)*

period of days or weeks. The frequency will depend on the situation. For instance, in myasthenia gravis we often use a course of six plasma exchanges over 2 weeks, possibly adding one or two more procedures if indicated. In contrast, treatment of a patient with a factor VIII inhibitor might involve plasma exchange daily for several days.

A beautiful model of the effect of plasma exchange was developed by Kellogg and Hester.[57] This model takes into account the size of the exchange relative to the patient's blood volume, the amount of material available to exchange, the amount of material in both the intravascular and extravascular compartments, the mobility of the material between the pools, and the production and catabolic rate of the material. When tested in patients with hyperbilirubinemia and hypercholesterolemia, the model showed good agreement with in vivo observations.[57]

Replacement Solutions

Managing the fluid balance of the patient during the exchange may be difficult, especially if the patient has compromised cardiovascular function or is hemodynamically unstable due to the clinical situation. Therefore, it is usually desirable to replace the plasma being removed with an equal volume of material with oncotic pressure similar to plasma. The most common of these solutions is 5% normal serum albumin. In some situations, it is not necessary to replace the plasma removed with an equal volume of

albumin. Instead, some saline (crystalloid) can be used, but this should be no more than 25% to 30% of the replacement volume and must depend on the patient's specific condition. If the patient has an elevated protein level or is quite stable from a cardiovascular standpoint, some mixture of saline and albumin can be used. On the other hand, if the patient is hemodynamically unstable, it is best to maintain the intravascular volume unless a decrease or increase is indicated to correct the instability.

Usually albumin alone or albumin plus saline is used as the replacement solution. This avoids the possibility of disease transmission and allergic reactions from fresh frozen plasma. As discussed below, the loss of coagulation or other proteins is not so extreme that replacement with fresh frozen plasma is necessary in patients who have a normal coagulation system. Fresh frozen plasma should be used only when there is a need to replace coagulation factors or other unknown but essential constituents such as in the therapy of thrombotic thrombocytopenic purpura. An example of the relative amount of replacement solutions is available from Canada, where data are obtained on a national scale about replacement solutions. Approximately 8,000 L of albumin, 3,000 L of fresh frozen plasma, and 275 L of liquid plasma were used during the period from 1981 to 1991.[3] Thus, albumin was used about two and a half times as much as fresh frozen plasma. In an assessment of TPE in another country, albumin was used for replacement in about 50% of exchanges, fresh frozen plasma in about 22%, and a combination of albumin and fresh frozen plasma in 22%.[4]

Biochemical Changes Following Plasma Exchange

Removal of such a large volume of plasma has several biochemical effects.[58–60] Because some platelets are in the plasma being removed, there is about a 30% decrease in the platelet count, which takes about 3 days to return to baseline. The changes in the proteins IgG, IgM, IgA, factor V, ferritin, transferrin, lactic dehydrogenase, serum glutamic oxaloacetic transaminase, and alkaline phosphatase follow closely the decrease expected based on the volume of plasma removed.[58,59] When no fresh frozen plasma is used for replacement, coagulation test results are quite abnormal at the end of the plasma exchange. For instance, the prothrombin time is usually 20 seconds or more, the partial thromboplastin time is more than 180 seconds, and the fibrinogen is decreased by about 70%.[58,61] These test values return to baseline in about 24 hours, except fibrinogen, which normalizes in 72 hours[58,59] (Fig. 19.2).

Complement components C3, C4, and CH50 can be depleted when albumin is used as the replacement fluid. Because of its rapid rate of synthesis, however, complement is not depleted unless plasma exchange is done daily for several days.[62]

There are no clinically important changes in electrolytes as a result of plasma exchange. Because citrate is usually used as the anticoagulant, and it exerts its effect by binding calcium, an important consideration is the ionized calcium level. If fresh frozen plasma is used for replacement, this provides additional citrate. Citrate toxicity is the result of the hypocalcemia, not the citrate itself. The hypocalcemia may cause symptoms of paresthesia, muscle cramping, tremors, shivering, lightheadedness, and anxiety; when more severe, it can cause grand mal seizures, tetany, and most dangerous of all, electrocardiographic abnormalities. Studies of citrate and calcium metabolism during normal-

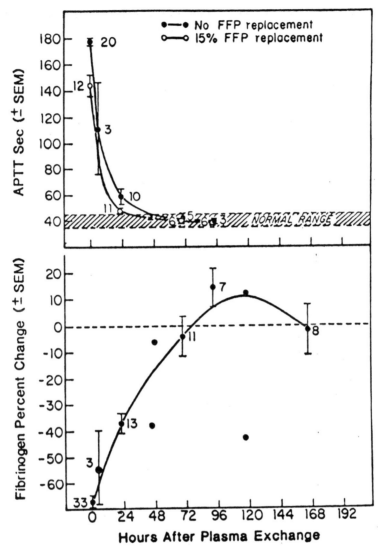

Figure 19.2. Normalization of fibrinogen level and activated partial thromboplastin time after plasma exchange using albumin for replacement. *(Source: Chopek M, McCullough J. Therapeutic plasma exchange. Lab Med 1981;12:745–753.)*

donor plateletpheresis have established that symptoms only begin to occur when the rate of citrate infusion exceeds 60 mg/kg/hour.[63,64] Although there is some reduction in ionized calcium levels even when albumin is used as the replacement solution,[58,65] the citrate infusion rates are below 60 mg/kg/hour and only approach this rate when fresh frozen plasma is used and the flow rates are substantial. Thus, routine supplementation with calcium during plasma exchange is not recommended.

Table 19.2 Comparison of changes induced by plasma exchange of 1.0 to 1.5 plasma volumes with equal volume replacement

	Albumin replacement	FFP replacement
Hematology	↓ platelets (30% to 50%) ↑ granulocytes (2,000 to 3,000/μL) ↓ hemoglobin (10% to 15%)	↓ platelets (30% to 50%) ↑ granulocytes (2,000 to 3,000/μL) No change in hemoglobin
Proteins	↓ pathological antibodies (60% to 75%) ↓ all other proteins (60% to 75%) Long-term effects depend upon TER, FCR, and S (see text)	↓ pathological antibodies (60% to 75%) All other proteins change to approximate levels present in FFP
Coagulation	↓ individual factors (60% to 75%) transient coagulopathy (24 to 48 hr)	All factors approximate levels in FFP
Electrolytes	Slight ↓ potassium Albumin: ↓ bicarbonate (6 mEq/L) ↑ chloride (4 mEq/L) PPF: ↑ bicarbonate ↓ chloride	↓ potassium (0.7 mEq/L) ↑ bicarbonate (3 mEq/L) ↓ chloride (6 mEq/L)
Citrate and calcium	Slight ↑ citrate (0.2 mM/L) ↓ total calcium (1.4 mg/dL) ↓ ionized calcium (0.5 mEq/L)	↑ citrate (1.1 mM/L) Slight ↓ total calcium (0.3 mg/dL) ↓ ionized calcium (0.6mEq/L)

Source: Chopek M, McCullough J. Protein and biochemical changes during plasma exchange. In: Therapeutic Hemapheresis. Arlington, VA: American Association of Blood Banks, 1980:13.

FCR, Fractional catabolic rate; FFP, fresh frozen plasma; PPF, plasma protein fraction; S, synthesis; TER, transcapillary escape rate.

The differences between albumin and fresh frozen plasma as replacement solutions are summarized in Table 19.2.

COMPLICATIONS OF PLASMA EXCHANGE

Apheresis of normal donors for the production of blood components is well tolerated with few side effects and only very rare serious complications. However, therapeutic apheresis is carried out in ill patients who should not be expected to react the same as a healthy donor.[66] It has been estimated that at least 59 deaths have occurred due to therapeutic apheresis, and the mortality rate is 3 per 10,000 procedures.[66,67] Most deaths have resulted from cardiac or respiratory arrest, but deaths due to anaphylaxis, pulmonary embolus, and vascular perforation have also been reported (Table 19.3).[67,68] The nature and incidence of complications will depend somewhat on the condition of the patient prior to plasma exchange. For instance, a stable patient with myasthenia gravis might have fewer complications than an actively bleeding hemophilia patient with a factor VIII inhibitor. In one comprehensive report of complications of plasma exchange, side effects occurred during 12% of procedures and involved 40% of

Table 19.3 Complications of plasma exchange

Mild
  Muscle cramps
  Perioral paresthesias
  Urticaria
  Metabolic changes
  Coagulation changes
Moderate
  Hypotension
  Vasovagal reaction
  Nausea
  Vomiting
Severe
  Pneumothorax
  Catheter-related bacteremia
  Sternocleidomastoid hematoma

patients.[69] The incidence of severe complications was 0.5% of procedures. A national registry of therapeutic apheresis procedures in the former East Germany reported complications in 22% of 1,945 procedures in 419 patients.[4] There were severe complications in 2%, including cardiac arrhythmia, bronchospasm, adult respiratory distress syndrome (ARDS), and thromboembolic problems. Of the 419 patients, 87 died; of these, 64 died of their underlying disease, and 19 of related causes not thought to be due to the plasma exchange. Twelve patients died during or immediately after the plasma exchange, and four of these fatalities were thought to be due to the apheresis procedure.[4] Two of these fatalities resulted from ARDS, one from myocardial infarction, and one from pulmonary embolus. The complication rate was almost twice as great when fresh frozen plasma was used as the replacement solution compared to albumin, although the nature of the complications was not described.[4] The Canadian Apheresis Study Group reported that adverse reactions occurred in about 9% of 58,000 procedures.[3] About two-thirds of these were mild, and only 8% were severe, resulting in a severe reaction rate of 7 per 1,000 procedures.[3]

In general, plasma exchange is reasonably safe if it is used in appropriate clinical circumstances where there is a rational expectation of benefit to the patient and in which proper nursing care is available for the patient. The complications of plasma exchange can be categorized as those related to (*a*) vascular access, (*b*) replacement solutions, or (*c*) the procedure itself.

Vascular Access

The most severe complications of plasma exchange are sometimes related to the vascular access devices.[51] In one study of 391 procedures in 63 patients, the only four severe complications were bacterial sepsis due to an infected catheter, a sternocleidomastoid hematoma, a pneumothorax, and a hemopneumothorax, all resulting from placement of a subclavian catheter. An additional patient exsanguinated from an artery

that was lacerated during placement of a subclavian catheter. In another study of vascular access in patients undergoing TPE, there were three severe catheter-related complications in 23 patients who received 28 venous catheters.[52] The complications were a pneumothorax during placement of the catheter, acute respiratory failure due to an air embolus after removal of a catheter, and bacteremia from an infected catheter. Thus, the necessity of using venous catheters is an important part of the risks of plasma exchange.

Replacement Solutions

Complications related to replacement solutions include citrate-induced hypocalcemia, coagulation factor depletion, depletion of other functional proteins, electrolyte abnormalities, and transfusion reactions or disease transmission when plasma is used. Allergic reactions such as urticaria or mild fevers are rather common even when albumin is the replacement solution. Progenic reactions can occur to specific lots of albumin.[70] An unusual case of hemolysis due to infusion of hypotonic replacement solution has been reported.[71] The 25% albumin was diluted to 5% in sterile water rather than saline, resulting in the hypotonic solution. Depletion of coagulation factors leading to a bleeding diathesis should not occur, because this can be prevented by using fresh frozen plasma as the replacement solution. The same is true for other functional proteins and electrolytes. If fresh frozen plasma is used, febrile or allergic reactions are more common because of the proteins in the plasma. Antibodies in the plasma may cause transfusion-related acute lung injury (see Chapter 14), and ABO-incompatible plasma can cause hemolysis.

Apheresis Procedure

Mild reactions are rather common during plasma exchange; they are usually chills (possibly due to infusion of room-temperature replacement solutions) or lightheadedness (possibly due to a vasovagal reaction). These can also be symptoms of hypocalcemia due to citrate infusion, and so when the symptoms begin the operator often slows the blood flow rate and the symptoms subside. Another procedure-related complication is hypotension or hypertension due to fluid imbalance. Hypotension can be caused by hypovolemia resulting from the blood required to fill the extracorporeal circuit. This can be a substantial volume if the Haemonetics equipment is used, because plasma is continually removed until the bowl is filled with red cells. Thus, the volume of the circuit in relation to the patient's blood volume must be considered, and for smaller patients it may be desirable to prime the circuit with albumin. If this is done, the dilutional effect of the priming solution must also be considered. Hypertension can occur if the volume of fluid returned exceeds that removed. Thus, it is important that the operator closely monitor the fluid balance during the procedure. Other types of reactions include hypersensitivity to ethylene oxide and anaphylactoid reactions consisting of flushing, hypotension, bradycardia, and dyspnea occurring in patients taking angiotensin-converting enzyme (ACE) inhibitors for hypertension. It has been speculated that during plasma exchange, vasoactive substances are produced and the ACE inhibitor prevents their catabolism, resulting in the symptoms.[72,73]

RED CELL EXCHANGE OR ERYTHROCYTAPHERESIS

Red cell exchange is done when removal of a large proportion of the patient's circulating red cells is desired. Use of a blood cell separator makes it possible to rapidly remove a patient's red cells and replace them with normal-donor cells while maintaining hemostasis and fluid balance. Red cell exchange transfusion is used to treat or prevent sickle cell crisis[74,75] and to treat severe malaria.[76] The objectives of the therapy for patients with sickle cell disease are discussed more fully in Chapter 12. The exchange transfusion procedure is carried out similarly to plasma exchange, except that the red cells instead of the plasma are diverted into a waste bag and donor red cells are recombined with the plasma for return to the patient.

THERAPEUTIC CYTAPHERESIS

In some patients with hematologic proliferative disorders, symptoms and severe complications can occur because of the high levels of circulating cells. Symptomatic vascular slugging due to high levels of circulating leukemia cells can be a medical emergency. In one study, leukemic cellular aggregates were the cause of death in 24% of patients with acute myelogenous leukemia and 60% of patients with chronic myelogenous leukemia.[77] All patients who died with leukocyte counts greater than 200,000/μL and half of those who died with leukocyte counts between 50,000 and 200,000/μL had prominent cellular aggregates and thrombi in their tissues. Central nervous system leukostasis can lead to cerebral vascular neurosis with intracranial hemorrhage or thrombosis,[78] pulmonary insufficiency,[79] or coronary artery occlusion.[80] Patients with acute myelogenous leukemia and blast counts above 100,000/μL are likely to experience acute respiratory distress or fatal intracranial hemorrhage. Thus, emergency therapeutic leukapheresis may be used in conjunction with chemotherapy when the blast count is greater than 50,000/μL or approaches 100,000/μL.

Blood cell separators can be used to accomplish this by removing abnormal accumulations of leukocytes, platelets, or red cells (Table 19.1). In therapeutic cytapheresis, the blood cell separator instrument is operated similarly to collection of the particular blood component from a normal donor. The procedure is usually lengthened to process more blood and thus remove a large number of cells. The number of cells removed depends on the initial level but can be 10^{11} or even 10^{12}. The peripheral leukocyte or platelet count may be reduced by 20% to 80% depending on the initial level.[81] Several instruments are available for therapeutic cytapheresis. One study directly compared the COBE Spectra and the Haemonetics V-50 for therapeutic plateletpheresis and leukapheresis.[82] The V-50 provided a greater platelet reduction in therapeutic plateletpheresis; the leukocyte reduction in therapeutic leukapheresis was similar for both instruments. There was greater hemoglobin loss and a larger extracorporeal volume during cytapheresis with the V-50.

In general, there are fewer complications from cytapheresis than from plasma exchange because in cytapheresis the small volume of cells removed is replaced by saline and/or anticoagulant. However, patients undergoing therapeutic cytapheresis are

often quite ill, and the cytapheresis procedure may be risky because of other factors such as bleeding or central nervous system problems. Reaction rates of 8% to 10% have been reported for therapeutic plateletpheresis and 14% to 21% for therapeutic leukapheresis.[82]

As in therapeutic plasma exchange, very few controlled trials of therapeutic cytapheresis have been carried out. There is no doubt that cytapheresis can be used to rapidly lower the elevated cell levels in acute or chronic leukemia and thrombocytosis. Sometimes the procedure is done to prevent potential problems such as central nervous system vascular slugging in patients with chronic myelogenous leukemia, reduction of metabolic problems due to cell lysis during chemotherapy of acute myelogenous leukemia, or prevention of thrombotic episodes in patients with thrombocytosis. In other situations, cytapheresis is done to attempt to treat existing problems such as central nervous system symptoms in acute or chronic myelogenous leukemia patients with high leukocyte counts.

The medical literature is helpful in establishing the general indications for these procedures, but it is often difficult to decide for specific patients whether cytapheresis is necessary and, if done, whether it was helpful. The following is a summary of the value of therapeutic cytapheresis in specific situations:

Chronic Myelogenous Leukemia

Symptoms of leukostasis may develop when the leukocyte count exceeds 100,000/µL. If the clinical condition warrants, one or two cytapheresis procedures can be used to rapidly lower the leukocyte level. Chemotherapy should also be started, because cytapheresis is not effective maintenance therapy.

Chronic Lymphocytic Leukemia

It is not clear that high leukocyte levels in these patients create problems. Although the count can be lowered rapidly by cytapheresis, this is not recommended unless the patient has symptoms due to high levels of circulating lymphocytes.

Acute Myelogenous Leukemia

Patients who present with leukocyte counts greater than 100,000/µL (usually mostly myeloblasts) may have serious problems during the first few days of chemotherapy. These problems—which include leukostasis, hyperuricemia, renal failure, and disseminated intravascular coagulopathy—are thought to be partly due to the lysis of a large number of leukemia cells. The problems may be reduced or prevented by lowering the leukocyte count by cytapheresis. Usually one or two cytapheresis procedures suffice.

Thrombocytosis

Thrombocytosis that occurs as part of myeloproliferative diseases can lead to hemorrhage or thrombosis, especially in the central nervous system. Platelet counts of

1,000,000/μL or more may occur. Cytapheresis can be used to lower the platelet count rapidly[81,83] with the expectation that complications of thrombocytosis would be prevented.

PHOTOPHERESIS

Photopheresis is a form of adoptive immunotherapy (see also Chapter 18) involving the combination of photochemotherapy and leukapheresis. In photopheresis, the patient is given a dose of 8-methoxypsoralen, and 1 to 2 hours later leukapheresis is performed. A mononuclear cell concentrate is collected containing approximately 1 to 2 $\times$ 10^{10} cells, or about 10% to 15% of the patient's total circulating lymphocytes. After the mononuclear cell concentrate has been collected, it is removed from the instrument, heparinized, and diluted with the patient's plasma and saline. The mononuclear cell concentrate is then passed for about 2 to 3 hours through a disposable clear plastic plate that rests between two banks of ultraviolet A lights. The ultraviolet irradiation activates the psoralen to become an alkylating agent, but this is only temporary because the effect only persists while the cells are exposed to the ultraviolet light. The ultraviolet-treated mononuclear cell concentrate is then transfused to the patient as a form of adoptive immunotherapy. It is important that the mononuclear cell concentrate has a low hematocrit, because red cells absorb the light and thus interfere with the effect of the ultraviolet light on the mononuclear cells.

There are several possible mechanisms of action of photopheresis, but in general it is believed that the process somehow directs an immune response against expanded disease-producing clones. Suggested possible mechanisms of action of photopheresis include (a) stimulation of the development of anticlonotypic response against clones of pathogenic T lymphocytes; (b) stimulation of the development of clone-specific suppressor cells; (c) activation of monocytes; (d) release of cytokines, including interleukins 1 and 6 and tumor necrosis factor; and (e) presentation of intact but inactivated cells to the immune system, enabling development of an immune response to the cells. It seems likely that more than one mechanism of action occurs, because photopheresis appears to be beneficial in several clinical situations.

Photopheresis has been used in the treatment of cutaneous T-cell lymphoma, autoimmune disease, and allograft rejection.[84,85] The initial success of photopheresis—and the only situation in which this is accepted therapy—was in cutaneous T-cell lymphoma when at the advanced stage.[86] Early stages of cutaneous T-cell lymphoma have survival rates of 8 years, and this has not been improved by photopheresis. However, for patients with advanced disease, a response rate of 75% was reported and the median survival was extended from about 30 months to well beyond 60 months.[87] These results applied to patients with both Sézary syndrome and mycosis fungoides. The skin disease improves and the leukocyte counts decrease, usually into the normal range. Photopheresis is given as a course of treatment. Usually two treatments are given on consecutive days each month for 1 year. After patients have stabilized, the interval between treatments is lengthened. Some patients develop fever following transfusion of their mononuclear cells and the erythrodermia usually becomes more severe, although this diminishes as the treatments progress.

Photopheresis has been used or is under investigation in the treatment of the autoimmune diseases pemphigus vulgaris, scleroderma, rheumatoid arthritis, and systemic lupus erythematosus, but its benefit has not yet been established in any of these conditions.[84] Photopheresis has reversed acute rejection of transplanted hearts and reduced chronic rejection in a few patients.[88,89] It has been used to reverse rejection of a transplanted kidney in at least one patient.[90] Thus, photopheresis shows promise as an adjunct to anti-rejection therapy for solid organ transplants. It seems likely that this form of adoptive immunotherapy will be used increasingly and that studies of the scientific basis for its actions will be very interesting. The long-term role of this therapy in immunologic diseases and malignancy other than advanced cutaneous T-cell lymphoma remains to be established.

THERAPEUTIC APHERESIS USING IMMUNOADSORPTION COLUMNS

Familial Hypercholesterolemia

Apheresis can be used to treat familial hypercholesterolemia. The general approaches involve (a) immunoadsorbent affinity columns using antilipoprotein B, (b) chemical adsorbent affinity columns using dextran sulfate, (c) chemical precipitation with heparin, and (d) secondary filtration.[91] In the procedures, blood cell separators are used to produce plasma, which is then passed over the columns in a continuous flow. About 3 to 4 L of plasma is usually treated during 2 hours.[91] The patient is usually treated every 2 weeks. Adverse reactions, which are most commonly chills and/or hypotension, are mild and occur in fewer than 5% of procedures.[92] These methods can produce a decrease in LDL cholesterol of 130 to 170 mg/dL or 44% to 81%.[93,94] This is associated with prevention of the progression of carotid or aortotibial vascular disease.[92] There is no doubt that extracorporeal therapy using LDL-specific apheresis is safe and efficacious,[95] but it is very costly and involves a substantial commitment by the patient.

Autoimmune Disease Treated with Dextran Sulfate Columns

Dextran sulfate columns such as those used to treat hypercholesterolemia have also been used for selective immunoadsorption of anti-DNA from the blood of patients with systemic lupus erythematosus.[96,97] The clinical value of this therapy is not established.

Immune Disease Treated with Staphylococcal Protein A Columns

Staphylococcal protein A binds IgG—especially IgG classes 1, 2, and 4—and also immune complexes. Staphylococcal protein A (SPA) cannot be infused because of severe toxicity, but plasma exposed to SPA bonded to silica beads, sepharose, or polyacrylamide can be transfused to patients with few side effects. During the 1970s, it was thought that in the immunity of cancer, blocking antibodies of the IgG type might interfere with the body's natural defenses against the tumor. Thus, removal of the blocking antibodies was a possible strategy for treating cancer. As a result, considerable interest

developed in using SPA to remove these antibodies, and some clinical studies were carried out in patients with carcinoma of the colon and breast.[98–101] Although initial experience was promising, these encouraging results were not sustained, as illustrated by the lack of subsequent reports of success.

This flurry of activity did, however, result in the production of a clinically useful column system over which plasma could be perfused and returned to the patient. Columns were developed and made available for investigational use. The SPA procedure can be carried out in two ways. A small volume of blood (approximately 500 mL) is withdrawn as for an ordinary blood donation, then the plasma is separated and passed over the column in the laboratory. The treated plasma is then transfused to the patient. Alternatively, a larger volume of plasma (approximately 1,000 to 2,000 mL) can be processed through the column by placing it in the plasma line of a blood cell separator. Any blood cell separator used for plasma exchange can be used for SPA column processing. The instrument is operated as for plasma exchange but the SPA column is placed in the plasma line. The plasma is recombined with red cells and returned to the patient continuously throughout the procedure.

As clinical studies of the SPA column in malignancy were under way, interest developed in using the SPA system in other malignant and immunologic diseases. Since the first area of activity was malignant disease, SPA treatment was also attempted in multiple myeloma,[102] acute myeloid or lymphocytic leukemia,[103,104] and chronic lymphocytic leukemia.[105] Although some of these patients seemed to improve, this therapy clearly was not a major breakthrough. During the late 1970s and the 1980s, the autoimmune nature of idiopathic thrombocytopenia was becoming more clear, and the SPA columns were used to treat refractory ITP by removing the antiplatelet IgG antibody. Patients underwent six treatments over about 2 weeks. SPA treatment was very effective, providing an increase in platelet count in 46% to 66% of patients refractory to other therapies.[106,107] As a result, the SPA column is licensed by the U.S. Food and Drug Administration for the treatment of autoimmune thrombocytopenia (idiopathic thrombocytopenic purpura, or ITP). Another immunologic condition for which there were no good treatment strategies in the late 1970s and early 1980s was inhibitors to coagulation factors VIII and IX in hemophilia A and B. Since the inhibitors were known to be IgG antibodies, the removal of these antibodies by SPA treatment was a logical approach. This was effective[108] and was used until activated coagulation factor concentrates became available to bypass the inhibited portion of the coagulation system. SPA columns have also been used for removal of IgG antibodies in patients who are alloimmunized and refractory to platelet transfusions,[109,110] patients with hemolytic- uremic syndrome, and patients experiencing rejection of transplanted organs. In most of these situations, other than ITP, the results have been mixed. Occasional individual patients seem to benefit from the therapy, but many do not. The continued production of antibody and/or the presence of the antigen makes treatment by physical removal of IgG antibody of limited effectiveness.

Because of the special need to avoid immunosuppressive therapy for ITP in AIDS patients, plasma exchange (see above) and the SPA column have been used. Preliminary experience with SPA column treatment was encouraging,[106,111] but this therapy has not been widely pursued in the past few years. A trial of the SPA column in an AIDS patient who has ITP unresponsive to other therapies or in whom the usual ITP therapies are not

effective is appropriate. Recently the manufacture of the SPA columns was transferred to a new company. Thus, a new phase of studies may be undertaken to determine whether other clinical indications can be defined.

Another consideration in the use of the SPA columns is the side effects of the treatment. Although several reports contended that the side effects were modest, some side effects have been severe and have included generalized pain, fever, rigors, sweating, hypotension, nausea, abdominal pain, dyspnea, cyanosis, disorientation, arthralgia, skin rash, vasculitis, purpura, thrombosis, renal failure, urticaria edema, and chest pain.[112] Some of these effects may result from the SPA-caused binding of immune complexes liberating free antibody, complement activation, and increased helper T cell activity.[112] As clinical trials of the SPA columns are carried out in the future, it will be important to define the side effects as well as the benefits of the therapy.

THERAPEUTIC APHERESIS IN CHILDREN

Therapeutic plasma exchange or cytapheresis can be performed on even very small children.[113,114] The major consideration is that the instruments are designed for adults and thus the extracorporeal volume may be too large for small patients. This can be overcome by priming the instrument with red cells, albumin, or other combinations of fluids. The blood flow rates through the instrument are not high for adults but may represent a large portion of a small child's blood volume. Therefore, problems can arise quickly if there are difficulties with the lines or blood flow. Also, the rate of return of blood and solutions can be much greater in relation to the total blood volume of a small child, and thus citrate or other complications can occur more frequently than in adults if adjustments in blood flow are not made to reflect the small patient's blood volume.

REFERENCES

1. American Society for Apheresis Standards and Education Committee. Organizational guidelines for therapeutic apheresis facilities. J Clin Apheresis 1996;11:42–45.
2. Consensus Conference. The utility of therapeutic plasmapheresis for neurological disorders. JAMA 1986;256:1333–1337.
3. Rock G, Herbert CA, and members of the Canadian Apheresis Study Group. Therapeutic apheresis in Canada. J Clin Apheresis 1992;7:47–48.
4. Schmitt E, Kundt G, Klinkmann H. Three years with a national apheresis registry. J Clin Apheresis 1992;7:58–62.
5. Council on Scientific Affairs. Current status of therapeutic plasmapheresis and related techniques—report of the AMA panel on therapeutic plasmapheresis. JAMA 1985;253:819–825.
6. The safety, efficacy, and cost effectiveness of therapeutic apheresis—excerpts from Congressional Office of Technology Assessment study. Contemp Dial Nephrol, July 1985:32–36.
7. Shumak KH, Rock GA. Therapeutic plasma exchange. N Engl J Med 1984;310:76–81.
8. McKhann GM, Griffin JW, Cornblath DR, Quaskey SA, Mellits ED. Role of therapeutic plasmapheresis in the acute Guillain-Barré syndrome. J Neuroimmunol 1988;20:297–300.
9. The Guillain-Barré Syndrome Study Group. Plasmapheresis and acute Guillain-Barré syndrome. Neurology 1985;335:1096–1104.
10. Kunze K, Emskotter T. The value of plasmapheresis in the treatment of acute and chronic Guillain-Barré syndrome. J Neuroimmunol 1988;20:301–303.

11. McKhann GM, Griffin JW, Cornblatch DR, et al. Plasmapheresis and Guillain-Barré syndrome: analysis of prognostic factors and the effect of plasmapheresis. Ann Neurol 1988;23:347–353.

12. van der Meche FGA, Schmitz PIM, and the Dutch Guillain-Barré Study Group. A randomized trial comparing intravenous immune globulin and plasma exchange in Guillain-Barré Syndrome. N Engl J Med 1992;326:1123–1129.

13. Dau PC, Lindstrom JM, Cassel CK, et al. Plasmapheresis and immunosuppressive drug therapy in myasthenia gravis. N Engl J Med 1977;297:1134–1140.

14. Behan PO, Shakir RA, Simpson JA, et al. Plasma-exchange combined with immunosuppressive therapy in myasthenia gravis. Lancet 1979;1:438–440.

15. Plasma exchange for neurological disorders. Lancet 1986;1:1313–1319. Editorial.

16. Khatri BO, McQuillen MP, Harrington GJ, et al. Chronic progressive multiple sclerosis: double-blind controlled study of plasmapheresis in patients taking immunosuppressive drugs. Neurology 1985;35:312–319.

17. Vamvakas EC, Pineda AA, Weinshenker BG. Meta-analysis of clinical studies of the efficacy of plasma exchange in the treatment of chronic progressive multiple sclerosis. J Clin Apheresis 1995;10:163–170.

18. Tindall R. A closer look at plasmapheresis in multiple sclerosis: the cons. Neurology 1988;38:53–56

19. Khatri BO. Experience with use of plasmapheresis in chronic progressive multiple sclerosis: the pros. Neurology 1988;38:50–52.

20. Newsom-Davis J, Murray MMF. Plasma exchange and immunosuppressive treatment in the Lambert-Eaton myasthenic syndrome. Neurology 1984;34:480–485.

21. Dyck PJ, Low PA, Windebank AJ, et al. Plasma exchange in polyneuropathology associated with monoclonal gammopathy of undetermined significance. N Engl J Med 1991;325:1482–1486.

22. Rosenblatt SG, Knight W, Bannayan GA, Wilson CB, Stein JH. Treatment of Goodpasture's syndrome with plasmapheresis—a case report and review of the literature. Am J Med 1979;66:689–696.

23. Johnson JP, Whitman W, Briggs WA. Plasmapheresis and immunosuppressive agents in antibasement membrane antibody-induced Goodpasture's syndrome. Am J Med 1978;64:354–359.

24. Lockwood CM, Rees AJ, Pearson TA, Evans DJ, Peters DK, Wilson CB. Immunosuppression and plasma-exchange in the treatment of Goodpasture's syndrome. Lancet 1976;1:711–715.

25. Lockwood CM, Pinching AJ, Sweny P, et al. Plasma-exchange and immunosuppression in the treatment of fulminating immune-complex crescentic nephritis. Lancet 1977;1(8002):63–67.

26. Gilcher RO, Strauss RG, Ciavarella D, et al. Management of renal disorders. J Clin Apheresis 1993;8:258–269.

27. Misiani R, Remuzzi G, Bertani T. Plasmapheresis in the treatment of acute renal failure in multiple myeloma. Am J Med 1979;66:684–688.

28. Feest TG, Burge PS, Cohen SL. Successful treatment of myeloma kidney by diuresis and plasmapheresis. Br Med J 1976;1:503–504.

29. Zucchelli P, Pasquali S, Cagnoli L, Rovinetti C. Plasma exchange therapy in acute renal failure due to light chain myeloma. Trans Am Soc Artif Intern Organs 1984;30:36–39.

30. Zucchelli P, Pasquali S, Cagnoli L, Ferrari G. Controlled plasma exchange trial in acute renal failure due to multiple myeloma. Kidney Int 1988;33:1775–1780.

31. Rubinstein MA, Kagan BM. Unusual remission in a case of thrombotic thrombocytopenic purpura syndrome following fresh blood exchange transfusions. Ann Intern Med 1959;51:1409–1416.

32. Bukowski RM, Hewlett JS. Exchange transfusions in the treatment of thrombotic thrombocytopenic purpura. Semin Hematol 1976;13:219–223.

33. Byrnes JJ, Khurana M. Treatment of thrombotic thrombocytopenic purpura with plasma. N Engl J Med 1977;297:1386–1389.

34. Bukowski RM, Hewlett JS, Reimer RR, Grappe CW, Weick JK, Livingston RB. Therapy of thrombotic thrombocytopenia purpura: an overview. Semin Thromb Hemost 1981;7:1–8.

35. Kwaan HC, Soff GA. Management of thrombotic thrombocytopenic purpura and hemolytic uremic syndrome. Semin Hematol 1997;34:159–166.

36. Byrnes JJ, Moake JL, Klung P, Periman P. Effectiveness of the cryosupernatant fraction of plasma in the treatment of refractory TTP. Am J Hematol 1990;34:169–174.

37. Rock G, Shuman KH, Sutton DMC, Buskard NA, Nair RC, and the Members of the Canadian Apheresis Group. Cryosupernatant as replacement fluid for plasma exchange in thrombotic thrombocytopenic purpura. Br J Haematol 1996;94:383–386.

38. Berkman EM, Orlin JB. Use of plasmapheresis and partial plasma exchange in the management of patients with cryoglobulinemia. Transfusion 1980;20:171–178.
39. Reinhart WH, Lutolf O, Nydegger U, Mahler F, Werner Straub P. Plasmapheresis for hyperviscosity syndrome in macroglobulinemia Waldenstrom and multiple myeloma: influence on blood rheology and the microcirculation. J Lab Clin Med 1992;119:69–76.
40. Taft EG, Propp RP, Sullivan SA. Plasma exchange for cold agglutinin hemolytic anemia. Transfusion 1977;17:173–176.
41. Wallace DJ, Goldfinger D, Gatti R, et al. Plasmapheresis and lymphoplasmapheresis in the management of rheumatoid arthritis. Arthritis Rheum 1979;22:703–710.
42. Wallace D, Goldfinger D, Lowe C, et al. A double-blind, controlled study of lymphoplasmapheresis versus sham apheresis in rheumatoid arthritis. N Engl J Med 1982;306:1406–1418.
43. Berkman E. Issues in therapeutic apheresis. N Engl J Med 1982;306:1418–1420.
44. Dwosh IL, Giles AR, Ford PM, et al. Plasmapheresis therapy in rheumatoid arthritis—a controlled, double-blind, crossover trial. N Engl J Med 1983;308:1124–1129.
45. Report from NCHCT. Evaluation of therapeutic apheresis for rheumatoid arthritis. JAMA 1981;246:1053.
46. Roujeau JC, Kalis B, Lauret P, et al. Plasma exchange in corticosteroid-resistant pemphigus. Br J Dermatol 1982;106:103.
47. Stricker RB. Hematologic aspects of HIV disease: diagnostic and therapeutic considerations. J Clin Apheresis 1991;6:106–109.
48. Cardella J, Sutton D, Uldall PR, de Veber GA. Intensive plasma exchange and renal- transplant rejection. Lancet 1977;1:264.
49. Kurland J, Franklin S, Goldfinger D. Treatment of renal allograft rejection by exchange plasma-lymphocytapheresis. Transfusion 1980;20:337–340.
50. Noseworthy JH, Shumak KH, Vandervoort MC, the Canadian Cooperative Multiple Sclerosis Study Group. Long-term use of antecubital veins for plasma exchange. Transfusion 1989;29:610–613.
51. Couriel D, Weinstein R. Complications of therapeutic plasma exchange: a recent assessment. J Clin Apheresis 1994;9:1–5.
52. Grishaber JE, Cunningham MC, Rohret PA, Strauss RG. Analysis of venous access for therapeutic plasma exchange in patients with neurological disease. J Clin Apheresis 1992;7:119–123.
53. Thompson L. Central venous catheters for apheresis access. J Clin Apheresis 1992;7:154–57.
54. Pineda AA, Brzica SM, Taswell HF. Continuous- and semicontinuous-flow blood centrifugation systems: therapeutic applications, with plasma-, platelet-, lympha-, and eosinapheresis. Transfusion 1977; 17:407–416.
55. Derksen RHWM, Schuurman HJ, Gmelig-Meyling FHJ, Struyvenberg A, Kater L. Rebound and overshoot after plasma exchange in humans. J Lab Clin Med 1984;104:35–43.
56. Derksen RHWM, Schuurman HJ, Gmelig-Meyling FHJ, Struyvenberg A, Kater L. The efficacy of plasma exchange in the removal of plasma components. J Lab Clin Med 1984;104:346–354.
57. Kellogg RM, Hester JP. Kinetics modeling of plasma exchange: intra- and post-plasma exchange. J Clin Apheresis 1988;4:183–187.
58. Chopek M, McCullough J. Protein and biochemical changes during plasma exchange. In: Therapeutic Hemapheresis. Arlington, VA: American Association of Blood Banks, 1980:13.
59. Orlin JB, Berkman EM. Partial plasma exchange using albumin replacement: removal and recovery of normal plasma constituents. Blood 1980;56:1055–1059.
60. Keller AJ, Urbaniak SJ. Intensive plasma exchange on the cell separator: effects on serum immunoglobulins and complement components. Br J Haematol 1978;38:531–540.
61. Flaum MA, Cuneo RA, Appelbaum FR, et al. The hemostatic imbalance of plasma-exchange transfusion. Blood 1979;54:694–702.
62. Keller AJ, Urbaniak SJ. Intensive plasma exchange on the cell separator: effects on serum immunoglobulins and complement components. Br J Haematol 1978;38:531.
63. Olson PR, Cox C, McCullough J. Laboratory and clinical effects on the infusion of ACD solution during plateletpheresis. Vox Sang 1977;33:79–87.
64. Szymanski IO. Ionized calcium during plateletpheresis. Transfusion 1978;18:701–708.
65. Watson DK, Penny AF, Marshall RW, Robinson EAE. Citrate induced hypocalcaemia during cell separation. Br J Haematol 1980;44:503–507.

66. Huestis DW. Risks and safety practices in hemapheresis procedures. Arch Pathol Lab Med 1989;113:273–278.
67. Strauss RG. Mechanism of adverse effects during hemapheresis. J Clin Apheresis 1996;11:160–164.
68. Ziselman EM, Bongiovanni MB, Wurzel HA. The complications of therapeutic plasma exchange. Vox Sang 1984;46:270–276.
69. Sutton DMC, Nair RC, Rock NG, Canadian Apheresis Study Group. Complications of plasma exchange. Transfusion 1989;29:124.
70. Pool M, McLeod BC. Pyrogen reactions to human serum albumin during plasma exchange. J Clin Apheresis 1995;10:81–84.
71. Danielson C, Parker C, Watson M, Thelia A. Immediate gross hemolysis due to hypotonic fluid administration during plasma exchange: a case report. J Clin Apheresis 1991;6:161–162.
72. Fried MR, Eastlund T, Christie B, Mullin GT, Key NS. Hypotensive reactions to white cell-reduced plasma in a patient undergoing angiotensin-converting enzyme inhibitor therapy. Transfusion 1996;36:900–903.
73. Brecher ME, Own HG, Collins ML. Apheresis and ACE inhibitors. Transfusion 1993;33:963–964.
74. Miller DM, Winslow RM, Klein HG, Wilson KC, Brown FL, Statham NJ. Improved exercise performance after exchange transfusion in subjects with sickle cell anemia. Blood 1980;56:1127–1131.
75. Green M, Hall RJC, Huntsman RG, et al. Sickle cell crisis treated by exchange transfusion—treatment of two patients with heterozygous sickle cell syndrome. JAMA 1975;231:948–950.
76. Wong RD, Murthy AR, Mathisen GE, Glover N, Thornton PJ. Treatment of severe falciparum malaria during pregnancy with quinidine and exchange transfusion. Am J Med 1992;92:561–562.
77. McKee LC, Collins RD. Intravascular leukocyte thrombi and aggregates as a cause of morbidity and mortality in leukemia. Medicine 1974;53:463.
78. Freireich EJ, Thomas LB, Frei E, Fritz RD, Forkner CE. A distinctive type of intracerebral hemorrhage associated with "blastic crisis" in patients with leukemia. Cancer 1960;13:146–154.
79. Lokich JJ, Moloney WC. Fatal pulmonary leukostasis following treatment of acute myelogenous leukemia. Arch Intern Med 1972;130:759–762.
80. Roberts WC, Bodey GP, Wertlake PT. The heart in acute leukemia: a study of 420 autopsy cases. Am J Cardiol 1968;21:388–412.
81. Steeper TA, Smith JA, McCullough J. Therapeutic cytapheresis using the Fenwal CS-3000 blood cell separator. Vox Sang 1985;48:193.
82. Burgstaler EA, Pineda AA. Therapeutic cytapheresis: continuous flow versus intermittent flow apheresis systems. J Clin Apheresis 1994;9:205–209.
83. Greenberg BR, Watson-Williams EJ. Successful control of life-threatening thrombocytosis with a blood processor. Transfusion 1975;15:620–622.
84. Rook AH, Wolfe JT. Role of extracorporeal photopheresis in the treatment of cutaneous T-cell lymphoma, autoimmune disease, and allograft rejection. J Clin Apheresis 1994;9:28–30.
85. Edelson RL. Photopheresis. J Clin Apheresis 1990;5:77–79.
86. Edelson RL, Berger CL, Gasparro FP, et al. Treatment of cutaneous T cell lymphoma by extracorporeal photochemotherapy. N Engl J Med 1987;316:297–303.
87. Christensen I, Heald P. Photopheresis in the 1990s. J Clin Apheresis 1991;6:216–220.
88. Costanzo-Nordin MR, Hubbell EA, O'Sullivan EJ, et al. Successful treatment of heart transplant rejection with photopheresis. Transplantation 1992;53:808–815.
89. Rose EA, Barr ML, Xu H, et al. Photochemotherapy in human heart transplant recipients at high risk for fatal rejection. J Heart Lung Transplant 1992;11:746–750.
90. Wolfe JT, Tomaszewski JE, Grossman RA, et al. Reversal of acute renal allograft rejection by extracorporeal photopheresis: a case presentation and review of the literature. J Clin Apheresis 1996;11:36–41.
91. Burgstaler EA, Pineda AA. Plasma exchange versus an affinity column for cholesterol reduction. J Clin Apheresis 1992;7:69–74.
92. Kroon AA, van Asten WNJC, Stalenhoef AFH. Effect of apheresis of low-density lipoprotein on peripheral vascular disease in hypercholesterolemic patients with coronary artery disease. Ann Intern Med 1996;125:945–954.
93. Gordon BR, Saal SD. Low-density lipoprotein apheresis using the liposorber dextran sulfate cellulose system for patients with hypercholesterolemia refractory to medical therapy. J Clin Apheresis 1996;11:128–131.

94. Jovin IS, Taborski U, Muller-Berghaaus G. Comparing low-density lipoprotein apheresis procedures: difficulties and remedies. J Clin Apheresis 1996;11:168–170.

95. Thompson GR, Maher VM, Matthews S, et al. Familial hypercholesterolaemia regression study: a randomized trial of low-density-lipoprotein apheresis. Lancet 1995;345:811–816.

96. Matsuki Y, Suzuki K, Kawakami M, et al. High-avidity anti-DNA antibody removal from the serum of systemic lupus erythematosus patients by adsorption using dextran sulfate cellulose columns. J Clin Apheresis 1996;11:30–35.

97. Suzuki K, Hara M, Harigai M, et al. Continuous removal of anti-DNA antibody, using a new extracorporeal immunoadsorption system, in patients with systemic lupus erythematosus. Arthritis Rheum 1991;34:1546–1552.

98. Terman DS, Young JB, Shearer WT, et al. Preliminary observations of the effects on breast adenocarcinoma of plasma perfused over immobilized protein A. N Engl J Med 1981;305:1195–1200.

99. Terman DS, Yamamoto T, Tillquist RL, et al. Tumoricidal response induced by cytosine arabinoside after plasma perfusion over protein A. Science 1980;209:1257–1259.

100. Ray PK, Idiculla A, Mark R, et al. Extracorporeal immunoadsorption of plasma from a metastatic colon carcinoma patient by protein A-containing nonviable staphylococcus aureus—clinical, biochemical, serologic, and histologic evaluation of the patient's response. Cancer 1982;49:1800–1809.

101. Ray PK, McLaughlin D, Mohammed J, et al. Ex vivo immunoadsorption of IgG or its complexes—a new modality of cancer treatment. In: Serrou B, Rosenfeld C, eds. Immune Complexes and Plasma Exchange in Cancer Patients. New York: Elsevier/North Holland Publishers, 1981;1:197–208.

102. Ray PK, Besa E, Idiculla A, et al. Efficient removal of abnormal immunoglobulin G from the plasma of a multiple myeloma patient—description of a new method for treatment of the hyperviscosity syndrome. Cancer 1980;45:2633–2638.

103. Branda RF, Miller WJ, Soltis RD, McCullough JJ. Immunoadsorption of human plasma with protein A-sepharose columns. Transfusion 1986;26:471–477.

104. Carpentier NA, Fiere DM, Schuh D, et al. Circulating immune complexes and the prognosis of acute myeloid leukemia. N Engl J Med 1982;307:1174–1180.

105. Besa EC, Ray PK, Swami V. Specific immunoadsorption of IgG antibody in a patient with chronic lymphocytic leukemia and autoimmune hemolytic anemia—a new form of therapy for the acute critical stage. Am J Med 1981;71:1035–1040.

106. Bertram JH, Snyder HW Jr, Gill PS, Shulman I, Henry DH, Jenkins D, Kiprov DD. Protein A immunoadsorption therapy in HIV-related immune thrombocytopenia: a preliminary report. Artif Organs 1988;12:484–490.

107. Snyder HW, Cochran SK, Balint J, et al. Experience with protein A-immunoadsorption in treatment-resistant adult immune thrombocytopenic purpura. Blood 1992;79:2237–2245.

108. Nilsson IM, Jonsson S, Sundqvist SB, Ahlberg A, Bergentz SV. A procedure for removing high titer antibodies by extracorporeal protein-A-Sepharose adsorption in hemophilia: substitution therapy and surgery in a patient with hemophilia B and antibodies. Blood 1981;58:38–44.

109. Howe RB, Christie DJ. Protein A immunoadsorption treatment in hematology: an overview. J Clin Apheresis 1994;9:31–32.

110. Christie DJ, Howe RB, Lennon SS, Sauro SC. Treatment of refractoriness to platelet transfusion by protein A column therapy. Transfusion 1993;33:234–242.

111. Mittelman A, Bertram J, Henry DH, et al. Treatment of patients with HIV thrombocytopenia and hemolytic uremic syndrome with protein A (Prosorba column) immunoadsorption. Semin Hematol 1989;26:15–18.

112. Morrison FS, Huestis DW. Toxicity of the staphylococcal protein A immunoadsorption column. J Clin Apheresis 1992;7:171–172.

113. Kasprisin DO. Techniques, indications, and toxicity of therapeutic hemapheresis in children. J Clin Apheresis 1989;5:21–24.

114. Kevy SV, Fosburg M. Therapeutic apheresis in childhood. J Clin Apheresis 1990;5:87–90.

.

APPENDIX

QUALITY PROGRAMS IN BLOOD BANKING AND TRANSFUSION MEDICINE

During the past decade, the nation's blood supply system has undergone extensive and fundamental change. This has occurred primarily in response to the AIDS epidemic and has focused on improving the safety of the blood supply.[1] Retrospective review of the initial responses to the AIDS epidemic have been critical of the blood supply system,[2] and this has led to a new regulatory climate.[1,3,4] One aspect of this new regulatory climate is the expectation that the blood supply will be produced in a manner more similar to the production of pharmaceuticals than has been true in the past.[1,3,5,6] One result is the development and implementation of fundamental new ways of operating blood centers and also the development of new quality assurance programs and systems.[1,5,6]

Specific examples of changes introduced by blood banks and blood centers include new donor eligibility criteria, direct questioning of donors about high-risk behavior (see Chapter 4), and new laboratory tests of donated blood (see Chapter 8). These are specific operational changes that enhance traditional blood center functions. Possibly more important has been a change in the organizational philosophy to introduce new concepts of quality and process control.[6]

The need for such programs and systems is also driven by scientific and medical developments that will have a substantial impact on blood centers in the future. The impact may involve (*a*) new transfusion strategies that could alter the demand for existing blood components, (*b*) new techniques that could lead to the production of new kinds of blood components, or (*c*) innovations that could alter the methods of producing existing blood components. The scientific and medical developments that will bring about these new impacts include the use of hematopoietic growth factors such as

erythropoietin, granulocyte colony-stimulating factor (G-CSF), granulocyte-macrophage colony-stimulating factor (GM-CSF), or thrombopoietin to stimulate blood cell production, eliminate the need for transfusion, or reduce the period of cytopenia following chemotherapy or bone marrow transplantation (see Chapter 17). Hematopoietic growth factors and cytokines and advances in cell culture technology are being combined to create innovative ways to prepare blood cells in the laboratory for new therapeutic uses (see Chapter 18). Umbilical cord blood cells are now being used for transplantation, and cord blood banks are being established in the United States and other countries. Adoptive immunotherapy is the use of peripheral blood mononuclear cells as a specific blood component in new transfusion strategies for the treatment of malignancy, for the prevention of graft versus host disease, for the restoration of immunity against viruses, and possibly as treatment for autoimmune diseases. Research developments in gene therapy are moving rapidly, and this therapy is now being used for several inherited diseases and cancer. It is clear that blood transfusion has an immunomodulatory effect, and there is a likely an association of blood transfusion with postoperative infection or recurrence of cancer (see Chapter 14). As the mechanism becomes more clearly defined, it will be necessary to alter the preparation of blood components to avoid unwanted immunologic effects. System and regulatory changes of the past few years are designed to deal with HIV, hepatitis, HTLV, and syphilis. However, a number of other infectious agents and diseases can be transmitted by blood transfusion (see Chapter 15). One approach to these challenges is to implement more complex and sophisticated test methods such as polymerase chain reaction to detect the infectious agent. Another approach is the use of methods to treat blood or its components to inactivate viruses or bacteria after the blood has been collected. These viral inactivation procedures will probably become part of the routine processing of blood in blood centers, thus adding another new level of complexity to blood center operations. All of these medical and scientific developments will greatly increase the complexity of blood center operations. Blood centers must be prepared to implement these processes effectively and to carry them out accurately to produce a high-quality blood component. This will require a level of quality assurance and process control beyond that used by most blood centers in the past.

Quality programs and systems within transfusion medicine take two different general forms. One involves the blood supply system, as described above, and the other involves the patient transfusion system. The approach used to ensure the highest quality of the blood components in the blood supply system is similar to that used in the manufacture of pharmaceuticals, whereas the approach used to ensure that patients receive the highest quality transfusion therapy incorporates some of this but also is part of a hospital's overall quality-of-care program. Both of these categories of quality activities have been expanded in the past few years; in particular the quality systems used in the production of blood have undergone fundamental change.

One important measure of quality is the safety of the blood supply. This is described in more detail in Chapter 15. Several strategies have been used to accomplish this improved safety, but the purpose of this appendix is to describe specific activities targeted toward improving the quality of the blood operation and of transfusion practice.

QUALITY AND QUALITY ASSURANCE SYSTEMS

In contemporary manufacturing practices, quality is usually the most important standard. Not only is it valuable in itself, but it contributes to productivity by eliminating wastage, redundancy, and the costs of troubleshooting failed products, and it also maintains customer loyalty. Traditionally, the detection model has been used to achieve quality in a manufactured product. In this approach, a random sample of the final product is tested for certain desirable and undesirable characteristics.[6] This selective testing accepts that some defective products will be produced, move through the system, and be distributed. Theoretically, the customer finds the defective product and returns it to the manufacturer. "Reliance on inspection as a mechanism of quality control was discredited long ago in industry."[7] In the case of transfusion therapy and blood components, the detection approach means that some patients receive a product of less than desirable quality, since there is usually no effective way to detect a "poor-quality" component before it is transfused. Other reasons that the detection approach is not ideal for blood components is that the "raw material" or donated blood is variable and cannot be standardized like chemicals in a manufacturing process;[1,6,8] and since each donation becomes a "lot," it is impossible to carry out quality control testing on a random sample of material from each lot.[6] A more contemporary approach to quality is the prevention model.[6] This model assumes that errors will occur and attempts to minimize them by rigidly controlling the process.[6,8] This approach is especially suited for blood and components. While this discussion and terminology may seem like jargon or concepts applicable only to traditional assembly-line manufacturing, these principles can be extremely valuable in the production of blood components. The U.S. Food and Drug Administra-tion (FDA) requires demonstration of the safety, potency, purity, and efficacy of licensed blood components. For the patient and the practicing physician, it is essential to be as certain as possible that the component is exactly that desired and expected. Thus, the effect of the transfusion can be attributed to the product itself. If the patient has the expected beneficial effect, this is a good outcome. If the expected effect does not occur, this can be attributed to patient-related factors, and the next steps in diagnosis or therapy can be taken because the lack of benefit is not the result of a poor-quality component or unknown adventitious agents in the component. In addition, adverse effects of the transfusion can be more easily investigated if the component is assuredly standard and meets all expected criteria for quality.

The quality assurance system is ". . . the sum of the activities planned and performed to provide confidence that all systems and their elements that influence the quality of the product are working as expected."[5] The goals of the quality assurance system (program) are to decrease errors, obtain credible results consistently, improve product safety, and improve product quality.[5] The quality program should provide predictable, high-quality, and cost-effective collection, processing, and distribution of blood and components.[8] To achieve this, "all parts of an organization work together to create the cultural environment and infrastructure necessary to support the program."[8]

There are two general approaches to ensuring quality: control of the process and control of the product. It is presumed that good control of the process provides better

Table A.1 The elements of total process control

Process maps
Standard operating procedures (SOPs)
Performance-based training
Competency assessment
Records

control of the final products and leads to a relatively standardized product. In other types of manufacturing this control is achieved using "total process control" (TPC). TPC includes five elements (Table A.1). In this approach, the process map identifies the critical steps of the process, the standard operating procedures (SOPs) define the procedures to be used, the training is based on the SOPs, and assessment is used to determine that employees understand and can carry out the SOPs.[6,8] A similar approach to process control is "process analysis and management" (PAM). PAM includes seven steps (Table A.2). These involve deciding that PAM will be used, educating participants about PAM, developing a new or revised process including new SOPs, validating the process, training the staff to carry out the process, determining whether staff members are trained satisfactorily and how this will be monitored, and finally implementing the new process.

QUALITY ASSURANCE IN THE BLOOD SUPPLY SYSTEM

The FDA has over the years defined in the Code of Federal Regulations their expectations of process control. These are called Good Manufacturing Practices (GMPs) (Table A.3). Zuck describes these in a more expanded form (Table A.3) based on the common requirements to comply with the Code of Federal Regulations.[6] Each item in the GMPs is applied to each blood center operation whether it be blood collection, infectious disease testing, or the production of components. There are eight parts or components of good manufacturing practices as defined in the Code of Federal Regulations (Table A.3). The GMPs describe the organization and requirements for personnel responsible for different aspects of the operation; the buildings, equipment, and facilities necessary for different aspects of the operation; the production and process control requirements; requirements for controlling and releasing the finished product; laboratory controls; and the records and reports that should be maintained.

Table A.2 Process analysis and management

Define the work output
Understand the process
Develop a prototype process
Validate the process
Train to comply with process SOPs
Assess competency
Implement the process

Table A.3 Good manufacturing practices

Code of Federal Regulations	Zuck modification*
General	
Organization and personnel	Personnel management
Buildings and facilities	Facilities
Equipment	Equipment
Production and process controls	Process controls
Finished product control	Labeling
Laboratory controls	Quality control and auditing
Records and reports	Record keeping
	Calibration
	Error management
	SOPs

*From Zuck TF. Current good manufacturing practices. Transfusion 1995;35:955–966.

Personnel

The director of the processing activity should have the authority necessary to ensure the overall quality of the operation. The qualifications of personnel carrying out processing should be defined. There should be a written training program that should include training in concepts of good manufacturing practices as well as training in the specific processing and testing methods. There should be a written description of the competency required before an individual can begin working on actual production for patient use. Thereafter, the individual's continued competence should be demonstrated through an ongoing program of monitoring or proficiency testing. Capabilities of personnel should be commensurate with their responsibilities.

Facilities

The principles governing the facility operation are that production areas should be separate from other activities such as research or testing; access to the production area should be limited; equipment used for production should not be shared with nonproduction activities; there should be procedures for responding to spills or accidents; and environmental testing should demonstrate adequate control of the area used for processing.[5] An environmental testing program for air quality and pest control should be in place to establish the quality of air and the absence of rodents or other pests. There should be adequate space so that overcrowding leading to errors is avoided. Space should be adequate to allow proper storage of materials and quarantine of products not ready for patient use. In addition, wall coverings, floors, and countertops should be such that adequate cleanliness can be maintained and that there are smooth surfaces designed for aseptic processing. The flow of people, incoming materials, and material in processing should be organized to avoid or minimize the likelihood of microbial contamination, introduction of adventitious agents, or cross contamination among cells from different individuals. Security of the area should be such that unauthorized personnel are excluded.

Equipment

Equipment should be selected so as to be optimally effective for its desired function and to minimize the likelihood of microbial contamination, introduction of adventitious agents, or cross contamination of cells among different individuals. Initially, all equipment should be calibrated, making sure that calibration is done in the critical operating range of the instrument. There should be an ongoing program of calibration to ensure that the equipment is maintained in a satisfactory performance range. The equipment must be maintained in a clean state.

All supplies and reagents should be recorded and should be stored under proper conditions.

Production and Process Controls

Total process control is the concept that quality, safety, and effectiveness are built into the product.[6,8] Each step in the process must be controlled to meet quality standards. The expectation is that this approach provides a predictable outcome or product from the process. This results in a final product with a minimum of variability and as close as practical to the desired product every time it is produced. The two important parts of total process control are the use of standard operating procedures and critical control points.

Standard operating procedures   All procedures should be carried out using written instructions or standard operating procedures (SOPs). First it is essential to determine where SOPs are necessary, then who will develop them. These procedures should be developed in a systematic way, use a standard format, and be readily available to the staff. All steps should be carried out exactly as specified in the SOPs. There should be a specific policy and procedure for changing procedures (change control), including definition of personnel authorized to make changes. A permanent record of all outdated SOPs should be maintained so that in the future there can be no doubt as to how each specimen was processed.

Critical control points   A separate part of process control is the use of "critical control points." This involves defining the critical steps in each method where clinically important errors might occur and establishing systems or check steps to minimize the likelihood of an error occurring or being undetected.

Laboratory Controls

Laboratory controls must be used to ensure that reagents are working properly and that the blood components have the expected composition. The tests for reagents are not usually specified in the Code of Federal Regulations but are established locally as part of each institution's quality program. Testing of the components or final product is specified in the Code of Federal Regulations. This defines the test to be done, the proportion or frequency of testing, and acceptable limits of results.

Labeling

There should be written definition of the information to be contained on the label of each container of cells intended for patient therapy. This prevents mix-ups of components and provides information regarding the proper handling of the cellular product. The material to be specified on the label is defined in the GMPs.

Records Management

There should be written description of the records to be maintained and the length of retention. Records retained should at least make it possible to determine the source (donor) of the cells, donor-related information, all manipulations to which the blood or components were subjected, and key quality control tests related to the safety, purity, and potency of the cellular product. The records should make it possible to trace all steps clearly; they should be indelible; and they should identify the person who performed the work. Record keeping should be performed concurrently with the work; it is unacceptable to complete records after the work is completed.

Computers

A new requirement related to quality is the declaration by the FDA that computer software is considered a device.[9] The FDA has taken this position because computers and the software that controls them now play a key role in the control of the operation of the blood center and thus are major contributors to the safety of the blood. This position by the FDA has major implications, however. It means that the software must be developed, tested, validated, and maintained in a manner similar to the development of a medical device. Computer software then must go through the process of becoming licensed by the FDA under device licensing procedures. While this process should improve the quality of computer software, it adds to the cost and time necessary to develop these systems. Some companies that provided this software in the past will probably discontinue doing so.

Internal Quality Audits

For the manufacture of biologics and blood, it is recommended that a program of internal audits be carried out. Quality audits should be focused on systems, not on specific procedures. For instance, in addition to counseling a staff member who makes an error, the factors that made the error possible should be identified to determine whether corrective action is indicated. Corrective action should focus on the systems involved. Examples of systems to consider are (*a*) donor suitability and blood collection; (*b*) incoming material testing, quarantine, and release; (*c*) cell processing or testing procedures; (*d*) storage and shipping; (*e*) staffing and personnel competency; (*f*) reagents and materials management; (*g*) quality control testing and outcome actions; (*h*) equipment maintenance and calibration; and (*i*) error, accident, and adverse reaction reporting systems.

Error and Accident System and Error Management

An error and accident detection and management system is part of GMPs. The program should be written and appropriate portions should have SOPs and be part of the laboratory's SOP system. Errors or accidents that occur during cell processing or testing should be documented and investigated to determine whether this indicates any shortcoming in the processing method. In addition to any action in response to a particular error or accident, there should be periodic review of these errors and accidents to determine whether systemic or process changes are indicated. Thus, there should be a system of corrective action that will define the actions to be taken as a result of errors, accidents, or adverse reactions. An excellent description of a comprehensive program and its use were provided by transfusion medicine professionals from the Mayo Clinic in a recent workshop sponsored by the American Association of Blood Banks (AABB).[10]

Adverse Reaction Files

A record of adverse reactions to the transfusion of blood or components should be maintained. The adverse reactions should be reviewed at the time they are reported and also periodically to determine whether they suggest that any shortcomings exist in the processing methods or that modifications of methods or procedures should be made.

Organization and Quality Assurance Personnel

In the quality assurance program recommended by the FDA,[5] the personnel responsible for the program report separately from those responsible for the "manufacturing" operation. In this way, the operation is separate from the quality activity and those responsible for quality have equal authority over the production activities. The principle of separation of authority for quality from production is key, as it establishes that the quality function is equally as important as the production function.

QUALITY ASSURANCE IN THE TRANSFUSION SERVICE

Quality as it relates to the transfusion service can be considered as (*a*) quality of the blood and components, (*b*) quality of the blood bank operations, (*c*) quality of the transfusion procedure, and (*d*) quality of the transfusion practice. The blood and components must be as safe as possible, provide the expected potency, be readily available as needed, and be stored and handled properly within the hospital; the patient testing must be carried out in a timely and accurate manner; and the blood and components must be transfused to patients safely and effectively. The therapeutic uses of blood and components should reflect good medical practice and the record systems should be adequate to document all of the activities mentioned here. The medical practice activities will be discussed separately below. Before going into these specific areas, it is appropriate to consider quality programs as they apply to hospital blood banks. The descriptions of quality programs in the previous sections of this chapter were directed more to organizations

that collect blood and prepare components. Some of the issues and critical control points are the same for a blood production organization and a hospital transfusion service, but some are different. The next section is a general discussion of the approach to quality in a hospital transfusion service.

General Quality Program for Hospital Blood Banks and Transfusion Services

The AABB has developed a quality program, the modules of which are listed in Table A.4.[11] The program contains the elements of total process control and good manufacturing practices. It begins with general organizational issues such as the statement of the goals of the program and the organizational structure, in which there is independent reporting of the quality unit to top management separate from operations personnel. Personnel elements include position descriptions, evidence of training, and systems to ensure that adequate training is provided and that competency is monitored. The validation element includes procedures for validation, calibration, and preventive maintenance of equipment and records of this. Supplier qualification is an important concept. Specifications or product requirements are provided to suppliers, and there is a system to determine that suppliers meet these specifications continually. In process analysis control and management, critical control points are defined, SOPs written, and controls put in place to monitor specified conditions for each critical step. The documentation program includes the format for records, lists of pertinent documents, and the change process. Label control involves written procedures for handling labels, preventing mix-ups, revising labels, and discarding obsolete labels. Procedures for the identification of all errors, adverse events, or accidents are an essential part of a quality program. This process is used to identify shortcomings in the operation and make improvements. An internal audit or assessment program is also valuable; when carried out by staff members who do not directly perform the procedures it provides another way of identifying potential shortcomings so that corrective action can be initiated. All of this program is based on the concept of continuous improvement, which involves constant vigilance for shortcomings in the operation, collection of baseline data, development of solutions to

Table A.4 Critical control points of the American Association of Blood Banks quality system for blood banks

Organizational issues
Personnel selection/training/education
Validation/calibration/preventive maintenance/proficiency testing
Supplier qualification
Total process control and good manufacturing practices
Documentation/record keeping/record review
Label control
Incident/error /accident review
Internal assessment
Process improvement

improve the operation, implementing the solutions, and monitoring the impact. This is a very thorough program and will take a considerable effort to develop and implement. The AABB will probably make it a requirement for accreditation that some form of this plan be implemented.

Another way of thinking about quality programs divides the activities into four categories: (1) processes, (2) people, (3) material and equipment, and (4) management.[12] Another way of thinking about this is what is being done, who is doing it, the tools they use to carry out their tasks, and the overall systems and leadership of the program. In the program, flow charts are used to demonstrate the process, policies are developed defining the expected outcomes at different steps, and SOPs are written to provide step-by-step instructions to carry out the process. Within the process there may be some particularly important points that determine the outcome. These are established as "critical control points," and systems are established to check the process at these points. Before putting any process into operation, it is necessary to "validate" it to ensure that the process in fact produces the intended result. Equally important as a sound, clearly defined process is the people who carry it out. Important steps in the acquisition of a competent staff are selection, training, work assignment, validation of competency, and maintenance of skills and competency.[12] The necessity that materials and equipment function as expected has been mentioned above in the description of quality programs for blood production. This applies equally to the hospital blood bank operation. It is essential that reagents have the potency and accuracy expected and that equipment functions as expected so that test results will be valid. In order for a quality program to be effective it is necessary that the leaders of the organization be committed to this. It will not be possible to develop and implement a program without the support and leadership of top management. In addition, for a successful ongoing quality program, there must be a commitment from the organization's leaders to search for continuous improvements. Some of the activities that provide this are internal audits of the processes, people, materials, and equipment; the follow-up on adverse events or errors; and the commitment to maintaining a knowledgeable staff.

Berte[13] has categorized the tools for improving quality in a transfusion service as those dealing with quality control, quality assurance, and quality systems. Examples of quality control are equipment maintenance, calibration, and reagent testing. Quality assurance tools are the use of quality indicators, or teams, and tools for systems include vendor certification, corrective action plans, and internal audits. These and many other activities she describes are nice examples of a rather comprehensive quality program. Another example of a practical approach to the use of this type of quality assurance program is described by Galel and Richards.[14] In addition, computers can be used to provide better structure for data capture and thus facilitate monitoring quality.[15]

Blood Supply

The quality of the transfusion service begins with ensuring an adequate supply of safe and high-quality blood components. Some hospital blood banks produce a portion of their supply themselves, while many purchase their blood and components from a community

blood center. If the hospital produces some of its supply, then the above description of quality in programs for the blood supply apply and the hospital will have its own blood production quality program.

However, even if the hospital does not produce its supply, the transfusion service professionals have a responsibility to ensure the adequacy and quality of the components that make up the hospital's inventory. This involves close interaction with the supplier to determine that a suitable quality program exists and that the blood and components being provided contain the expected potency and meet the safety expectations of the hospital. This becomes a form of "vendor qualification" similar to that used for the purchase of other supplies.

Hospital Blood Bank Operations

There are several types of activities that should be considered part of the quality program in the operation of the hospital blood bank (Table A.5). The first of these begins with the collection and labeling of the patient specimen and steps to ensure the quality of the specimen. One of the most common errors in clinical laboratories is mislabeling of specimens. This can cause a fatal hemolytic transfusion reaction due to ABO incompatibility, and so it is an important part of a quality program designed to minimize these specimen labeling errors. Of course it seems obvious that it is essential to carry out the correct tests in each situation for each specimen, but errors do occur and it is important to ensure that the proper test is ordered, that the records reflect this, and that the laboratory staff actually perform the test requested. It is expected that all tests will be done correctly according to the laboratory SOPs and that all test results will be reported timely and accurately. Complete, accurate, and legible records of all steps must be maintained. An adequate supply of safe, high-quality blood components has already been mentioned as an important part of the quality of the operation of the hospital blood bank and transfusion service. The blood and components must be stored under conditions that maintain optimum quality and effectiveness at the time of transfusion, and the procedures for release of blood from the blood bank must be sufficiently detailed to minimize the likelihood that blood will be dispensed to the wrong patient.

Table A.5 Activities of a hospital blood bank subject to quality programs

Specimen collection, labeling, and quality
Carrying out the correct tests in each situation for each specimen
Carrying out all tests correctly according to the laboratory SOPs
Reporting all test results timely and accurately
Maintaining complete, accurate, and legible records
Acquiring an adequate supply of safe, high-quality blood components
Storing the blood components under conditions that maintain optimum quality and
    effectiveness at the time of transfusion
Providing blood components requested for patient care timely and accurately

Transfusion of Blood and Components

Most of the activities in the actual transfusion of blood and components occur outside of the blood bank and are not carried out by blood bank personnel. Thus, the quality assurance program for these activities is a joint one usually involving both the blood bank and the nursing service. It is essential that the blood bank and transfusion medicine staff be very involved in the program, because they have special knowledge and an approach that adds to the quality program. The particular activities in the transfusion process that lend themselves to inclusion in the quality program are described below (Table A.6).

Ensuring that the blood components are transfused correctly so as to provide the maximum effectiveness while minimizing the chance for an adverse effect is another important aspect of quality in the transfusion service. This begins with release of the blood components from the blood bank and continues with the transport of the blood components from the blood bank to the patient care area. Systems should be in place to ensure that the proper unit is released from the blood bank. Although there will be subsequent checks of the identity of the unit and the patient, this is one of the redundant steps to minimize the likelihood that a patient will receive the incorrect unit. Administration of the incorrect unit, leading to ABO incompatibility and a hemolytic transfusion reaction, is the most common cause of transfusion-related fatality.[16] Thus, redundancies are built into the system to prevent these errors. The unit must be handled properly to avoid damaging it during transport. If the unit is exposed to extreme temperatures or prolonged storage at improper conditions, the potency of the component may be reduced or cells may be damaged, resulting in a transfusion reaction (see Chapters 13 and 14). When the blood component arrives at the patient care area, it should not be stored but administered to the patient as soon as possible. Patient care areas do not have proper equipment to store blood components. When preparing to transfuse a blood component, it is essential to correctly identify the unit and the patient. As mentioned above, the most common reason for a transfusion-related fatality is a hemolytic transfusion reaction due to ABO incompatibility resulting from transfusing the patient with an incorrect unit of blood.[16] Next it is important to select the proper intravenous route and vascular access device. Ordinarily, peripheral veins are used, but other

Table A.6 Activities in the transfusion of blood and components that are part of the transfusion medicine quality program

Release of the blood components from the blood bank
Transportation of the blood components from the blood bank to the patient care area
Identification of the unit and the patient prior to initiating the transfusion
Selection of the proper intravenous route and vascular access device
Administration of solutions used during transfusion of the blood component
Operation of devices used during the transfusion
Nursing care before, during, and after the transfusion
Documentation of all steps in the process and the nursing care information

venous access such as catheters may also be used. This will in turn determine the type of vascular access device used for the transfusion. The route and device must be large enough to permit administration of the volume of blood within the time desired or the maximum time allowable (see Chapter 13). However, transfusing red cells through small-bore needles, especially under pressure, can cause hemolysis, and so the nature of the transfusion device is important. If other solutions are to be administered along with the blood component, it is essential to determine that these solutions are safe and will not jeopardize the effectiveness of the blood by damaging the cells (see Chapter 13). There is a similar responsibility to ensure the safety and effectiveness of devices used during the transfusion. Examples of such devices are filters, blood warmers, and infusion pumps. These are valuable devices that assist with the transfusion, but each of these can also lead to problems if not used correctly (see Chapter 13). The nursing care provided to the patient before, during, and after the transfusion is an important part of ensuring quality and safety. The nurse confirms that the proper unit of the proper component is being transfused, that all the techniques and devices are proper and functioning, and that the patient's condition does not preclude starting the transfusion. The nurse can determine that the patient has given consent for the transfusion and provide reassurance by answering questions the patient may have about the transfusion. The vital signs obtained before transfusion provide a baseline for comparison if the patient develops any signs or symptoms during the transfusion. Observing the patient, especially during the early minutes of the transfusion, can identify a transfusion reaction early so that the complications can be minimized and proper care instituted quickly. An overall essential part of all of these activities is thorough, legible documentation. This is an invaluable part of the quality program, as it provides the record of exactly what is done and how it is done. This is the basis for the continuous review to maintain quality and also is the basis for problem solving and corrective action when this is necessary.

PATIENT THERAPY

There is general evidence indicating that the medical use of blood and components is not ideal. Consensus development conferences for the use of platelets, albumin, and fresh frozen plasma have all concluded that some inappropriate use occurs and have provided recommendations for more suitable indications (see Chapters 11 and 12). One study of blood use in coronary artery bypass surgery at 18 different hospitals found a 10-fold difference in the number of red cells and a 40-fold difference in the total number of components transfused and that 43% of these transfusions were unnecessary.[17] Other transfusion medicine professionals are concerned that undertransfusion might represent another form of inappropriate transfusion therapy.[18] Several approaches have been taken to continually improve transfusion practice. The major approach is continuing education of physicians. This is done in a wide variety of settings such as general and specialty medical meetings, medical societies, hospital medical staff meetings, publications in the medical literature, audio tapes, teleconferences, and written materials provided by blood suppliers. In addition, the use of blood within the hospital has been

monitored in an effort to determine the quality of transfusion practice and form the basis of changing physicians' behavior. These several approaches are described in more detail below.

Transfusion Committee

This committee of the medical staff is required by the Joint Commission on Accreditation of Healthcare Organizations (JCAHO). Sometimes the committee is chaired by the blood bank medical director, but often another member of the medical staff holds this responsibility. The transfusion committee is a key part of the overall quality program for the hospital transfusion service. The committee should be aware of and possibly approve the blood supplier and thus can influence the quality and availability of the blood supply. In addition, the committee should have some kind of system to monitor blood utilization using the data and reports prepared by the blood bank staff. The committee also would monitor adverse events, errors, and accidents and approve the blood bank's overall quality plan. The committee would be aware of the results of inspections and accreditation findings and use its influence to ensure that the blood bank has the resources needed to carry out the responsibilities. Thus, the transfusion committee can be a major force in the quality of the blood bank and transfusion service operation.

Medical Indications

The indications for transfusion are changing (see Chapters 11, 12, and 15), resulting in decreased blood utilization and thus improved safety for patients. In addition, the changes in donor selection and testing and in the organization of blood banks has reduced the infectivity of blood and made the blood supply safer than ever (see Chapter 15). All of these approaches are resulting in improvements in the overall quality of transfusion practice. As blood transfusion has become more directly linked to specific indications, its use has decreased, with an attendant decrease in the complications of transfusion. Changed indications have been developed in response to patients' concerns about blood safety and also to reduce the costs of patient care by avoiding unnecessary therapies. At the same time, however, medical and scientific knowledge is accumulating that forms the basis for altering the indications for some blood components. Examples of this are improvements in the management of acute blood loss and anemia, thus lowering the hemoglobin indication for routine transfusion; the use of erythropoietin to avoid red cell transfusions; and reduction in the platelet count indication for prophylactic platelet transfusion. Another factor that plays into the changing indications is the increased use of practice guidelines in health care.[19] As practice guidelines are developed for diseases or treatments involving transfusion, indications for transfusion are included, thus bringing some standardization and consistency to transfusion practice. For some situations, practice guidelines specifically related to transfusion are used.[20] The indications for blood and component use are implemented in several ways. Transfusion medicine professionals provide education through medical staff meetings or other medical education forums. Lectures by transfusion medicine professionals can improve compliance with the transfusion guidelines,[21] but the durability of the improve-

ment is not known. In general, educational programs are necessary and provide some benefit but do not accomplish the extent of change desired.

Transfusion Audit

In 1985 the JCAHO began to require that the medical staff audit the appropriateness of all transfusions. Usually this is done through the transfusion committee. The transfusion audit relates to the transfusion therapy guidelines established by the medical staff. In the transfusion audit, the criteria for the use of the different blood components established by the medical staff are compared with the use of blood components. All or a selected number of transfusions are reviewed to determine whether the use of the blood components is consistent with the medical staff guidelines. Transfusion audit can become a complex and time-consuming activity because, depending on the criteria, a rather extensive amount of information may be needed about each transfusion to determine whether it meets the indications specified for that component. In addition, such a review is by necessity retrospective. Thus, the transfusion has already occurred and the information is used to attempt to alter physicians' behavior in the future but not to prevent what might be an inappropriate therapy at the time. In the early experience with transfusion audits, some improvement was shown in the reduction of the number of transfusions that did not conform to hospital guidelines. Examples were the decline in the number of single-unit transfusions, considered at the time to be inappropriate. It appears that the gains that can be obtained by this retrospective audit method have been achieved, and the process may no longer be contributing to further improvements.[22,23]

Blood Ordering Practices

Another approach to improving both the quality of transfusion practice and the operational efficiency of the blood bank was the establishment of standard or maximum blood orders for common surgical procedures. This makes it possible for the surgeon to know the amount of blood that will always be available for particular types of operations and enables the blood bank to avoid the excess inventory and blood wastage that results from setting aside excessive amounts of blood for elective surgical procedures.[24–27] This program, which is described in more detail in Chapter 10, has been very effective in reducing blood wastage and improving blood availability for patients undergoing elective surgery. The standardization of blood ordering practices becomes part of medical care guidelines and the transfusion audit program and is then an important part of the quality program in transfusion therapy.[28]

Quality in Transfusion Therapy

Increased requirements by accrediting agencies, more medical knowledge, the increasing use of practice guidelines, improved methods of managing some patient situations,

the availability of drugs that avoid transfusion, the public and patient concerns about blood safety, and cost containment efforts are all interacting to strengthen the need for quality improvement in transfusion practice.

REFERENCES

1. McCullough J. The nation's changing blood supply system. JAMA 1993;269:2239–2245.
2. Leveton LB, Sox HC, Stoto MA, eds. HIV and the Blood Supply: An analysis of crisis decisionmaking. Committee to Study HIV Transmission Through Blood and Blood Products: Division of Health Promotion and Disease Prevention, National Institute of Medicine. Washington, DC: National Academy Press, 1995.
3. Solomon JM. The evolution of the current blood banking regulatory climate. Transfusion 1994;34:272–277.
4. Sayers MH. Whither the blood products advisory committee? Transfusion 1996;36:932–934.
5. Guideline for Quality Assurance in Blood Establishments. Docket No. 91N-045. Rockville, MD: U.S. Food and Drug Administration, June 17, 1993.
6. Zuck TF. Current good manufacturing practices. Transfusion 1995;35:955–966.
7. Leape LL. Error in medicine. JAMA 1994;272:1851–1857.
8. Callery MF, Nevalainen DE, Kirst TM. Quality systems and total process control in blood banking. Transfusion 1994;34:899–906.
9. Draft Guideline for the Validation of Blood Establishment Computer Systems. Docket No. 93N-0394. Rockville, MD: Center for Biologics Evaluation and Research, U.S. Food and Drug Administration, October 28, 1993.
10. Motschman TL, Santrach PJ, Moore SB. Error/incident management and its practical application in quality in action. In: Duckett JB, Woods LL, Santrach PJ, eds. Quality in Action. Bethesda, MD: American Association of Blood Banks, 1996:37–67.
11. Quality Plan Manual. In: Quality Program. Bethesda, MD: American Association of Blood Banks, 1994, vol. 1.
12. Chambers LA. Concepts of quality. In: Duckett JB, Woods LL, Santrach PJ, eds. Quality in Action. Bethesda, MD: American Association of Blood Banks, 1996;1–12.
13. Berte LM. Tools for improving quality in the transfusion service. Am J Clin Pathol 1997;107:S36–S42.
14. Galel SA, Richards CA. Practical approaches to improve laboratory performance and transfusion safety. Am J Clin Pathol 1996;106(Suppl 1):S33–S49.
15. Butsch SH. Practical use of computerized hospital information systems to improve blood transfusion. Am J Clin Pathol 1996;106(Suppl 1):S50–S56.
16. Sazama K. 355 reports of transfusion-associated deaths. Transfusion 1990;30:583.
17. Goodnough LT, Soegiarso RW, Birkmeyer JD, Welch HG. Economic impact of inappropriate blood transfusions in coronary artery bypass graft surgery. Am J Med 1993;94:509–514.
18. Mintz PD. Undertransfusion. Am J Clin Pathol 1992;98:150–151.
19. Reinertsen JL. Algorithms, guidelines, and protocols: can they really improve what we do? Transfusion 1994;34:281–282.
20. Silberstein LE, Kruskall MS, Stehling LC, et al. Strategies for the review of transfusion practices. JAMA 1989;262:1993–1997.
21. Soumerai SB, Salem-Schatz S, Avorn J, Casteris CS, Ross-Degnan D, Popovsky MA. A controlled trial of educational outreach to improve blood transfusion practice. JAMA 1993;270:961–966.
22. Lam HTC, Schweitzer SO, Petz L, et al. Are retrospective peer-review transfusion monitoring systems effective in reducing red blood cell utilization? Arch Pathol Lab Med 1996;120:810–816.
23. Goodnough LT, Audet AM. Utilization review for red cell transfusions—are we just going through the motions? Arch Pathol Lab Med 1996;120:802–803.
24. Friedman BA, Oberman HA, Chadwick AR, Kingdon KI. The maximum surgical blood order schedule and surgical blood use in the United States. Transfusion 1976;16:380–387.

25. Boyd PR, Sheedy KC, Henry JB. Use and effectiveness in elective surgery. Am J Clin Pathol 1980;73:694–699.
26. Mintz PD, Lauenstein K, Hume J, Henry JB. Expected hemotherapy in elective surgery. JAMA 1978;239:623–625.
27. Boral LI, Dannemiller FJ, Standard W, et al. A guideline for anticipated blood usage during elective surgical procedures. Am J Clin Pathol 1979;71:680–684.
28. Campbell JA. Appropriateness of blood product ordering: quality assurance techniques. Lab Med 1989;20:15–18.

Index

Page numbers in italics denote figures; those followed by "t" denote tables.

ISBN 0-07-045113-3

90000

9 780070 451131